Life Cycle Nutrition
An Evidence-Based Approach

Editors
Sari Edelstein, PhD, RD
Judith Sharlin, PhD, RD
Simmons College Faculty

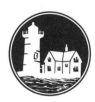

JONES AND BARTLETT PUBLISHERS

Sudbury, Massachusetts

BOSTON   TORONTO   LONDON   SINGAPORE

World Headquarters

Jones and Bartlett Publishers
40 Tall Pine Drive
Sudbury, MA 01776
978-443-5000
info@jbpub.com
www.jbpub.com

Jones and Bartlett Publishers
Canada
6339 Ormindale Way
Mississauga, Ontario L5V 1J2
Canada

Jones and Bartlett Publishers
International
Barb House, Barb Mews
London W6 7PA
United Kingdom

Jones and Bartlett's books and products are available through most bookstores and online booksellers. To contact Jones and Bartlett Publishers directly, call 800-832-0034, fax 978-443-8000, or visit our website www.jbpub.com.

Substantial discounts on bulk quantities of Jones and Bartlett's publications are available to corporations, professional associations, and other qualified organizations. For details and specific discount information, contact the special sales department at Jones and Bartlett via the above contact information or send an email to specialsales@jbpub.com.

The authors, editor, and publisher have made every effort to provide accurate information. However, they are not responsible for errors, omissions, or for any outcomes related to the use of the contents of this book and take no responsibility for the use of the products and procedures described. Treatments and side effects described in this book may not be applicable to all people; likewise, some people may require a dose or experience a side effect that is not described herein. Drugs and medical devices are discussed that may have limited availability controlled by the Food and Drug Administration (FDA) for use only in a research study or clinical trial. Research, clinical practice, and government regulations often change the accepted standard in this field. When consideration is being given to use of any drug in the clinical setting, the health care provider or reader is responsible for determining FDA status of the drug, reading the package insert, and reviewing prescribing information for the most up-to-date recommendations on dose, precautions, and contraindications, and determining the appropriate usage for the product. This is especially important in the case of drugs that are new or seldom used.

Production Credits
Publisher: Michael Brown
Production Director: Amy Rose
Associate Editor: Katey Birtcher
Production Editor: Tracey Chapman
Marketing Manager: Wendy Thayer
Manufacturing and Inventory Control Supervisor: Amy Bacus
Composition: Auburn Associates, Inc.
Cover Design: Kate Ternullo
Associate Photo Researcher and Photographer: Christine McKeen
Cover Image: © Photos.com; © Anna Chelnokova/ShutterStock, Inc.; © Losevsky Pavel/ShutterStock, Inc.;
© Oshvintsev Alexander/ShutterStock, Inc.; © iofoto/ShutterStock, Inc.
Printing and Binding: Malloy, Inc.
Cover Printing: Malloy, Inc.

Library of Congress Cataloging-in-Publication Data
Life cycle nutrition : an evidence-based approach / editors, Sari Edelstein, Judith Sharlin.
    p. ; cm.
  Includes bibliographical references and index.
  ISBN-13: 978-0-7637-3810-5 (pbk.)
  ISBN-10: 0-7637-3810-7 (pbk.)
  1. Nutrition. 2. Evidence-based medicine. I. Edelstein, Sari. II. Sharlin, Judith.
  [DNLM: 1. Nutrition Physiology. 2. Evidence-Based Medicine. 3. Longitudinal Studies. QU 145 L7206 2008]
  QP141.L53 2008
  612.3′99—dc22
                                2007046087
6048
Printed in the United States of America
12 11 10 09 08   10 9 8 7 6 5 4 3 2 1

Dedication

We thank our husbands, Marc and David, and children, Hillel, Staci, Jodi, and Sebastien, for inspiring us to conduct this personally and professionally fulfilling project.

Acknowledgment

We thank our teaching assistants at Simmons College, Christina Barnes and Nicole Gillis, for their assistance, as well as the staff at Jones and Bartlett Publishers.

Contents

SECTION **1** **Evidence-Based Nutrition in the Life Cycle; Prenatal to the Adolescent . . . 37**

CHAPTER **2** Nutritional Requirements During Pregnancy and Lactation and
Normal Infant Nutrition 39
Jennifer L. Bueche, PhD, RD, CDN, and Rachelle Lessen, MS, RD, IBCLC

CHAPTER **15** **Special Topics in Nutrition and Ethics: Nutritional and Ethical**
Issues at the End of Life
Judith Sharlin, PhD, RD, and I. David Todres, MD

Karlyn Grimes, MS, MPH, RD

Contributors

Claire Blais, RD, LDN, CNSD
Massachusetts General Hospital

Jennifer L. Bueche, PhD, RD, CDN
State University of New York

Victoria Hammer Castellanos, PhD, RD
Florida International University

Karen Chapman-Novakofski, RD, LDN, PhD
University of Illinois at Urbana-Champaign

Harriet H. Cloud, MS, RD, FADA
Nutrition Matters

Rachel Colchamiro, MPH, RD, LDN
Boston Department of Public Health

Sari Edelstein, PhD, RD
Simmons College

Karen M. Funderburg, MS, RD, LD
University of Oklahoma Health Sciences Center

Karlyn Grimes, MS, MPH, RD
Simmons College

Laura Harkness, PhD, RD
Nestle

Edna Harris-Davis, MS, MPH, RD, LD
Georgia East Central Health District

Roschelle Heuberger, PhD, RD
Central Michigan University

Pamela S. Hinton, PhD
University of Missouri

Sari Kalin, MS
Simmons College

Jan Kallio, MS, RD, LDN
Boston Department of Public Health

Anne R. Lee, MSEd, RD
Columbia University

Rachelle Lessen, MS, RD, IBCLC
The Children's Hospital of Philadelphia

Reed Mangels, PhD, RD
University of Massachusetts

Virginia L. Marchant-Schnee, BS
Writer

Migy K. Mathew, MD
The Donald W. Reynold Department of
    Geriatric Medicine
University of Oklahoma Health Sciences Center

Elizabeth Metallinos-Katsaras, PhD, RD
Simmons College

Yeemay Su Miller, MS, RD
Simmons College

Shideh Mofidi, MS, RD, CSP
Maria Fareri Childrens Hospital

Theresa A. Nicklas, DrPH
Baylor College of Medicine

Liesje Nieman, RD, CNSD, LDN
The Children's Hospital of Philadelphia

Carol O'Neil, PhD, MPH, LDN, RD
Louisiana State University

Aaron Owens, MS, RD
ECI Infant Development Program

Barbara Robinson, MPH, RD, CNSD
Hasbro Children's Hospital
Brown Medical School

Jennifer Sabo, RD, LDN, CNSD
The Children's Hospital of Philadelphia

Angela Sader, RD, LD, MBA
Beverly Enterprises Inc.

Judith Sharlin, PhD, RD
Simmons College

Inger Stallmann-Jorgensen, MS, RD, LD
Medical College of Georgia

Sara Snow, MS, RD
Nestle

I. David Todres, MD
Massachusetts General Hospital
Harvard Medical School

Stella Lucia Volpe, PhD, RD, LDN, FACSM
University of Pennsylvania

Preface

Life Cycle Nutrition: An Evidence-Based Approach provides a unique learning experience, a unique reference, and a unique start for graduate students learning about nutrition throughout the life cycle. It also provides a comprehensive reference for those of us already in practice. The book stands alone in its interwoven coverage of public health nutrition, with subjects as diverse as media influences on eating, skipping breakfast, sociodemographic moderators of dietary intake, tobacco use and nutritional status, and clinical nutrition; it includes a wide array of diverse topics, including parenteral nutrition and biochemical monitoring in neonates, inborn errors of metabolism, and cancer. Contemporary issues such as fruit juice consumption, nutritional needs of athletes, and dietary supplements as ergogenic aids are addressed across the life cycle as well as by using a multidisciplinary approach. This book gives students current knowledge, helps them evaluate emerging knowledge, and prepares them to uncover new knowledge for the public, their clients, and themselves as they journey together throughout the life cycle.

The book is divided into two sections. The first chapter covers epidemiologic research—how to do it and a review of landmark studies in children and adults. With this foundation students then journey through infancy, childhood, and adulthood. Along the way, knowledge and knowledge gaps, problems and solutions, and challenges and opportunities are presented and students learn to make a positive difference.

This section brings us from infancy to adolescence and covers virtually every topic imaginable. Chapter 2 gives students insight into the growth, development of normal infants, along with some of their nutrition "issues" such as food safety and the effect of early diet on health outcomes. As outlined in Chapter 3, toddlers have different issues as they begin to explore their world and express food preferences; food habits begin to be formed and are influenced by caregiver behaviors. Chapter 4 emphasizes that

school-aged children have different needs and are influenced by a wide variety of outside forces, including role models and television and other media. Although caregivers have a large influence, these children begin to make their own food choices and may be grazers or picky eaters. Adolescents, discussed in Chapter 4, are an understudied group with many nutrition issues; they, too, are influenced by media but also by their peers. Adolescents also make many of their own food choices and may skip breakfast or consume fast food and added sugars, often in the form of sweetened beverages. Poor food choices contribute to rising obesity and the appearance of nutrition-related chronic diseases formerly seen only in adults, such as metabolic syndrome and type 2 diabetes. As students learn about nutritional needs of infants, children, and adolescents, they also learn how to help these groups improve their nutritional status.

Chapters 5 through 8 discuss special nutrition considerations of infants, children, and adolescents. Eating disorders, failure to thrive, food allergies, and the nutrition needs of children with disabilities are all covered in these chapters. Highlighted are pediatric vegetarianism, childhood obesity, and dietary needs of athletes. Very specialized topics, such as inborn errors of metabolism and nutrition support of the neonate, are also included.

Section 2 covers adults. Chapters 9 to 11 include information on chronic nutrition-related diseases, such as coronary heart disease, hypertension, diabetes, kidney disease, cancer, osteoporosis, HIV/AIDS, and obesity. Evidence analysis for evidence-based practice in these diseases is included, as are prevention strategies. Chapter 11 is devoted to physical activity and weight management issues. Chapters 12 and 13 are dedicated to nutritional issues of the elderly; all topics ranging from special nutritional needs to nutritional problems, from activities of daily living to polypharmacy, and from risks of malnutrition to nutrition intervention are included in these chapters. Chapters 14 and 15 discuss professionalism and ethical issues, the final preparation for students to join us as colleagues.

This book has many exciting features that not only enhance its usefulness as a teaching tool but also pave the way in developing future clinicians and scientists at the cutting edge of nutritional sciences:

Evidence-Based Practice: This section contains articles where readers can transform the written word into a peer-reviewed study or clinical trial. I tell my students that I don't want to know their opinion, I want to know their informed opinion. But how do they shape these opinions? Only by reading about evidence-based studies and medicine and by conducting studies themselves can students learn the importance of evidence-based practice. With their Evidence Analysis Library, the American Dietetic Association is a leader in presenting practitioners with the concept of evidence-based practice. This text complements this effort and enhances our students' familiarity with this important subject.

Cultural Diversity Sidebar: Cultural differences that involve the nutrition and health differences and similarities among ethnic groups are highlighted. This is a wonderful opportunity for students to learn more about what I call "diseases that discriminate": Obesity, cardiovascular disease, and diabetes are all most common in minority populations. Why? Are differences genetic or are they related to lifestyle or to health care? What are the gaps in nutrition research in different groups? How do you work with people from cultures/ethnicities that are different from your own to improve their health or nutritional status? This feature will help students answer these questions, develop their professionalism, and improve their practice.

Critical Thinking Sidebar: Found throughout the chapters, the points considered assist the reader in critical thinking concepts of different sections of the text. Perhaps the most important thing a student can learn is to analyze and evaluate, examine and reason, reflect and decide. Why? So they can solve complex real-world problems, weigh evidence and make conclusions, learn to ask the right questions, and develop informed opinions to share with others.

Case Studies and Nutritional Management: These sections are provided to demonstrate chapter concepts. Case studies actively involve students in learning and simulate or represent actual problems they will face as professionals. Students can work alone or in groups to develop solutions, as they would in the workplace. Thus case studies help develop knowledge and skills of students in a wide variety of subjects and improve critical thinking skills, public speaking, and group interactions.

Issues to Debate: These issues include withholding and withdrawing nutrition, the ethical implications of nutritional care, and right to die case law. It is critical that students learn the physiologic, moral, ethical, and legal issues surrounding these emotionally charged issues. Debate and discussion with others help students understand these issues as they apply across the life span; it also helps nutrition students learn how they will interact with other health professionals.

Web Site Resources: Web sites are provided not only for present use as students work through the material presented, but also for use by the students when they become the teachers. The Internet has opened virtually all information to all people at all times. No health professional can work without it. However, there are no filters on or standard for materials posted on the Web. It is important to help students understand this and to help them use appropriate materials. The Web sites provided in this book provide reliable and accurate information.

For students, *Reader Objectives* guide them step-wise through the chapter, and *Key Terms* sidebars throughout the chapters assist with new terminology and concepts. Also included are *Special Sections*, which are designed to heighten curiosity and give insight to a particular issue. *Chapter Summaries* crystallize the most important elements of the chapters and help bring the chapter contents into perspective.

For instructors, there is a separate *Instructor's Manual* with *multiple choice questions* and *answers to case studies*, as well as *PowerPoints* available electronically as for all chapters.

Carol E. O'Neil, PhD, MPH, LDN, RD
Theresa A. Nicklas, DrPH

List of Tables

List of Figures

About the Editors

Sari Edelstein, PhD, RD

Assistant Professor of Nutrition
BS Florida State University
MS Florida International University
PhD University of Florida

Dr. Sari Edelstein's present position is as Assistant Professor in the Nutrition and Dietetics Department at Simmons College. She presently teaches both Food Science and Food Service classes. Before coming to Simmons College, Dr. Edelstein was previously in private practice and served as a hospital Food Service Director and Chief Dietitian. She is the author of many research articles, inclusive of topics on ethics, yoga, the glycemic index, and athletic performance, as well as the author or editor of multiple books, including *The Healthy Young Child* (Wadsworth Publishing, 1995), *Nutrition in Public Health,* 2nd ed. (Jones & Bartlett Publishers, 2005), *Nutrition: Rapid References for Nurses* (Jones & Bartlett Publishers, 2007), and *Managing Food and Nutrition Services: For Hospitality, Culinary and Dietetics Professionals* (Jones & Bartlett Publishers, 2007).

Judith Sharlin, PhD, RD

BA University of California, Berkeley
BS University of California, Berkeley
MS Boston University
PhD Tufts University

Dr. Judith Sharlin is a lecturer in the Nutrition and Dietetics Department at Simmons College. Before coming to Simmons College, Dr. Sharlin codirected the Graduate Nutrition Communications Program at Boston University and owned and operated a catering and baking business. She is the author of a national award-winning cookbook and nutrition guide and of many research articles and chapters, including topics on public health nutrition, weight management, cardiovascular nutrition, and consumer behavior; she has lectured nationally on these topics. Dr. Sharlin competes as a U.S. Masters swimmer and ranks as a "Top Ten" record-holder in New England.

CHAPTER

Interpreting Evidence-Based Research: Major Pediatric and Adult Nutrition Studies

Carol E. O'Neil, PhD, MPH, LDN, RD, Theresa A. Nicklas, DrPH, Elizabeth Metallinos-Katsaras, PhD, RD, and Sari Kalin, MS

CHAPTER OUTLINE

Reader Objectives

After studying this chapter and reflecting on the contents, you should be able to

1. Discuss the rationale for protection of human subjects in research.
2. Explain specific legal issues relating to research with children, such as the distinction between assent, consent, and permission.
3. Argue for and against giving incentives to study participants or their parents or guardians.
4. Discuss the strengths and weaknesses of different types of epidemiologic studies.
5. Explain the contribution of epidemiologic studies.
6. Explain why longitudinal studies are often referred to as hypothesis-generating studies and intervention studies as hypothesis-testing studies.
7. Discuss examples of health interventions, and how we can assess their impact on the target population.
8. Describe recent changes in the field of nutritional epidemiology and the impact of these changes.
9. Summarize key findings of major epidemiologic studies that have contributed to the research underlying current chronic disease prevention efforts.
10. Describe the strengths, weaknesses, and limitations of these studies, and describe how these studies have contributed to the nutrition guidelines in the United States.

Research Involving Children

Carol E. O'Neil, PhD, MPH, LDN, RD, and Theresa A. Nicklas, DrPH

Historically, research involving children has reflected societal views of children (Glantz, 1998; Meaux & Bell, 2001; Kopelman, 2006). Under traditional English common law children were seen as chattel. Early experiments with infectious diseases and vaccines were often conducted on children of slaves or servants or on poor, institutionalized, or mentally challenged children. The latter provided a controlled environment and a "captive subject pool" (Meaux & Bell, 2001). Children were intentionally infected with leprosy, syphilis, gonorrhea, tuberculosis, or yellow fever and then used to study diagnostic tests or vaccines to detect or prevent these diseases. In the 1800s Edward Jenner used his own children before moving on to institutionalized children to test his smallpox vaccine; all children were then challenged with smallpox to determine the efficacy of the vaccine. Other vaccines, such as pertussis (Burns, 2003), were also tested in this manner. These trials constituted a grave risk, and not all were successful. In the 1930s children were used in clinical trials of a live virus polio vaccine; the deaths associated with these trials underscored the necessity of protecting children in research studies. As recently as the 1970s institutionalized mentally challenged children were infected deliberately with hepatitis in an attempt to develop a vaccine. Although "consent" was obtained, it is unclear whether parents actually recognized the risks involved (Jonsen, 1983).

In 1941 this acceptance of using children in research began to change when Francis Payton Rous, the editor of the *Journal of Experimental Medicine*, rejected a manuscript and wrote to the author, "the inoculation of a twelve month old infant with herpes . . . was an abuse of power, an infringement of the rights of an individual, and not excusable because the illness which followed had implications for science. The fact that a child was 'offered as a volunteer'—whatever that may mean—does not palliate the action" (quoted in Glantz, 1998).

It was, however, the public knowledge of the atrocities conducted under the guise of scientific experiments perpetrated by the Nazis that ultimately led to regulations that protected the rights of children in research studies. The 1964 Nuremberg Code clearly mandated the need for "informed, uncoerced, voluntary consent" by all research subjects; however, this effectively excluded the use of children in research because they cannot legally give consent. The Declaration of Helsinki (1964) gave parents the authority to consent for their children; it also stipulated that when minor children were able, they must also provide consent. The Belmont Report—Ethical Principles and Guidelines for the Protection of Human Subjects, or *Common Rule*, underscored the importance of children being able to choose if they wanted to participate in a research project. The Belmont Report established the three fundamental ethical principles that apply to research using human subjects—respect for persons, beneficence, and justice—and provides the philosophical underpinnings for the current federal laws governing human subjects research: Title 45 Code Federal Regulations, Part 46, Protection of Human Subjects (45 CFR Part 46).

> ● **Learning Point** Before you continue, complete the tutorial, "Human Participant Protections Education for Research Teams," and print out your certificate: http://cme.cancer.gov/c01/intro_02.htm

As researchers strove to protect children from abuses in research, there was increasing concern that children were not benefiting from medical advances, especially important research on drugs. Society continues to view children as vulnerable and in need of protection (Christensen, 1997), but care must be taken not to exclude children from research on new vaccines, pharmaceuticals, and medical devices that would benefit them (Morrow & Richards, 1996). The legal status of children has evolved from that of chattel to persons with limited autonomy (Grodin & Alpert, 1988). Today, the use of children as research participants reflects respect for the child and parents, a balance of risks and benefits, and distributive justice (Nelson, 1998).

Ethics and Regulations Regarding Research with Children

Institutional Review Board

Every organization that conducts biomedical or behavioral research with human subjects is federally mandated to have an institutional review board (IRB). The purpose of the IRB is to review the scientific merits and ethical principles of studies involving human research before the research is conducted.

An IRB must have at least 5 members with varied backgrounds; however, an IRB should include as many members as needed to perform a complete review of research involving human subjects, and membership may include 20 to 30 members. At least one member must be a "scientist" and at least another, a "nonscientist." One member must be unaffiliated with the institution housing the IRB; this member is considered so important that many IRBs will not review protocols if that person is not present. Diversity in race, gender, cultural heritage, and sensitivity to issues, such as community attitudes, should be considered when considering IRB membership. If the IRB regularly reviews research involving vulnerable subjects, including children or physically or mentally challenged persons, someone who is knowledgeable about and experienced with these subjects should be included in membership. IRB review is guided by The Belmont Report and the Federal Policy for the Protection of Human Subjects.[1] Although federal guidelines are in place, regulations are flexible and there is a broad spectrum of interpretation by different IRBs.

Children have many unique issues with respect to research and the IRB. First, what defines a child needs to be determined. The legal definition is clear, but cognitive abilities of children vary, and a child who has a chronological age of 7 may be unable to understand complexities that a similarly aged child can. Thus, despite individual regulations of the IRB, the individual abilities of the child should also be considered.

Parental Permission and Child Assent

Enrolling children and adolescents in research studies raises ethical concerns because they lack the legal status to provide consent; thus regulations require both parental permission and child assent (Broome & Stieglitz, 1992; Glantz, 1996; Field & Behrman, 2004). Parents provide consent out of beneficence, and assent is obtained from the child to respect his or her autonomy (Rossi, Reynolds, & Nelson, 2003). Generally, if a parent gives permission to participate in a research study but the child does not assent, the child's wishes supersede the parents' (Koren, 2003). Child assent, as defined by federal regulations, means "a child's affirmative agreement to participate in research. Mere failure to object should not, absent affirmative agreement, be construed as assent." Adequate provisions for assent must be provided, unless waived under limited circumstances, for example, if the child is judged incapable of providing assent. Individual IRBs are responsible for setting the exact criteria for assent, but generally the child must (1) demonstrate a developmentally appropriate understanding of the nature of the procedures to be performed, (2) freely choose to undergo

the procedure(s), (3) communicate his or her choice unambiguously, and (4) understand that he or she can withdraw at any time without penalty.

Factors affecting the ability of a child to provide assent are divided into two categories: individual factors, such as age, developmental level, and health status, and environmental factors, such as role constraints, family factors, and consent-seeker factors (Weithorn & Scherer, 1994; Meaux & Bell, 2001). The American Academy of Pediatrics (AAP) recommends obtaining assent from children 7 years and older; however, the capacity for assent should be viewed as a continuum as the child matures and as cognitive ability increases. Information for children should be age appropriate. Decision-making ability in children improves with increasing grade level (Lewis, 1998).

Use of Incentives in Pediatric Research Studies

Giving financial or other compensation to research volunteers is a common (Levine, 1979; Vere, 1991; Dickert, Emanuel, & Grady, 2002; Grady, Dickert, Jawetz , Gensler, & Emanuel, 2005) although questionable practice in the United States. Although little empirical data explore the impact of incentives on participation, critics propose that low income populations may be exploited, prospective participants may overlook potential risks associated with the study for financial gain, and altruistic motives may be undermined (Russell, Moralejo, & Burgess, 2000; Dresser, 2001; Kuczewski, 2001; Viens, 2001; Weise, Smith, Maschke, & Copeland, 2002). Giving payment to children and adolescents or their parents is even more debatable (Glantz, 1998; Fernhoff, 2002; Weise et al., 2002; Wendler, Rackoff, & Emanuel, 2002; Field & Behrman, 2004; American Academy of Pediatrics [AAP], 2005). Even seemingly small amounts of money may coerce children and adolescents to overlook the risks associated with a study or may deter them from withdrawing voluntarily. The AAP states that "serious ethical questions arise when payment is offered to adults acting on behalf of minors in return for allowing minors to participate as research subjects" (AAP, 1995). The AAP suggests that any payment be limited to a token gesture and that payment for reimbursement of costs for time or travel should be low enough that it does not become an inducement (AAP, 1995). They further recommend that if the recipient of the payment is a child, the discussion should occur after the completion of the study, not before, as recommended by federal guidelines.

Table 1.1 provides Internet resources on legal and ethical issues concerning children in research. Table 1.2

---

1. http://www.cdc.gov/nchs/nhanes.htm

TABLE 1.1	Internet Resources for Ethics and Human Research

American Society for Bioethics and Humanities http://www.asbh.org

Belmont Report http://www.cdc.gov/od/ads/ethcodes/belm-eng.pdf

Bioethics Databases http://www.nlm.nih.gov/pubs/cbm/hum_exp.html#300

Bioethics Resources on the Web http://www.nih.gov/sigs/bioethics

Center for Cancer Research Institutional Review Board: The Process of Informed Consent http://home.ccr.cancer.gov/irb/informed.html

Council for International Organizations of Medical Sciences http://www.cioms.ch

Declaration of Helsinki http://www.wma.net/e/policy/b3.htm

Food and Drug Administration http://www.fda.gov

Health Insurance Portability and Accountability Act (HIPAA) http://www.hhs.gov/ocr/hipaa

HIPAA Privacy Rule http://privacyruleandresearch.nih.gov

Information about National Institutes of Health (NIH)/National Cancer Institute cancer research studies http://cancertrials.nci.nih.gov

International Guidelines for Ethical Review of Epidemiologic Studies http://www.cdc.gov/od/ads/intlgui3.htm

National Bioethics Advisory Commission http://www.georgetown.edu/research/nrcbl/nbac

NIH Ethics Program http://ethics.od.nih.gov

NIH Infosheets, Forms, Checklists http://ohsr.od.nih.gov/info

NIH Office of Extramural Research http://grants.nih.gov/grants/oer.htm

NIH Office of Human Subjects Research http://ohsr.od.nih.gov

National Library of Medicine Bibliography—Ethical Issues in Research Involving Human Participants http://www.nlm.nih.gov/pubs/cbm/hum_exp.html

Nuremberg Code http://ohsr.od.nih.gov/guidelines/nuremberg.html http://www.fda.gov

Office for Human Research Protections (OHRP) http://www.hhs.gov/ohrp

OHRP Guidance Topics by Subject http://www.hhs.gov/ohrp/policy/topics.html

President's Council on Bioethics http://www.bioethics.gov

Public Responsibility in Medicine and Research http://www.primr.org

provides information on the requirement under the U.S. Department of Health and Human Services Regulations 45 CFR 46, Subpart D based on the risks and benefits to children who participate in research.

Nuturition Monitoring of Infants, Children, and Adolescents

The Centers for Disease Control and Prevention (CDC) has several health monitoring studies of infants, children, and adolescents. The best known is the National Health and Nutrition Examination Survey[2] (NHANES), which is part of the National Center for Health Statistics (NCHS).[3] Other important studies are the Pediatric Nutrition Surveillance System (PedNSS)[4] and the Pregnancy Surveillance System (Table 1.3). NHANES I and II and the PedNSS were initiated in the 1970s. In 1990 the National Nutrition Monitoring and Related Research Program (PL 101-445) established a comprehensive coordinated program for nutrition monitoring and related research to improve health and nutrition assessment in U.S. populations. The National Nutrition Monitoring and Related Research Program requires a program to coordinate federal nutrition monitoring efforts and assists states and local governments in participating in a nutrition monitoring network to create an interagency board to develop and implement the program, to create a nine-member advisory council to provide scientific and technical advice, and to evaluate program effectiveness.

● **Learning Point** NHANES data are available to researchers to help them understand the data set and how to work with it. The CDC has a tutorial that can be found at http://www.cdc.gov/nchs/tutorials/index.htm. Why not take the tutorial to see how NHANES data can help you with your research?

NHANES

The NHANES cohort is selected to comprise a nationally representative sample. The current NHANES has a special accent on adolescents and the elderly; accordingly, these groups are oversampled. The emphasis for adolescents is nutrition and fitness. New measures of physical fitness can improve our understanding of the impact that physical activity has on health. African-Americans and

---

2. http://www.cdc.gov/nchs/nhanes.htm
3. http://www.cdc.gov/nchs/Default.htm

4. http://www.cdc.gov/pednss/index.htm

TABLE 1.2

Requirements Under the U.S. Department of Health and Human Services (DHHS) Regulations 45 CFR 46, Subpart D Based on the Risks and Benefits to Children Who Participate in Research

Types of Research	Requirements	Examples
§46.404 Research not involving greater than minimal risk	Assent of child and permission of at least one parent. **Note:** An advantage to this type of research is that it enables investigators to obtain expedited review, modify or waive consent, and allow vulnerable populations, like children, to be enrolled in studies (Kopelman, 2004).	Surveys, blood drawing, x-rays, chart reviews, educational interventions, growth and development studies
§46.405 Research with greater than minimal risk but with the prospect of direct benefit to the individual subjects	Assent of child and permission of at least one parent. Anticipated benefit justifies the risk AND Anticipated benefit is at least as favorable as that of alternative approaches	Randomized clinical trials; comparison of the efficacy and safety of standard treatments of asthma
§46.406 Research with greater than minimal risk and no prospect of direct benefit to the individual subjects but likely to yield generalizable knowledge about the subject's condition or disease	Assent of child and permission of both parents. Only a minor increase over minimal risk. Likely to yield generalizable knowledge about the child's disorder or condition that is of vital importance for the understanding or amelioration of the disorder or condition AND The intervention or procedure presents experiences to the child that are reasonably commensurate with those in the child's actual or expected medical, dental, psychological, social, or educational situations.	Bone marrow aspiration, lumbar puncture, skin punch biopsy—all with suitable pain control
§46.407 Research not otherwise approvable, which presents an opportunity to understand, prevent, or alleviate a serious problem affecting the health or welfare of children	Assent of child and permission of both parents. IRB finds that the research presents a reasonable opportunity to further the understanding, prevention, or alleviation of a serious problem affecting the health or welfare of children AND The Secretary of DHHS, after consultation with a panel of experts in pertinent disciplines (e.g., science, medicine, education, ethics, law) and following publication and public comment, determines the research will be conducted in accordance with sound ethical principles. **Note:** The United States alone has a provision for this type of research on children (Kopelman and Murphy, 2004).	

From http://grants.nih.gov/grants/guide/notice-files/not98-024.html Accessed May 19, 2006.

TABLE 1.3 Other Epidemiologic Studies Looking at Health and Nutrition of Infants, Children, and Adolescents

Study	Population	Purpose	Comments/Important Findings
Gerber Feeding Infants and Toddlers Study (FITS)	3,000 4- to 24-month-old children	To investigate infant and toddler eating habits and nutrient intakes, to determine whether IOM recommendations are being met, and to examine the relationship between food intake and self-feeding	Collaboration among researchers in diet and food, statisticians, and the food industry. Results can be found in the January 2006 supplement of the *Journal of the American Dietetic Association*.
Northern Ireland Young Hearts Project (YH 1990) (1989–1990)	~2,000 boys and girls 12–15 years of age	To identify major modifiable coronary risk factors with a randomly selected cohort of adolescents in Northern Ireland	Risk factors for cardiovascular disease tend to cluster (Twisk et al., 1999). Ttracking of nutrients in adolescents was inconsistent (Robson et al., 2000). Although socioeconomic status is defined, it is not yet lined with cardiovascular risk factors (Van Lenthe et al., 2001).
Northern Ireland Young Hearts Project (YH 2000) (1999–2000)	~2,000 boys and girls 12–15 years of age	To identify the prevalence of risk factors for cardiovascular disease present in this population and to identify modifiable life-style factors associated with bone mineral density in the participants To be able to examine secular trends in these factors by comparing data to YH 1990	Decreases in blood pressure between the studies (Watkins et al., 2004); high intake of fruit is associated with increased bone health in girls (McGartland et al., 2004), whereas carbonated beverage intake is associated with lower bone health (McGartland et al., 2003).
Growing up in Australia	Cohort 1: 5,000 infants aged less than 12 months in 2003–2004 followed until 6–7 years old Cohort 2: 5,000 children aged 4 years followed until 10–11 years old	To determine critical periods to provide social and welfare support and to determine individual, family, and broader social impacts on children's development and change	There are a limited number of published papers available at this time, but some include descriptions of the study (Nicholson and Sanson, 2003; Harrison and Ungerer, 2005).
Amsterdam Growth and Health Longitudinal Study—initiated in 1977	500 healthy 13-year-old boys and girls	Until ~age 17 annual assessments included anthropometrics, physiologic and psychological parameters, life-style characteristics (activity, diet, smoking), and health parameters (Kemper et al., 1997). Subsequent testing was done at ages 21, 27, 32, and 36, allowing investigators to track health and life-style variables from early adolescence into young adulthood.	No differences were observed for high and mid-level calcium intake at a threshold of approximately 800 mg/day above which calcium intake has no additional beneficial effect (Boon et al., 2005). A 14-year follow-up showed both stability coefficients and tracking for subjects at risk for life-style risk factors were low (except for smoking), indicating low predictability of early measurements for values later in life. For cardiopulmonary fitness and blood pressure tracking was also low, whereas for the lipoproteins and body fatness tracking was much better, indicating good predictability (Twisk et al., 1997).
PNSS	Convenience sample of low-income high-risk pregnant women	To assess the demographics, pregravid weight and maternal weight gain, anemia, behavioral risk factors, birth weight, and formula-feeding data as risk factors for the mother and infant. PNSS provides surveillance reports to help with	Begun in 1973 and continuing

Study	Population	Purpose	Comments/Important Findings
		priority setting, planning, implementing, and evaluating public health policy.	
Early Childhood Longitudinal Study	Two overlapping cohorts—birth (*n* = 10, 688 born in 2001) to be followed to kindergarten and kindergarten (*n* = 22,000 from 1,000 programs) to be followed to the eighth grade	Provides national data on children's status from birth on children's transitions to nonparental care, early education programs, and school and children's experiences and growth through the eighth grade. Data are also provided to test hypotheses about a wide range of family, school, community, and individual variables on children's development, early learning, and school performance.	http://nces.ed.gov/ecls/index.asp is the best way to learn about this study. One recent article using these data showed that WIC mothers are less likely to breast-feed than noneligible participants (Jacknowitz et al., 2007).

IOM, Institute of Medicine; PNSS, Pregnancy Surveillance System: WIC, Special Supplemental Nutrition Program for Women, Infants, and Children.

Mexican-Americans are also over-sampled to get a more representative cohort.

Data are collection for NHANES at three levels: a brief household screener interview, an in-depth household survey interview, and a medical examination. Because detailed interviews and clinical, laboratory, and radiologic examinations are conducted, participants' response burden is significant. For the years 1999–2000 and 2001–2002 the interview sample size was 21,004, and the Mobile Examination Center sample size was 19,759.

Data from the NCHS was used to establish the CDC pediatric growth charts[5] in 1977; when these growth charts were revised in 2000 most of the data came from NHANES. The most obvious change in the growth charts is the substitution of body mass index (BMI) for weight for height measures. These charts can be used when the child is 2 years old and a standing height can be obtained. Other changes involved infants, including revision of head circumference standards; NHANES provided the national data needed for these charts. These charts have been adapted and adopted for worldwide use. Another major effect on the health of children is the monitoring of blood lead levels. Early NHANES studies documented a high percentage (77.8%) of children aged 1 to 5 years with high blood lead levels. This information was instrumental in using legislation to remove the lead from gasoline and food and soft drink cans. NHANES 1991/1994 showed a steep decline in the percentage (4.4%) of children with blood lead levels of at least 10 µg/dL (Centers for Disease Control and Prevention [CDC], 2005). Information from NHANES can be used to monitor the impact that fortification of foods has on nutrient intake of children, which in turn can lead to policy change.

It is difficult to quantify the tremendous impact that NHANES and related surveys have had on health policy and health research in the United States (Woteki, 2003). A recent PubMed search using NHANES with the key words "English," "Human," and "All Children" produced 3,780 articles. Research as diverse as late bottle weaning and obesity, alcohol consumption

GROUP Project

NHANES is an ongoing survey, and new questions can be added if investigators need the information; for example, dietary supplement use was recently added to the surveys. Look at the survey contents (http://www.cdc.gov/nchs/about/major/nhanes/nhanes2003-2004/questexam03_04.htm) and at the proposal guidelines for new survey content (the deadline is past, but there will be another; http://www.cdc.gov/nchs/about/major/nhanes/research_proposal_guidelines.htm). What would you add to the NHANES survey and why? Include in your answer the knowledge gap your new question(s) is designed to fill and how you will use the information. It may help you to understand the power of NHANES if you review some of the literature and explore the website before completing this project.

---

5. http://www.cdc.gov/growthcharts

and periodontal disease, and blood pressure trends in children and adolescents was found. NHANES also showed ethnic differences in dietary intake (Ford & Ballew, 1998; Arab, Carriquiry, Steck-Scott, & Gaudet, 2003), food sources for different nutrients are different in separate ethnic groups (Looker, Loria, Carroll, McDowell, & Johnson, 1993), cardiovascular risk factors cluster according to socioeconomic status (Sharma, Malarcher, Giles, & Myers, 2004), and hypertension varies according to geographic region (Hicks, Fairchild, Cook, & Ayanian, 2003). These findings demonstrate that data cannot be generalized for state or local areas without considering age, gender, ethnicity, or socioeconomic status in the particular area and that these data have important implications for public policy and intervention strategies. The findings underscore the importance of looking at nationally representative data.

Youth Risk Behavior Surveillance System

Initiated in 1990 by the CDC, the Youth Risk Behavior Surveillance System (YRBSS) is a large-scale biennial survey of 9th through 12th grade students at national, state, and local levels that studies behaviors linked to the leading causes of morbidity and mortality—chronic disease and unintentional injury. This self-reported survey looks at tobacco use, unhealthy dietary behaviors, and physical activity levels. Purposes include determining the prevalence of risk-taking behaviors, providing national and state data, monitoring levels of risk-taking behavior, and assessing progress toward the goals outlined in *Healthy People 2010*. The most recent survey assessed the national data, 40 state surveys, and 21 local surveys throughout the period from October 2004 to January 2006. That survey used sampling strategies to over-sample African-American and Hispanic youth. The full report is available online,[6] but, briefly, 79.9% had not eaten five or more servings of fruits and vegetables per day in the 7 days preceding the survey,

16.2% consumed three or more glasses of milk per day, 67% did not attend daily physical activity classes, and 13.1% were overweight. These data clearly indicate that most adolescents are not meeting current recommendations for diet and physical activity.

A Middle School RBSS was initiated by the CDC to assess health risk behaviors in students in sixth to eighth grade. The 2003 report is also available online.[7]

The advantages of the YRBSS are that the study is anonymous, encouraging youth to be truthful in their answers, and the large sample size—data generated for the 2005 report were from 13,953 surveys and the national representation. Limitations are that the survey only reaches those in school and the data are self-reported. Although test/retest reliability is good, BMI may be underreported.

PedNSS

The PedNSS is a child-based public health monitoring system that describes the nutritional status of low income children in federally funded maternal and child health and nutrition programs, including Special Supplemental Nutrition Program for Women, Infants, and Children; Early and Periodic Screening, Diagnosis, and Treatment Program; and Title V Maternal and Child Health Program. The goal of PedNSS is to provide data on the prevalence and trends of nutrition-related indicators and to disseminate information that would help establish policy.

Epidemiologic Surveys of Children and Adolescents

In addition to the NCHS data, a number of long-term, primarily government-funded, epidemiologic studies on children and adolescents have provided critical information used to guide the nation's health policies. The Bogalusa Heart Study (BHS) and the National Longitudinal Study of Adolescent Health are leading examples, as is the new National Children's Study.

Most governments, either autonomously or through universities, track the health and nutrition status of their population. Many of the studies listed below, such as the Young Finns Study and the Amsterdam Growth and Health Longitudinal Study, were not done in the United States. As global health problems, notably obesity and its recognized comorbid conditions, invade not only developed countries but also undeveloped

CRITICAL **Thinking**

You may have participated in the YRBSS when you were in high school. If not, you can see what this study is about. The 2007 survey (http://www.cdc.gov/HealthyYouth/yrbs/pdf/questionnaire/2007 HighSchool.pdf) and the Middle School Behavioral Risk Survey (http:// www.cdc.gov/HealthyYouth/yrbs/pdf/questionnaire/2007Middle School.pdf) are available online. How can these new data be used?

6. http://www.cdc.gov/mmwr/PDF/SS/SS5505.pdf

7. http://www.cdc.gov/healthyyouth/yrbs/middleschool2003/pdf/fullreport.pdf

ones, it is important to understand more fully the universality that diet, physical activity, and other life-style factors have on the development of chronic disease.

BHS

The BHS was designed initially to examine the early natural history of coronary heart disease and essential hypertension in a biracial (African-American and white) pediatric population (Berenson et al., 1980; Berenson, Wattigney, Bao, Srinivasan, & Radhakrishnamurthy, 1995; Berenson, 1986). Today, the BHS population consists of approximately 5,000 individuals studied at various growth phases and followed for as long as 15 years. The mixed epidemiologic design of the study included **cross-sectional** and longitudinal surveys to provide information on three questions:

> **Cross-sectional surveys:** Look at individuals with respect to both exposure and disease at a point in time. Because both exposure and disease are assessed at the same time, it can be difficult to determine whether exposure predated disease.

1. What is the distribution and prevalence of cardiovascular disease risk factors in a defined pediatric population, and how are abnormal serum lipid levels, blood pressure, and other risk factors defined?
2. Do cardiovascular risk factors track and change over time?
3. What is the interrelationship among these risk factors?

Other questions—notably, what is the interaction of genetics and the environment—were also posed.

Data from the BHS have contributed significantly to our knowledge and understanding of cardiovascular risk factors in children. More than 800 publications have been generated from this study. Information on children, adolescents, and young adults from birth to 31 years of age has provided the framework to establish desirable cholesterol levels in children and has led investigators to recommend screening of cardiovascular risk factors for all children, not only those with a parental history of cardiovascular disease, beginning at preschool age. Data have also suggested that risk factors for cardiovascular disease "track," that is, they remain in a rank relative to peers. For example, children with elevated serum total cholesterol or low-density lipoprotein (LDL) cholesterol levels are likely to become adults with dyslipidemia. Recently it was shown that children with BMIs in the 99th percentile may be at risk for biochemical anomalies and severe adult obesity (Freedman, Kettel-Khan, Srinivasan, & Berenson, 2000).

BHS data have been used to characterize children's diets and secular trends in children's diets for more than 20 years (Nicklas et al., 2004) and were used by the AAP as part of the rationale for its recommendation that the Dietary Guidelines for Americans could apply to healthy children aged 2 years and older. Data were also used to develop the American Dietetic Association's position paper on dietary guidance for healthy children aged 2 to 11 years (Nicklas & Johnson, 2004). This rich data set has also provided the opportunity to examine the link between cardiovascular risk factors and genotypes in individuals who had been evaluated from 2 to 12 times (Hallman, Srinivasan, Chen, Boerwinkle, & Berenson, 2004; Chen, Li, Srinivasan, Boerwinkle, & Berenson, 2005).

Another major accomplishment of the BHS comes not from the epidemiologic data per se but from autopsy studies of participants (Berenson et al., 1992), usually children and adolescents killed in accidents. BHS data confirmed and extended earlier studies (Strong & McGill, 1962) that showed fatty streaks in the aorta are evident in the first decade of life and that the extensiveness of these lesions is highly correlated with serum total cholesterol and LDL cholesterol levels.

The strengths of the BHS include its length, which allowed children to be followed into young adulthood; a large well-characterized biracial cohort; and excellent relations with the community that allowed ancillary studies, such as the autopsy study described above. Early in the BHS study it was demonstrated that BHS dietary data were similar to national data (Nicklas, 1995; Nicklas, Johnson, Myers, Webber, & Berenson, 1995). Limitations of the BHS are that data were collected from a restricted semirural geographic area and may not be representative of the country as a whole; although a biracial (African-American and white) population was studied, African-Americans were underrepresented in some surveys and no other ethnic groups were considered. Many of the dietary studies are based on a single dietary recall. Because the BHS has a mixed study design, many of the publications present cross-sectional data only; thus cause and effect relationships cannot be determined. Finally, physical activity data were not collected on the children.

The Framingham Children's Study

The Framingham Children's Study is a longitudinal study looking at diet and physical activity patterns in childhood. In 1987, 106 two-parent families who were third- or fourth-generation offspring of the original Framingham Heart Study[8] cohort with a healthy biological child between 3 and 5 years of age (mean age, 4.0) were enrolled. Diet was assessed using a 3-day food diary. This study showed that tracking of nutrient intake begins in children as young as 3 years of age (Singer, Moore, Garrahie, & Ellison, 1995). Further, children ($n = 95$) who consumed four or more servings of fruit and vegetables or two or more servings of dairy had smaller yearly increases in systolic blood pressure than those who did not (Moore et al., 2005).

The Framingham Children's Study examined the relationship of life-style factors to measures of adiposity in children and underscored the contribution of physical activity to weight in children. Preschool children who were not physically active gained more subcutaneous fat than those who were not (Moore, Nguyen, Rothman, Cupples, & Ellison, 1995). Moore et al. (2003) also showed that higher levels of physical activity in early childhood ($n = 103$) led to lower levels of body fat in early adolescence. By age 11 ($n = 106$), children who watched 3 or more hours of television a day had a higher mean sum of five skinfold measurements than those who did not. The effect of television viewing was greater in children who were sedentary and had a high-fat diet (Proctor et al., 2003). Further, parents displaying high levels of disinhibited eating, especially when coupled with high dietary restraint, fostered the development of excess body fat in their children ($n = 92$) (Hood et al., 2000). Together, these studies suggest that obesity in children is multifactorial and that when planning intervention studies a multidisciplinary approach should be taken.

Advantages of the Framingham Children's Study are that this is a longitudinal study and there has been a high retention rate, possibly because this is such a well-studied population. However, a major limitation is its small sample size; thus all data should be interpreted with caution.

Healthy Passages

Healthy Passages is a 10-year study, begun in 2004, that looks at individual, family, peer, and community influences on health risk factors of preteens and teens (Windle et al., 2004). Although the primary focus is to examine influences on substance abuse, mental health, sexual behaviors, and school achievement, the study also looks at factors that contribute to diet and physical activity and how race, ethnicity, gen-

If you want to know more about adolescent health, the monograph "Reducing the Risk: Connections That Make a Difference in the Lives of Youth" is available online (http://allaboutkids.umn.edu/cfahad/Reducing_the_risk.pdf).

der, family income, and parental behavior affect behaviors and health. This multicenter study enrolled 5,250 fifth-grade students and will collect data every other year from the children and their parents. Participants are from 75 schools in Houston, Texas, Birmingham, Alabama, and Los Angeles, California, and the population is approximately divided among white, African-American, and Hispanic children. Although this study has barely begun, investigators are designing a follow-up study to continue monitoring the population. The strengths of this study are that it is multicentered and has a large and ethnically diverse sample. Healthy Passages has the potential to provide the basis for adolescent health recommendations and interventions.

National Longitudinal Study of Adolescent Health

The National Longitudinal Study of Adolescent Health[9] is the largest and most comprehensive survey of adolescents ever undertaken. It was created in response to a federal mandate as part of the National Institutes of Health Revitalization Act of 1993 (Public Law 103-43, Title X, Subtitle D, Section 1031). Initiated in 1994, this study explores the causes of health-related behaviors of adolescents in grades 7 through 12 and their outcomes in young adulthood. The impact of three potential influences on adverse health—social environment, behaviors, and "strengths and vulnerabilities"—are being studied. Information collected includes diet, physical activity, sexual practices, substance use, and suicidal thoughts. Complementary information collected includes height, weight, physical development, mental status, and any chronic health conditions.

There were 80 high schools and 52 middle schools in the core study, and in wave I (1994–1995) 12,105 adolescents were interviewed as part of the core sample. The cohort had an oversampling of certain ethnic/socioeconomic status groups: 1,038 African-Americans with at least one parent with a college education, 334 Chinese, 450 Cubans, 437 Puerto Ricans, and 1,500 Mexican-Americans, and other Hispanics and Asians. Further, 589 students described themselves as disabled. This provides an ethnically diverse data set that is lacking in many

---

8. http://www.nhlbi.nih.gov/about/framingham

9. http://www.cpc.unc.edu/projects/addhealth

of the other cohorts, and, not surprisingly, this study has provided a rich data set for study. Wave II (1996) interviewed nearly 15,000 of the original cohort. Wave III (2001 and 2002) interviewed the original participants and their partners and collected saliva and urine to test for sexually transmitted diseases and the human immunodeficiency virus. Wave IV has been funded through 2010 and will study developmental and health trajectories across adolescents into young adulthood.

More than 1,700 publications and dissertations have used data generated from this study, and the list is available online.[10] Virtually every aspect of adolescent life is covered in these publications, including but certainly not limited to clustering of behavior problems (Bartlett, Holditch-Davis, & Belyea, 2005), perceptions of weight management (Kilpatrick, Ohanessian, & Bartholomew, 1999), and the accuracy of teen reporting of BMI (Goodman et al., 2000).

Cardiovascular Risk in Young Finns Study

The purpose of this multicenter study[11] was to determine the effects that childhood life-style as well as biological and psychological measures have on the risk of cardiovascular diseases in adulthood. Begun in 1980, the original cohort of 3,596 (83.2% of those invited to participate) children and adolescents aged 3, 6, 9, 12, 15, and 18 years were followed at 3-year intervals. Risk factor assessment included laboratory measures of serum lipoproteins, insulin, markers of inflammation (e.g., C-reactive protein), and homocysteine; adiposity measures; blood pressure; life-style factors, including diet, physical activity, smoking status, and alcohol use; psychological factors, such as depressive symptoms; and socioeconomic status. Genetic studies were also conducted. In 2001 the 21-year follow-up was conducted on over 2,283 (63.5% of the original cohort) young adults (aged 24 to 30 years). In addition to the risk factors mentioned, noninvasive ultrasound examinations were performed to assess carotid artery intima-media thickness, carotid artery elasticity, and brachial artery flow-mediated endothelium-dependent dilatation.

The Young Finns Study confirmed and extended data on the tracking of risk factors for cardiovascular disease generated by the BHS. For example, the study showed that systolic blood pressure tracks into

adulthood but also demonstrated that low socioeconomic status in early life influences blood pressure later in life, in part due to its effect on blood pressure in childhood (Kivimaki et al., 2006a, 2006b). This study demonstrated that the diet of young Finns has improved over time but that it fell short of recommendations (Mikkilä, Räsänen, Raitakari, Pietinen, Viikari, 2004). Other diet intake studies used pattern analysis to show changes over time and identified two food patterns—a traditional one and a health-conscious pattern, which was associated with other healthy behaviors (Mikkilä, Räsänen, Raitakari, Pietinen, & Viikari, 2005). The studies with ultrasound at the 21-year follow-up provide important information on the relationship of subclinical atherosclerosis and other risk factors. The study suggested that endothelial dysfunction is an early event in atherosclerosis, and systemic endothelial function may modify the association between risk factors and atherosclerosis (Juonala et al., 2004). Moreover, there were geographic differences in greater carotid intima-media thickness and lower brachial flow-mediated dilation, suggesting genetic influences (Juonala et al., 2005).

The strengths of the Young Finns Study include the long follow-up period, large sample size (it is one of the largest longitudinal studies of children, adolescents, and young adults), inclusion of physical activity, use of a 48-hour recall to assess diet, and innovative approach with ultrasound to detect early changes associated with atherosclerosis. To date, there are over 200 publications from data collected during this study. Study limitations are that the sample was all white and all limited to a single group. Further, a high percentage of the cohort was lost to follow-up.

Avon Longitudinal Study of Parents and Children

The Avon Longitudinal Study of Parents and Children was initiated in 1990 (Golding, 1990). It is the largest longitudinal study of childhood in the world, aiming to reveal how physical and social environment interact with genetic inheritance to affect all aspects of a child's health and development. This birth study has the advantage of long-term follow-up. The core sample consisted of 14,541 pregnancies (1991–1992), with 14,062 live births (13,971 alive at 12 months). There are comprehensive data on nearly 10,000 children and their parents, from early pregnancy to ages 8 and 9. These data appear very comparable with national United Kingdom data, increasing the generalization of the

10. http://www.cpc.unc.edu/projects/addhealth/pubs?func=viewandwid=1257andfolderId=1009
11. http://vanha.med.utu.fi/cardio/youngfinnsstudy

findings. The goal of the study is to continue to collect detailed data on the children as they go through puberty, noting in particular changes in anthropometry, attitudes and behavior, fitness and other cardiovascular risk factors, bone mineralization, allergic symptoms, and mental health.

There are several important findings from the Avon Longitudinal Study of Parents and Children: childhood bone mass is related to maternal diet in pregnancy (Tobias et al., 2005), breast-feeding is associated with lower blood pressure in children born at term (Martin et al., 2004), and habitual physical activity was associated with improved bone size and bone mineral density (Tobias, Steer, Mattocks, Riddoch, & Ness, 2007). It is obvious that this rich data set will continue to be assessed and other important publications will be forthcoming; to date, more than 270 peer-reviewed journal articles have appeared.

This study is presented because it is an example of a birth study—newborns and their parents can be followed over time, providing insight into the development of physical, physiologic, and psychosocial changes and their relationship to chronic disease. The large sample size adds statistical power to the variety of studies performed. Limitations include a limited racial/ethnic diversity and a small geographic area from which subjects were recruited.

The German Dortmund Nutritional and Anthropometric Longitudinally Designed Study

The Dortmund Nutritional and Anthropometric Longitudinally Designed (DONALD) study is an observational longitudinal open **cohort study** began in 1985 that examines diet, metabolism, growth, and development from healthy subjects between infancy and adulthood (Kroke et al., 2004). This study has approximately 1,000 children, 1,000 mothers, and 1,000 fathers participating. Approximately 40 to 50 healthy infants are enrolled yearly. Participants are studied every 3 months in year 1, twice in year 2, and once a year thereafter. A 3-day diet record kept either by the parents or by older children is used to assess dietary intake. Urine sampling and urinalysis, anthropometry, and physical examinations are also conducted. Participants are interviewed using age-specific questions on sleeping habits, dejection, sports activities,

Cohort studies: Classify participants based on the presence or absence of exposure and follow them over time to assess disease development. An example of this type of study is the Nurses Health Study. In a *retrospective cohort study,* the disease of interest has already occurred at the time the study begins; in a *prospective cohort study,* the disease has not yet occurred.

and use of medical preventative services. One of the unique aspects of the DONALD study is attention to dietary supplementation. The DONALD study has shown that on average German children meet nutritional recommendations without supplements, with the exception of folate and vitamin D (Sichert-Hellert, Kersting, Alexy, & Manz, 2000). The study also showed that 56% of fortified foods consumed had added sugar. However, the positive effect of food fortification was stronger than the negative effect of added dietary sugars, suggesting that fortification of foods masks nutrient dilution (Alexy, Sichert-Hellert, & Kersting, 2002). Other diet studies suggest that an energy-based approach should be used when setting dietary recommendations for children (Alexy, Kersting, & Sichert-Hellert, 2006). Findings like these are important in setting nutrition policy with regard to food fortification and dietary recommendations for individual countries.

The DONALD study also defined adequate intake of water (Manz, Wentz, & Sichert-Hellert, 2000) and the role of nutritional status in the regulation of adrenarche (Remer & Manz, 1999). Subsets of the population have participated in the Euro Growth Study (van't Hof, Haschke, & the Euro-Growth Group, 2000) and a study to determine the circadian rhythms of urine osmolality and renal excretion rates (Ballauff, Rascher, Tolle, Wember, & Manz, 1991). Studies like these suggest the flexibility of the data set.

Advantages of the DONALD study are that the food consumed was recorded for 3 days, leading to greater accuracy in estimating intake, and special care was taken to collect information on fortified food and supplements. Disadvantages are its use of a convenience sample and that no blood was collected, so the relationship of diet or obesity cannot be related to genetic or other biomarkers of chronic disease. Another limitation is the study's relatively small sample size, with a limited ethnic variety residing in a limited geographic area.

| Intervention Studies

Large-scale long-term diet or physical activity **intervention studies** are relatively uncommon in healthy children. The two discussed in this chapter were chosen because they illustrate interventions at different times in the life cycle—infancy

Intervention studies: A type of prospective cohort study where the exposure is controlled by the investigator. These studies can be considered therapeutic (secondary prevention) or preventative. Dietary Approaches to Stop Hypertension (DASH) and DASH-sodium are intervention studies.

Think about it. What elements of an intervention study are needed to make it successful? What can be done to maintain the population over time?

(Special Turku Coronary Risk Factor Intervention Project for Babies) (Lapinleimu et al., 1995; Simell et al., 2000) and childhood and adolescence (Child and Adolescent Trial for Cardiovascular Health [CATCH]).

Special Turku Coronary Risk Factor Intervention Project for Babies

This study was designed to test the effect of a low saturated fat, low cholesterol diet on infants. The argument for doing this was that atherosclerotic mechanisms, including foam cells in the arterial intima (Strong, Malcom, Newman, & Oalmann, 1992), are already active in children; lesion development depends in part on serum cholesterol levels (Newman et al., 1986) in childhood. Studies also show that if earlier cholesterol levels can be lowered, the prognosis is better (Law, Wald, & Thompson, 1994). The argument against an intervention like this is that altering dietary fat in the diets of children would interfere with growth and development (Lifshitz & Moses, 1989; AAP, 1992).

CRITICAL Thinking

The Special Turku Coronary Risk Factor Intervention Project for Babies study is a well-conceived and carefully controlled intervention. Do you believe the results from this study should be used to make policy changes in dietary recommendations for infants and young children? Why or why not? Do additional studies need to be performed? If so, what kind of studies should be done?

Originally, 1,062 seven-month-old infants in Turku, Finland were recruited and randomly assigned to a low saturated fat, low cholesterol diet ($n = 540$) to meet the Nordic dietary recommendations for individuals 3 years and older or to a control group ($n = 522$). Twice yearly, the intervention group received intensive health education aimed at reducing risk of atherosclerosis and individual dietary counseling from a physician and a dietitian; after weaning of the infants, families kept food records for 4 consecutive days, including a weekend day. The control group received standard health education given to well babies at clinics, but they did not receive individual dietary counseling. Serum lipids, lipoproteins, and apolipoproteins were measured, as were weight and length or standing height (depending on the age of the child). There was no difference in baseline parameters between the two groups.

At 36 months of age, 426 children (79%) remained in the intervention group and 417 children (80%) remained in the control group (Simell et al., 2000). At that time total serum and high-density lipoprotein (HDL) cholesterol levels were lower in the intervention group than in the control group; further, there was no evidence of delayed growth, and height and weight increases were comparable with Finnish standards (Simell et al., 2000). At 5 years of age the children in the intervention group consumed less saturated fat, had lower total and LDL cholesterol levels (Salo et al., 1999), and had no delays in neurodevelopment (Rask-Nissila et al., 2002). The conclusion of this study was that there were no ill effects of the low saturated fat, low cholesterol diet in these children.

CATCH (1987–2000)

CATCH was a National Heart Lung and Blood Institute funded multicenter randomized trial of a school-wide intervention to improve cardiovascular disease–related behaviors, including diet, physical activity, and smoking, of elementary schoolchildren. CATCH provides an excellent example of how information from a natural history study like the BHS, that identified risk factors for cardiovascular disease present in childhood, can be used as the basis for an intervention study. CATCH was the largest and one of the most comprehensive school-based intervention studies and included an educational curriculum along with a behavioral component, modification of the school environment—including modifying school meals and family-oriented interventions (Perry et al., 1990). The overarching goal was to reduce dietary fat and sodium, increase physical activity, and prevent smoking in children. Initially, 5,100 racial and ethnically diverse third- to fifth-grade students attending 96 elementary schools in California, Louisiana, Minnesota, and Texas constituted the cohort; schools were randomized to intervention ($n = 56$) or control ($n = 40$) schools. Follow-up surveys were conducted in 1996–1997 (Osganian et al., 1999) and in 2000–2001 (Osganian et al., 2003a), when students were in grades 8 and 12, respectively.

CATCH participants provided information about diet and health behaviors; BMI and serum lipid levels were determined. CATCH demonstrated the following: cardiovascular risk factors in children varied by gender and ethnicity (Webber et al., 1995); physiologic variables, including serum lipid levels, tracked into the eighth grade, and tracking was stronger in boys and in African-Americans (Kelder et al., 2002); a school food service–based intervention could modify school lunch, health behaviors, and physical activity programs (Luepker et al., 1996); and changes resulting from the intervention could be maintained (Nader et al., 1999).

The success of CATCH as an intervention study can be seen by its widespread adoption in school systems. For example, by autumn 2000, 728 elementary schools in Texas had adopted CATCH materials (Hoelscher et al., 2001), and it is clear that the program has been successful (Hoelscher et al., 2004). What makes an intervention program successful and adaptable to other school systems is not clear. Because CATCH was adopted by so many other schools, it was important to use this program as a model of a program that can be institutionalized—the CATCH-ON study was designed to do this (Osganian, Parcel, & Stone, 2003b). The physical activity component appeared to have the highest level of institutionalization (Lytle, Ward, Nader, Pedersen, & Williston, 2003), whereas the educational curriculum and the family components had the lowest level. Factors that facilitated maintenance of the CATCH Eat Smart Program (the school food service component of CATCH) included satisfaction of school food service personnel and perceived student satisfaction with the program (McCullum-Gomez, Barroso, Hoelscher, Ward, & Kelder, 2006). Identification of barriers to and enablers for program institutionalization are key elements of a successful program.

Comment on Epidemiologic Studies in Children and Adolescents

Many of these studies have followed children from birth into young adulthood and, in some cases, into middle adulthood. This provides a smooth transition through the life cycle and allows us to understand more fully the changes that occur in chronic disease risk factors and the occurrence of chronic disease throughout the life cycle. Over time, studies have become more complex. As more biological risk factors for disease have been identified and the understanding of risk factors for chronic diseases has improved, investigators have been able to include additional questionnaires or laboratory tests to garner still more information.

Study results can be compared and trends can be identified and targeted for intervention. NHANES data have allowed us to follow the pediatric obesity epidemic. Using 1999–2002 data, 23% of children aged 2 to 5 years were overweight or at risk of becoming overweight (BMI ≥ 85th percentile) and 10.3% were overweight (BMI ≥ 95th percentile). The percentage of children who were overweight increased compared with data from NHANES III (1988–1994), which showed 7.2% of children aged 2 to 5 years were overweight. These data were confirmed by the YRBSS and by longitudinal studies from all over the world. Additional studies confirmed risk factors that are amenable to modification through intervention, so clearly the universality of these data clear the way for policy change and intervention studies.

A number of challenges had to be met when conducting research with children. The first, as discussed above, revolved around issues of informed consent. Although these issues have not been fully resolved, solutions have been found for individual studies to allow research to go forward. Other challenges include how to collect information on children because, for instance, young children cannot complete a 24-hour recall or fill out a food frequency questionnaire (FFQ). Investigators in pioneering studies, like BHS, painstakingly worked to develop methods to obtain diet information on children (Frank, Berenson, Schilling, & Moore, 1977). BHS set the standard for working with children in longitudinal studies: Their quality controls included a standardized protocol for the collection, calculation, and editing of 24-hour dietary recalls (from the BHS nutrition staff: "In-house Dietary Studies Methodology" [editions 1–8], 1978–1988); graduated food models for quantification of amounts of foods and beverages consumed (Moore, Judlin, & Kennemur, 1967); a product identification notebook for snack probing; a school lunch (Nicklas, Forcier, Webber, & Berenson, 1991); and a family recipe collection of actual food preparation, recipes, brand names of foods, and actual serving sizes of school meal food items served.

A major limitation of many of these studies described herein is that most examined white children and adolescents only. This is also true of the international studies. Even in studies where children of other racial and ethnic groups were included, they were often underrepresented, making it difficult to statistically factor race or ethnicity into any analysis—especially in small studies. It is critical that studies look at the impact that life-style factors have on different races and ethnicities. The BHS study showed clear differences with regard to weight, especially in African-American girls (Freedman et al., 2000); with regard to physiologic parameters such as birth weight and blood pressure (Cruickshank et al., 2005); and with regard to diet (Demory-Luce et al., 2004) of African-American children when compared with white children. It is clear that when Asian and Hispanic children and adolescents were studied, there were differences in health behaviors (Allen et al., 2007), suggesting a need for different intervention strategies.

Many of the studies are regional with comparatively small sample sizes. These studies have provided important information on diet and other life-style behaviors, health parameters such as blood pressure, and biomarkers of disease such as serum lipid levels. Multiple studies demonstrated that these risk fac-

tors track into adulthood and suggest that early intervention is important to reduce the risk of childhood and adult disease. It is important to replicate these findings in nationally representative samples.

Finally, when assessing these and other studies, it is vital to evaluate the strength of the body of scientific evidence, by taking the following into account:

1. The quality of the studies, including the extent to which bias was minimized
2. The quantity of the studies, including the magnitude of effect, the number of studies, and the *sample size* and *statistical power* of the study
3. The consistency of results (i.e., do similar studies produce similar results)
4. The study design (i.e., what type of study was used to produce the test results and the relevance to the disease under study)

The National Heart, Lung, and Blood Institute uses a four-point scale to grade the scientific evidence from different study types (Table 1.4). Other types of evidence may also be available, but they are weaker and should be considered less definitive.

Cooper and Zlotkin (2003) outlined a six-step framework by which nutrition guidelines can be developed. Their method is similar to that of the National Heart, Lung, and Blood Institute but emphasizes nutrition information. The Agency for Healthcare Research and Quality[12] provides additional information about evidence-based practice, outcomes and other types of research, technology assessment, and clinical practice guidelines to professionals and to the public. A review of systems to rate the strength of sci-

TABLE 1.4 National Heart, Lung, and Blood Institute's Evidence Categories

Category	Sources of Evidence	Definition
A	Randomized controlled trials (rich body of data)	Well-designed randomized clinical trials that provide a consistent pattern of findings in the population for which the recommendation is made. Category A requires substantial numbers of studies involving substantial numbers of participants.
B	Randomized controlled trials (limited body of data)	Limited randomized trials or interventions, post-hoc subgroup analyses, or meta-analyses of randomized clinical trials are used when there are a limited number of existing trials, study populations are small or provide inconsistent results, or when the trials were undertaken in a population that differs from the target population.
C	Observational or nonrandomized studies	Evidence is from outcomes of uncontrolled or nonrandomized trials or from observational studies.
D	Panel consensus judgment	Expert judgment is based on the panel's synthesis of evidence from experimental research described in the literature or derived from the consensus of panel members based on clinical experience or knowledge that does not meet the criteria described in the above categories. This category is used only where the provision of some guidance was deemed valuable but an adequately compelling clinical literature addressing the subject of the recommendation was deemed insufficient to place in one of the other categories.

Source: Adapted from the National Heart, Lung, and Blood Institute, available at http://www.nhlbi.nih.gov/guidelines/obesity/ob_gdlns.pdf

12. http://www.ahrq.gov

entific evidence is also available from the National Library of Medicine.[13]

Future of Epidemiologic Studies in Children

National Children's Study

Perhaps the most exciting epidemiologic study of children is one that has not yet begun—the National Children's Study.[14] Authorized by Congress as part of the Children's Health Act of 2000,[15] this study will examine the environmental influences on health and development on a nationally representative cohort of 100,000 children from before birth to age 21.

Priority health and disease outcomes are pregnancy outcomes, neurodevelopment and behavior, childhood injury, asthma, obesity, and physical development. "Environment" is broadly defined and will include natural and man-made environmental factors, biological and chemical factors, physical surroundings, social factors, behavioral influences and outcomes, genetics, cultural and family influences, and differences among geographic locations. This study is predicted to be one of the richest information sources available on children's health and should form the basis for interventions, policy, training future researchers, and a "comprehensive blueprint for

disease prevention in children" (Trasande et al., 2006; Landrigan et al., 2006).

In 2005 contracts were awarded to seven Vanguard Centers in universities, hospitals, and health departments located in Orange County, California; New York City (Queens); Duplin County, North Carolina; Montgomery County, Pennsylvania; Brookings County, South Dakota; Lincoln, Pipestone, and Yellow Medicine Counties, Minnesota (cluster site); Salt Lake City, Utah; and Waukesha County, Wisconsin. The lead federal agencies involved (the U.S. Department of Health and Human Services, the Environmental Protection Agency, the CDC, and the National Institute for Environmental Health Sciences) anticipate 30 to 40 study sites that will involve 105 sites, of which 79 are metropolitan counties and 26 are rural nonmetropolitan areas, as defined by the U.S. Census Bureau. The 79 metropolitan sites include populous counties and smaller urban and suburban areas. Each site has the goal of enrolling at least 250 newborns each year for 5 years. Initial enrollment is planned for 2008.

The National Children's Study will be the first to evaluate environmental exposures before and early in pregnancy and to then track participants into adulthood. Pregnant women and their partners, couples planning pregnancy, and women who are of childbearing age but are not planning a pregnancy will constitute the initial cohort. Although other studies have assessed prenatal exposures on children, they have either started in the first trimester of pregnancy or stopped tracking at birth.

Centers for Children's Environmental Health and Disease Prevention Research

Two of the lead federal agencies for the National Children's Study are the Environmental Protection Agency and the National Institute for Environmental Health Sciences, who funded the Centers for Children's Environmental Health and Disease Prevention Research (Children's Centers).[16] Recently, a minimonograph about the Children's Centers was published that was intended to serve as a "primer" for the National Children's Study (Kimmel, Collman, Fields, & Eskenazi, 2005), including topics on methodology on conducting birth cohort studies (Eskenazi et al., 2005) and community participatory research (Israel et al., 2005) as well as issues in studying air pollution (Gilliland et al., 2005), pesticide exposure (Fenske, Bradman, Whyatt, Wolff, & Barr,

---

13. http://www.nlm.nih.gov/nichsr/hta101/ta10107.html
14. http://www.nationalchildrensstudy.gov/index.cfm
15. http://frwebgate.access.gpo.gov/cgi-bin/getdoc.cgi?dbname=106_cong_billsanddocid=f:h4365enr.txt

---

16. http://www.niehs.nih.gov/translat/children/children.htm

2005), asthma (Eggleston et al., 2005), and neurobehavioral toxicity (Dietrich et al., 2005). In *Life of Reason* (1905, p. 284) George Santayana says, "Progress, far from consisting in change, depends on retentiveness. Those who cannot remember the past are condemned to repeat it." This "lessons learned" philosophy should also be applied to research, and these authors should be applauded for sharing this information.

The impact that the National Children's Study and other future studies will have on the understanding of health and disease is extraordinary, and it is questionable whether they could have been attempted previously. There has been a growing public concern over the link between health, genetics, and environmental exposures (Israel et al., 2005) because of the mounting evidence of increasing morbidity and mortality in children from health problems, including those from environmental exposures, including asthma (Akinbami & Schoendorf, 2002), neuropsychological and developmental disorders (Hertz-Picciotto et al., 2006), and cancer (Daniels, Olshan, & Savitz, 1997). The rising prevalence of pediatric overweight and obesity, coupled with the appearance of adult comorbidities, such as type 2 diabetes, metabolic syndrome, and nonalcoholic fatty liver disease, in pediatric populations (Cruz et al., 2005) has fueled public interest in children's health. From a scientific standpoint these adult disease risk factors include health behaviors such as diet (Mikkilä et al., 2005; Lake, Mathers, Rugg-Gunn, & Adamson, 2006) and physical activity (Telama et al., 2005); anthropometric markers, notably weight (Deshmukh-Taskar et al., 2006); and health measures such as plasma lipid (Webber, Srinivasan, Wattigney, & Berenson, 1991; Bao, Srinivasan, Wattigney, & Berenson, 1994), C-reactive protein levels (Juonala et al., 2006), insulin levels (Bao et al., 1994), and blood pressure (Bao, Threefoot, Srinivasan, & Berenson, 1995).

Thus strong public interest in health research coupled with technologic advances, including sequencing the human genome, public health genomics, and the creation of the Human Genome Epidemiology Network[17]; advances in assessing biomarkers, including markers of human environmental exposures; public health informatics; statistical advances in data modeling; and improved communications have led to the conceptualization of such ambitious projects. This is not to say that these studies will be without problems. The diversity of the population

and growing health disparities in the United States are major challenges (Gupta, Carrion-Carire, & Weiss, 2006; Selden, 2006). Medical–legal issues, such as those revolving around the use of vulnerable populations, including children and adolescents (Diaz et al., 2004; Summers et al., 2006), and the financial support of investigators, are becoming more complex (Davidoff et al., 2001). Finally, research standards have risen, and the way research studies are evaluated has changed.

Research Involving Adults

Elizabeth Metallinos-Katsaras, PhD, RD and Sari Kalin, MS

The purpose of this section is to provide an overview of some of the major adult epidemiologic studies that have contributed to the research-based underlying prevention efforts and the development of nutrition guidelines. The following major nutrition-related adult studies are summarized and, where applicable, links are made to dietary recommendations:

- Framingham Heart Study, original and offspring cohorts
- Nurses Health Study I
- Nurses Health Study II
- Health Professionals Follow-Up Study
- Physicians' Health Study I
- Physicians' Health Study II
- Iowa Women's Health Study
- Dietary Approaches to Stop Hypertension (DASH) and DASH-sodium
- Women's Health Initiative
- OmniHeart

Each study is reviewed regarding the following aspects:

1. History and original purpose
2. Sample characteristics
3. Types of data collected (nutrition related)
4. Example of a major contribution
5. Study strengths and limitations

Studies are classified according to design, emphasizing how the selected design elucidated the association between nutrition and the development of chronic diseases.

Prospective Cohort Studies

A cohort study is a type of observational study in which the researcher defines two or more groups of people who are disease free and differ with respect

---

17. http://www.cdc.gov/genomics/hugenet/default.htm

to their degree of exposure to a possible cause of the disease in question (Rothman & Greenland, 1998). Prospective cohort studies are those in which the subjects are free of the disease at the initiation of the study and the relevant exposure may or may not have occurred (Hennekens & Buring, 1987). This design is rigorous and is second only to the randomized controlled trial. A major strength of this study design is that exposure data are collected before disease diagnosis. Thus the presence of the disease does not bias the reporting of the exposure data. Limitations of this design are that it is not good for studying rare diseases and there is significant potential for confounding bias because subjects have self-selected their exposure.

Framingham Heart Study

The Framingham Heart Study, one of the longest running prospective cohort studies, started in 1948 with the goal of understanding the causes of heart disease. The original cohort of 5,209 men and women, ranging from ages 30 to 62 years, was randomly selected from the adult population of Framingham, Massachusetts (Framingham Heart Study, 2005). Every 2 years since the study's inception participants received a thorough physical examination (including medical history interviews and laboratory tests) (Framingham Heart Study, 2005). The study has grown into a multigenerational enterprise, one that is now using molecular techniques to yield information about the genetic underpinnings of chronic disease. In 1971 study investigators began the Framingham Offspring Cohort, which includes 5,124 sons and daughters of the original cohort participants who are examined approximately every 4 years (Millen et al., 1996; Framingham Heart Study, 2005). Moreover, in 2005 investigators launched the Generation III Cohort with 4,095 third-generation descendants of the original study participants; by September of that year 299 of the 472 surviving original participants received their 28th medical examinations (Framingham Heart Study, 2005).

One critique of the Framingham study is that the original and offspring cohorts are predominantly white, reflecting the homogenous demographic makeup of the Framingham community at the study's launch. Framingham has since become a more diverse community, and study investigators began the multiethnic Omni Cohort in 1994, with 506 men and women (Framingham Heart Study, 2005). At baseline, Omni cohort members were between the ages of 40 and 74, and they received a thorough physical and laboratory examination identical to that of the Framingham Offspring Cohort (Quan et al., 1997).

Framingham's nutritional assessment methods have evolved throughout the decades. Some of the earliest inquiries, in the early 1960s, used Burke-style hour-long interviews (Mann, Pearson, Gordon, & Dawber, 1962). Single 24-hour recalls were collected at various time points (e.g., in 1966–1969 from the original cohort and in 1984–1988 from the offspring cohort), as were 3-day diet records, yielding insights on the relationship between diet and heart disease (Gordon et al., 1981; Millen et al., 1996). Framingham investigators also developed a 145-item FFQ (a modified version of the Willett semiquantitative FFQ) and validated it with the offspring cohort (Posner et al., 1992). Cluster analysis of the offspring cohort's FFQ data has been used to identify distinct dietary patterns (e.g., the "heart healthy" and "empty calorie" patterns in women) and relate these patterns to overweight, metabolic syndrome, and chronic disease outcomes (Millen et al., 2001, 2002, 2005a, 2005b; Sonnenberg et al., 2005). This type of pattern analysis could be useful for target health promotion messages to prevent chronic disease.

Credited with coining the term "risk factor," the Framingham Heart Study is best known for providing decades of evidence that smoking, high blood cholesterol, high blood pressure, sedentary life-styles, obesity, and diabetes dramatically increase the risk of heart disease (Framingham Heart Study, 2005). Doctors now use the Framingham Point Score prediction algorithm to predict patients' 10-year risk of coronary heart disease; this risk prediction helps guide clinical decision making on LDL targets and management (National Cholesterol Education Program, 2001). Over the years the Framingham cohorts have yielded insights on nutrition and life-style relationships for other disease end points, including cancer (Radimer et al., 2004), osteoporosis (Tucker et al., 2006), and Alzheimer's disease (Seshadri et al., 2002).

Nurses Health Studies

There are two prospective cohort studies based solely on female registered nurses. These are, in chronological order, the Nurses Health Study (NHS) and the NHS II. The first NHS was initiated in 1976 with the express purpose of studying the long-term consequences of oral contraceptive use (Nurses Health Study [NHS] I, n.d.). The NHS I was begun by Dr. Frank Speizer and was designed to study oral contraceptives and also to investigate diet and life-style risk factors in the population (Nurses Health Study [NHS] II, n.d.).

Originally, registered nurses were selected as the target population because their degree of education would facilitate accurate responses to technically worded health-related questions (NHS I, n.d.). Moreover, it was anticipated that they would be more motivated than the average person in the population to participate over the long term. This was substantiated in relatively high response rates reported, 71% for the 1976 questionnaire (Meyers et al., 1987) and 90% for each 2-year period thereafter (NHS I, n.d.).

NHS originally included 121,700 female nurses who were between the ages of 30 and 55 in 1976. They were sampled from the most populous states whose nursing boards agreed to supply the member's names and addresses; this yielded a representation from 11 states (NHS I, n.d.). The original cohort was 96.8% white (G. Chase, Data Manager, NHS, personal communication, August 16, 2006). Dietary assessment for the NHS was conducted in 1980, 1984, and 1986 and every 4 years thereafter, using a semi-quantitative FFQ developed for the study (HFFQ). Three different versions of the HFFQ were developed ranging from the inclusion of 61 items to 126 items (NHS, n.d.). Validity and reliability was examined using these HFFQs among nurses using two or four 1-week food records; most of the adjusted correlations for macro- and selected micronutrients were between 0.5 and 0.7 (Willett & Lenart, 1998). These are considered relatively good for epidemiologic measures of risk (Willett & Lenart, 1998).

Toenail (1982 and 1984) and blood samples (1989–1990 and 2000–2001) were also obtained on a subset of the original cohort; the former is useful for mineral analyses, and the latter can be used to identify potential biomarkers, such as hormone levels and genetic markers, although blood samples can also be used to assess the status of some vitamins and minerals (Gibson, 1990).

The NHS II was established in 1989 by Dr. Walter Willett to study oral contraceptives and to investigate effects of diet and life-style risk factors in a population younger than the original NHS cohort (NHS II, n.d.). The target age group was between 25 and 42 in 1989 with a sample size goal of 125,000 female registered nurses. In NHS II the sampling consciously aimed to enroll only those most enthusiastic about participating in this study to maximize future long-term participation. A single mailing was done to 517,000 women in 14 states, and

those who responded to that first questionnaire were enrolled. Twenty-four percent of those sampled responded to that first questionnaire, with 22.6% in the final sample due to exclusions for incomplete forms or not meeting inclusion criteria, yielding a sample size of 116,686 women. Response rates to subsequent questionnaires were 90% for each 2-year cycle. Similar to the original NHS, the HFFQ was administered every 4 years beginning in 1991. Blood and urine samples were also collected on a subset of the sample (about 30,000 nurses) (NHS II, n.d.). Similar to the NHS I, this sample was predominately white (95.8%) (G. Chase, Data Manager, NHS, personal communication, August 16, 2006).

An example of the influence the NHS I and II had on the 2005 Dietary Guidelines for Americans is in the limiting of trans fatty acids in the diet, specifically the guideline "Limit intake of fats and oils high in saturated and/or trans fatty acids, and choose products low in such fats and oils" (U.S. Department of Health and Human Services and the U.S. Department of Agriculture [DHHS and USDA], 2005). The NHS was one of the early studies providing evidence that a high intake of trans fatty acids was associated with a significantly higher risk of myocardial infarction (Willett et al., 1993). Moreover, the NHS I and II were specifically cited in the 2005 Dietary Guidelines Advisory Committee report (DHHS and USDA, n.d.) as showing that trans fat intake was positively associated with the systemic inflammatory markers (i.e., soluble tumor necrosis factor receptors and C-reactive protein) for cardiovascular disease (Mozaffarian et al., 2004).

The strengths of both of these studies lie in their large sample sizes, their long follow-up period, their meticulous collection of dietary data using an instrument that produces a good relative measure of long-term (versus short-term) diet for the purposes of predicting disease outcomes (Caan et al., 1998; Wirfalt et al., 1998), and the high sample retention over the course of the studies. As previously mentioned, the prospective cohort design is one of the stronger epidemiologic designs (Rothman & Greenland, 1998); however, the potential that residual confounding may account for reported results is a real threat to internal validity in this design because the subjects self-select their behaviors and diets. Another potential limitation of both studies is their predominantly white cohort of women. This affects external validity, that is, to whom the results may be applied. Results may not be applicable to other diverse populations if the biological mechanisms underlying the cause and effect relationships are different for different race and ethnic groups. For example, in the case of diet and breast cancer, the association between dietary factors and breast cancer has been shown to vary as a function of whether the cancer occurs pre- or postmenopausally and whether the cancer is estrogen positive or negative and other factors; ethnic or racially specific factors (biological or cultural practices) may also interact with dietary factors to affect breast cancer rates; however, there is no way to elucidate these if the sample is not racially or ethnically diverse.

Health Professionals Follow-Up Study

The Health Professionals Follow-Up Study is an all male prospective cohort study begun in 1986 that intended to complement the all female NHS (Health Professionals Follow-Up Study, n.d.). The hypotheses under investigation centered on the relationship between nutritional factors and the development of chronic diseases such as cardiovascular disease, cancer, and other vascular diseases. The study sample of 51,529 male health professionals (excluding medical doctors) was aged between 40 and 75 years who in 1986 were free of these diseases (Health Professionals Follow-Up Study, n.d.). The justification for examining this group was that, like the nurses, these health professionals would presumably be motivated to participate in a long-term study and would be committed to accurately responding to the questions asked of them. A small percentage of the sample was African-American (1.0%) or Asian-American (1.7%). Study participants received questionnaires about their health-related behaviors and diseases. Dietary data were collected every 4 years using the HFFQ previously described (Health Professionals Follow up Study, n.d.); both validity and reliability of this instrument were assessed using the Health Professionals Follow-Up Study sample (Jensen et al., 2004). Supplemental information on micronutrient supplements and cooking methods were also collected more frequently, some every 2 years (Health Professionals Follow-Up Study, n.d.).

One example of the study's use in the development of the 2005 Dietary Guidelines (DHHS and USDA, 2005) was in the area of the relationship between whole grain intake and risk of coronary heart disease. One of the major studies (DHHS and USDA, n.d.) cited the Health Professionals Follow-Up Study, in which it was found that for every 20-g increase in whole grain consumption there was a 6% risk reduction in coronary heart disease (Jensen et al., 2004).

The strengths and limitations of this prospective cohort study mirror those of the NHS because the design, instruments used, and implementation are so similar. Moreover, both used predominately white participants with very little diversity.

Physicians' Health Studies

The Physicians' Health Studies (PHS) are two studies, one completed and one ongoing, designed as randomized placebo-controlled trials and whose study samples are solely male medical doctors (Physicians' Health Studies II [PHS], 2006). Pertinent nutrition research that emerged from this study is primarily related to the further analyses of the data collected prospectively on these cohorts. PHS I was funded in 1980, and its original intent was to assess the effects of aspirin on cardiovascular outcomes and of beta-carotene on cancer (PHS I, 2002; PHS II, 2006). The original intent of PHS II was to investigate the effects of vitamin E, ascorbic acid, beta-carotene, and/or multivitamins on prevention of prostate cancer, other cancers, and cardiovascular disease in healthy older male doctors; however, beta-carotene was no longer given as of March 8, 2003 (PHS II, 2006). Because this study is a randomized controlled trial, it is discussed further under Randomized Controlled Trials, below. However, it should be noted that because of the long-term follow-up of these physicians (i.e., 8 years for the clinical trail [PHS II, 2002]), it is likely that this study's data will also be analyzed further as a prospective cohort study and therefore results will likely be published using this design.

Physicians were selected as the population from which to draw the samples because of their ability to accurately report data on their health status, medical conditions, and side effects of the intervention. In addition, given their strong interest in health, their compliance, an essential factor in the success of any randomized trial, was anticipated to be high (PHS I, 2002).

In PHS I physicians between the ages of 40 and 84 living in the United States and registered with the American Medical Association were contacted and screened. Of the 33,223 physicians who were willing and eligible to participate, 22,071 (66.4%) were enrolled in the randomized trial after participation in an 18-week run-in phase. Physicians were randomized to one of four interventions: 325 mg aspirin and beta-carotene placebo ($n = 5,517$), 325 mg aspirin and 50 mg beta-carotene ($n = 5,520$), aspirin placebo and 50 mg beta-carotene ($n = 5,519$), and aspirin placebo and beta-carotene placebo ($n = 5,515$) (PHS I, 2002).

The PHS sample was primarily non-Hispanic white with 7.5% of the sample composed of ethnic or racial minorities (Howard et al., 2006). Data related to nutritional status were collected via administration of an abbreviated version of the HFFQ, which included questions on breakfast cereals and alcohol (Liu, Sesso, Manson, Willett, & Buring, 2003). Multivitamin use was also assessed as well as self-reported weight and height. Questionnaires were administered annually. In addition, on a subset (*n* = 14,916) baseline blood specimens were collected and archived (PHS I, 2002). The selection of physicians as study participants in PHS I did indeed yield both a high level of compliance (greater than 80%) and minimal loss to morbidity and mortality follow-up (less than 1%) (PHS I, 2002).

In addition to finding that aspirin significantly reduced the risk of first myocardial infarction by 44% (*p*<0.0001) and that there was no benefit or harm from 13 years of beta-carotene supplementation, this study was used to address a multitude of other research questions related to other risk factors for a variety of chronic diseases, including cardiovascular disease, stroke, diabetes, macular degeneration, and cataract (PHS I, 2002). Over 250 articles have been published using this study, many of which used the study as a prospective cohort to examine effects of other risk factors independent of the intervention (PHS I, 2002). These included other nutritional related factors such as weight status (Ajani et al., 2004), homocysteine (Bowman, Gaziano, Stampfer, & Sesso, 2006), breakfast cereal intake (Liu et al., 2003), multivitamin intake (Muntwyler, Hennekens, Manson, Buring, & Gaziano, 2002), and alcohol intake (Gaziano et al., 2000).

An example of how the results of the prospective data analyses were used in the development of dietary recommendations is in the area of alcohol consumption and mortality, in which the advisory committee concluded that research supported the contention that among middle-aged adults one or two drinks per day was associated with the lowest overall mortality (DHHS and USDA, n.d.). Although the PHS I study results in conjunction with other studies were used to support this reduction in mortality in males (Gaziano et al., 2000), research from other studies was used to support this finding in females.

Although the original design of the PHS I was a randomized controlled trial, most of the nutrition-related findings stemmed from the prospective cohort design. Strengths and limitations of this type of design were previously mentioned. Similar to both the NHS and the Health Professionals Follow-Up Study, the PHS I was a well-carried-out prospective cohort study that had a high response rate and low loss to follow-up. In addition, PHS I collected a broad range of nutrition-related data that are important for elucidating the relationship between diet and disease development.

Iowa Women's Health Study

In 1986, the Iowa Women's Health Study began following more than 41,000 postmenopausal women (Bisgard, Folsom, Hong, & Sellers, 1994). The study's initial aim was to explore life-style and exposure risk factors related to cancer in a prospective population-based cohort of older women. Over time, the study has broadened its scope to include other chronic diseases (A. Folsom, University of Minnesota, School of Public Health, personal communication, 2006), among them type 2 diabetes (Pereira, Parker, & Folsom, 2006), heart disease (Ellsworth, Kushi, & Folsom, 2001), and rheumatoid arthritis (Merlino et al., 2004).

Researchers randomly selected study participants from a list of women with Iowa driver's licenses who were between the ages of 55 and 69 years (Folsom et al., 1993). The baseline and five follow-up surveys gathered self-reported information on life-style, medical history, and other factors, including waist-to-hip ratio (the study subjects were mailed a paper tape measure and written instructions on how to have a friend take body circumference measurements) (University of Minnesota Cancer Center, 2006). The most recent questionnaire was completed in 2004, with a response rate of roughly 70% (A. Folsom, University of Minnesota, School of Public Health, personal communication, 2006). Diet was only assessed twice: at baseline (using a modified version of the Willett semiquantitative FFQ) (Hunger, Folsom, Kushi, Kaye, & Sellers, 1992) and in 2004.

A linkage to the Iowa Cancer Registry provides annual data on cancer incidence in the cohort; a linkage to the National Death Index provides information on mortality. At this writing, study investigators are working to link to the Center for Medicare and Medicaid Services Database, which will enable them to collect information on additional chronic diseases and exposures (University of Minnesota Cancer Center, 2006).

The study has yielded more than 200 publications addressing risk factors for cancer and chronic disease, such as body fat distribution, diet, smoking, and other life-style factors. The 2005 Dietary

Guidelines for Americans recommendation to increase whole grain consumption (DHHS and USDA, 2005) was based, in part, on findings from the Iowa Women's Health Study. These findings confirmed the findings of the NHS (Liu et al., 1999, 2000), the Health Professionals Follow-Up Study (Fung et al., 2002), and the Framingham Offspring Study (McKeown, Meigs, Liu, Wilson, & Jacques, 2002; McKeown et al., 2004) that suggested whole grain consumption protects against type 2 diabetes and heart disease (Jacobs, Meyer, Kushi, & Folsom, 1998; Meyer et al., 2000).

The strengths of the Iowa Women's Health Study include the size of the cohort and the two decades of follow-up, which provided data on more than 7,800 incident cancer cases and more than 10,000 deaths (University of Minnesota Cancer Center, 2006). Limitations include the population's lack of ethnic diversity (99% of participants are white) and that the published dietary analyses to date have been based on one FFQ (at this writing no analyses have been published based on the 2004 dietary data). In addition, early diet exposures have not been assessed, and these exposures may play an important role in cancer etiologies.

Randomized Controlled Trials

Randomized controlled trials are studies in which subjects are randomly assigned either to a treatment/intervention or a placebo/no intervention. Ideally, the group not assigned to the intervention is assigned to a placebo or sham intervention that is unrecognizable from the actual intervention; however, this kind of blinding of the participants (and researchers) is not always possible. The **randomized design**, particularly if placebo controlled and blinded, is the gold standard for providing evidence for a cause and effect relationship. Possible limitations of this study design are the timing of the intervention in relation to the development of the disease (if the intervention does not take place during the time in which the exposure occurs), then null findings may occur because there is no intervention effect. Another possible limitation is the question of whether results seen in a controlled research setting will occur in free-living populations.

Randomized design: When individuals are randomly assigned to a treatment or control group.

Dietary Approaches to Stop Hypertension

The original Dietary Approaches to Stop Hypertension (DASH) study was a multicenter random-

ized feeding study to examine the effects of dietary patterns on blood pressure (Appel, Moore, Obarzanek, & Vollmer, 1997). The sample consisted of 459 adults 22 years of age or older not taking any antihypertensive medications and with systolic blood pressure less than 160 mm Hg and diastolic blood pressure between 80 and 95 mm Hg. About two-thirds of the sample was a racial or ethnic minority, with African-American the most common race reported (about 60% of the sample). There were three phases to the trial: screening, run-in (3 weeks), and intervention (8 weeks). At the beginning of the intervention phase subjects were randomly assigned to one of three diets all of which contained 3,000 mg of sodium:

1. Control diet: typical of the American diet, with potassium, magnesium, and calcium levels approximately at the 25th percentile of the U.S. consumption and macronutrient levels and fiber content at the average U.S. consumption
2. Fruit and vegetable diet: provided more fruits and vegetables and fewer snacks and sweets, with a commensurate level of potassium and magnesium that were at the 75th percentile of U.S. consumption
3. Combination diet: rich in fruits and vegetables, low-fat dairy, and lower in saturated fat, total fat, and cholesterol, with potassium, magnesium, and calcium levels approximately at the 75th percentile of U.S. consumption.

All food was provided by the researchers with research kitchens doing all preparation, including all meals and snacks on weekdays and weekend days, although lunch was eaten at the research centers on weekdays. The combination diet was associated with significantly greater declines in both systolic (5.5 mm Hg, $p < 0.001$) and diastolic (3.0 mm Hg, $p < 0.001$) blood pressure than the control diet. Those with hypertension benefited the most from this diet, with average declines exceeding 11 mm Hg for systolic and 5 mm Hg for diastolic blood pressure after 8 weeks. Although significant effects of lowering both systolic and diastolic blood pressure was also seen among those on the fruit and vegetable diet, these effects were not as dramatic as on the combination diet and not as significant in men or nonminority groups (Appel et al., 1997). The aforementioned combination diet henceforth became known as the DASH diet. However, it was unknown what effects sodium restriction would have while subjects were following the DASH diet, and it was not known what the DASH diet's effects on blood pressure would be when sodium intake was restricted (Svetkey et al., 1999). Thus the DASH-sodium study was developed.

DASH-sodium was also a randomized controlled intervention study in which subjects were assigned to either a control diet (previously described) or the DASH diet. Then, using a crossover design, subjects were fed three different levels of sodium daily: low (1,150 mg/2,100 kcal), intermediate (2,300 mg/2,100 kcal), and high (3,450 mg/2,100 kcal) each for a 30-day period (Svetkey et al., 1999). The sodium-varied diets were fed in random order separated by a 3- to 5-day break (Svetkey et al., 1999). The sample of 412 subjects was again about 60% African-American (Sacks et al., 2001).

Implementation of this study was similar to that of the original DASH study in terms of providing all food, requiring that subjects ate lunch at the research center on the weekdays, and using standardized methods of collecting blood pressure data. In addition, weight was kept constant. The results showed that the subjects on the DASH diet had significantly lower mean systolic blood pressure at every level of sodium compared with that of the control subjects and lower diastolic blood pressure at the high and intermediate sodium levels than the control group. As compared with the high sodium control diet, the DASH diet combined with a low sodium level resulted in systolic blood pressure that was 7.1 mm Hg lower in those without hypertension and 11.5 mm Hg lower in those with hypertension. Conversely, diastolic blood pressure was not different for DASH versus control diet when subjects' sodium consumption was at the lowest sodium level. The implications of this study according to the authors (Sacks et al., 2001) was that the DASH diet effectively lowers blood pressure at different levels of sodium and that reducing sodium intake does result in declines in blood pressure, not only among those with hypertension but also among those without it even when using the typical diet consumed in the United States.

One aspect, however, not mentioned is that the 11.5 mm Hg difference between the low sodium DASH diet and the high sodium control diet among those with hypertension is similar to that found in the original DASH study in which the DASH diet at a 3,000-mg level of daily sodium was associated with a 11.4mm Hg greater decline in blood pressure than the 3,000-mg control diet. The fact that both DASH and DASH-sodium were well-implemented randomized controlled trials with high adherence (over 93% to 95% completed the studies and biochemical markers corroborated dietary adherence)

and that blinded measurements of blood pressure used a standardized methodology are all strengths of these intervention studies. Moreover, the ethnic diversity of the samples implies that extrapolation of these results to the very groups with high risk (i.e., ethnic minorities) of developing hypertension is appropriate. The limitation of both studies, however, is that it is unknown whether the effects seen under these highly controlled research conditions with all food provided can be replicated in a free-living U.S. population.

Both DASH and DASH-sodium have had tremendous influence on the 2005 Dietary Guidelines. This is illustrated in the declaration in the Dietary Guidelines for Americans that the DASH eating plan is an example of a healthy eating plan promoted by the dietary guidelines. In fact, several of the key recommendations in the 2005 Dietary Guidelines for Americans name the DASH diet specifically (DHHS and USDA, 2005). For example, one of the key recommendations in the section on adequate nutrients within energy needs is "Meet recommended intakes within energy needs by adopting a balanced eating pattern, such as the USDA Food Guide or the DASH Eating Plan" (DHHS and USDA, 2005). Moreover, the results of the DASH-sodium study guided the recommendation of the lower sodium levels (<1,500 mg) among those with hypertension (DHHS and USDA, n.d.). Given the pervasiveness of the DASH studies' influence on the 2005 Dietary Guidelines and the fact that through our national nutrition surveillance systems the dietary intake of the U.S. population is tracked, the effectiveness of the DASH diet in a free-living population may be ascertained through this natural experiment.

Women's Health Initiative

The Women's Health Initiative (WHI) study was launched in 1991 to investigate major diseases affecting postmenopausal women, including heart disease, breast and colorectal cancers, and osteoporosis. The 15-year study includes 161,000 women aged 50 to 79 years at baseline in a total of three clinical trials and one observational trial conducted across 40 clinical centers in the United States. One of its most striking findings was that postmenopausal hormone replacement therapy with estrogen–progestin increases the risk of breast cancer (Writing Group, 2002).

Two of the WHI's clinical trials tested two of the most widely recommended nutrition therapies aimed at preventing chronic disease: low-fat diets and calcium–vitamin D supplements. The dietary modification trial examined the effect of a low-fat high-carbohydrate diet on breast cancer, colorectal cancer, heart disease, and stroke. The calcium plus vitamin D trial looked at the effect of taking daily supplements of 1,000 mg calcium and 400 IU vitamin D on osteoporosis-related fractures and colorectal cancer. Overall, both trials failed to demonstrate that these preventive regimens had a protective effect, prompting controversy about the studies' merits and flaws as well as their implications for future nutrition recommendations.

In the dietary modification trial, 48,835 women were randomly assigned to the intervention group or the control group (Prentice et al., 2006). Women in the intervention group were instructed to adopt a low-fat diet (20% of total calories from fat) that was high in grains (at least six servings a day) and fruits and vegetables (at least five servings a day). The intervention subjects also received extensive dietary counseling, including personalized fat intake goals and nutritionist-led group counseling sessions (18 during the first year and quarterly follow-up meetings during subsequent years). Women in the control group were given general information on healthy diets but were instructed not to make any changes in their diets.

Dietary intake was assessed via FFQ (administered to everyone at baseline and then to a third of subjects each year thereafter), 4-day food records (collected from everyone at baseline and from ~5% of subjects after year 1), and single 24-hour recalls (collected from ~5% of subjects in year 3 and 6 and from an additional 1% of subjects every year). Serum samples were also analyzed for biomarkers of dietary intake, such as carotenoids, lipids, and glucose. During yearly clinic follow-up visits investigators measured subjects' height, weight, waist circumference, and blood pressure. Outcomes were assessed by self-report and medical record examination.

Overall, after roughly 8 years of follow-up the study found that the low-fat dietary pattern did not significantly decrease risk of invasive breast cancer, colorectal cancer, heart disease, or stroke (Beresford et al., 2006; Howard et al., 2006; Prentice et al., 2006). Although breast cancer incidence was 9% lower in the intervention group compared with the control group, this difference was not statistically significant (Hazard Ratio (HR) = 0.91; 95% confidence interval, 0.83–1.01; $p = 0.07$). Secondary analyses, however, suggested that the low-fat dietary pattern had a protective effect in women who had the highest baseline fat intake.

The study authors suggested that the lack of statistically significant overall findings could be due to several factors. Only a small percentage of women in the intervention group achieved the 20% of calories from fat dietary goal; furthermore, the differences in fat intake and fruit and vegetable intake between the intervention and control groups were lower than anticipated by the original study design (Prentice et al., 2006). The authors pointed to the secondary findings as evidence that the intervention did have a protective effect against breast cancer. Other observers, however, suggested that the slight decrease in breast cancer incidence could be due to modest weight loss among intervention group subjects (Lagiou, Trichopoulos, & Adami, 2006). Although the intervention phase of the study has ended, study participants will be followed for another 5 years, so it is possible that further differences between the intervention and control groups will emerge over time.

The calcium plus vitamin D trial, which followed 36,282 postmenopausal women for an average of 7 years, had similarly mixed results. The study found that daily supplementation with 1,000 mg of calcium and 400 IU vitamin D slightly increased hip bone density but did not lead to a decrease in hip fractures and that supplementation was linked with a higher risk of kidney stones. Secondary subgroup analyses did show a protective effect in the most adherent women (Jackson et al., 2006). The supplementation regimen also had no effect on the women's risk of colorectal cancer (Wactawski-Wende et al., 2006). The authors and other observers suggested several explanations for the bone findings, among them that the dose of vitamin D may not have been sufficient (600 IU or higher of supplementation may be required to reduce fracture risk), that many women in the control group had a high daily intake of calcium from diet and supplements (800 mg calcium and 400 IU vitamin D a day), and that more than half of the women in the intervention and control groups were receiving hormone replacement therapy (some as part of the WHI trial) (Finkelstein, 2006). The lack of a protective effect on colorectal cancer could be because such cancers are slow growing and a 7-year follow-up may not be enough time to show evidence of benefit. It remains to be seen whether any effects emerge during the planned postintervention 5-year follow-up (Wactawski-Wende et al., 2006).

The strengths of the WHI nutrition investigations include the enrollment of a large number of women drawn from diverse ethnic and socioeconomic groups across the country as well as the careful long-term follow-up of outcomes. Potential limitations include the postmenopausal study population itself and the timing of the interventions; breast and colorectal cancer, heart disease, and osteoporosis outcomes may be determined by exposures or preventive measures taken earlier in life.

The ultimate effect of the WHI findings on nutrition recommendations remains to be seen. Government dietary recommendations have already moved away from advocating a uniformly low-fat diet, focusing instead on reducing saturated and trans fat to prevent chronic disease. The Institute of Medicine's latest recommendations, echoed by the 2005 Dietary Guidelines for Americans, suggest a daily fat intake for adults between 20% and 35% of total calories. There is also increasing evidence that the current daily recommended intake for vitamin D is too low and that at least 1,000 IU/day of vitamin D may be needed to promote optimum blood levels for prevention of hip fractures (Bischoff-Ferrari, Giovannucci, Willett, Dietrich, & Dawson-Hughes, 2006).

Optimal Macro-Nutrient Intake Trial to Prevent Heart Disease (OmniHeart)

The Optimal Macro-Nutrient Intake Trial to Prevent Heart Disease (OmniHeart) study was designed to determine whether altering the DASH diet's macronutrient composition could further lower heart disease risk (Appel et al., 2005; Carey et al., 2005). The feeding study used a randomized, three-period, crossover design to examine the effect of three healthy diets—high carbohydrate, high protein, and high unsaturated fat—on blood pressure, LDL, HDL, triglycerides, and overall cardiovascular disease risk in men and women. The subjects ($n = 164$) were healthy adults with prehypertension or stage 1 hypertension; in light of the higher prevalence of cardiovascular disease among African-Americans, the study investigators sought to recruit a cohort that was 50% African-American (the final cohort was 55% African-American and 40% non-Hispanic white).

Like DASH, all three study diets were low in saturated fat (6% of total energy), sodium (2,300 mg/day), and cholesterol (<150 mg/day). Furthermore, the diets emphasized vegetables, fruit, grains, and low-fat dairy products; had similar levels of potassium (4,700 mg/day), magnesium (500 mg/day), and calcium (1,200 mg/day); and used commonly available foods. The carbohydrate diet was most similar to the DASH diet, with 58% of total energy from

carbohydrate, 15% from protein, and 27% from fat (6% saturated fatty acid, 13% monounsaturated fatty acid, 8% polyunsaturated fatty acid). The protein diet substituted 10% of carbohydrate with primarily nonmeat sources of protein, for a final dietary composition of 48% carbohydrate, 25% protein, and 27% fat. The unsaturated fat diet substituted 10% of carbohydrate with primarily monounsaturated fat, for a final dietary composition of 48% carbohydrate, 15% protein, and 37% fat (21% monounsaturated fatty acid, 10% polyunsaturated fatty acid, 6% saturated fatty acid).

Each subject was randomly assigned to follow one of six feeding period sequences (e.g., carbohydrate, unsaturated fat, protein; unsaturated fat, protein, carbohydrate; and so on). Each feeding period lasted 6 weeks, with a short washout period in between; 97% of subjects completed all three feeding periods.

The study found that compared with the carbohydrate diet, the protein and unsaturated fat diets further decreased mean systolic blood pressure; the protein diet also lowered LDL, slightly lowered HDL (an unexpected finding), and lowered triglycerides, whereas the unsaturated fat diet had no effect on LDL, increased HDL, and lowered triglycerides. When compared with baseline, the carbohydrate, protein, and unsaturated fat diets all lowered estimated 10-year coronary heart disease risk (by 16.1%, 21.0%, and 19.6%, respectively); when compared with the carbohydrate diet, the protein diet and unsaturated fat diets further decreased coronary heart disease risk (by 5.8% and 4.2%, respectively).

The strengths of the study include subjects' high adherence to the study diets and the fact that study participants maintained their body weight over the course of the study (so that weight loss or gain was not a confounding factor). Limitations include the fact that subjects were on each study diet for only 6 weeks and that the measured outcomes were risk factors for cardiovascular disease rather than cardiovascular disease events.

PHS II

The PHS II, previously noted, is an ongoing **double-blind placebo-controlled** primary prevention trial of vitamin E, ascorbic acid, beta-carotene, and/or multivitamins on prevention of prostate cancer, other cancers, or cardiovascular disease in healthy older male doctors. It is actually the only such prevention

Double-blind placebo-controlled design: When neither the individuals nor the investigator know whether participants are assigned to a treatment or a placebo group. This study design is usually considered to provide the most compelling evidence of a cause and effect relationship.

trial of its kind on apparently healthy men (Christen, Gaziano, & Hennekens, 2000). Since August 1997, 14,642 men have been randomized into 1 of 16 possible combinations of vitamin C (500 mg synthetic ascorbic acid), vitamin E (400 IU of synthetic alpha-tocopherol), beta-carotene (50 mg Lurotin), a multivitamin (Centrum Silver), or their placebos. Vitamin C and the multivitamin or their placebos are taken daily, whereas vitamin E and beta-carotene or their placebos are taken every other day (PHS II, 2002). Ethnic minorities comprise 9.4% of the sample, with the primary minority group being Asian (5.1%) (Howard et al., 2006); thus this sample, like PHS I, is primarily non-Hispanic white.

The trial is scheduled to end in December 2007 (PHS II, 2002); however, the beta-carotene portion was discontinued in 2003 (PHS II, 2006). Baseline blood samples were obtained on 76% of the sample (PHS II, 2002), and questionnaires are administered annually with questions about compliance with the study treatments, use of nonstudy medications, occurrence of major illnesses or adverse effects, and other risk factor information (PHS II, 2002). Although not stated in the description of the study design, some of these risk factors may include dietary information (Christen et al., 2000). The strengths of this study lie in its strong design, enabling researchers to attribute cause and effect to the treatment(s) and apply such results to an older healthy male population. However, like many of the other studies previously described, the external validity of applying these results to racial ethnic minority populations is limited because of the sample's homogeneity.

Conclusion

This section reviewed several epidemiologic studies, some that have been important contributors to dietary recommendations that have been promulgated and some that have potential for informing future recommendations. Although all have limitations, as the perfect study has yet to be conducted, these designs have strong internal validity. Nevertheless, many do not include samples that represent ethnic minorities, and this appears to be the "Achilles' heel" of chronic disease prevention research. Looking to the future, therefore, this gap needs to be filled with more studies that include a larger proportion of ethnic minorities (like DASH and OmniHeart) so that national nutrition policy, which currently is considered to apply to all, can be grounded in research that was not conducted on a primarily white non-Hispanic samples.

As the evolution of national dietary guidelines on fat has illustrated, it takes many years for research findings to be applied to the transformation of nutrition policy. Early studies on trans fat were published in 1993, but the U.S. Food and Drug Administration regulations on labeling to include trans fat did not begin until January 2006. Nevertheless, the studies described herein, although not exhaustive, exemplify that well-conducted epidemiologic research has made important contributions to national dietary guidelines. Broadening such research to diverse populations and other innovative nutrition-related research questions will likely help shape future dietary recommendations.

References

Research Involving Children

Akinbami, L. J., & Schoendorf, K. C. (2002). Trends in childhood asthma: Prevalence, health care utilization, and mortality. *Pediatrics, 110*, 315–322.

Alexy, U., Kersting, M., & Sichert-Hellert, W. (2006). Evaluation of dietary fibre intake from infancy to adolescence against various references—results of the DONALD Study. *European Journal of Clinical Nutrition, 60*, 909–914.

Alexy, U., Sichert-Hellert, W., & Kersting, M. (2002). Fortification masks nutrient dilution due to added sugars in the diet of children and adolescents. *Journal of Nutrition, 132*, 2785–2791.

Allen, M. L., Elliott, M. N., Morales, L. S., Diamant, A. L., Hambarsoomian, K., & Schuster, M. A. (2007). Adolescent participation in preventive health behaviors, physical activity, and nutrition: Differences across immigrant generations for Asians and Latinos compared with Whites. *American Journal of Public Health, 97*, 337–343.

American Academy of Pediatrics (AAP). (1995). American Academy of Pediatrics, Committee on Bioethics: Informed consent, parental permission, and assent in pediatric practice. *Pediatrics, 95*, 314–317.

American Academy of Pediatrics, Committee on Nutrition. (1992). Statement on cholesterol. *Pediatrics, 90*, 469–473.

Arab, L., Carriquiry, A., Steck-Scott, S., & Gaudet, M. M. (2003). Ethnic differences in the nutrient intake adequacy of premenopausal US women: Results from the Third National Health Examination Survey. *Journal of the American Dietetic Association, 103*, 1008–1014.

Ballauff, A., Rascher, W., Tolle, H. G., Wember, T., & Manz, F. (1991). Circadian rhythms of urine osmolality and renal excretion rates of solutes influencing water metabolism in 21 healthy children. *Mineral and Electrolyte Metabolism, 17*, 377–382.

Bao, W., Srinivasan, S. R., Wattigney, W. A., & Berenson, G. S. (1994). Persistence of multiple cardiovascular risk clustering related to syndrome X from childhood to young adulthood. The Bogalusa Heart Study. *Archives of Internal Medicine, 154*, 1842–1847.

Bao, W., Threefoot, S. A., Srinivasan, S. R., & Berenson, G. S. (1995). Essential hypertension predicted by tracking of elevated blood pressure from childhood to adulthood: The Bogalusa Heart Study. *American Journal of Hypertension, 8*, 657–665.

Bartlett, R., Holditch-Davis, D., & Belyea, M. (2005). Clusters of problem behaviors in adolescents. *Research in Nursing and Health, 28*, 230–239.

The Belmont Report. (n.d.). Retrieved May 22, 2006, from http://www.cdc.gov/od/ads/ethcodes/belm-eng.pdf

Berenson, G. S. (1986). *Causation of Cardiovascular Risk Factors in Childhood: Perspectives on Cardiovascular Risk in Early Life*. New York: Raven Press.

Berenson, G. S., McMahan, C. A., Voors, A. W., Webber, L. S., Srinivasan, S. R., Frank, G. C., et al. (1980). *Cardiovascular Risk Factors in Children—The Early Natural History of Atherosclerosis and Essential Hypertension*. New York: Oxford University Press.

Berenson, G. S., Wattigney, W. A., Bao, W., Srinivasan, S. R., & Radhakrishnamurthy, B. (1995). Rationale to study the early natural history of heart disease: The Bogalusa Heart Study. *American Journal of the Medical Sciences, 310*(Suppl. 1), S22–S28.

Berenson, G. S., Wattigney, W. A., Tracy, R. E., Newman, W. P., Srinivasan, S. R., Webber, L. S., et al. (1992). Atherosclerosis of the aorta and coronary arteries and cardiovascular risk factors in persons aged 6 to 30 years and studied at necropsy (The Bogalusa Heart Study). *American Journal of Cardiology, 70*, 851–858.

Centers for Disease Control and Prevention. (2005). Blood lead levels—United States 1999–2002. *Morbidity and Mortality Weekly Report, 54*, 513–516.

Boon, N., Koppes, L. L., Saris, W. H., & Van Mechelen, W. (2005). The relation between calcium intake and body composition in a Dutch population: The Amsterdam Growth and Health Longitudinal Study. *American Journal of Epidemiology, 162*, 27–32.

Broome, M. E., & Stieglitz, K. A. (1992). The consent process and children. *Research in Nursing and Health, 15*, 147–152.

Burns, J. (2003). Research in children: Research ethics—scientific reviews. *Critical Care Medicine, 31*, S131–S136.

Chen, W., Li, S., Srinivasan, S. R., Boerwinkle, E., & Berenson, G. S. (2005). Autosomal genome scan for loci linked to blood pressure levels and trends since childhood: The Bogalusa Heart Study. *Hypertension, 45*, 954–959.

Christensen, P. H. (1997). Difference and similarity: How children's competence is constructed in illness and its treatment. In I. Hutchby & J. Moran-Ellis (Eds.), *Children and social competence: Arenas of action* (pp. 187–210). London: Falmer.

Cooper, M. J., & Zlotkin, S. H. (2003). An evidence-based approach to the development of national dietary guidelines. *Journal of the American Dietetic Association, 103*(Suppl. 2), S28–S33.

Cruickshank, J. K., Mzayek, F., Liu, L., Kieltyka, L., Sherwin, R., Webber, L. S., et al. (2005). Origins of the "black/white" difference in blood pressure: Roles of birth weight, postnatal growth, early blood pressure, and adolescent body size: The Bogalusa heart study. *Circulation, 111*, 1932–1937.

Cruz, M. L., Shaibi, G. Q., Weigensberg, M. J., Spruijt-Metz, D., Ball, G. D., & Goran, M. I. (2005). Pediatric obesity and insulin resistance: Chronic disease risk and implications for treatment and prevention beyond body weight modification. *Annual Review of Nutrition, 25*, 435–468.

Daniels, J. L., Olshan, A. F., & Savitz, D. A. (1997). Pesticides and childhood cancer. *Environmental Health Perspectives, 105*, 1068–1077.

Davidoff, F., DeAngelis, C. D., Drazen, J. M., Nicholls, M. G., Hoey, J., Hojgaard, L., et al. (2001). Sponsorship, authorship, and accountability. *New England Journal of Medicine, 345*, 825–827.

The Declaration of Helsinki. (1964). Retrieved July 7, 2006, from http://www.cirp.org/library/ethics/helsinki

Demory-Luce, D., Morales, M., Nicklas, T., Baranowski, T. Zakeri, I., & Berenson, G. (2004). Changes in food group consumption patterns from childhood to young adulthood: The Bogalusa Heart Study. *Journal of the American Dietetic Association, 104*, 1684–1691.

Deshmukh-Taskar, P., Nicklas, T. A., Morales, M., Yang, S. J., Zakeri, I., & Berenson, G. S. (2006). Tracking of overweight status from childhood to young adulthood: The Bogalusa Heart Study. *European Journal of Clinical Nutrition, 60*, 48–57.

Diaz, A., Neal, W. P., Nucci, A. T., Ludmer, P., Bitterman, J., & Edwards, S. (2004). Legal and ethical issues facing adolescent health care professionals. *Mount Sinai Journal of Medicine, 71*, 181–185.

Dickert, N., Emanuel, E., & Grady, C. (2002). Paying research subjects: An analysis of current policies. *Annals of Internal Medicine, 136*, 368–373.

Dietrich, K. N., Eskenazi, B., Schantz, S., Yolton, K., Rauh, V. A., Johnson, C. B., et al. (2005). Principles and practices of neurodevelopmental assessment in children: Lessons learned from the Centers for Children's Environmental Health and Disease Prevention Research. *Environmental Health Perspectives, 113*, 1437–1446.

Dresser, R. (2001). Payments to research participants: The importance of context. *American Journal of Bioethics, 1*, 47.

Eggleston, P. A., Diette, G., Lipsett, M., Lewis, T., Tager, I., McConnell, R., et al. (2005). Lessons learned for the study of childhood asthma from the Centers for Children's Environmental Health and Disease Prevention Research. *Environmental Health Perspectives, 113*, 1430–1436.

Eskenazi, B., Gladstone, E. A., Berkowitz, G. S., Drew, C. H., Faustman, E. M., Holland, N. T., et al. (2005). Methodologic and logistic issues in conducting longitudinal birth cohort studies: Lessons learned from the Centers for Children's Environmental Health and Disease Prevention Research. *Environmental Health Perspectives, 113*, 1419–1429.

Fenske, R. A., Bradman, A., Whyatt, R. M., Wolff, M. S., & Barr, D. B. (2005). Lessons learned for the assessment of children's pesticide exposure: Critical sampling and analytical issues for future studies. *Environmental Health Perspectives, 113*, 1455–1462.

Fernhoff, P. M. (2002). Paying for children to participate in research: A slippery slope or an enlightened stairway. *Journal of Pediatrics, 141*, 153–154.

Field, M. J., & Behrman, R. E. (2004). *Committee on Clinical Research Involving Children Board on Health Sciences Policy: Institute of Medicine Ethical Conduct of Clinical Research Involving Children.* Washington, DC: The National Academies Press.

Ford, E. S., & Ballew, C. (1998). Dietary folate intake in US adults: Findings from the third National Health and Nutrition Examination Survey. *Ethnicity and Disease, 8*, 299–305.

Frank, G. C., Berenson, G. S., Schilling, P. E., & Moore, M. C. (1977). Adapting the 24-hr dietary recall for epidemiologic studies of school children. *Journal of the American Dietetic Association, 71*, 26–31.

Freedman, D. S., Kettel-Khan, L., Srinivasan, S. R., & Berenson, G. S. (2000). Black/white differences in relative weight and obesity among girls: The Bogalusa Heart Study. *Preventive Medicine, 30*, 234–243.

Gilliland, F., Avol, E., Kinney, P., Jerrett, M., Dvonch, T., Lurmann, F., et al. (2005). Air pollution exposure assessment for epidemiologic studies of pregnant women and children: Lessons learned from the Centers for Children's Environmental Health and Disease Prevention Research. *Environmental Health Perspectives, 113*, 1447–1454.

Glantz, L. H. (1996). Conducting research with children: Legal and ethical issues. *Journal of the American Academy of Child and Adolescent Psychiatry, 35*, 1283–1291.

Glantz, L. H. (1998). Research with children. *American Journal of Law and Medicine, 24*, 213–244.

Golding, J. (1990). Children of the nineties: A longitudinal study of pregnancy and childhood based on the population of Avon (ALSPAC). *West of England Medical Journal, 105*, 80–82.

Grady, C., Dickert, N., Jawetz, T., Gensler, G., & Emanuel, E. (2005). An analysis of U.S. practices of paying research participants. *Contemporary Clinical Trials, 26*, 365–375.

Grodin, M. A., & Alpert, J. J. (1988). Children as participants in medical research. *Pediatric Clinics of North America, 35*, 1389–1401.

Gupta, R. S., Carrion-Caire, V., & Weiss, K. B. (2006). The widening black/white gap in asthma hospitalizations and mortality. *Journal of Allergy and Clinical Immunology, 117*, 351–358.

Hallman, D. M., Srinivasan, S., Chen, W., Boerwinkle, E., & Berenson, G. S. (2004). The beta(2)-adrenergic receptor Arg16-gly polymorphism and interactions involving beta(2)- and beta(3)-adrenergic receptor polymorphisms are associated with variations in longitudinal serum lipid profiles: The Bogalusa Heart Study. *Metabolism, 53*, 1184–1191.

Harrison, L., & Ungerer, J. (2005). What can the longitudinal study of Australian children tell us about infants' and 4 to 5 year olds' experiences of early childhood education and care? *Family Matters, 72*, 26–35.

Hertz-Picciotto, I., Croen, L. A., Hansen, R., Jones, C. R., van de Water, J., & Pessah, I. N. (2006). The CHARGE study: An epidemiologic investigation of genetic and environmental factors contributing to autism. *Environmental Health Perspectives, 114*, 1119–1125.

Hicks, L. S., Fairchild, D. G., Cook, E. F., & Ayanian, J. Z. (2003). Association of region of residence and immigrant status with hypertension, renal failure, cardiovascular disease, and stroke, among African-American participants in the third National Health and Nutrition Examination Survey (NHANES III). *Ethnicity and Disease, 13*, 316–323.

Hoelscher, D. M., Feldman, H. A., Johnson, C. C., Lytle, L. A., Osganian, S. K., Parcel, G. S., et al. (2004). School-based health education programs can be maintained over time: Results from the CATCH Institutionalization study. *Preventive Medicine, 38*, 594–606.

Hoelscher, D. M., Kelder, S. H., Murray, N., Cribb, P. W., Conroy, J., & Parcel, G. S. (2001). Dissemination and adoption of the Child and Adolescent Trial for Cardiovascular Health (CATCH): A case study in Texas. *Journal of Public Health Management and Practice, 7*, 90–100.

Hood, M. Y., Moore, L. L., Sundarajan-Ramamurti, A., Singer, M., Cupples, L. A., & Ellison, R. C. (2000). Parental eating attitudes and the development of obesity in children. The Framingham Children's Study. *International Journal of Obesity and Related Metabolic Disorders, 24*, 1319–1325.

Israel, B. A., Parker, E. A., Rowe, Z., Salvatore, A., Minkler, M., Lopez, J., et al. (2005). Community-based participatory research: Lessons learned from the Centers for Children's Environmental Health and Disease Prevention Research. *Environmental Health Perspectives, 113*, 1463–1471.

Jacknowitz, A., Novillo, D., & Tiñe, L. (2007). Special supplemental nutrition program for women, infants, and children and infant feeding practices. *Pediatrics, 119*, 281–289.

Jonsen, A. (1983). Research involving children. In T. Silber (Ed.), *Ethical Issues in the Treatment of Children and Adolescents* (pp. 123–131). Thorofare, NJ: Slack.

Juonala, M., Viikari, J. S., Kahonen, M., Taittonen, L., Ronnemaa, T., Laitinen, T., et al. (2005). Geographic origin as a determinant of carotid artery intima-media thickness and brachial artery flow-mediated dilation: The Cardiovascular Risk in Young Finns Study. *Arteriosclerosis, Thrombosis, and Vascular Biology, 25*, 392–398.

Juonala, M., Viikari, J. S., Laitinen, T., Marniemi, J., Helenius, H., Ronnemaa, T., et al. (2004). Interrelations between brachial endothelial function and carotid intima-media thickness in young adults: The Cardiovascular Risk in Young Finns Study. *Circulation, 110,* 2918–2923.

Juonala, M., Viikari, J. S., Ronnemaa, T., Taittonen, L., Marniemi, J., & Raitakari, O. T. (2006). Childhood C-reactive protein in predicting CRP and carotid intima-media thickness in adulthood: The Cardiovascular Risk in Young Finns Study. *Arteriosclerosis, Thrombosis, and Vascular Biology, 26,* 1883–1888.

Kelder, S. H., Osganian, S. K., Feldman, H. A., Webber, L. S., Parcel, G. S., Leupker, R. V., et al. (2002). Tracking of physical and physiological risk variables among ethnic subgroups from third to eighth grade: The Child and Adolescent Trial for Cardiovascular Health cohort study. *Preventive Medicine, 34,* 324–333.

Kemper, H. C., van Mechelen, W., Post, G. B., Snel, J., Twisk, J. W., van Lenthe, F. J., et al. (1997). The Amsterdam Growth and Health Longitudinal Study. The past (1976–1996) and future (1997–?). *International Journal of Sports Medicine, 18,* S140–S150.

Kilpatrick, M., Ohanessian, C., & Bartholomew, J. B. (1999). Adolescent weight management and perceptions: An analysis of the National Longitudinal Study of Adolescent Health. *Journal of School Health, 69,* 148–152.

Kimmel, C. A., Collman, G. W., Fields, N., & Eskenazi, B. (2005). Lessons learned for the National Children's Study from the National Institute of Environmental Health Sciences/U.S. Environmental Protection Agency Centers for Children's Environmental Health and Disease Prevention Research. *Environmental Health Perspectives, 113,* 1414–1418.

Kivimaki, M., Lawlor, D. A., Smith, G. D., Keltikangas-Jarvinen, L., Elovainio, M., Vahtera, J., et al. (2006a). Early socioeconomic position and blood pressure in childhood and adulthood: The Cardiovascular Risk in Young Finns Study. *Hypertension, 47,* 39–44.

Kivimaki, M., Smith, G. D., Elovainio, M., Pulkki, L., Keltikangas-Jarvinen, L., Talttonen, L., et al. (2006b). Socioeconomic circumstances in childhood and blood pressure in adulthood: The Cardiovascular Risk in Young Finns Study. *Annals of Epidemiology, 16,* 737–742.

Kopelman, L. M. (2004). What conditions justify risky nontherapeutic or "no benefit" pediatric studies: A sliding scale analysis. *Journal of Law, Medicine and Ethics, 32,* 749–758.

Kopelman, L. M. (2006). Children as research subjects: Moral disputes, regulatory guidance, and recent court decisions. *Mount Sinai Journal of Medicine, 73,* 596–604.

Kopelman, L. M., & Murphy, T. F. (2004). Ethical concerns about federal approval of risky pediatric studies. *Pediatrics, 113,* 1783–1789.

Koren, G. (2003). Healthy children as subjects in pharmaceutical research. *Theoretical Medicine, 24,* 149–159.

Kroke, A., Manz, F., Kersting, M., Remer, T., Sichert-Hellert, W., Alexy, U., et al. (2004). The DONALD Study. History, current status and future perspectives. *European Journal of Nutrition, 43,* 45–54.

Kuczewski, M. (2001). Is informed consent enough? Monetary incentives for research participation and the integrity of biomedicine. *American Journal of Bioethics, 1,* 49–51.

Lake, A. A., Mathers, J. C., Rugg-Gunn, A. J., & Adamson, A. J. (2006). Longitudinal change in food habits between adolescence (11–12 years) and adulthood (32–33 years): The ASH30 Study. *Journal of Public Health (Oxford, England), 28,* 10–16.

Landrigan, P. J., Trasande, L., Thorpe, L. E., Gwynn, C., Lioy, P. J., D'Alton, M. E., et al. (2006). The National Children's Study: A 21-year prospective study of 100,000 American children. *Pediatrics, 118,* 2173–2186.

Lapinleimu, H., Viikari, J., Jokinen, E., Salo, P., Routi, T., Leino, A., et al. (1995). Prospective randomized trial in 1062 infants of diet low in saturated fat and cholesterol. *Lancet, 345,* 471–476.

Law, M. R., Wald, N. J., & Thompson, S. G. (1994). By how much and how quickly does reduction in serum cholesterol lower risk of ischaemic heart disease? *British Medical Journal, 308,* 367–373.

Levine, R. (1979). What should consent forms say about cash payment? *Institutional Review Board, 1,* 7–8.

Lewis, C. C. (1998). How adolescents approach decisions: Changes over grades seven to twelve and policy implications. *Child Development, 52,* 538–544.

Lifshitz, F., & Moses, N. (1989). Growth failure. A complication of dietary treatment of hypercholesterolemia. *American Journal of Diseases of Children, 143,* 537–542.

Looker, A. C., Loria, C. M., Carroll, M. D., McDowell, M. A., & Johnson, C. L. (1993). Calcium intakes of Mexican Americans, Cubans, Puerto Ricans, non-Hispanic whites, and non-Hispanic blacks in the US. *Journal of the American Dietetic Association, 93,* 1274–1279.

Luepker, R. V., Perry, C. L., McKinlay, S. M., Nader, P. R., Parcel, G. S., Stone, E. J., et al. (1996). Outcomes of a field trial to improve children's dietary patterns and physical activity. The Child and Adolescent Trial for Cardiovascular Health. CATCH collaborative group. *Journal of the American Medical Association, 275,* 768–776.

Lytle, L. A., Ward, J., Nader, P. R., Pedersen, S., & Williston, B. J. (2003). Maintenance of a health promotion program in elementary schools: Results from the CATCH-ON study key informant interviews. *Health Education and Behavior, 30,* 503–518.

Manz, F., Wentz, A., & Sichert-Hellert, W. (2000). The most important nutrient: Defining the adequate intake of water. *Journal of Pediatrics, 14,* 587–592.

Martin, R. M., Ness, A. R., Gunnell, D., Emmett, P., Davey Smith, G., & ALSPAC Study Team. (2004). Does breastfeeding in infancy lower blood pressure in childhood? The Avon Longitudinal Study of Parents and Children (ALSPAC). *Circulation, 109,* 1259–1266.

McCullum-Gomez, C., Barroso, C. S., Hoelscher, D. M., Ward, J. L., & Kelder, S. H. (2006). Factors influencing implementation of the Coordinated Approach to Child Health (CATCH) Eat Smart School Nutrition Program in Texas.

Journal of the American Dietetic Association, 106, 2039–2044.

McGartland, C., Robson, P. J., Murray, L., Cran, G., Savage, M. J., Watkins, D., et al. (2003). Carbonated soft drink consumption and bone mineral density in adolescence: The Northern Ireland Young Hearts project. *Journal of Bone and Mineral Research, 18*, 1563–1569.

McGartland, C. P., Robson, P. J., Murray, L. J., Cran, G. W., Savage, M. J., Watkins, D. C., et al. (2004). Fruit and vegetable consumption and bone mineral density: The Northern Ireland Young Hearts Project. *American Journal of Clinical Nutrition, 80*, 1019–1023.

Meaux, J. B., & Bell, P. L. (2001). Balancing recruitment and protection: Children as research subjects. *Issues in Comprehensive Pediatric Nursing, 24*, 241–251.

Mikkilä, V., Räsänen, L., Raitakari, O. T., Pietinen, P., & Viikari, J. (2004). Longitudinal changes in diet from childhood into adulthood with respect to risk of cardiovascular diseases: The Cardiovascular Risk in Young Finns Study. *European Journal of Clinical Nutrition, 58*, 1038–1045.

Mikkilä, V., Räsänen, L., Raitakari, O. T., Pietinen, P., & Viikari, J. (2005). Consistent dietary patterns identified from childhood to adulthood: The Cardiovascular Risk in Young Finns Study. *British Journal of Nutrition, 93*, 923–931.

Moore, L. L., Gao, D., Bradlee, M. L., Cupples, L. A., Sundarajan-Ramamurti, A., Proctor, M. H., et al. (2003). Does early physical activity predict body fat change throughout childhood? *Preventive Medicine, 37*, 10–17.

Moore, L. L., Nguyen, U. S., Rothman, K. J., Cupples, L. A., & Ellison, R. C. (1995). Preschool physical activity level and change in body fatness in young children. The Framingham Children's Study. *American Journal of Epidemiology, 142*, 982–988.

Moore, L. L., Singer, M. R., Bradlee, M. L., Djousse, L., Proctor, M. H., Cupples, L. A., et al. (2005). Intake of fruits, vegetables, and dairy products in early childhood and subsequent blood pressure change. *Epidemiology, 16*, 4–11.

Moore, M. C., Judlin, B. C., & Kennemur, P. M. (1967). Using graduated food models in taking dietary histories. *Journal of the American Dietetic Association, 51*, 447–450.

Morrow, V., & Richards, M. (1996). The ethics of social research with children: An overview. *Children and Society, 10*, 90–105.

Nader, P. R., Stone, E. J., Lytle, L. A., Perry, C. L., Osganian, S. K., Kelder, S., et al. (1999). Three-year maintenance of improved diet and physical activity: The CATCH cohort. Child and Adolescent Trial for Cardiovascular Health. *Archives of Pediatrics and Adolescent Medicine, 153*, 695–704.

Nelson, R. (1998). Children as research subjects. In J. Kahn, A. Mastroianni, & J. Sugarman (Eds.), *Beyond Consent: Seeking Justice in Research* (pp. 47–68). New York: Oxford University Press.

Newman, W. P., Freedman, D. S., Berenson, G. S., Gard, P. D., Srinivasan, S. R., Cresanta, J. L., et al. (1986). Relation of serum lipoprotein levels and systolic blood pressure to early atherosclerosis. *New England Journal of Medicine, 314*, 138–144.

Nicholson, J. M., & Sanson, A. (2003). A new longitudinal study of the health and wellbeing of Australian children: How will it help? *Medical Journal of Australia, 178*, 282–284.

Nicklas, T., & Johnson, R. (2004). Dietary guidance for healthy children aged 2 to 11 years. *Journal of the American Dietetic Association, 104*, 660–677.

Nicklas, T. A. (1995). Dietary studies of children: The Bogalusa Heart Study experience. *Journal of the American Dietetic Association, 95*, 1127–1133.

Nicklas, T. A., Demory-Luce, D., Yang, S. J., Baranowski, T., Zakeri, I., & Berenson, G. (2004). Children's food consumption patterns have changed over two decades (1973–1994): The Bogalusa Heart Study. *Journal of the American Dietetic Association, 104*, 1127–1140.

Nicklas, T. A., Forcier, J. E., Webber, L. S., & Berenson, G. S. (1991). School lunch assessment to improve accuracy of 24-hour dietary recall for children. *Journal of the American Dietetic Association, 91*, 711–713.

Nicklas, T. A., Johnson, C. J., Myers, L., Webber, L. S., & Berenson, G. S. (1995). Eating patterns, nutrient intakes and alcohol consumption patterns of young adults. The Bogalusa Heart Study. *Medicine, Exercise, Nutrition and Health, 4*, 316–324.

The Nuremberg Code. (n.d.). Retrieved July 7, 2006, from http://www.hhs.gov/ohrp/references/nurcode.htm

Osganian, S. K., Feldman, H. A., Hoelscher, D. M., Kelder, S. H., Steffen, L. M., Luepker, R. V., et al. (2003a). Serum homocysteine in US adolescents before and after universal folate supplementation. *Circulation, 107*, e7026.

Osganian, S. K., Parcel, G. S., & Stone, E. J. (2003b). Institutionalization of a school health promotion program: Background and rationale of the CATCH-ON study. *Health Education and Behavior, 30*, 410–417.

Osganian, S. K., Stampfer, M. J., Spiegelman, D., Rimm, E., Cutler, J. A., Feldman, H. A., et al. (1999). Distribution of and factors associated with serum homocysteine levels in children: The Child and Adolescent Trial for Cardiovascular Health. *Journal of the American Medical Association, 281*, 1189–1196.

Perry, C. L., Stone, E. J., Parcel, G. S., Ellison, R. C., Nader, P. R., Webber, L. S., et al. (1990). School-based cardiovascular health promotion: The Child and Adolescent Trial for Cardiovascular Health (CATCH). *Journal of School Health, 60*, 406–413.

Proctor, M. H., Moore, L. L., Gao, D., Cupples, L. A., Bradlee, M. L., Hood, M. Y., et al. (2003). Television viewing and change in body fat from preschool to early adolescence: The Framingham Children's Study. *International Journal of Obesity and Related Metabolic Disorders, 27*, 827–833.

Rask-Nissila, L., Jokinen, E., Terho, P., Tammi, A., Hakanen, M., Ronnemaa, T., et al. (2002). Effects of diet on the neurologic development of children at 5 years of age: The STRIP project. *Journal of Pediatrics, 140*, 328–333.

Remer, T., & Manz, F. (1999). Role of nutritional status in the regulation of adrenarche. *Journal of Clinical Endocrinology and Metabolism, 84*, 3936–3944.

Robson, P. J., Gallagher, A. M., Livingstone, M. B., Cran, G. W., Strain, J. J., Savage, J. M., et al. (2000). Tracking of nutrient intakes in adolescence: the experiences of the Young Hearts Project, Northern Ireland. *British Journal of Nutrition, 84*, 541–548.

Rossi, W. C., Reynolds, W., & Nelson, R. (2003). Child assent and parental permission in pediatric research. *Theoretical Medicine, 24*, 131–148.

Russell, M. L., Moralejo, D. G., & Burgess, E. D. (2000). Paying research subjects: Participant's perspectives. *Journal of Medical Ethics, 26*, 126–130.

Salo, P., Viikari, J., Rask-Nissila, L., Hamalainen, M., Ronnemaa, T., Seppanen, R., et al. (1999). Effect of low-saturated fat, low-cholesterol dietary intervention on fatty acid compositions in serum lipid fractions in 5-year-old children. The STRIP project. *European Journal of Clinical Nutrition, 53*, 927–932.

Santayana, G. (1905). *Life of Reason, Reason in Common Sense.* New York: Charles Scribner's Sons.

Schunemann, H. J., Fretheim, A., & Oxman, A. D. (2006). Improving the use of research evidence in guideline development. 1. Guidelines for guidelines. *Health Research Policy and Systems, 21*, 4 and 13.

Selden, T. M. (2006). Compliance with well-child visit recommendations: Evidence from the Medical Expenditure Panel Survey, 2000–2002. *Pediatrics, 118*, e1766–e1778.

Sharma, S., Malarcher, A. M., Giles, W. H., & Myers, G. (2004). Racial, ethnic and socioeconomic disparities in the clustering of cardiovascular disease risk factors. *Ethnicity and Disease, 14*, 43–48.

Sichert-Hellert, W., Kersting, M., Alexy, U., & Manz, F. (2000). Ten-year trends in vitamin and mineral intake from fortified food in German children and adolescents. *European Journal of Clinical Nutrition, 54*, 81–86.

Simell, O., Niinikoski, H., Ronnemaa, T., Lapinleimu, H., Routi, T., Lagstrom, H., et al. (2000). Special Turku Coronary Risk Factor Intervention Project for Babies (STRIP). *American Journal of Clinical Nutrition, 72*(5 Suppl.), 1316S–1331S.

Singer, M. R., Moore, L. L., Garrahie, E. J., & Ellison, R. C. (1995). The tracking of nutrient intake in young children: The Framingham Children's Study. *American Journal of Public Health, 85*, 1673–1677.

Strong, J. P., Malcom, G. T., Newman, W. P., & Oalmann, M. C. (1992). Early lesions of atherosclerosis in childhood and youth: Natural history and risk factors. *Journal of the American College of Nutrition, 11*, 51S–54S.

Strong, J. P., & McGill, H. C. (1962). The natural history of coronary atherosclerosis. *American Journal of Pathology, 40*, 37–49.

Summers, D., Alpert, I., Rousseau-Pierre, T., Minguez, M., Manigault, S., Edwards, S., et al. (2006). An exploration of the ethical, legal and developmental issues in the care of an adolescent patient. *Mount Sinai Journal of Medicine, 73*, 592–595.

Telama, R., Yang, X., Viikari, J., Valimaki, I., Wanne, O., & Raitakari, O. (2005). Physical activity from childhood to adulthood: A 21-year tracking study. *American Journal of Preventive Medicine, 28*, 267–273.

Tobias, J. H., Steer, C. D., Emmett, P. M., Tonkin, R. J., Cooper, C., & Ness, A. R. (2005). Bone mass in childhood is related to maternal diet in pregnancy. *Osteoporosis International, 16*, 1731–1741.

Tobias, J. H., Steer, C. D., Mattocks, C. G., Riddoch, C., & Ness, A. R. (2007). Habitual levels of physical activity influence bone mass in 11-year-old children from the United Kingdom: Findings from a large population-based cohort. *Journal of Bone and Mineral Research, 22*, 101–109.

Trasande, L., Cronk, C. E., Leuthner, S. R., Hewitt, J. B., Durkin, M. S., McElroy, J. A., et al. (2006). The National Children's Study and the children of Wisconsin. *Wisconsin Medical Journal, 105*, 50–54.

Twisk, J. W., Boreham, C., Cran, G., Savage, J. M., Strain, J., & van Mechelen, W. (1999). Clustering of biological risk factors for cardiovascular disease and the longitudinal relationship with lifestyle of an adolescent population: the Northern Ireland Young Hearts Project. *Journal of Cardiovascular Risk, 6*, 355–362.

Twisk, J. W. R., Kemper, H. C. G., van Mechelen, W., & Post, G. B. (1997). Tracking of risk factors for coronary heart disease over a 14-year period: A comparison between lifestyle and biologic risk factors with data from the Amsterdam Growth and Health Study. *American Journal of Epidemiology, 145*, 888–898.

U.S. Department of Health and Human Services. (n.d.). Regulations in Title 45, Part 46 of the Code of Federal Regulations. Retrieved May 22, 2006, from http://www.hhs.gov/ohrp/humansubjects/guidance/45cfr46.htm

Van Lenthe, F. J., Boreham, C. A., Twisk, J. W., Strain, J. J., Savage, J. M., & Smith, G. D. (2001). Socio-economic position and coronary heart disease risk factors in youth. Findings from the Young Hearts Project in Northern Ireland. *European Journal of Public Health, 11*, 43–50.

Van't Hof, M. A., Haschke, F., and the Euro-Growth Group. (2000). The Euro-Growth Study: Why, who, and how. *Journal of Pediatric Gastroenterology and Nutrition, 31*, S3–S13.

Vere, D. W. (1991). Payments to healthy volunteers—ethical problems. *British Journal of Clinical Pharmacology, 32*, 141–142.

Viens, A. M. (2001). Socio-economic status and inducement to participate. *American Journal of Bioethics, 1*, 1F–2F.

Watkins, D., McCarron, P., Murray, L., Cran, G., Boreham, C., Robson, P., et al. (2004). Trends in blood pressure over 10 years in adolescents: Analyses of cross sectional surveys in the Northern Ireland Young Hearts project. *British Medical Journal, 329*, 139.

Webber, L. S., Osganian, V., Luepker, R. V., Feldman, H. A., Stone, E. J., Elder, J. P., et al. (1995). Cardiovascular risk factors among third grade children in four regions of the United States. The CATCH Study. Child and Adolescent Trial for Cardiovascular Health. *American Journal of Epidemiology, 141*, 428–439.

Webber, L. S., Srinivasan, S. R., Wattigney, W. A., & Berenson, G. S. (1991). Tracking of serum lipids and lipoproteins from childhood to adulthood. The Bogalusa Heart Study. *American Journal of Epidemiology, 133*, 884–899.

Weise, K. L., Smith, M. L., Maschke, K. J., & Copeland, H. L. (2002). National practices regarding payment to research subjects for participating in pediatric research. *Pediatrics, 110*, 577–582.

Weithorn, L. A., & Scherer, D. G. (1994). Children's involvement in research participation decisions: Psychological considerations. In M. A. Grodin & L. H. Glantz (Eds.), *Children as Research Subjects: Science, Ethics, and Law* (pp. 133–180). New York: Oxford University Press.

Wendler, D., Rackoff, J. E., & Emanuel, E. J. (2002). The ethics of paying for children's participation in research. *Journal of Pediatrics, 141*, 166–171.

Windle, M., Grunbaum, J. A., Elliott, M., Tortolero, S. R., Berry, S., Gilliland, J., et al. (2004). Healthy passages. A multilevel, multimethod longitudinal study of adolescent health. *American Journal of Preventive Medicine, 27*, 164–172.

Woteki, C. E. (2003). Integrated NHANES: Uses in national policy. *Journal of Nutrition, 133*, 582S–584S.

Research Involving Adults

Ajani, U. A., Lotufo, P. A., Gaziano, J. M., Lee, I. M., Spelsberg, A., Buring, J. E., et al. (2004). Body mass index and mortality among US male physicians. *Annals of Epidemiology, 14*, 731–739.

Appel, L. J., Moore, T. J., Obarzanek, E., & Vollmer, W. (1997). A clinical trial of the effects of dietary patterns on blood pressure. *New England Journal of Medicine, 336*, 1117–1125.

Appel, L. J., Sacks, F. M., Carey, V. J., Obarzanek, E., Swain, J. F., Miller, E. R., et al. (2005). Effects of protein, monounsaturated fat, and carbohydrate intake on blood pressure and serum lipids: Results of the OmniHeart randomized trial. *Journal of the American Medical Association, 294*, 2455–2464.

Beresford, S. A., Johnson, K. C., Ritenbaugh, C., Lasser, N. L., Snetselaar, L. G., Black, H. R., et al. (2006). Low-fat dietary pattern and risk of colorectal cancer: The Women's Health Initiative Randomized Controlled Dietary Modification Trial. *Journal of the American Medical Association, 295*, 643–654.

Bischoff-Ferrari, H. A., Giovannucci, E., Willett, W. C., Dietrich, T., & Dawson-Hughes, B. (2006). Estimation of optimal serum concentrations of 25-hydroxyvitamin D for multiple health outcomes. *American Journal of Clinical Nutrition, 84*, 18–28.

Bisgard, K. M., Folsom, A. R., Hong, C. P., & Sellers, T. A. (1994). Mortality and cancer rates in nonrespondents to a prospective study of older women: 5-year follow-up. *American Journal of Epidemiology, 139*, 990–1000.

Bowman, T. S., Gaziano, J. M., Stampfer, M. J., & Sesso, H. D. (2006). Homocysteine and risk of developing hypertension in men. *Journal of Human Hypertension, 20*, 631–634.

Caan, B. J., Slattery, M. L., Potter, J., Quesenberry, C. P., Coates, A. O., & Schaffer, D. M. (1998). Comparison of the Block and the Willett self-administered semiquantitative food frequency questionnaires with an interviewer-administered dietary history. *American Journal of Epidemiology, 148*, 1137–1147.

Carey, V. J., Bishop, L., Charleston, J., Conlin, P., Erlinger, T., Laranjo, N., et al. (2005). Rationale and design of the Optimal Macro-Nutrient Intake Heart Trial to Prevent Heart Disease (OMNI-Heart). *Clinical Trials, 2*, 529–537.

Christen, W. G., Gaziano, J. M., & Hennekens, C. H. (2000). Design of Physicians' Health Study II—a randomized trial of beta-carotene, vitamins E and C, and multivitamins, in prevention of cancer, cardiovascular disease, and eye disease, and review of results of completed trials. *Annals of Epidemiology, 10*, 125–134.

Ellsworth, J. L., Kushi, L. H., & Folsom, A. R. (2001). Frequent nut intake and risk of death from coronary heart disease and all causes in postmenopausal women: the Iowa Women's Health Study. *Nutrition, Metabolism, and Cardiovascular Diseases, 11*, 372–377.

Finkelstein, J. S. (2006). Calcium plus vitamin D for postmenopausal women—bone appetit? *New England Journal of Medicine, 354*, 750–752.

Folsom, A. R., Kaye, S. A., Sellers, T. A., Hong, C. P., Cerhan, J. R., Potter, J. D., et al. (1993). Body fat distribution and 5-year risk of death in older women. *Journal of the American Medical Association, 269*, 483–487.

Framingham Heart Study. (2005). Retrieved December 20, 2006, from http://www.framinghamheartstudy.org

Fung, T. T., Hu, F. B., Pereira, M. A., Liu, S., Stampfer, M. J., Colditz, G. A., et al. (2002). Whole-grain intake and the risk of type 2 diabetes: A prospective study in men. *American Journal of Clinical Nutrition, 76*, 535–540.

Gaziano, J. M., Gaziano, T. A., Glynn, R. J., Sesso, H. D., Ajani, U. A., Stampfer, M. J., et al. (2000). Light-to-moderate alcohol consumption and mortality in the Physicians' Health Study enrollment cohort. *Journal of the American College of Cardiology, 35*, 96–105.

Gibson, R. (1990). *Principles of Nutritional Assessment*. New York: Oxford University Press.

Gordon, T., Kagan, A., Garcia-Palmieri, M., Kannel, W. B., Zukel, W. J., Tillotson, J., et al. (1981). Diet and its relation to coronary heart disease and death in three populations. *Circulation, 63*, 500–515.

Health Professionals Follow up Study. (2005). Retrieved July 18, 2006, from http://www.hsph.harvard.edu/hpfs/hpfs_about.htm

Hennekens, C. H., & Buring, J. E. (1987). *Epidemiology in Medicine* (pp. 16–29). Boston: Hennekens and Buring.

Howard, B. V., Van Horn, L., Hsia, J., Manson, J. E., Stefanick, M. L., Wassertheil-Smoller, S., et al. (2006). Low-fat dietary pattern and risk of cardiovascular disease: The Women's Health Initiative Randomized Controlled Dietary Modification Trial. *Journal of the American Medical Association, 295,* 655–666.

Hunger, R. G., Folsom, A. R., Kushi, L. H., Kaye, S. A., & Sellers, T. A. (1992). Dietary assessment of older Iowa women with a food frequency questionnaire: Nutrient intake, reproducibility, and comparison with 24-hour dietary recall interviews. *American Journal of Epidemiology, 136,* 192–200.

Jackson, R. D., LaCroix, A. Z., Gass, M., Wallace, R. B., Robbins, J., Lewis, C. E., et al. (2006). Calcium plus vitamin D supplementation and the risk of fractures. *New England Journal of Medicine, 354,* 669–683.

Jacobs, D. R., Meyer, K. A., Kushi, L. H., & Folsom, A. R. (1998). Whole-grain intake may reduce the risk of ischemic heart disease death in postmenopausal women: The Iowa Women's Health Study. *American Journal of Clinical Nutrition, 68,* 248–257.

Jensen, M. K., Koh-Banerjee, P., Hu, F. B., Franz, M., Sampson, L., Gronbaek, M., et al. (2004). Intake of whole grains, bran and germ and risk of coronary heart disease among men. *American Journal of Clinical Nutrition, 80,* 1492–1499.

Lagiou, P., Trichopoulos, D., & Adami, H. O. (2006). Low-fat diet and risk of breast cancer. *Journal of the American Medical Association, 296,* 278.

Liu, S., Manson, J. E., Stampfer, M. J., Rexrode, K. M., Hu, F. B., Rimm, E. B., et al. (2000). Whole grain consumption and risk of ischemic stroke in women: A prospective study. *Journal of the American Medical Association, 284,* 1534–1540.

Liu, S., Sesso, H. D., Manson, J. E., Willett, W. C., & Buring, J. E. (2003). Is intake of breakfast cereals related to total and cause-specific mortality in men? *American Journal of Clinical Nutrition, 77,* 594–599.

Liu, S., Stampfer, M. J., Hu, F. B., Giovannucci, E., Rimm, E., Manson, J. E., et al. (1999). Whole-grain consumption and risk of coronary heart disease: Results from the Nurses' Health Study. *American Journal of Clinical Nutrition, 70,* 412–419.

Mann, G. V., Pearson, G., Gordon, T., & Dawber, T. R. (1962). Diet and cardiovascular disease in the Framingham study. I. Measurement of dietary intake. *American Journal of Clinical Nutrition, 11,* 200–225.

McKeown, N. M., Meigs, J. B., Liu, S., Saltzman, E., Wilson, P. W., & Jacques, P. F. (2004). Carbohydrate nutrition, insulin resistance, and the prevalence of the metabolic syndrome in the Framingham Offspring Cohort. *Diabetes Care, 27,* 538–546.

McKeown, N. M., Meigs, J. B., Liu, S., Wilson, P. W., & Jacques, P. F. (2002). Whole-grain intake is favorably associated with metabolic risk factors for type 2 diabetes and cardiovascular disease in the Framingham Offspring Study. *American Journal of Clinical Nutrition, 76,* 390–398.

Merlino, L. A., Curtis, J., Mikuls, T. R., Cerhan, J. R., Criswell, L. A., & Saag, K. G. (2004). Vitamin D intake is inversely associated with rheumatoid arthritis: Results from the Iowa Women's Health Study. *Arthritis and Rheumatism, 50,* 72–77.

Meyer, K. A., Kushi, L. H., Jacobs, D. R., Jr., Slavin, J., Sellers, T. A., & Folsom, A. R. (2000). Carbohydrates, dietary fiber, and incident type 2 diabetes in older women. *American Journal of Clinical Nutrition, 71,* 921–930.

Millen, B. E., Franz, M. M., Quatromoni, P. A., Gagnon, D. R., Sonnenberg, L. M., Ordovas, J. M., et al. (1996). Diet and plasma lipids in women. I. Macronutrients and plasma total and low-density lipoprotein cholesterol in women: The Framingham Nutrition Studies. *Journal of Clinical Epidemiology, 49,* 657–663.

Millen, B. E., Quatromoni, P. A., Copenhafer, D. L., Demissie, S., O'Horo, C. E., and D'Agostino, R. B. (2001). Validation of a dietary pattern approach for evaluating nutritional risk: The Framingham Nutrition Studies. *Journal of the American Dietetic Association, 101,* 187–194.

Millen, B. E., Quatromoni, P. A., Nam, B. H., Pencina, M. J., Polak, J. F., Kimokoti, R. W., et al. (2005a). Compliance with expert population-based dietary guidelines and lower odds of carotid atherosclerosis in women: The Framingham Nutrition Studies. *American Journal of Clinical Nutrition, 82,* 174–180.

Millen, B. E., Quatromoni, P. A., Nam, B. H., O'Horo, C. E., Polak, J. F., & D'Agostino, R. B. (2002). Dietary patterns and the odds of carotid atherosclerosis in women: The Framingham Nutrition Studies. *Preventive Medicine, 35,* 540–547.

Millen, B. E., Quatromoni, P. A., Pencina, M., Kimokoti, R., Nam, B. H., Cobain, S., et al. (2005b). Unique dietary patterns and chronic disease risk profiles of adult men: The Framingham Nutrition Studies. *Journal of the American Dietetic Association, 105,* 1723–1734.

Mozaffarian, D., Pischon, T., Hankinson, S. E., Rifai, N., Joshipura, K., Willett, W. C., et al. (2004). Dietary intake of trans fatty acids and systemic inflammation in women. *American Journal of Clinical Nutrition, 79,* 606–612.

Muntwyler, J., Hennekens, C. H., Manson, J. E., Buring, J. E., & Gaziano, J. M. (2002). Vitamin supplement use in a low-risk population of US male physicians and subsequent cardiovascular mortality. *Archives of Internal Medicine, 162,* 1472–1476.

Myers, A. H., Rosner, B., Abbey, H., Willett, W., Stampfer, M. J., Bain, C., et al. (1987). Smoking behavior among participants in the Nurses Health Study. *American Journal of Public Health, 77,* 628–630.

National Cholesterol Education Program. (2001). Executive Summary of the Third Report of the National Cholesterol Education Program Expert Panel on Detection, Evaluation, and Treatment of High Blood Cholesterol in Adults (Adult Treatment Panel III). *Journal of the American Medical Association, 285,* 2486–2497.

Nurses Health Study (NHS) I. (n.d.). History. Retrieved July 18, 2006, from http://www.channing.harvard.edu/nhs/history/index.shtml#histII

Nurses Health Study (NHS) II. (n.d.). History. Retrieved July 18, 2006, from http://www.channing.harvard.edu/nhs/history/index.shtml#histII

Nurses Health Study (NHS). (n.d.). NHS questionnaires. Retrieved August 16, 2006, from http://www.channing.harvard.edu/nhs/questionnaires/index.html

Pereira, M. A., Parker, E. D., & Folsom, A. R. (2006). Coffee consumption and risk of type 2 diabetes mellitus: An 11-year prospective study of 28,812 postmenopausal women. *Archives of Internal Medicine, 166*, 1311–1316.

Physicians' Health Study (PHS). (2005). Retrieved July 18, 2006, from http://phs.bwh.harvard.edu/index.html

Physicians' Health Study (PHS) I. (2002). Retrieved July 18, 2006, from http://phs.bwh.harvard.edu/phs1.htm

Physicians' Health Study (PHS) II. (2002). Retrieved July 18, 2006, from http://phs.bwh.harvard.edu/phs2.htm

Physicians' Health Study (PHS) II. (2006). Vitamin E, ascorbic acid, beta carotene, and/or multivitamins in preventing cancer and cardiovascular disease in older healthy males. Retrieved August 17, 2006, from http://www.clinicaltrials.gov/ct/show/NCT00270647?order=1

Posner, B. M., Martin-Munley, S. S., Smigelski, C., Cupples, L. A., Cobb, J. L., Schaefer, E., et al. (1992). Comparison of techniques for estimating nutrient intake—the Framingham Study. *Epidemiology, 3*, 171–177.

Prentice, R. L., Caan, B., Chlebowski, R. T., Patterson, R., Kuller, L. H., Ockene, J. K., et al. (2006). Low-fat dietary pattern and risk of invasive breast cancer: The Women's Health Initiative Randomized Controlled Dietary Modification Trial. *Journal of the American Medical Association, 295*, 629–642.

Quan, S. F., Howard, B. V., Iber, C., Kiley, J. P., Nieto, F. J., O'Connor, G. T., et al. (1997). The Sleep Heart Health Study: Design, rationale, and methods. *Sleep, 20*, 1077–1085.

Radimer, K. L., Ballard-Barbash, R., Miller, J. S., Fay, M. P., Schatzkin, A., Troiano, R., et al. (2004). Weight change and the risk of late-onset breast cancer in the original Framingham cohort. *Nutrition and Cancer—An International Journal, 49*, 7–13.

Rothman, K. J., & Greenland, S. (1998). Types of epidemiologic studies. In Rothman, K. J., & Greenland, S. (Eds.), *Modern Epidemiology* (2nd ed., pp. 67–78). Philadelphia: Lippincott Raven.

Sacks, F. M., Svetkey, L. P., Vollmer, W. M., Appel, L. J., Bray, G. A., Harsha, D., et al. (2001). Effects on blood pressure of reduced dietary sodium and the Dietary Approaches to Stop Hypertension (DASH) Diet. DASH-Sodium Collaborative Research Group. *New England Journal of Medicine, 135*, 1019–1028.

Seshadri, S., Beiser, A., Selhub, J., Jacques, P. F., Rosenberg, I. H., D'Agostino, R. B., et al. (2002). Plasma homocysteine as a risk factor for dementia and Alzheimer's disease. *New England Journal of Medicine, 346*, 476–483.

Sonnenberg, L., Pencina, M., Kimokoti, R., Quatromoni, P., Nam, B. H., D'Agostino, R., et al. (2005). Dietary patterns and the metabolic syndrome in obese and nonobese Framingham women. *Obesity Research, 13*, 153–162.

Svetkey, L. P., Sacks, F. M., Obarzanek, E., Vollmer, W. M., Appel, L. J., Lin, P. H., et al. (1999). The Dash Diet, Sodium Intake and Blood Pressure Trial (DASH-sodium): Rationale and design. *Journal of the American Dietetic Association, S99*, S96–S104.

Tucker, K. L., Morita, K., Qiao, N., Hannan, M. T., Cupples, A., & Kiel, D. P. (2006). Colas, but not other carbonated beverages, are associated with low bone mineral density in older women: The Framingham Osteoporosis Study. *American Journal of Clinical Nutrition, 84*, 936–942.

University of Minnesota Cancer Center. (2006). Prevention and etiology program. Iowa Women's Health Study. Retrieved August 16, 2006, from http://www.cancer.umn.edu/research/programs/peiowa.html

U.S. Department of Health and Human Services and the U.S. Department of Agriculture. (n.d.). 2005 Dietary Guidelines Advisory Committee Report. Retrieved June 12, 2006, from http://www.health.gov/dietaryguidelines/dga2005/report/default.htm

U.S. Department of Health and Human Services and the U.S. Department of Agriculture. (2005). *Dietary Guidelines for Americans, 2005* (6th ed.). Washington, DC: U.S. Government Printing Office.

Wactawski-Wende, J., Kotchen, J. M., Anderson, G. L., Assaf, A. R., Brunner, R. L., O'Sullivan, M. J., et al. (2006). Calcium plus vitamin D supplementation and the risk of colorectal cancer. *New England Journal of Medicine, 354*, 684–696.

Willett, W., & Lenart, E. (1998). Reproducibility and validity of food-frequency questionnaires. In W. Willet (Ed.), *Nutritional Epidemiology* (2nd ed., pp. 101–147). New York: Oxford University Press.

Willett, W. C., Stampfer, M. J., Manson, J. E., Colditz, G. A., Speizer, F. E., Rosner, B. A., et al. (1993). Intake of trans fatty acids and risk of coronary heart disease among women. *Lancet, 341*, 581–585.

Wirfalt, E., Gulberg, B., Jeffery, R. W., et al. (1998). Response to Drs. Block and Willett. *American Journal of Epidemiology, 148*, 1162–1165.

Writing Group for the Women's Health Initiative Investigators. (2002). Risks and benefits of estrogen plus progestin in healthy postmenopausal women. *Journal of the American Medical Association, 288*, 321–333.

SECTION

1

Evidence-Based Nutrition in the Life Cycle; Prenatal to the Adolescent

CHAPTER 2

Nutritional Requirements During Pregnancy and Lactation and Normal Infant Nutrition

Jennifer L. Bueche, PhD, RD, CDN, and Rachelle Lessen, MS, RD, IBCLC

With Special Sections: Social and Cultural Aspects of Breast-Feeding
Yeemay Su Miller, MS, RD, and Virginia L. Marchant-Schnee, BS

Postpartum Depression and Maternal Nutrition
Rachelle Lessen, MS, RD, IBCLC

CHAPTER OUTLINE

Reader Objectives

After studying this chapter and reflecting on the contents, you should be able to

1. Articulate the nutritional impact of pregnancy and lactation.
2. Compare growth differences between breast-fed and formula-fed infants.
3. Describe the impact of early diet on later development of obesity, diabetes, and food allergies.
4. Discuss adequate intake of key nutrients in the first year of life, including energy, protein, fatty acids, iron, zinc, and vitamin D.
5. Describe caregiver behaviors that can impact normal transitioning from an all-milk infant diet to a diet of family foods.
6. Compare and contrast actual complementary feeding patterns with recommended guidelines.

The physiologic changes that occur during pregnancy and lactation affect nutritional requirements. These nutritional requirements include both macronutrients and micronutrients, which in turn affect the health of both mother and baby. After birth, early childhood is an important time for the development of food preferences and eating patterns. Establishment of lifelong eating habits begins in infancy and is based on a complex integration of physiologic and psychological events, including food preferences, food availability, parental modeling, praise or reward for food consumption, and peer behaviors (Stang, 2006).

Nutritional Requirements During Pregnancy and Lactation

Jennifer L. Bueche, PhD, RD, CDN

The physiologic changes that occur during pregnancy and lactation affect nutritional requirements. The Dietary Reference Intakes (DRIs) provide the reference standards for recommended nutrient requirements for pregnant and lactating females (see Appendix 2).

Energy Intake

Increased energy intake is needed during pregnancy and lactation. Increased energy is needed during pregnancy because of an increase in metabolic rate (+15%). Adequate energy intake is required for adequate weight gain during pregnancy to support the growth of the fetus, placenta, and maternal tissues. Energy needs for pregnant females in the first trimester are the same as their nonpregnant counterparts based on the 2002 DRIs. Energy requirements increase between 340 and 360 kcal/day in the second trimester and increase by 112 kcal/day in the third trimester (Institute of Medicine [IOM], Food and Nutrition Board, 2002). Energy requirements during lactation depend on whether the mother is breast-feeding exclusively or feeding a combination of human milk and formula. Energy needs are higher the first 6 months (500 kcal/day) as compared with the second 6 months (400 kcal/day) because the mother produces more milk in the first 6 months. It is important to note that some of the energy required to produce milk comes from the mobilization of maternal body fat (~170 kcal/day); thus the IOM recommends an additional 330 kcal/day above nonpregnant estimated energy requirements.

Carbohydrate

During pregnancy and lactation carbohydrates should continue to provide the primary energy source (45% to 65% of total kcal). The IOM established DRIs for carbohydrate intake during pregnancy and lactation to provide enough kilocalories in the diet, to prevent ketosis, and to maintain appropriate blood glucose levels during pregnancy (IOM, Food and Nutrition Board, 2002). The estimated average requirement is 160 g/day, and the adequate intake (AI) is 210 g/day.

Protein

Pregnant and lactating females require an additional 25 g of protein based on the current DRI/Recommended Daily Allowance (RDA) of 71 g compared with those who are not pregnant. Protein requirements can also be calculated based on 1.1 g/kg/day using prepregnant weight (IOM, Food and Nutrition Board, 2002). The additional protein is required to help form fetal and maternal tissues.

Fat

Dietary fats are an important contributor to total energy intake. Although there are no DRIs for total fat, AIs have been established for fatty acids. The AIs for linoleic and linolenic acid are 13 and 1.4 g/day, respectively, for pregnant females (IOM, Food and Nutrition Board, 2002). These are important fatty acids because they are used by the body to form other fatty acids: linoleic acid is converted to arachidonic acid (AA) and linolenic acid is converted to docosahexaenoic acid (DHA) and eicosapentaenoic acid (EPA). AA, DHA, and EPA are critical for fetal growth and development. In addition, DHA is particularly important for brain development and formation of the retina.

During lactation, the maternal diet has an impact on the amount and type of fat in breast milk. In cases of severe energy restriction, body fat is mobilized for energy and breast milk resembles maternal body fat stores. No DRI for lipids exists because energy requirements are highly variable; thus fat should contribute 20% to 35% of total calories (IOM, Food and Nutrition Board, 2002).

Micronutrient Intakes

The requirements for most micronutrients increase during pregnancy, although there are some, such as vitamins D, E, and K and the mineral calcium, that do not increase at all. Of concern is the association between excessively high intakes of preformed vitamin A consumed during pregnancy and fetal malformations. Pregnant females are cautioned to not exceed the UI of 3,000 µg/day. Surprisingly, calcium requirements do not increase during pregnancy because maternal physiology accommodates the extra needs by increasing absorption and reducing urinary calcium loss. Most females become pregnant with insufficient iron stores to meet the physiologic needs of pregnancy. The DRI/RDA for iron is 27 mg/day because iron is needed to form hemoglobin and for the growth and development of the fetus and placenta. This a substantial increase when compared with nonpregnant females (DRI/RDA is 18 mg/day). Without supplemental iron maternal anemia develops.

Supplemental iron therapy consists of 60 to 120 mg of ferrous iron in divided doses throughout the day. The consumption of iron supplements in excess of 56 mg per dose is not recommended because excessive iron consumption interferes with zinc absorption and should be avoided (Fairweather-Tait, 1995). The DRI/RDA for folate has been set at 600 μg/day during pregnancy because of the importance of folate in neural tube development. It is recommended that all females of childbearing age consume 400 μg/day of folic acid as a supplement or in fortified foods in addition to consuming folate naturally occurring in foods to achieve red blood cell folate concentrations considered optimal for protection against neural tube defects.

Recommendations for micronutrient intakes during lactation are similar to those during pregnancy except for vitamin C. The requirement for vitamin C increases substantially with lactation (120 mg/day) because a large amount of vitamin C is secreted in milk.

Water

It is important that pregnant and lactating females take in enough fluid. This is particularly important for females who are lactating because although increased fluid does not increase milk production, a lack of fluid can decrease milk volume.

Nutritional Assessment: Pregnancy and Lactation

A poor nutritional status before and during pregnancy increases the risk for a premature birth or low birth weight infants. "Low birth weight babies are 40 times more likely to die before 1 year of age compared to normal-weight infants" (Villar et al., 2003). Low birth weight and premature births are the leading causes of infant mortality. It has been theorized that inadequate growth during the prenatal period may have profound long-term effect (Rasmussen, 2000). This is known as the fetal origins hypothesis. The evidence suggests that nutrient inadequacies in the womb may cause permanent changes in the structure and/or function of organs and tissues, predisposing individuals to certain chronic diseases later in life (Barker, 1991).

Adequate weight gain during pregnancy is one of the most important determinants of fetal growth and development. The IOM developed current weight gain guidelines for pregnant females based on maternal prepregnancy body mass index (IOM, 2005).

Excessive weight gain is undesirable as well. Obesity increases the risk of gestational diabetes, pregnancy-induced hypertension, and cesarean section (Brost et al., 1997).

Evidence Analysis for Evidence-Based Practice: Pregnancy and Lactation

Adequate nutritional intake and an appropriate gestational weight gain are among the most important modifiable contributors to healthful outcomes for both mother and infant (IOM, National Academies of Science, 1990). Nutritional intervention may especially benefit high-risk groups such as pregnant teens, high-risk pregnancies (including multiple births), and those diagnosed with gestational diabetes given the need to individualize nutritional recommendations. There is much evidence in the literature to support the benefits of breast-feeding. Thus it is the position of the American Dietetic Association (2005) that "exclusive breastfeeding provides optimal nutrition and health protection for the first 6 months of life, and breastfeeding with complementary foods for at least 12 months is the ideal feeding pattern for infants." The new MyPyramid was not designed to provide nutritional recommendations for pregnant and lactating females; however, current nutritional recommendations for pregnant and lactating females are outlined in the 2005 U.S. dietary guidelines for Americans (U.S. Department of Agriculture and U.S. Department of Health and Human Services, 2005).

Normal Infant Nutrition
Rachelle Lessen, MS, RD, IBCLC

Growth

Adequate Growth in Infancy

In general, if a mother is well nourished and is exclusively breast-feeding, her milk will provide adequate nutrition for her infant to grow at an appropriate rate. Human milk has unique nutritional characteristics, such as a high ratio of whey to casein, a high proportion of nonprotein nitrogen, and fatty acids essential for brain and retinal development. It is not known at what point human milk is no longer sufficient for sustained growth, but it is unlikely that complementary foods are required before 6 months of age. Although it is commonly believed that insufficient calories and protein in human milk limit growth, it is probably more likely that other factors, such as iron and zinc, affect growth. This applies to infants in both disadvantaged and affluent populations (Dewey, 2001).

Feeding mode has been found to impact weight gain and body composition during the period of exclusive or predominant milk feeding in early infancy. In a prospective cohort study of 40 exclusively breast-fed infants and 36 exclusively formula-fed infants, weight gain was greater in the formula-fed group (Butte, Wong, Hopkinson, Smith, & Ellis, 2000b). Changes in body composition and weight were both age dependent and gender dependent. Daily intakes of energy, protein, fat, and carbohydrates were positively associated with weight gain and fat-free mass from birth through 12 months, but not after that. Formula-fed infants took in greater volumes and consumed significantly more energy, protein, fat, and carbohydrates.

Development of Growth Charts

The nutritional status of children is assessed by plotting height and weight on **growth charts** to determine adequacy of nutrient intake, particularly calories and protein. The growth charts currently in use by the Centers for Disease Control and Prevention (CDC) have been available since 2000 and are an improvement over the previous charts from 1977 (see Appendix 1). The growth charts for children from birth through 3 years are based on data from the National Health and Nutrition Examination Survey (NHANES III) with supplemental birth data from Wisconsin and Missouri. This national survey data represent the combined size and growth patterns of breast-fed and formula-fed infants in the U.S. general population from 1971 to 1994. It replaces data based on primarily formula-fed infants from 1929 to 1975 from the Fels Longitudinal Study that contained few breast-fed infants (National Center for Health Statistics, 2000). These data do not reflect differences in racial or ethnic groups that could affect growth and include all infants and children in the United States regardless of race and ethnicity. The most important influences on growth potential appear to be economic, nutritional, and environmental (National Center for Health Statistics, 2000).

Current growth charts do not accurately reflect the growth patterns of breast-fed infants (Dewey, 2001). During 1988 to 1994 when NHANES III data were collected, less than 50% of all infants born in the United States were exclusively breast-fed at birth

Growth charts: Used to assess nutritional status of children by plotting height and weight and comparing to reference data.

and only about 10% were exclusively breast-feeding at 6 months (Ryan, Wenjun, & Acosta, 2002). There is considerable evidence to show that growth rates differ for breast-fed and formula-fed infants. Formula-fed infants typically weigh 600 to 650 g more at 12 months than breast-fed infants. Average weight of breast-fed infants is noticeably lower than formula-fed infants from 9 to 12 months, whereas length is not significantly different. Thus breast-fed infants appear leaner and may even be classified as failure to thrive because of a downward trend in percentiles on the growth chart (Dewey, 2001). However, one study found no decrease in weight gain observed in exclusively breast-fed children in the first year of life (Kramer et al., 2002).

The World Health Organization (WHO) conducted a 6-year multicenter international study to develop new growth charts derived from the growth of exclusively or predominantly breast-fed infants based on the assumption that optimal infant growth occurs in infants from healthy populations who are exclusively breast-fed for the first 6 months of life with continued breast-feeding until 2 years of age. The new WHO Child Growth Standards (de Onis, Garza, Onyango, & Borghi, 2007) show how every child in the world should grow when free of disease and when their mothers follow healthy practices such as breast-feeding and not smoking. The standards depict normal human growth under optimal environmental conditions and can be used to assess children everywhere, regardless of ethnicity, socioeconomic status, and type of feeding (de Onis et al., 2007).

Early Feeding

Colic

Infantile colic is characterized by paroxysms of uncontrolled crying or fussing in an otherwise healthy and well-nourished infant. The crying and fussing behavior can be described by the rule of threes: It starts at 3 weeks of age, there is more than 3 hours of crying a day for at least 3 days a week, and it lasts for more than 3 weeks. Colic resolves spontaneously without any further sequelae. Some attribute this behavior to psychogenic causes from tension in the maternal–infant bond and to maternal smoking or alcohol consumption, whereas other models focus on possible allergens in breast milk or infant formula as the causative agent (Schach & Haight, 2002).

Colic can be particularly distressing for not only the infant, but for the parents as well. Colic occurs in both breast-fed and formula-fed infants. Breast-feeding is not protective against colic, and it is estimated that at 6 weeks the overall prevalence of colic in all infants is 24% (Clifford, Campbell, Speechley, & Gorodzinsky, 2002). Colic appears earlier and resolves earlier in formula-fed infants. Lucas and St. James-Robert (1998) reported that at 2 weeks 43% of formula-fed infants show signs of intense crying and colic behavior but only 16% of breast-fed infants demonstrated these symptoms. By 6 weeks distressed behavior was seen in 31% of breast-fed infants but only in 12% of formula fed infants.

In searching for a remedy for this stressful condition, attempts to modify the infant's diet may be implemented. Cow's milk protein may contribute to the etiology of colic, and removal of the protein may alleviate the symptoms. Use of a hypoallergenic formula for non–breast-fed infants may be recommended (Canadian Paediatric Society, 2003). Switching to a low lactose formula or a formula with fiber was not found to be helpful in reducing colic symptoms.

A hypoallergenic maternal diet for breast-feeding mothers may reduce colicky symptoms in some infants. For some, removal of all cow's milk from the mother's diet can provide relief for the colicky breast-fed infant. Other common allergens that may produce colicky symptoms in an infant include proteins from peanuts, eggs, soy, wheat, tree nuts, and strawberries. Hill et al. (2005) conducted a randomized controlled trial of breast-feeding infants less than 6 weeks of age with colic. Mothers in the experimental group excluded dairy, soy, wheat, eggs, peanuts, tree nuts, and fish. After 1 week 74% of mothers in the experimental group reported a 25% reduction in cry or fuss behavior versus 37% of the mothers in the control group.

Lust and colleagues (1996) hypothesized that maternal intake of cruciferous vegetables would cause colic symptoms in the breast-fed infant. A mailed questionnaire was used to collect information on maternal diet and colic in infants under 4 months of age. A positive relationship was seen between colic and consumption of cabbage, cauliflower, broccoli, cow's milk, onion, and chocolate. Symptoms were self-reported, and analysis failed to show a dose-response relationship between colic symptoms and frequency of the foods consumed by the mother. Mothers reported that they avoided cruciferous vegetables, milk, dried beans, spicy foods, chocolate, and caffeine either on the advice of a friend or because of a past experience related to the infant's perceived reaction to the food. Clifford et al. (2002)

> ## Research About Colic
> Studies have failed to show a clear link between dietary factors in either breast milk or formula as the cause of infant colic. Evidence suggests that dietary interventions may be helpful for some infants, especially those with a family history of atopic disease and severe colic. Most of the studies on the impact of dietary changes on colic have had a small sample size and were not blinded or controlled. Colic always improves over time, and any intervention is susceptible to a placebo effect affecting the outcome. Speculations as to the origins of colic abound, and treatment options are limited.

found that maternal intake of caffeinated beverages was not associated with colic symptoms.

Rather than transitioning an infant from breast milk to a hypoallergenic formula when symptoms persist, Schach and Haight (2002) reported a unique protocol treatment at the Davis Medical Center at the University of California that called for a maternal elimination diet followed by the use of Pancrease MT 4 enzymes with all meals and snacks. Pancrease is a digestive enzyme that further breaks down protein in the digestive track before it enters the bloodstream, thereby minimizing the potential for allergens to appear in human milk and eliciting an allergic reaction in the infant. Symptoms of colic, as well as blood in the stool, were reduced after the mothers began the treatment.

Food Safety

Safe Handling of Infant Formula

Infant formula should be prepared with careful attention to manufacturer's instructions for use and storage. Bottle-fed infants are at an increased risk for exposure to food-borne pathogens, particularly if the bottles are left at room temperature for several hours. Freshly expressed, but not previously frozen, breast milk contains live white cells that destroy pathogens and can remain at room temperature for up to 8 hours before feeding. All bottles, nipples, and other feeding equipment should be properly cleaned and disinfected between uses.

Powdered infant formula products are not sterile and can be a source of potentially devastating illness and infection in infants. At greatest risk are neonates in the first 28 days of life, premature infants, low birth weight infants, and immunocompromised infants. Intrinsic contamination of powdered infant formula products with *Enterobacter sakazakii* and *Salmonella* has been a cause of significant disease, causing severe developmental sequelae and death (MMWR, 2002). The Infant Formula Act of 1980 (revised 1986) requires formula makers to use "good manufacturing practice" but does not guarantee or require sterility

(Baker, 2002). Formula manufacturers are urged to develop a sterile powdered product for high-risk infants. Even low concentrations of *E. sakazakii* in powdered infant formula can cause serious harm due to the potential for exponential multiplication during preparation and holding at ambient temperatures. Good hygienic practices, such as hand washing, using sanitized containers, and preparing only the amount needed for one feeding and using immediately, have been recommended to minimize risk (European Food Safety Authority, 2004). The U.S. Food and Drug Administration (FDA) issued warnings regarding the use of powdered infant formula in neonatal intensive care units. No events have been reported for healthy full-term infants in home settings or involving the use of sterile liquid infant formula products (FDA Talk Paper, 2002).

Safe Handling of Complementary Foods

Infants are at risk of exposure to food-borne pathogens when complementary foods are not prepared using safe food-handling techniques. Contamination of food with microbes is recognized as the leading cause of diarrheal disease and ill health in infants. A wide range of symptoms, including diarrhea, vomiting, abdominal pain, fever, and jaundice, occurs with potentially severe and life-threatening consequences. Two particular areas of food preparation are of concern because they allow the survival and growth of pathogens to disease-causing levels. The first is preparation of food several hours before consumption along with storage at ambient temperatures favoring the growth of pathogens and/or toxins. The second concern is insufficient cooling of foods or inadequate reheating to reduce or eliminate pathogens (Motarjemi, 2000). General food safety guidelines for both commercially prepared and homemade infant food should be followed.

Nutrient Requirements

Energy

It is difficult to estimate energy requirements for infants and young children. The 1985 Food and Agriculture Organization/WHO/United Nations Organization (FAO/WHO/UNO) recommendations for energy intake were derived from the observed intakes of healthy thriving children. This assumes that the natural ad libitum feeding of infants and toddlers reflects desirable intake. However, the observed energy intake of infants and toddlers may not be optimal and may reflect outside influences such as type of feedings and caregiver behaviors. The FAO/WHO/UNO recommendations for energy were based on data compiled from the literature predating 1940 and up to 1980 and included an extra 5% allowance for presumed underestimation of energy intake (IOM, 2002).

Experts questioned the validity of the 1985 FAO/WHO/UNO recommendations for energy intake, and in 1996 experts concluded that the guidelines were too high. Energy requirements for infants and toddlers based on actual energy expenditure and energy deposition, rather than observed intake, would more accurately reflect true energy needs. Energy requirements of infants and young children need to support a rate of growth and body composition consistent with good health. Satisfactory growth is an indicator that energy needs are being met.

Butte et al. (2000a) used data obtained from doubly labeled water studies on infants aged 3 to 24 months to define energy requirements in the first 2 years of life based on total energy expenditure and energy deposition. They were able to demonstrate that total energy expenditure was greater in older infants than in younger infants, greater for males than for females, and greater for formula-fed infants than for breast-fed infants. After adjusting for body weight and fat-free mass, only feeding mode, not gender or age, influenced total energy expenditure. Breast-fed infants had lower rates of energy deposition in

Nitrates

Infant methemoglobinemia results in cyanosis in infants with few other clinical symptoms and is caused by nitrates in food or water that are converted to methemoglobin-producing nitrites before or after ingestion. The resulting compound, methemoglobin, cannot bind oxygen and results in hypoxemia. Absorbed nitrate that has not been converted to nitrite can be readily excreted in the urine without adverse effects. The greatest risk to infants comes from well water contaminated with nitrates (Greer, Shannon, the Committee of Nutrition, & the Committee on Environmental Health, 2005). It is estimated that 2 million families drink water from private wells that fail to meet federal drinking water standards for nitrate, and 40,000 infants younger than 6 months old live in homes that have nitrate-contaminated water supplies. Breast-fed infants whose mothers consume water with high nitrate nitrogen concentrations are not at increased risk, because nitrate concentration does not increase in human milk.

Nitrates also occur naturally in plants and may be concentrated in foods such as green beans, carrots, squash, spinach, and beets. Some commercially prepared infant foods are voluntarily monitored for nitrate content, and because of exceedingly high levels in spinach, this product is often labeled as not to be used for infants younger than 3 months of age. Concerns for home-prepared foods are unfounded because there is no nutritional indication for introduction of complementary foods before 6 months. The risk of methemoglobinemia decreases with age as the infant's gastric pH approaches lower levels typical of later childhood and fetal hemoglobin, which more readily oxidizes to methemoglobin, is replaced by adult hemoglobin after 3 months.

the first year of life, although differences between breast-fed and formula-fed infants diminished in the second year. The energy cost of growth is important in early infancy when energy deposition contributes significantly to energy requirements. At 3 months of age 22% of energy requirements are utilized for growth. This drops dramatically to 6% at 6 months and even further to 2% to 3% of total energy requirements in late infancy. Estimated energy requirements based on studies of total energy expenditure and energy deposition were 80% of the former recommendations, providing strong evidence that revisions were needed to lower the energy requirements for children in this age group.

The WHO/United Nations Children's Fund (UNICEF) compiled data from 21 studies of children in developing countries to estimate the amount of energy received from breast milk and to determine how much energy would be required from complementary foods to meet their needs for growth. To ensure that children receive sufficient calories, foods must be prepared with an adequate energy density and served an appropriate number of times per day. Both energy density and meal frequency independently affect the child's total energy consumption.

Dewey (2000b) expressed concern that the improper introduction of complementary foods has the potential to adversely affect breast milk intake and breast-feeding duration. Providing excess energy in the form of complementary foods can reduce the intake of breast milk. Breast-fed infants reduce their intake of human milk as non–breast milk foods and fluids are introduced. Although it appears that the timing of breast-feeding in relation to complementary foods (e.g., offering complementary foods before or after breast-feeding) does not seem to affect overall breast milk intake, there is a paucity of information on the effect of the introduction of complementary foods on breast-feeding.

Protein

It is not difficult to meet the protein needs of infants. Exclusively breast-fed infants receive adequate protein for at least the first 6 months of life. The most recent recommended AI of protein for infants from birth to 6 months is 1.5 g/kg/day and reflects the observed mean intake of infants who are fed mostly human milk (IOM, 2002). This value is calculated from various studies in which the volume of human milk consumed is measured by test weighing, and the average protein content of human milk was determined using values from several studies.

DuPont (2003) reported that total protein in breast milk varies greatly during the course of lactation, providing from less than 2.0 g/kg/day in the first weeks of life to approximately 1.15 g/kg/day at 4 months, less than the AI recommendations of the IOM. Dewey, Cohen, Rivera, Canahuati, and Brown (1996b) reported that protein intake of breast-fed infants decreases from 2.0 g/kg/day at 1 month to 1.0 g/kg/day at 6 months as protein concentration in milk decreases and average breast milk intake increases slightly. According to Dewey et al., estimated daily protein intake of a 6-month-old breast-fed infant is 8.0 to 8.4 g/day, lower than the calculated AI of 9.1 g/day.

Protein content of infant formula is greater than human milk, but no study has shown that the amount of protein in human milk has deleterious effects. Multiple studies have shown that infants fed human milk have improved immune function and fewer illnesses than formula-fed infants. The casein and whey in infant formula are different from those present in human milk; therefore the digestibility, absorption, and functionality of these proteins differ. The IOM (1990) states that digestibility and comparative protein quality need to be considered when determining the amount of protein to be included in infant formula based on various protein sources. Protein requirements for formula-fed infants may be greater due to less efficient utilization and retention of protein than breast-fed infants. Dewey et al. (1996b) found that adding extra protein to 4- to 6-month-old exclusively breast-fed infants did not improve weight or length gain despite an additional 20% protein to their diet, and no differences were found in growth rate based on protein intake.

The amount of protein required for growth is highest in early infancy and decreases over time. At 1 month of age 64% of protein intake is used for growth, decreasing to 24% at 6 to 12 months. Daily increments in body protein gains in male breast-fed infants decreased from 1.0 g/kg/day at 1 month to 0.2 g/kg/day at 6 months. Protein needs for growth in early infancy are influenced by birth weight as well. Infants with higher birth weights generally grow at a slower rate and would require less protein than infants born at a lower birth weight who experience faster rates of weight gain (Dewey, Beaton, Fjeld, Lonnerdal, & Reeds, 1996a). Protein requirements (both total protein and protein per kilogram body weight) for infants older than 6 months are lower than the requirements for younger infants. High protein follow-up formulas are not indicated or necessary for infants consuming a variety of foods (Dewey, 2000a).

Calculations for protein requirements for infants ages 7 through 12 months are based on the relationship between protein intake and nitrogen balance. Studies examining protein losses, requirements for maintenance, and protein deposition were used to derive the DRI/RDA for older infants of 1.5 g/kg/day, which do not differ greatly from the AI for younger infants. Higher protein intake would be indicated for a child requiring catch-up growth or recovery from an infection. Infants older than 6 months may receive a significant portion of their protein needs from complementary foods.

An adequate growth rate has traditionally been used as the determinant for sufficient protein intake. Dewey et al. (1996a) reported that other measures of protein intake, such as immune function and behavioral development, may become compromised long before growth falters. Observed differences in growth rates between infants who are breast-fed and formula-fed raise the question of whether maximal growth rate is synonymous with optimal growth rate. Higher intakes of protein in formula-fed infants have been a cause for concern, because the liver and kidney need to metabolize and excrete the increased levels of plasma amino acids and urea nitrogen, which could have long-term consequences on immature organs.

Fatty Acids

Both human milk and currently available infant formula contain generous amounts of the essential fatty acids, linoleic and alpha-linolenic acid. Cow's milk contains very little, and infants and toddlers who drink cow's milk often have low levels of these fatty acids. Corn, soybean, or safflower oil can be added to the diet of a child who has been weaned from breast milk or formula to provide these nutrients (Butte et al., 2004).

In addition to the essential fatty acids linoleic and alpha-linolenic acid, there is growing concern that

LCPUFA (long chain polyunsaturated fatty acids): A category of dietary fats important in brain and retinal growth; normally present in human milk, they are now added to infant formula.

infants also need long chain polyunsaturated fatty acids (**LCPUFAs**) in their diets. These fats, particularly AA and DHA, are vital for neural development and visual acuity. Infants fed formula containing only linoleic and alpha-linolenic acid, the precursors for AA and DHA, are able to synthesize only a limited amount of long chain fatty acids. When compared with breast-fed infants, formula-fed infants had less mature neurophysiologic maturation and brain function (Khedr, Farghaly, Amry Sel, & Osman, 2004).

These LCPUFAs are concentrated in the phospholipid bilayer of biologically active brain and retinal neural membranes during the periods of rapid brain and retinal growth from the last trimester of pregnancy until 2 years of age. During this critical period of rapid growth and maturation, the quantity and quality of the LCPUFAs may influence the efficiency of nerve cell signaling and have long-lasting effects on brain function. The rationale for adding these LCPUFAs to infant formula is based on the observation that they are present in large quantities in the brains and retinas of breast-fed children and are present in breast milk. In February 2002 term infant formula with added DHA and AA became readily available, and shortly thereafter DHA and AA were added to preterm infant formula. In 1998 an expert panel for the FDA in the United States and a working group for the Canadian authorities did not recommend the addition of LCPUFAs to infant formula because of the uncertainties related to product safety and efficacy (Koo, 2003). Maternal plasma and human milk DHA levels as well as the infant's plasma levels can be increased by adding DHA to the maternal diet at levels of 200 mg/day or greater. However, studies have not shown marked improvement in infant outcome related to visual function and neurodevelopment in breast-fed infants whose mothers received 200 mg/day DHA supplementation (Jensen et al., 2005).

A comparison of the multitude of studies on LCPUFA supplementation and visual acuity and neurodevelopmental outcomes in infants is hindered by the fact that many of the neurodevelopment tests were never designed to test normal healthy infants and lack predictive ability for long-term neurodevelopment outcomes. Although DHA and AA supplementation no doubt raises plasma levels in both infants and breast-feeding mothers, it remains highly controversial whether or not there is any functional benefit in visual acuity or neurodevelopment. The

Research Studies by Formula Companies

A study sponsored by Ross Products Division, Abbott Labs, makers of Similac, Neosure, and Isomil infant formulas, found that the addition of DHA and AA to infant formula increased DHA and AA plasma levels to those commonly seen in breast-fed infants without improvement in measures of visual acuity or other neurodevelopment tests (Auestad et al., 2001). A study sponsored by Mead Johnson Nutritionals, makers of Enfamil Lipil, found that when infants received a continuous supply of DHA and AA throughout the first year of life they had improved visual acuity at 1 year of age (Morale et al., 2005). Compared with women in other countries where greater intakes of fish are consumed, the DHA levels in the milk of mothers from the United States are much lower and do not meet the WHO recommendations.

safety of these additives is an additional concern, although there have been few reported adverse events. The oils used for the supplementation are new food products from Martek Biosciences and have been approved by the FDA as "Generally Recognized as Safe" and are approved for use in infant formula and baby food.

DHA is an oil derived from microalgae, and AA is an oil derived from soil fungi. An imbalance of omega-3 to omega-6 fatty acids could have biological effects such as prolonged bleeding time and diminished growth, and close monitoring of infants consuming infant formula with added LCPUFAs through scientific studies is indicated and indeed required by the FDA. Although families will embrace a new product promising to deliver a formula that is closer to human milk and is good for the brain and eyes, the cost of these products is a burden on the family budget and on public funding for nutrition programs. Justification of increased costs of up to 25% may prove difficult without substantial scientific evidence of improved clinical outcomes in vision and intelligence.

Iron

Iron deficiency anemia: The most common childhood deficiency resulting in motor and cognitive developmental deficits.

Iron deficiency anemia is the most common childhood nutritional deficiency worldwide, with consequences of delays in motor and cognitive development caused by irreversible brain injury. Developmental deficits occur when iron deficiency becomes severe and chronic enough to result in anemia. Although iron supplementation increases iron stores, poor developmental outcomes may persist with lower scores on mental and motor tests and functional impairment in school-aged children. A high prevalence of nutritional iron deficiency anemia was first noted in the United States in infants in the 1930s and has decreased dramatically since the 1960s when it was acknowledged as a public health problem. Interventions, including an increase in breast-feeding, the start of the Special Supplemental Nutrition Program for Women, Infants, and Children (**WIC**) in 1972, and education of physicians and the public, resulted in a dramatic decrease in iron deficiency anemia across all socioeconomic groups in the United States. The intervention was so successful that in the 1980s it was sug-

WIC: The Special Supplemental Nutrition Program for Women, Infants, and Children that serves to safeguard the health of low-income women, infants, and children up to age 5 who are at nutritional risk by providing nutritious foods to supplement diets, information on healthy eating, and referrals to health care.

gested that routine screening of all infants be replaced by selective screening of high risk patients.

It now appears that the prevalence of iron deficiency anemia is increasing in 1- to 3-year-olds (Kazal, 2002). Data from the 2001 Pediatric Nutrition Surveillance System indicated that 16.6% of 6- to 11-month-old infants and 15.3% of 12- to 17-month old children were anemic. The subjects in this national sample were largely from low-income populations, where 82% were enrolled in WIC (Altucher, Rasmussen, Barden, & Habicht, 2005). It is not unusual for children ages 1 to 3 years to have low intakes of iron. Most 12-month-olds receive 100% of the daily requirement for iron, but this declines to less than recommended intake by 18 months, likely due to cessation of breast-feeding and switching from iron-fortified infant formula to cow's milk and reduced intake of iron-fortified cereals (Kazal, 2002). Juice intake can decrease a child's appetite for other more nutritional solid foods, further contributing to iron deficiency.

Healthy, normal birth weight, full-term infants receive adequate iron from human milk for approximately the first 6 to 9 months of life. Reserves at birth are a critical factor for anemia. Total body iron is fairly stable in infants from birth through age 4 months as stored iron is gradually used to support growth. Between 4 and 12 months there is a significant increase in iron requirements as body size increases. These needs cannot be met through the iron available in human milk. The concentration of iron in human milk is 0.2 to 0.4 mg/L and remains stable throughout lactation. Although the absolute amount of iron in human milk is low, efficiency of iron absorption from human milk is quite high, at about 50%. Once iron stores are depleted, iron-related physiologic functions may become compromised with both cognitive and motor deficits even in the absence of anemia. After age 2 years when growth velocity decreases, iron stores start to accumulate and the risk for deficiency decreases (American Academy of Pediatrics [AAP], 2004).

The risk for anemia is much greater in low birth weight infants. In a study of low birth weight infants born in Honduras, infants with birth weights less than 3,000 g were at risk for anemia at 6 months even when iron-fortified complementary foods were introduced between ages 4 and 6 months (Dewey, Peerson, & Brown, 1998). It is recommended that low birth weight breast-fed infants receive iron drops beginning at ages 2 to 3 months.

Fomon (2001) stated that infants who are exclusively or predominantly breast-fed are at risk of becoming iron deficient by 8 to 9 months of age. Whereas Fomon recommended beginning iron supplementation of breast-fed infants at an early age to prevent depletion of body stores, the AAP notes that iron deficiency is rare in breast-fed infants due to increased absorption and the absence of microscopic blood loss in the intestinal tract that may occur with whole cow's milk. Supplementation of healthy term breast-fed infants with iron to prevent deficiency is controversial. Unnecessary supplementation can increase the prevalence of gastrointestinal infection, sepsis, and cancer because iron is essential for the growth of microorganisms and malignant cells. Gastrointestinal effects such as nausea, vomiting, constipation, and abdominal pain have been reported by individuals on iron supplementation. Routine iron supplementation of breast-fed infants with normal hemoglobin levels resulted in increased diarrhea and poor linear growth, possibly due to the pro-oxidant effect of iron on the intestinal mucosa. Reduction in zinc absorption leading to poor growth can occur from excessive iron intake (Dewey et al., 2002). Ermis and coworkers (2002) found that supplementation of breast-fed infants from ages 5 to 9 months with iron at a dose of 2 mg/kg every other day prevented iron deficiency and iron deficiency anemia. Every-other-day dosing improved compliance and reduced unpleasant side effects.

Domellof, Lonnerdal, Abrams, and Hernall (2002) found that regulation of iron absorption in breast-fed infants undergoes developmental changes from ages 6 to 9 months that enhances the ability of the infant to adapt to a low iron diet. Unlike iron absorption in adults that increases in states of iron depletion, iron absorption in infants was found to be directly related to the dietary intake rather than to iron status. Iron status as measured by serum ferritin was improved in infants given iron supplementation, but there was a significant inverse relationship between dietary iron provided and absorption of iron from human milk. Unsupplemented infants absorbed 37% of the iron in human milk compared with only 17% absorption in breast-fed infants supplemented with 1 mg/kg/day. Supplemental iron drops had a greater effect on decreasing iron absorption from human milk than iron in complementary foods. Domellof et al. concluded that breast-feeding with the addition of complementary foods containing adequate iron likely provides sufficient iron for some, but not all, healthy 9-month-old infants, possibly due to up-regulation of iron in response to low dietary intake, thus avoiding iron deficiency.

Iron absorption from foods varies greatly from less than 1% to 50% of available iron. About 4% of the iron in fortified infant formula is absorbed versus 50% of the iron in human milk. The AAP estimates that for infants consuming iron-fortified formula there is an 8% risk for iron deficiency and less than 1% risk for iron deficiency anemia. Infants drinking cow's milk have a 30% to 40% risk of iron deficiency by ages 9 to 12 months. Exclusively breast-fed infants have a 20% risk of iron deficiency by 9 to 12 months of age. Formula-fed infants should not be switched to whole cow's milk until after 1 year of age, and there is no medical indication for low iron formulas. The AAP has recommended that the manufacture of low iron formulas be discontinued because there is no scientific evidence to support the claim that iron-fortified formulas increase gastrointestinal distress in infants.

The main sources of iron from complementary foods in the infant diet are iron-fortified cereal and meats. Absorption of iron from infant cereal is only about 4%. The form of iron used in dry infant cereals is an insoluble iron salt or metallic iron powder that is used to reduce oxidative rancidity, and these forms have low bioavailability. Meat is a much better source of iron because the iron is in the heme form, with an absorption efficiency of 10% to 20%. Non-heme iron from plant foods and fortified products is less well absorbed. Plant-based foods have a high phytic acid, polyphenol, and/or dietary fiber content that can inhibit absorption of micronutrients. Ascorbic acid counteracts the effects of phytate on iron absorption by preventing it from binding with available iron.

Estimates for absorption of iron depend on the amount of animal or fish protein in a meal relative to plant-based foods. Consumption of meat, fish, or poultry enhances the absorption of non-heme iron from plant-based foods. Vitamin C in the form of fresh fruits such as cantaloupe, kiwi, or strawberries or vegetables such as broccoli and kale consumed at the same time as non-heme iron enhances absorption. Tea, bran, and milk inhibit non-heme iron absorption. Heme iron is absorbed in the intestines intact and is not affected by inhibitors of non-heme iron.

Engelmann and colleagues (1996) studied the effect of meat intake on hemoglobin levels in breast-fed infants. When healthy 8-month-old partially breast-fed infants were fed a high meat intake of 27 g/day for 2 months, they had only minimal decreases in hemoglobin of 0.6 g/L compared with a similar group of breast-fed infants with a low meat intake of 10 g/day who had decreases in hemoglobin of 4.9 g/L. The group with the low meat intake had overall greater intakes of iron (3.4 versus 3.1 mg/day) but lower intakes of iron from meat (0.1 versus 0.4 mg/day), suggesting that animal muscle protein has an iron absorption enhancing effect and can minimize decreases in hemoglobin that are typically observed from ages 8 to 10 months in breast-fed infants.

Heath, Tuttle, Simons, Cleghorn, & Parnell (2002) found that 9- to 18-month-old New Zealand breast-fed infants experienced low rates of iron deficiency anemia of 7% even while their intake of breast milk and infant formula declined. Their intake of highly bioavailable iron in the form of meat, poultry, and fish increased from 0 g/day at 9 months to 21 g/day at 12 months and 32 g/day at 18 months. Their intake of vitamin C was also high, at 52 to 96 mg/day, likely further enhancing iron absorption.

Kattelmann and coworkers (2001) found that the age of introduction of complementary foods to formula-fed infants did not affect iron status parameters. Infants introduced to complementary foods early, at 3 to 4 months of age, had greater iron intakes at age 6 months but no difference in hemoglobin levels at ages 12, 24, or 36 months than infants with later introduction to complementary foods at age 6 months. These infants were all formula fed and received at least the RDA for iron for the first 6 months of life.

Zinc

The AI for zinc for infants from birth to age 6 months reflects the usual zinc intake of infants fed exclusively human milk. Human milk alone is inadequate to meet infants' needs for zinc after 6 months of age (IOM, 2001). **Zinc deficiency** is prevalent in undernourished children and is linked to reduced activity and play with subsequent poor developmental outcomes. Zinc deficiency is associated with poor growth as well as diarrheal disease. It is estimated that 12- to 24-month-olds only meet 50% to 60% of the DRI/RDA for zinc (Krebs, 2000). Meeks Gardner et al. (2005) found that when poor undernourished Jamaican children ages 9 to 30 months were supplemented with 10 mg zinc daily and also participated in a weekly program to improve mother–child interactions, the developmental quotient and hand and eye coordination improved. Diarrheal morbidity was

Zinc deficiency: Prevalent in undernourished children and associated with poor growth, poor developmental outcomes, and diarrheal disease.

reduced, but there were no improvements in the children's growth.

Zinc concentration in human milk is low, but bioavailability is high. Neonatal stores are likely sufficient to maintain zinc homeostasis until 6 months of age. The young infant has a relatively high zinc requirement to support the rapid growth of early infancy. Zinc concentration in human milk decreases throughout lactation, but as the infant's growth rate declines with increasing age so does the requirement for zinc (Lawrence, 1999). The concentration of zinc in human milk decreases rapidly from 4 mg/L at 2 weeks to 2 mg/L at 2 months and to 1.2 mg/L at 6 months (Krebs, Reidinger, Robertson, & Hambridge, 1994). Despite an increased intake in volume over the first 6 months, this steep decline in zinc concentration in human milk results in a decline in zinc intake. Zinc concentration in human milk of well-nourished mothers is resistant to changes in the maternal diet. Although zinc supplementation is associated with improved growth, exclusively breast-fed infants grow well without additional zinc. Dewey et al. (1998) found that when breast-fed children received complementary foods fortified with zinc to double their average zinc intake there was no significant increase in weight or length.

Zinc absorption is greater from a diet high in animal protein, and the best source of zinc is red meat. Plant-based foods containing phytic acid bind with zinc in the intestines and reduce absorption. Vegetarians who rely on a plant-based diet may need to increase their zinc intake by 50% due to decreased bioavailability of zinc from phytic acid. Complementary foods based on unrefined cereals and legumes have a high phytate-to-zinc ratio and can compromise zinc status, whereas rice has a lower phytate-to-zinc ratio (Gibson & Holtz, 2000). Offering infants complementary foods of animal origin such as red meat and fish improves zinc intake and bioavailability. Supplementation with a combination of micronutrients can lead to problems of interaction and limitations of absorption. A zinc supplement given in water interferes with absorption of iron but not when both are added to food (Rossander-Hulten, Brune, Sandstrom, Lonnerdal, & Hallberg, 1991).

Vitamin D

Rickets was almost universally seen in African-American infants living in the northern United States at the turn of 20th century. With the dis-

Rickets: Vitamin D deficiency resulting in growth deficits, developmental delay, failure to thrive, short stature, tetany, seizures, and skeletal deformities.

covery of vitamin D and a public health campaign to fortify infant foods and supplement breast-fed infants with cod liver oil, rickets were nearly eradicated (Rajakumar & Thomas, 2005). Once again, nutritional rickets is a public health concern. Breast-fed infants are at risk for vitamin D deficiency due to limited amounts of vitamin D in breast milk and the current trend to limit sun exposure (Fomon, 2001). Vitamin D deficiency rickets can cause significant morbidity, including delays in growth and motor development, failure to thrive, short stature, tetany, seizures, and skeletal deformities. A review of published reports from 1986 to 2001 found 166 cases of rickets in children in North Carolina, Texas, Georgia, and the mid-Atlantic region (Weisberg, Scablon, Li, & Cogswell, 2004). Most cases (83%) were African-American, and 96% were breast-fed. Only 5% of the breast-fed infants received vitamin D supplementation, and most were weaned from the breast to a diet low in vitamin D and calcium.

Dark-skinned infants who are exclusively breast-fed are at particular risk. From 1990 to 1999 in North Carolina 30 cases of nutritional rickets were seen in African-American children who were breast-feeding without supplemental vitamin D, even though infants living in sunny southern states were believed to be at low risk (Kreiter et al., 2000). Vitamin D deficiency rickets is common in infants in Pakistan, Saudi Arabia, and the United Arab Emirates where breast-feeding women have limited sun exposure and a diet low in vitamin D. Infants are not routinely supplemented with vitamin D while breast-feeding, and many mothers avoid consumption of fortified dairy products. Despite abundant sunshine only rural women who spent more time working outdoors had adequate serum levels of vitamin D (Dawodu, Adarwal, Hossain, Kochiyil, & Zayed, 2003).

Guidelines from the AAP, based on recommendations of the National Academy of Sciences, state that all infants, including those exclusively breast-fed, require a minimum intake of 200 IU of vitamin D per day beginning the first 2 months of life to prevent vitamin D deficiency rickets (Gartner, Greer, & the Section on Breastfeeding and Committee on Nutrition, 2003). Universal supplementation of all breast-fed infants is controversial and not endorsed by all practitioners (Henderson, 2005). Implicit in this recommendation is that human milk is inferior and does not meet all the infant's nutritional requirements, reducing the mother's confidence in her choice to breast-feed her infant. Concerns for oral supplementation of the breast-fed infant include aspiration and possible changes in the pH and flora of the gut, altering absorption of other nutrients and affecting rates of infection. The only infant vitamin D supplements readily available either contain other vitamins not required by healthy full-term infants or are available in highly concentrated forms that increase the risk of overdose.

Vitamin D synthesis occurs in the skin from exposure to ultraviolet B light from sunlight. Dietary sources include fish liver oils, fatty fish, and foods fortified with vitamin D, particularly cow's milk, infant formula, and breakfast cereals. Sunlight exposure may not be sufficient at higher latitudes, during winter months, or with sunscreen use. Individuals with dark skin pigmentation have limited vitamin D synthesis with sunlight exposure. Human milk typically contains 25 IU/L of vitamin D, not enough to meet the recommended requirement. Infant formula has at least 400 IU/L; therefore an infant consuming more than 500 mL/day of infant formula receives the recommended 200 IU/day.

Maternal vitamin D status has a direct effect on the vitamin D content in human milk. Traditionally, sunlight exposure provided adequate vitamin D for both mothers and breast-feeding infants. For instance, in light-skinned individuals 10 to 15 minutes of total body peak sunlight exposure endogenously produces and releases into circulation 20,000 IU of vitamin D. The daily recommended intake for vitamin D for lactating women is 400 IU, an amount unlikely to provide for optimal vitamin D levels in human milk. Wagner and colleagues (2006) found that by supplementing lactating mothers with 6,400 IU/day of vitamin D they were able to increase maternal vitamin D levels sufficiently to increase the amount of vitamin D in human milk from 82 to 873 IU/L and to significantly improve circulating vitamin D in both the mother and the breast-fed infant.

Supplemental Nutrients

Human milk continues to provide many nutrients in the second half of the first year of life during the period of **complementary feeding**. Human milk intake of infants ages 9 to 11 months meets the estimated needs for vitamin C, folate, vitamin B_{12}, selenium, and iodine. After 6 months complementary foods are needed to provide 12% of vitamin A; 25% to 50% of copper; 50% to 75% thiamin, niacin, and

> **Complementary feeding:** The period that begins with the introduction of the first nonmilk food and ends with the cessation of breast or formula feeding.

manganese; and up to 98% of iron and zinc (Gibson & Holtz, 2000).

Despite the fact that most young children receive adequate vitamins and minerals from their diet, many families supplement their child's diet with additional vitamins and minerals. Eichenberger Gilmore, Hong, Broffitt , & Levy (2005) studied trends in children under age 2 years in Iowa and found that by 24 months 31.7% used some type of supplement. In the first 6 months of life 3.5% to 6.3% of non–breast-fed infants received supplements compared with 18.3% to 29.2% of breast-fed infants. After 6 months of age use of multiple vitamin supplement and multiple vitamin with minerals increased with age. Diet alone provided AI of most vitamins and minerals, and with additional supplementation intake of vitamin A exceeded the recommended upper limit. Hypervitaminosis A is a concern because reports associate excessive vitamin A intake with decreased bone mineral density and increased risk of fracture. The long-term adverse effects of high intakes of vitamin A during early life are not clear.

Milner and coworkers (2004) reported that early use of multivitamins increased the risk of developing food allergies and asthma. There was an association between infant multivitamin supplementation within the first 6 months of life and an increased risk of developing asthma by 3 years of age among black children. In addition, multivitamin supplementation in the first 6 months of life was associated with increased risk for food allergies by 3 years of age in both formula-fed and breast-fed infants. Early infancy may be a sensitive time for exposure to exogenous stimuli that influence the differentiation of naive T cells into either proinflammatory or anti-inflammatory cells. Vitamins may be a potent stimulus for the differentiation of T cells that promote allergic response when encountering specific antigens. Recommendations for routine vitamin supplementation, including vitamin D supplementation for breast-fed infants, may need reevaluation in light of these findings.

Fortified foods provide a significant portion of nutrient needs, reflecting a limited intake of nutritious foods such as fruits and vegetables (Fox, Reidy, Novak, & Ziegler, 2006c). As infants move into the toddler stage, a decrease in naturally occurring vitamin A from vegetables is replaced by vitamin A from cereals and supplements. At the same time, two of three of the leading sources of vitamin C are fortified juices and fortified sweetened beverages rather than fruits and vegetables. Consumption of a wide variety of foods to meet nutrient needs, rather than reliance on fortified foods and supplements, is optimal. There is potential for excess intake and toxicity when vitamin A, zinc, and folate are consumed through fortified foods and supplements.

Vegetarianism

A vegetarian diet during infancy and childhood can be adequate in all essential nutrients, with normal growth and nutritional status expected unless the diet is severely restricted. A breast-fed infant of a well-nourished vegetarian mother receives adequate nutrition, particularly if the mother pays close attention to her own intake of iron, vitamin B_{12}, and vitamin D. Women who consume three or more servings of dairy products receive sufficient vitamins D and B_{12} from their diet. Women following a vegan diet need to supplement with foods fortified with vitamin B_{12} such as nutritional yeast or soy milk. Vegan infants who are not breast-fed need to receive soy infant formula until 1 year of age. Soy milk, rice milk, or homemade formulas do not provide adequate nutrition for infants less than 1 year old and should not be used to replace breast milk or commercial infant formula (American Dietetic Association, 2003).

A variety of protein-rich vegetarian foods is available for the older infant and toddler, including tofu, legumes, soy or dairy yogurt and cheese, eggs, and cottage cheese. These foods can be easily pureed or mashed for increased acceptance when the child is first introduced to complementary foods. Later, soft cooked beans, bean spreads, or nut butters on toast, chunks of tofu, or cheese and soy burgers can be offered as finger foods. Fat is an important source of energy and should not be restricted in children under 2 years of age. Vegan infants need a supplementary source of vitamin B_{12} when they are weaned from breast milk or infant formula. Read more about vegetarianism in Chapter 7.

Complementary Feeding

Transitioning from All Milk to Family Foods

Complementary feeding is defined as the period extending from the first introduction of nonmilk feeds to the cessation of breast or formula feeding (Weaver, 2000). Any food that provides energy and displaces breast milk is considered a complementary food. A gradual progression from an exclusive milk diet to a variety of complementary foods allows the infant's gastrointestinal function to accommodate new types of foods, including starch, sucrose, and fiber. In many other mammals there are abrupt and well-defined changes to the intestinal mucosa and enzyme activity as weaning occurs. However, in humans these changes are less obvious and more gradual. Human milk contains many bioactive substances, including digestive enzymes such as bile salt-stimulated lipase, amylase, and protease, that may be involved in the digestion of complementary foods.

The timing of complementary feeding varies according to cultural practices and the personal beliefs of the mother as well as guidance she receives from her pediatrician. In some instances pediatricians may suggest adding cereal to the infant's diet before age 4 months when a mother is concerned about the baby's sleeping patterns or growth. Child nutrition experts agree that there is no reason to introduce complementary foods before 4 months of age. At least 60 countries have policies in place to introduce complementary foods after 6 months of age. Earlier introduction of complementary foods can affect immune function and immunotolerance, development of chronic disease, and risk of atopy.

At birth the gut of a full term infant may be anatomically and functionally mature, but subtle immaturities in luminal digestion, mucosal absorption, and protective function could predispose the infant to gastrointestinal and systemic disease during the first 6 months of life. It is not known exactly when the period of immature immune function ends and when it is safe to feed foreign proteins. Early introduction can cause protein-induced enteropathies, leading to mucosal inflammation, villous atrophy, diarrhea, and failure to thrive (Muraro et al., 2004). The question of when the normal term infant is developmentally ready to discontinue **exclusive breast-feeding** and begin the intake of solid and semisolid complementary foods is an important one. There probably is not a single optimal age for introduction of complementary foods but rather optimal ages that are determined by factors such as infant birth weight, maternal nutrition while breast-feeding, and environmental conditions.

Exclusive breast-feeding: Infant receiving only breast milk and no other foods or drinks for the first 6 months.

Feeding Guidelines

From 1979 until 2001 the WHO recommended that normal full-term infants be exclusively breast-fed for 4 to 6 months. Later, it was found that discontinuing exclusive breast-feeding before 6 months increased infant morbidity and mortality, and the WHO rec-

ommendations were revised to encourage exclusive breast-feeding for 6 months. Early introduction of complementary foods and exposure to pathogens in food could result in symptomatic infection and illness in the infant and reduced sucking at the breast, followed by a decrease in the amount of milk and immune substances consumed as well as decreased maternal milk production from reduced demand. Exclusive breast-feeding for 6 months results in greater immunologic protection and limits exposure to pathogens at an early age when the immune system is immature. Energy and nutrients that are valuable for normal growth and development can be used for their intended purpose rather than diverted for immunologic function.

Malnutrition is the leading cause of death in children under 1 year of age worldwide. Inappropriate feeding practices include early cessation of exclusive breast-feeding, introducing complementary foods too early or too late, and providing nutritionally inadequate or unsafe foods. Malnourished children who survive are frequently sick and may suffer lifelong consequences. Overweight and obesity are increasing at alarming rates throughout the world and are associated with poor feeding practices that often begin in early childhood. Global strategies for infant and young child feeding can impact social and economic development.

The WHO feeding guidelines (World Health Organization [WHO], 2003) are for generally healthy breast-fed infants. These guidelines target primarily low income countries where most children are breast-fed and safe low-cost alternatives to breast milk are not readily available. No information is included for feeding premature infants or children with infections or other acute or chronic diseases that could affect nutritional status. No information is provided on feeding non–breast-fed infants. An important goal of the WHO is to improve complementary feeding practices in terms of timeliness, quality, quantity, and safety to ensure adequate global nutrition. It is difficult to make recommendations regarding the optimal age for introduction of complementary foods. Ideally, the appropriate time to introduce complementary foods and the optimal duration of breast-feeding consider infant outcomes, such as growth, behavioral development, micronutrient status, the risks of infection, allergy, and impaired intestinal function, as well as those of the mother, such as general health and nutritional status and return to fertility.

The AAP states that there is no evidence for harm when safe, nutritious, complementary foods are introduced after 4 months when the infant is developmentally ready. The AAP Section on Breastfeeding (2005) recommends that complementary foods rich in iron be introduced gradually around 6 months of age, but due to the unique needs of individual infants the need to introduce complementary foods could occur as early as 4 months or as late as 8 months of age. Exclusive breast-feeding in the first 6 months is defined by the AAP as consumption of human milk with no supplementation of any type (no water, no juice, no nonhuman milk, and no foods) except for vitamins, minerals, and medications. During the first 6 months water, juice, or other liquids are unnecessary, even in hot climates, and can introduce contaminants or allergens. Exclusive breast-feeding provides protection from many acute and chronic diseases. Breast-feeding is also more likely to continue for at least the first year of life when infants are exclusively breast-fed for the first 6 months. For optimal health benefits breast-feeding should continue for 12 months or longer. The recommendations of the WHO are to breast-feed for at least 2 years, and the AAP states that there is no upper limit to the duration of breast-feeding and no evidence of psychological or developmental harm from breast-feeding into the third year of life or longer (AAP, Section on Breastfeeding, 2005). Indeed, in late infancy breast milk provides significant amounts of energy and micronutrients and is a key source of PUFAs crucial for brain development and neurologic function (Villalpando, 2000).

A partnership of the Agricultural Research Service (ARS) at the U.S. Department of Agriculture-Children's Nutrition Research Center at the Baylor College of Medicine in Houston, Texas and the American Dietetic Association, funded by Gerber Food Products Company, developed the "Start Healthy Feeding Guidelines for Children Ages 0–24 Months." The expert panel realized that guidance was needed to help parents through the transition period from an all-milk diet to the first introduction of solids foods by adding variety and texture throughout the weaning process and to establish healthy eating patterns. These new guidelines are an effort to address the growing problem of childhood obesity and inappropriate food choices at an early age. They are intended to complement and expand on already existing guidelines from the AAP, CDC, and other expert groups. These evidence-based guidelines answer the important questions "when, what, and how" complementary foods should be introduced (Butte et al., 2004). Where scientific evidence was limited or unavailable, expert opinion was referenced. For instance, there is only limited evidence to suggest any order for introduction of textures, and expert opinion suggests a general progression based on the child's readiness for and acceptance of different food textures.

Complementary Foods and Growth

Introducing complementary foods to the exclusively breast-fed infant before 6 months does not increase total calorie intake or improve growth. A breast-fed infant who receives complementary foods at 4 months decreases his or her intake of human milk to maintain the same level of calories. Complementary foods displace human milk, and the infant receives fewer immune factors and is at greater risk for infection. No significant improvement in weight or length was observed by Dewey (2001) in infants up to 12 months of age when they received complementary foods at 4 months compared with infants who received exclusive human milk until 6 months.

Despite recommendations to exclusively breast-feed for the first 6 months of life, this practice may be uncommon. Carruth, Skinner, Houck, & Moran (2000) found that in a study of 94 mothers, 60 added solid food by 4 months and 8 were feeding cereal in a bottle. The median age for introduction of cereal was 4 months and for juice 4½ months. Thirteen mothers introduced cereal, juice, or fruit as early as 2 months. In looking at the growth of the children who had early solids, there was no association between the age of introduction of complementary foods and change in weight or length from 2 to 8 months or from 12 to 24 months. These results were similar to the WHO data (WHO Working Group, 2002) showing only minor differences in growth among infants receiving complementary foods at different ages. The WHO data was based on a unique longitudinal seven-country study of predominantly breast-fed infants. They found little evidence of risk or benefit related to growth based on timing of introduction or types or frequency of complementary foods in healthy infants living in environments without major economic restraints and with low rates of illness.

The amount of energy and nutrients needed from complementary foods depends on the amount of breast milk or formula the infant is consuming. Although it is possible for an infant to receive adequate nutrition for the first year solely from iron-fortified formula, all infants need complementary foods for exposure to novel tastes and textures and to develop appropriate feeding skills. A variety of flavors and foods is important in the first 2 years of life and may increase the likelihood that children will try new foods.

Meal Patterns and Nutrient Intakes

During infancy and early childhood, lifelong patterns of eating are formed that can influence later eating habits and overall health. As the child makes the transition from an all-milk diet to sharing foods from the family table, meeting nutritional guidelines may become more problematic for families. Families strive to follow nutrition recommendations to provide the best for their children, particularly in the year after birth when the infant is eating mostly jarred baby foods. As the infant matures and begins to incorporate more of the family foods into his or her diet, less than optimal nutrition becomes evident. Transitioning from baby food to table food has been associated with a decreased intake of vitamin A, iron, and folate at meals as baby food fruits, vegetables, and meats are not replaced with equivalent table foods.

Children imitate what others around them are eating, and if no one else eats fruits or vegetables, the young child will quickly abandon these foods. When other family members drink sweetened carbonated beverages and eat high calorie low nutrient dense foods, such as French fries, donuts, and potato chips, the young child will happily join in. As rates of obesity, excess weight, and type 2 diabetes are increasing in children, it is evident that the influence of early diet needs to be addressed. At a surprisingly young age many infants and toddlers do not receive a variety of fruits and vegetables and instead are consuming high calorie, high fat, salty snacks and sweetened drinks. It is the parent's responsibility to offer nutritious foods to infants and toddlers. Although a preference for sweet foods is innate, repeated exposure at an early age and observing other family members eating these foods increases the likelihood that young children will develop preference for these foods. The disappearance of the family meal and the increase in the number of meals eaten outside the home and from fast food establishments has concerned experts as the prevalence of snacking and the quantity and quality of foods consumed by children and adolescents in recent years has changed.

Food Trends and Preferences

The Feeding Infants and Toddlers Study (**FITS**) was a cross-sectional telephone study using a national random sample of 3,022 infants and toddlers between 4 and 24 months of age and a subsample of 703 two-day dietary recalls. The sample size was sufficiently large to categorize data by age groups: 4 to 6 months, 7 to 11 months, and 12 to 24 months. Conducted in 2002, it consisted of up to three telephone interviews to collect data on growth, development, and feeding patterns. The study had a large sample size and was representative of ethnicity of the general population. It also included a large proportion of breast-fed infants. The FITS survey collected data on food choices and their nutritional impact, feeding practices and patterns, and infant and toddler growth and developmental milestones (Devaney et al., 2004a). The study was sponsored by Gerber Products Company and provided in-depth nutritional information about feeding behaviors of infants and toddlers and compared intakes with the newly developed DRIs (see Appendix 2).

FITS: The Feeding Infants and Toddlers Study conducted on a large random sample of infants and toddlers to collect data on food choices and feeding practices and their impact on growth and development.

Some new trends were noted in infant nutrition. The unhealthy practice of early introduction of unmodified cow's milk before 6 months of age has been nearly eradicated, but the fact that some infants under 24 months of age drank little or no milk in a day is concerning. Overall, the FITS study found that most infants and toddlers in the United States were receiving adequate nutrition without getting excessive amounts of nutrients. Even infants whose motor skills lagged or those who were described by parents as picky eaters were receiving adequate nutrients. In fact, the data suggested that many children were being overfed (Dwyer, Suitor, & Hendricks, 2004).

Energy intake reported by parents was often greater than those recommended using the new DRI standard for energy, called the estimated energy requirement. The mean energy intake exceeded the estimated energy requirement by 10% for infants ages 4 to 6 months, by 23% for infants ages 7 to 12 months, and by 31% for ages 12 to 24 months (Devaney, Ziegler, Pac, Karwe, & Barr, 2004b). For infants under 6 months of age, the largest discrepancies were for those receiving complementary foods in addition to breast milk or formula. The FITS infants and toddlers consumed more energy than recommended on average for all age groups. Over-reporting of food intake by caregivers is possible because parents may perceive the amount of food consumed reflects their success as providers. Parents may also have difficulty accurately assessing food intake because of spillage and a discrepancy between foods offered and foods consumed. However, with 10% of 2- to 5-year-old children considered overweight, it is plausible that overfeeding is occurring in infants and toddlers. Early exposures to fruits and vegetables or to foods high in energy, sugar, and fat at this critical time period can influence food preferences and dietary habits later in life.

Complementary foods continue to be introduced at ages earlier than recommended by experts, and 29% of all infants were introduced to infant cereals or pureed foods before 4 months of age (Briefel, Reidy, Karwe, & Devaney, 2004a). There was no significant difference in the mean age of introduction of complementary foods or cow's milk according to income level or ethnicity or in children ever breast-fed compared with those never breast-fed. The contribution of commercial baby foods and beverages to energy consumption peaks at ages 7 to 8 months and declines as table food intake increases (Briefel, Reidy, Karwe, Jankowski, & Hendricks, 2004b).

The FITS study revealed disturbing trends regarding the food consumption of infants and toddlers. Early food preferences can predict future eating behaviors, and an alarming percentage of young children have already developed suboptimal food consumption patterns. Not surprisingly, food consumption patterns in infants and toddlers reflect the typical eating patterns of older children and adults, such as diets lacking in fruits and vegetables with high intakes of readily available low nutrient snacks and beverages. Daily consumption of fruits and vegetables are the cornerstone of a healthy diet, and a wide variety is encouraged. Many infants and toddlers do not meet the Five a Day for Better Health program's recommendation for fruits and vegetables. Fruit was not consumed daily by more than 25% of infants and toddlers (Skinner, Ziegler, Pac, & Devaney, 2004a). About 50% do not have fruit for breakfast or lunch, and 60% do not have fruit at dinner. Fruit was even more uncommon for snacks. Similar patterns of vegetable consumption were observed, with 50% not having a vegetable at lunch, and 30% not having a vegetable with dinner. Less than 5% had vegetables for breakfast or snacks (Skinner et al., 2004a). Among infants aged 9 to 11 months old, 27% consumed no vegetables in a day, and French fries were among the most commonly eaten vegetable

in all age groups above 9 months (Fox, Pac, Devaney, & Jankowski, 2004). Fewer than 10% of infants and toddlers consumed dark leafy vegetables at any age. Intake of deep yellow vegetables decreased as infants transitioned from commercial baby food to table food. Commercial baby food was the main source of fruits and vegetables until 9 months of age when children were offered a greater percentage of cooked vegetables and fresh fruits. Bananas were the most commonly consumed fruit, followed by apples, and few children received citrus, melon, or berries.

Establishment of healthy patterns of beverage consumption including milk with meals is important for adequate calcium intake during the years of active bone growth in childhood and adolescents. Water is a better choice for quenching thirst than sweetened juice drinks or carbonated beverages. The FITS study found that colas, fruit-flavored carbonated drinks, and carbonated mineral water were consumed by an increasing percentage of children from ages 4 through 24 months. Substitution of fruit drinks or carbonated beverages for milk at lunch, dinner, and snacks was evident after 15 months (Skinner, Ziegler, & Ponza, 2004b). Fruit juice is not a necessary component of the diet of infants and toddlers and, if used at all, should be introduced after 6 months of age and limited to 8 ounces per day (Kleinman, 2000a). Adverse gastrointestinal reactions to pear or apple juice are possible because of poor absorption of fructose and sorbitol (Fomon, 2001). Offering juice in a bottle after teeth have erupted can increase the risk of dental caries and should be avoided.

According to the AAP, limited amounts of 100% juice amounting to 4 to 6 ounces per day can be offered after 6 months of age, yet Skinner et al. (2004b) found from the FITS study that 22% of infants were introduced to juice earlier. Juice consumption increases dramatically with age. Ten percent of toddlers ages 15 to 24 months consume more than 14 ounces of juice per day. Fruit drinks are also popular, and 5% of toddlers consume more than 16 ounces of fruit drinks a day. The AAP does not provide recommendations for limitations on fruit drinks or carbonated beverages but states that they are not equivalent to 100% juice and should not be considered a fruit serving. Most fruit juices and fruit drinks contain added vitamin C and provide 20% to 30% of the daily vitamin C requirements, but apple juice, the most commonly consumed juice, contains little vitamin A and folate, nutrients commonly obtained from fruits and vegetables. Overfeeding juice and juice drinks can displace more nutritious beverage options such as milk and water and can be associated with excessive calorie intake and risk of obesity in older children.

Desserts and sweets are introduced at a surprisingly early age, with 10% of 4- to 6-month-olds already consuming a dessert, sweet, or sweetened beverage daily. These numbers increased dramatically after age 6 months, when nearly half were consuming one or more foods in this category. Younger infants consume commercial baby food desserts or cookies marketed specifically for infants, but after age 9 months children are offered many of the foods that other family members eat, such as cakes, cookies, doughnuts, ice cream, candy, fruit-flavored drinks, and salty snacks, foods that are low in important nutrients but high in fat and calories. Parents should offer age-appropriate finger foods such as soft fresh fruits, diced canned fruit, well-cooked vegetables, and easily dissolvable fortified grains such as unsweetened ready-to-eat cereals.

There are no controlled studies addressing the practical aspects of introducing foods for the first time. Although feeding guidelines for parents abound, there is no evidence for a benefit of introducing one particular food first or at any particular rate. The AAP suggests that when complementary food introduction is initiated after 6 months of age, the order of the specific food introduction is not critical. Mixing cereal with breast milk may enhance acceptance of solid foods by breast-fed infants. Foods commonly consumed by infants at 1 year of age include cereals and fruits. FITS data showed that infant cereal was the most common source of grains in young infants, but even by ages 7 to 8 months many infants were consuming ready-to-eat cereals, crackers, pretzels, rice cakes, breads, and rolls (Fox et al., 2004). After 9 to 11 months, the number of infants receiving infant cereal declined. This was replaced by other noninfant ready-to-eat and cooked cereals, including presweetened cereals. Many presweetened cereals are comparable in vitamins and minerals with unsweetened ready-to-eat cereals but their use in this age group may lead to preference for sweetened foods.

Infants rarely consume meat. Krebs (2000) suggested that meat intake for breast-fed infants at 6 months would adequately support both iron and zinc requirements in this age group. Introduction of red meat is desirable by ages 5 to 6 months because of the high bioavailability of iron (Fomon, 2001). Offering plain single meats promotes the goals of com-plementary feeding, which is to gradually increase the variety of flavors and textures in the diet. The formula-fed infant is less reliant on complementary foods for iron and zinc. The addition of cereal to complement the intake of protein and energy from formula is considered adequate (Wharton, 2000). In the FITS study few infants were receiving any type of meat, and often the meat appeared in commercially prepared baby food dinners. Fewer than 5% of infants in any age group received plain baby food meats. After 9 to 11 months of age non–baby food meats were offered, with chicken or turkey the most common, followed by beef and hot dogs, sausages, and cold cuts. By 12 months of age less nutritious high-fat deli meats were the second most commonly consumed source of meat. Pork, ham, fish, shellfish, and beans were consumed by only a small number of infants and toddlers on a regular basis. Popular nonmeat protein sources include cheese, eggs, and yogurt (Skinner et al., 2004a). Peanut butter, seeds, and nuts were rarely offered before 1 year of age, and only about 10% of toddlers consumed any peanut butter daily.

Cow's milk and cow's milk products make a significant contribution to nutritional intake during the period of complementary feeding. If breast-feeding continues into the second year of life and the diet contains a reasonable amount of animal protein in the form of meat, fish, poultry, or eggs, most infants thrive without the addition of dairy products to their diet (Michaelsen, 2000).

In the FITS study nearly all children under 24 months of age consumed some form of milk daily. The average duration of breast-feeding was 5½ months (Briefel et al., 2004a). Exclusive breast-feeding was uncommon, and more than half of 4- to 6-month-old infants currently breast-feeding also received infant formula daily. At 6 to11 months the percentage of breast-fed infants receiving infant formula increased to 70%. Overall, 9 of 10 infants who were ever breast-fed also had received infant formula.

Infant formula was consumed by 82% of 7- to 8-month-olds and decreased as cow's milk was introduced. Over 90% of infant formula consumed was iron fortified, and about 10% consumed soy-based formula. At ages 9 to 11 months 33% had received cow's milk and 20% were receiving cow's milk daily, increasing the potential for iron deficiency. Cow's milk has an undesirably high renal solute load compared with infant formula and is a significant concern for children at risk of dehydration. Iron in cow's milk is low and poorly absorbed, and feeding non–heat-treated cow's milk can cause microscopic gastrointestinal bleeding in infants, resulting in loss of iron and anemia. Cow's milk is low in essential fatty acids, zinc, vitamin C, and niacin and is high in saturated fats. Recommendations to delay cow's milk introduction until 12 months of age are mainly focused on prevention of iron deficiency anemia (Michaelsen, 2000).

Feeding Skills and Neuromuscular Development

Reflexes

A normal progression of sucking and feeding reflexes is necessary for the child to advance from a milk-only diet to consumption of foods from the family diet. Swallowing is present in early fetal life at the end of the first trimester. The fetus has ample opportunities to practice by swallowing amniotic fluid even before the development of the **sucking reflex**, which appears by the middle of the second trimester. The sucking reflex is quite strong in the newborn and can be easily elicited by stroking the infant's lips, cheeks, or inside the mouth. By about 3 months of age sucking becomes less automatic and more voluntary. The **gag reflex** is present in the third trimester and is stimulated by contact of the posterior two-thirds of the tongue. This reflex gradually diminishes to one-fourth of the posterior tongue by 6 months of age. The **rooting reflex**, which assists the infant to locate the breast and nipple by turning the head side to side and opening the mouth wide when the skin surrounding the mouth is stroked, disappears by 3 months of age.

Sucking reflex: Strong reflex present in the newborn elicited by stroking the infant's lips, cheeks, or inside the mouth.

Gag reflex: Reflex stimulated by contact with the tongue that gradually diminishes over the first 6 months.

Rooting reflex: Reflex present from birth to age 3 months that assists the infant to locate the breast and nipple by turning the head side to side and opening the mouth wide when the mouth is stroked.

Advanced Motor Skills

Infants need new oral motor skills to transition from a full liquid milk-based diet to a more solid diet of complementary foods. Disappearance of the rooting and sucking reflexes and the accompanying changes in anatomy help prepare the infant for this transition. Phasic biting, resulting in the rhythmic opening and closing of the jaw when the gums are stimulated, disappears between 3 and 4 months of age. Between 6 and 9 months it becomes possible for the infant to receive a bolus of food without reflexively pushing it out of the mouth. By 12 months of age rotary chewing is well established, along with sustained controlled biting that permits the infant to consume a variety of foods (Kleinman, 2000c).

During the first 2 years of life there is increasing head and torso control that permits a child to achieve developmental milestones required for proper self-feeding abilities. Finger coordination to permit self finger feeding usually is adequate by 6 to 7 months of age. The infant must be able to sufficiently stabilize the head and balance the trunk before he or she can sit without support and use arm and hand movements for self-feeding. Carruth and colleagues (2004) found that one-third of 4- to 6-month-old infants and 99% of 9- to 11-month-olds can sit alone without support. Stability of the trunk is crucial in the process of progressing to complementary foods, and by 6 months most infants have achieved greater strength in the trunk, shoulder, and neck muscles. There is a wide range of ages when feeding skills emerge, and it is crucial that caregivers allow amble opportunities for appropriate exploratory activities. Offering the child a variety of nutritious foods and allowing them to self-feed when they have sufficiently developed this skill is appropriate and will not jeopardize adequate nutrient intake.

Beginning at 6 months most infants are ready for pureed, mashed, and semisolid foods. By 7 months soft foods that can be pressed down by the infant's tongue can be introduced, and at 9 months the infant can handle foods that can be compressed by the gums. Teeth are not necessary for chewing of soft lumpy foods. The ability to handle advanced textures increases day by day, and children require multiple opportunities to practice new feeding skills. By 8 months they can progress to finger foods they can pick up and feed themselves. By 12 months of age most children can transition to the same diet as the rest of the family, keeping in mind the need for calorically and nutrient-dense foods because of the smaller portion size. Infants possessing self-feeding skills are reported to have higher energy and nutrient intakes (Carruth et al., 2004). Foods that are a choking risk that can lodge in the trachea, such as grapes, nuts, hard raw vegetables and fruits, and popcorn, should be avoided. Introduction to a cup usually occurs after 6 months, and by 12 months most infants are drinking from a "sippy cup."

Chewing Ability

Advances in gross motor skills parallel advances in dentition as the first primary teeth erupt at 7 to 8 months and continue throughout the first 2 years, with approximately 15 teeth by 19 to 24 months of age. Carruth et al. (2004) found the ability to consume foods that required chewing increases with age. Nutrient intakes of energy, fat, protein, vitamin B_6, vitamin B_{12}, folate, zinc, thiamin, niacin, and magnesium were greater for infants under 1 year of age who were able to eat foods that required chewing. Individual differences in the age of eruption of teeth can influence the ability to chew certain foods, especially meat and fibrous vegetables.

Feeding difficulties, particularly difficulty with chewing tough or fibrous foods, in Japanese children are thought to be caused by inappropriate transition from a milk-based diet to a diet of family foods. Sakashita and coworkers (2004) found that at 2 years of age many preschool children swallowed without chewing or were unable to chew and swallow certain foods and that many kindergarten children did not chew properly, retained food in the side of their mouth, or frequently spit food out (Sakashita et al., 2004). A transitional diet containing very soft and pureed foods for an extended period has been suspected of preventing children from developing proper masticatory system and chewing and swallowing ability. Leafy vegetables were usually offered early as a weaning food but were not well accepted because the fiber makes it difficult to chew. Meats were often introduced later than recommended, possibly due to parental concerns related to food allergies (Sakashita, Inoue, & Tatsuki, 2003). In Japan foods were specially cooked and fed to children from a spoon, inhibiting the proper development of the masticatory system and mature chewing and swallowing behavior.

Determinants of Food Acceptance

Sakashita et al. (2004) found that acceptance of new foods was greatest in children who were offered food prepared from the family table and was lowest in children fed jarred baby food. Offering infants foods prepared from the family table promotes feeding progress by giving the infant an opportunity to experience a variety of food textures from an early age. Infants first offered lumpy solid foods between ages 6 and 9 months had fewer feeding difficulties and improved acceptance than infants not introduced to these foods until after age 10 months. Observing other family members eating at the family table and having the opportunity to try new foods is also an important component of transitioning an infant to family foods. Sakashita et al. (2004) found that first-born children experience more feeding difficulties

than second- or third-born children. This may be a result of limited opportunities to observe other family members eating and to learn feeding behavior from older siblings.

The number of accepted foods increases rapidly from 6 months to 1 year and continues to increase throughout the first 2 years. Foods requiring significant chewing before swallowing, such as leafy vegetables and sliced meat, may be poorly accepted. Processed sliced deli meats are often more readily accepted when offered. Because chewing ability affects ability to swallow and therefore food acceptance, breast-fed infants who have more opportunity to develop the masticatory system have a higher rate of food acceptance than bottle-fed infants. Exposure to food flavors through mother's milk also prepares the infant for a variety of flavors. Breast-feeding seems to facilitate increased acceptance of different foods due to the greater variation in breast milk flavors compared with infant formula.

Other causes of food refusal include dislike of the taste or smell and an unfamiliar appearance. Often, a child's food preference reflects those of other family members. Early food experiences can be imprinted on the memory, and when children refuse to eat vegetables at an early age, these food preferences may remain throughout the childhood and adolescent years with significant health consequences. Child-feeding practices contribute to the development of food intake controls and energy balance and can affect childhood obesity. Obese individuals tend to prefer fatty foods to fruits and vegetables and dislike tough or fibrous texture. Exposure to fruits and vegetables in infancy and early childhood should be encouraged to reduce risk factors for obesity and obesity-related diseases.

Caregiver Behaviors

Although early childhood malnutrition can be attributable to poverty and lack of resources, family and caregiver characteristics, such as education and household management or coping skills of the mother, can determine normal growth and development. Lack of knowledge regarding appropriate foods and feeding practices can contribute to malnutrition to a greater degree than lack of food. Not only is providing the appropriate combination of complementary foods to meet the child's nutritional needs important, feeding practices such as frequency of feeds and feeding style need to be considered. Caregiving behaviors that have been identified as promoting normal growth and development are (1) active or interactive feeding, (2) selecting foods appropriate to the child's motor skills and taste preferences, (3) feeding in response to the child's hunger cues, (4) feeding in a nondistracting safe environment, and (5) talking and playing with the child in the context of the meal. This type of responsive parenting has been described as sensitive and supportive caregiving associated with good growth and development. Feeding interactions should include the caregiver observing the infant's intake and nonverbal cues and responding accordingly (Pelto, 2000). If children refuse many foods, parents should be encouraged to be creative and experiment with different food combinations, tastes, and textures. Parents should be taught to encourage children to eat, but never to force, because this can lead to aversion to food and behavioral problems.

Effect of Feeding Mode in Infancy

In early infancy parents choose whether the child will be breast-fed or bottle fed and whether human milk or formula will be consumed. They may also control the timing of the feedings and the volume consumed, although this is less likely when the infant is breast-fed. When a mother breast-feeds and her infant's sucking slows or stops, the mother assumes the child is satisfied and is finished eating. The amount of milk consumed is primarily under the infant's control. Breast-fed infants are able to adjust the amount of milk consumed to maintain a constant energy intake. Formula-feeding mothers may rely on visual cues of formula remaining in the bottle and encourage the infant to continue feeding after he or she has exhibited signs of satiety.

Taveras et al. (2004) found that the longer a mother breast-fed, the less likely she was to restrict her child's intake at 1 year. Compared with mothers who formula fed, mothers who exclusively breast-fed for 6 months were less likely to restrict their child's intake. Breast-feeding for at least 12 months was associated with lower levels of controlling feedings and resulted in improved intake by toddlers (Orlet Fisher, Birch, Smiciklas-Wright, & Picciano, 2000). Breast-feeding may protect against obesity by allowing the infant to naturally regulate energy intake based on hunger cues and by preventing parents from overriding these cues by controlling the feeding. Mothers who breast-feed may be more responsive to their infants' signals regarding the timing and volume of feedings.

Feeding Relationship

As the child transitions to a variety of family foods, the need to be independent and autonomous will be evident in the feeding relationship as the child assumes more control of his or her eating. The feeding relationship reflects the overall parent–child relationship, and feeding struggles may be indicative of other difficulties involving parent–child interactions. Feeding is a major area of frequent daily exchanges between the parent and the child, reflecting the characteristics of both the parent and the child that can either support or hinder the child's development. Feeding involves more than providing the correct mix of calories and vitamins to ensure adequate nutrition. The feeding relationship itself is crucial for the child's growth and development (Slaughter & Bryant, 2004). Feeding is a blend of nutrition, parenting, and human development and provides an opportunity for parents to be present and to provide love, support, and attention that can affect the child's physical, social, and emotional health.

As infants progress from a milk-based diet to sharing family foods, they develop unique likes and dislikes regarding the foods they are offered and will communicate these preferences to their parents. How the parents respond to this assertiveness can impact the child's developing sense of self and autonomy. The ability to refuse food and have this be accepted by the parents is paramount to future interactions between the child and the parents and provides a base for all future social interactions. It is important for the child's development to be able to say "no" and still be unconditionally loved and supported. If the parent withholds love from the child or forces or pressures the child to eat, the child feels helpless and abandoned. Furthermore, the child learns that he or she does not have the ability to say "no" and be respected, which can have far-reaching effects. By allowing a child to refuse to eat a certain food or to not eat at all because he or she is not hungry, parents are giving the child permission to express his or her needs without fear of repercussions.

High levels of maternal control over when and what children eat are associated with increased adiposity and an increased desire to consume restricted foods. Maternal restrictive feeding practices have been found to increase the child's preference for the restricted food and to promote overeating when the restricted foods are available and are counterproductive in preventing obesity (Birch, Orlet Fisher, & Krahnstoever Davison, 2003). In place of restricting desirable foods, parents should be taught skills that help children learn how to consume appropriate portion sizes, to like healthy foods, and to recognize hunger and satiety cues to determine when and how much to eat.

Portion Size

Children demonstrate an innate ability for self-regulation of energy intake. They can compensate for changes in energy density by adjusting the quantity of food they consume. Parents and caregivers potentially interfere with this natural hunger-driven mechanism by coercing children to eat when they are not hungry or by directing them to "finish their plate" or to "take one more bite" when they have demonstrated signs of satiety. Over-restriction of intake to prevent overeating in infants and toddlers can have negative consequences by preventing the natural development of feeding self-regulation. Table 2.1 indicates food types and corresponding development infants usually demonstrate; some variances should be expected.

The presence of self-regulation of dietary intake in infants and toddlers was confirmed by analysis of the relationship between portion size, number of eating occasions, number of unique foods, and energy density (Fox, Devaney, Reidy, Razafindrakoto, & Ziegler, 2006a). Children who ate less often during the day consumed larger portions, and children who ate more often ate smaller portions. For infants, energy density was negatively associated with portion size. As the energy density increased, portion size decreased, and as energy density decreased, portion size increased. The number of different foods consumed by 6- to 11-month-olds was also positively associated with portion size, indicating that infants with a more varied diet consume larger portions.

Children under 2 years of age typically eat seven times a day, although the number of meals and snacks reported ranges from 3 to 15. It is appropriate for infants and

TABLE 2.1	Infant Feeding by Age and Development	
Age	Development	What to Feed
Birth to 6 mo	Baby can suck and swallow. Baby should be held for feeding.	Breast milk is best. Use formula if not breast-feeding. No water or juice.
6–8 mo	Baby can sit with support and control head movement. Spoon feeding begins. No honey entire first year.	Breast-fed infants: begin pureed meats first and then eggs, pureed fruits and vegetables, and infant cereal. Formula-fed infants: begin infant cereals and then pureed fruits, vegetables, and meats and eggs. Wait 3–5 days between new foods. Watch for signs of food allergies such as rash, vomiting, or diarrhea.
7–9 mo	Baby can chew, grasp, and hold items. Finger feeding begins. Introduce a cup with water, juice, breast milk, or formula.	Try well-cooked carrots, sliced bananas, unsweetened dry cereals, graham crackers, soft cheeses, pancake bits, and well-cooked pasta.
9–12 mo	Baby can eat with a spoon and will feed self more often. Expect baby to eat with hands and make a mess.	Offer new tastes and textures such as plain yogurt, cottage cheese, tofu, and refried beans. Offer soft foods from the family meal. Limit juice to 4 oz/day. Offer fewer pureed foods and more foods from the family meal. Always try to eat together as a family. Parents should set a good example by eating fruits and vegetables. Avoid dangerous foods that are a choking hazard: raw vegetables, nuts, seeds, whole grapes or cherry tomatoes, hot dogs, popcorn, and spoonfuls of peanut butter.
1 year and beyond	Encourage self-feeding. Continue breast-feeding. Wean from bottle. Begin offering whole cow's milk in cup. No low-fat or skim milk until 2 years of age.	Infant should eat three meals and two to three snacks each day. Feeding should be a happy time for the entire family. Let infant decide when enough is enough. Never force infant to eat or drink. No sweetened drinks or soda. Avoid sweets. Offer fruit for dessert.

toddlers to consume many small meals and snacks because of their small stomachs and high energy demands. Snacks often provide about 25% of toddler's energy intake (Skinner et al., 2004a). The breakfast, lunch, dinner, and snacks pattern emerges at ages 7 to 8 months and is well established by 9 to 11 months.

Special Supplemental Nutrition Program for Women, Infants, and Children (WIC)

Food supplements have been available for more than 30 years for low-income women, infants, and children under 5 years of age through WIC of the U.S. Department of Agriculture. Pregnancy, infancy, and early childhood are critical periods of rapid growth and development. Nutritional insult during this time can have far-reaching consequences on cognitive and emotional health and can adversely impact health outcomes. Millions of families have benefited from the WIC program, and it has successfully improved the nutrient intakes of its participants, particularly by reducing the prevalence of iron deficiency anemia and improving physical, emotional, and cognitive development. Almost half of all infants and one-fourth of children ages 1 to 4 years old participate in the WIC program. Mothers of infants and toddlers participating in WIC are more likely to be teenagers, Hispanic, or black and less likely to have completed high school, to be married, or to be employed than nonparticipants (Ponza, Devaney, Ziegler, Reidy, & Squatrito, 2004).

Promoting breast-feeding as the norm for infant feeding is a major goal of the WIC program to ensure successful breast-feeding initiation and continuation of breast-feeding throughout the first year of life. Despite evidence that infants participating in WIC have improved dietary outcomes when compared with nonparticipating low-income infants, such as higher intakes of iron, zinc, and vitamin C, and improved compliance with recommendations not to feed cow's milk in the first 6 months, there is concern that WIC participation leads to less breast-feeding. Historically, WIC infants lag behind the national rates of breast-feeding for the general population, but encouraging trends have been seen since the early 1990s. Breast-feeding initiation rates for WIC infants increased from 34% in 1990 to 59% in 2002 (National WIC Association, 2004). WIC helps low-income at-risk families overcome barriers to breast-feeding by educating women and their families about the benefits of breast-feeding, training WIC staff and peer counselors, providing appropriate food packages, and providing support throughout the postpartum period. However, some critics view the provision of free infant formula as a deterrent to breast-feeding.

In the FITS study more than two-thirds of WIC infants had ever breast-fed, but by ages 4 to 6 months 95% had received infant formula. WIC infants were less likely than nonparticipants to have ever breast-fed, and only 21% were still breast-feeding at 4 to 6 months compared with 48% of nonparticipants. By 7 to 11 months of age almost one-fifth of WIC infants received cow's milk (Ponza et al., 2004). WIC infants and toddlers were more likely to consume sweets, desserts, and sweetened beverages than nonparticipants, and they consumed less baby food fruit, non–baby food fruit, fresh fruit, or canned fruit but consumed more 100% juice than nonparticipants. Overall, the diets of infants and children participating in WIC are nutritionally adequate, and the mean usual intake of calcium, vitamin A, iron, vitamin C, and protein, the nutrients targeted by the WIC program, exceeded recommended intakes. Reported energy intakes are higher for WIC participants than nonparticipants, and this should be addressed in light of the risk of obesity. Fruits and vegetables should be emphasized, and use of juice and low nutrient sweetened drinks should be avoided or minimized.

In early 2004 the IOM reviewed WIC's supplemental food package and made revisions based on dietary guidelines for infants and young children and nutrition concerns from WIC staff and participants (IOM, 2005). The new package attempts to reduce the prevalence of inadequate and excessive nutrient intakes, encourages consumption of fruits and vegetables, and emphasizes whole grains and lower saturated fat. The food packages are designed to be attractive for breast-feeding mothers and infants and to provide incentives for breast-feeding, especially full breast-feeding. Infants whose mothers intend to breast-feed will not routinely receive formula during the first month of life. After the first month partially breast-fed infants receive 12 to 14 ounces of formula per day. The previous food package provided 26 ounces of formula per day to all infants whether they were breast-fed or not. Exclusively formula-fed infants will continue to receive appropriate amounts of infant formula for the first year of life.

Women who are providing at least half of the infant's feedings as breast milk will receive an expanded food package from 1 month through 11 months after delivery that includes vitamin C–rich juice, fresh or canned fruits and vegetables, low-fat milk, whole-grain cereal, whole-grain bread, eggs, beans, and peanut butter. Fully breast-feeding women receive an additional 30 ounces of canned tuna or salmon, two dozen eggs, and 1 pound of cheese per month.

New WIC recommendations have changed the age of introduction of complementary feedings from 4 months to 6 months, and the amount of formula offered is decreased accordingly as more complementary foods are offered. Juice has been removed from all infant food packages and replaced with baby fruits and vegetables. The package for fully breast-fed infants older than 6 months includes 2½ ounces per day of baby food meats, 8 ounces a day of fruits and vegetables, and iron-fortified cereal. For partially breast-fed infants the revised package offers 10 ounces of infant formula a day along with 4 ounces of fruits and vegetables and iron-fortified infant cereal. Formula-fed infants older than 6 months receive 20 ounces a day of formula compared with 26 ounces a day in the previous package, and the 3 ounces a day of juice has been changed to 4 ounces a day of baby fruits and vegetables. Families receive cash-value vouchers to purchase fresh fruits and vegetables for older children and pregnant and lactating women, and if fresh produce is not available, choices of canned, dried, or frozen fruits or vegetables are permitted. Whole-grain options such as ready-to-eat cereals, whole-wheat bread, brown rice, corn tortillas, oatmeal, and barley will be offered to children ages 1 to 4 years. Children ages 1 to 2 years will receive 2 cups per day of whole milk, and women and children over age 2 years will only receive milk or yogurt that is less than 2% milk fat. Pregnant and lactating mothers will also have the option of choosing enriched soy products as a substitute for dairy milk. The nutrition messages here are clear. The emphasis is on establishing healthier eating habits during the very first year of life.

Effect of Early Diet on Health Outcomes

It is well known that a relationship exists between many chronic diseases and nutrition. It has been postulated that the diet during infancy and early childhood can impact the progression of chronic diseases that develop later in life, such as cancer, obesity, diabetes, hypertension, allergy, and osteoporosis. Whereas Kleinman (2000b) reported that little evidence exists to support the claim that early eating behaviors and patterns or consumption of specific nutrients can influence the development of some chronic illnesses in adulthood, studies have examined the link between obesity, allergies, and diabetes and diet early in life.

OBESITY

Increasing trends in childhood obesity, with its associated comorbidities and the likelihood of persistence of obesity into adulthood, compelled researchers to investigate preventive strategies. Treatment of childhood obesity is costly and rarely effective. Childhood obesity is associated not only with adult obesity, but also with adverse health outcomes in adulthood independent of weight status. One of the critical periods of attainment of excess weight is in infancy. A study by Stettler et al. (2005) found that in formula-fed infants, weight gain in the first week of life may be a critical determinant for the development of obesity in later life. Formula feeding is associated with a more rapid increase in weight gain in early infancy and an increased risk for obesity in childhood and adolescence.

An earlier multicenter cohort study by Stettler, Zemel, Kumanyika, & Stallings (2002) demonstrated that a pattern of rapid weight gain during the first 4 months of life was associated with an increased risk of overweight status at 7 years, independent of birth weight and weight at 1 year. For each 100 g of weight gain increase per month, the risk of overweight status at 7 years was increased by 30%. There was a clear association between the rate of early weight gain and childhood overweight status. The greatest proportional weight gain in postnatal life occurs during the time when birth weight is doubled by 4 to 6 months, and this may correspond with a critical period for energy balance regulation mechanisms.

Martorell and colleagues (2001) reviewed and critiqued the literature to determine whether nutrition in early life predisposes individuals to be overweight later in life. They looked at three plausible hypotheses: (1) overnutrition increases the risk of later excess weight; (2) undernutrition, at the other extreme, also is a risk for excess weight; and (3) optimal nutrition during infancy represented by breast-feeding is protective of future obesity. They found the link between undernutrition in infancy and later obesity contradictory and inconsistent. Intrauterine overnutrition, high birth weight, and gestational diabetes were found to be associated with later obesity. Breast-feeding was found to have an enduring influence on the development of subsequent obesity.

According to the AAP (2003), the extent and duration of breast-feeding is associated with a reduction in obesity risk later in life, possibly due to physiologic factors in human milk as well as the feeding and parenting patterns associated with breast-feeding. Increasing initiation and duration of breast-feeding may provide a low-cost readily available strategy to help prevent childhood and adolescent obesity (Dietz, 2001).

Owen, Martin, Whincup, Davey Smith, and Cook (2005) published a quantitative review of the effects of infant feeding on the risk of obesity later in life. Initial breast-feeding protected against obesity later in life, and the association was stronger with prolonged breast-feeding. The consistency of the association they found with increasing age suggested a protective effect of early breast-feeding that was independent of dietary and physical activity patterns later in life. Confounding by maternal factors such as social class and obesity, both of which are associated with childhood obesity and a tendency to formula feed, was a limitation of the observational studies.

Hediger and colleagues (2001) found a reduced risk of obesity for ever breast-fed 3- to 5-year-olds compared with those never breast-fed, but found a much stronger association with maternal obesity. Kries et al. (1999) studied 9,357 German children at the time they entered school at ages 5 and 6 years. They found a remarkably consistent, protective, and dose-dependent effect of breast-feeding on excess weight and obesity. This cross-sectional study found that obesity was reduced by 35% when children were breast-fed for 3 to 5 months. This protective effect was not attributable to social class or life-style factors and remained significant after adjusting for potential confounding factors. Gillman et al. (2001) found that adolescents who were mostly or only fed breast milk in the first 6 months of life were at a 22% lower risk of being overweight than adolescents who were only formula fed. They found an estimated 8% reduction in the risk of adolescent obesity for every 3 months of breast-feeding.

Bergmann et al. (2003) found that maternal obesity, bottle-feeding, maternal smoking during pregnancy, and low socioeconomic status were risk factors for becoming overweight and adiposity at age 6 years in a longitudinal study of German children from birth. At age 3 months body mass index and triceps skin-fold thickness were already significantly higher in the children who were formula fed. Children who were formula-fed continued to have a higher prevalence of excess weight and obesity, and the findings remained stable after adjusting for maternal weight, maternal smoking, and socioeconomic status.

Questions regarding the optimal duration of exclusive breast-feeding or whether combining breast-feeding with formula supplementation may weaken the preventive influence of breast-feeding need to be addressed. Gillman et al. (2001) found that infants who received more breast milk than formula in the first 6 months of life had a lower risk of obesity in older childhood and adolescence than children who received mostly or only formula. In a retrospective cohort study Bogen and coworkers (2004) found that in a population of low-income families breast-feeding was associated with a reduced risk of obesity at age 4 years only among whites whose mothers did not smoke in pregnancy and only when breast-feeding continued for at least 16 weeks without formula or at least 26 weeks with formula.

Several explanations are offered for the protective effect of breast-feeding against obesity. Breast milk production is stimulated by the infant's sucking, and it is unlikely that rapid weight gain in an exclusively breast-fed infant is a result of overfeeding. A breast-fed infant establishes a point of satiety based on internal physiologic cues rather than on external social cues. Children can naturally regulate their energy intake, but parents' behavior can override the child's appetite signals. It is possible that during bottle feeding parents exhibit more control of the feeding and prevent self-regulation by the child. Parents who do not recognize the child's hunger and satiety cues may contribute to the risk of later obesity. Overfeeding in infancy may increase adipose number and fat content at a critical time period and prevent development of lifelong patterns of healthy appetite regulation that would protect against the risk of obesity.

Metabolic consequences of ingesting human milk may help regulate appetite and food consumption. Leptin, a hormone that regulates food intake and energy metabolism, is present in human milk. In a study by Savino, Costamagna, Prino, Oggero, & Silvestro (2002) serum leptin levels were higher in breast-fed infants than in formula-fed infants. Breast-feeding may help to program the infant against later energy imbalance (Gillman et al., 2001). Owen et al. (2005) suggested that breast-feeding affects intake of calories and protein, insulin secretion, and modulation of fat deposition and adipocyte development. A higher protein to nitrogen content of infant formula might induce a metabolic response of increased insulin production in formula-fed infants, leading to excessive weight gain. Protective mechanisms of breast-feeding are difficult to identify because many of the same factors associated with obesity, such as race, ethnicity, maternal education, social status, and maternal obesity, are also associated with the initiation and duration of breast-feeding or the decision to formula feed. The effects of breast-feeding on the later development of obesity can be sustained and persist into adulthood either through learned behavior or perhaps through a more complex programming mechanism. Read more about childhood obesity in Chapter 7.

ALLERGIES

Most food allergies are acquired in the first year or two of life. Sensitization often occurs with the first exposure to an antigen. The prevalence of food allergy peaks at 6% to 8% at 1 year of age and then gradually decreases to 1% to 2% in later childhood. Foods that account for most allergic reactions in children are cow's milk protein, eggs, peanuts, soy, tree nuts, fish, and wheat. Symptoms manifest as urticaria, angioedema, anaphylaxis, atopic dermatitis, respiratory symptoms, or gastrointestinal disorders. Food allergies can be classified as (1) IgE mediated, with symptoms such as angioedema, urticaria, wheezing, rhinitis, vomiting, eczema, and anaphylaxis reactions; (2) mixed gastrointestinal syndromes involving both IgE-and T-cell mediated components, such as eosinophilic esophagitis; or (3) non–IgE-mediated allergies, such as protein-induced enterocolitis. Public health strategies for primary prevention of food allergies are necessary, but results of studies to determine the etiology of food allergies are conflicting. Breast-feeding is presumed to be protective, but study results vary and the size of the effect is controversial.

Early introduction of foreign proteins, including cow's milk, wheat, soy, rice, eggs, fish, and chicken, could induce a T-cell–mediated immune reaction of the intestinal mucosa associated with inflammation, villous atrophy, diarrhea, and failure to thrive (Schmitz, 2000). The earlier these foods are introduced to the infant, the greater the risk of developing enteropathy. These enteropathies are linked to the immaturity of the gut's immune system, leading to sensitization rather than to tolerance when exposed to foreign proteins. It is unknown precisely when the gut has matured sufficiently to accept foreign protein, although it is unlikely to occur in the first few months of life. Infants with dietary-induced proctocolitis, a non–IgE-mediated allergy, appear healthy but have visible specks or streaks of blood in their stool. Blood loss is minimal, and anemia is rare. This type of allergy is not usually associated with vomiting, diarrhea, or growth failure and is often caused by sensitivity to cow's milk or soy protein, often through the maternal diet while breast-feeding (Sicherer, 2003).

Atopic dermatitis is a chronic skin condition often seen in young children and is often the first sign of allergic sensitization in infants. The pathophysiology remains unclear, but it is increased in families with a history of atopic disorders, suggesting a genetic component. In infancy, atopic dermatitis is closely related to both IgE- and non–IgE-mediated food hypersensitivities that occur in formula-fed and breast-fed infants. Intact food allergens, particularly from cow's milk, eggs, and peanuts, may be secreted in small quantities by the mammary gland epithelium, causing a reaction with the mucosal immune system in the infant's intestinal lumen (Heine, Hill, & Hosking, 2004).

Use of soy or hypoallergenic infant formula as primary prevention of milk allergy is controversial, and the AAP Committee on Nutrition (2000) has established guidelines for the use of hypoallergenic infant formulas. The actual prevalence of milk protein allergy in infancy is only 2% to 3%. Because of the increased costs of using a hypoallergenic formula, their use should be limited to infants with well-defined clinical symptoms. Infants with cow's milk allergies should not be fed milk from goats, sheep, or other animals because of the likelihood of allergic reaction to other mammalian milk. Soy milk is often used as a substitute for cow's milk infant formula and may be well tolerated. Soy formula feeding is not recommended for primary prevention of allergies in high-risk infants. Infants with IgE-mediated cow's milk allergies may have better tolerance to soy than infants with non–IgE-mediated symptoms. Eight percent to 14% of infants with IgE-mediated cow's milk allergies have adverse reactions to soy, although anaphylaxis is rare. A higher prevalence of concomitant reactions (25% to 60%) is seen when soy is fed to infants with non–IgE-mediated cow's milk allergies; therefore soy is not recommended as a substitute for infants with proctocolitis and enterocolitis reactions. For these children an extensively hydrolyzed protein formula or a free amino-acid-based infant formula should be used. Benefits should be seen within 2 to 4 weeks, and the formula should be continued until the infant is at least 1 year of age.

A family history of allergy, defined as both parents or one parent and one sibling with **allergic disease**, is the strongest predictor of allergic disease in children. In high-risk infants up to 6% of exclusively breast-fed infants developed food-specific IgE allergies with symptoms occurring with the first reported direct food exposure. How-

ever, in the general population food allergy in exclusively breast-fed infants ranges from 0.04% to 0.5% (Zeiger, 2003).

Bottle feeding and early exposure to potential food allergens are risk factors for atopic disease. Studies suggest that combined maternal avoidance of food allergens while breast-feeding and infant avoidance of allergens for at least the first 6 months may reduce eczema and food allergy in early childhood (Zeiger, 2003). Data supporting a protective effect on respiratory allergy and asthma in later childhood are less compelling. Exclusive, rather than partial, breast-feeding for at least 4 months appears to have a significant impact on the occurrence of atopic dermatitis, allergic rhinitis, and respiratory symptoms (Kill, Wickman, Lilja, Nordvall, & Pershagen, 2002). High-risk infants should be breast-fed throughout the first year of life or longer or, alternately, fed with a hypoallergenic formula. Breast milk contains immunomodulating properties to regulate the immune system and also contains milk-specific IgA to bind cow's milk allergens and prevent allergies.

Food antigens have been detected in the milk of mothers after consumption of allergenic foods such as cow's milk, eggs, wheat, and peanuts, and the concentrations are sufficient to trigger reactions in allergic children (Zeiger, 2003). Concentrations of antigens in human milk depend on the amount consumed by the mother and appear in human milk 1 to 6 hours after ingestion. Peanut protein may be quickly cleared from the milk within 3 hours after ingestion. Secretion of antigens into human milk is variable. In a study by Vadas and coworkers (2001), only 48% of lactating women secreted peanut protein in their milk after ingestion of peanuts. Similarly, approximately two-thirds of women secrete cow's milk and egg protein into their milk after ingestion.

Characteristics of women who secrete food antigens into their milk have not been accounted for, making it difficult to determine preventive strategies. One study from Finland found that a maternal diet high in saturated fat and low in vitamin C while breast-feeding was associated with an increased risk of atopic sensitization in the infant (Joppu, Kalliomaki, & Isolauri, 2000). Allergic disease has also been linked to a maternal diet with a high ratio of omega-6 to omega-3 fatty acids, typical of Western diets containing processed and fried foods (Koletzko, 2000). Fish oil supplementation to provide omega-3 fatty acids during pregnancy and to infants older than 6 months has been shown to reduce the severity of atopic disease (Upham & Holt, 2005).

Gut microflora may play a role in immunomodulation in infants, reducing the risk of early atopic disease. Probiotics have successfully been used to reduce atopic eczema in high risk children by having mothers take Lactobacillus GG (GG refers to a healthy strain) 2 to 4 weeks before delivery and 6 months postnatally while breast-feeding (Kalliomaki et al., 2001).

The AAP provides guidelines for introduction of complementary foods for primary prevention of food allergy in high-risk children. They recommend avoiding cow's milk protein until 12 months, eggs until 24 months, and peanut, tree nut, and fish until 3 years. The AAP advises lactating mothers of high-risk infants to eliminate peanuts and tree nuts and to consider eliminating eggs, cow's milk, and fish while breast-feeding. Because of incomplete scientific data to support this, the European committees have decided on more general feeding recommendations, suggesting adding a limited number of foods with low allergenicity when starting solid foods, and they do not recommend modifications of the maternal diet while breast-feeding (Zeiger, 2003). There are no well-designed studies that demonstrate a clear benefit of avoiding potentially allergenic foods in the first year of life as a preventive measure against the development of atopic disease.

A study of British children recruited at birth for a population-based prospective birth cohort study to explore whether late introduction of solids is protective against the development of asthma, eczema, and atopy found, contrary to feeding guidelines, that late introduction of eggs after 8 months was associated with an increase in preschool wheezing, atopy, and eczema at age 5½ years and that the introduction of milk after 6 months was associated with an increase in eczema. The authors concluded that their study of 642 children did not support feeding recommendations to delay introduction of solid foods to protect against the development of asthma and allergy (Zutavern et al., 2004).

Allergic disease: Sensitization to allergens manifested by urticaria, angioedema, anaphylaxis, atopic dermatitis, respiratory symptoms, or gastrointestinal disorder.

The prevalence of peanut allergy is increasing and the cause is elusive as there are few known risk factors. Data from the Avon Longitudinal Study of Parents and Children were collected prospectively from early pregnancy throughout childhood to investigate possible causes of peanut allergy. Researchers found a positive association with consumption of soy infant formula (Fox et al., 2003). In the total cohort of 13,971 children, 8.3% consumed soy milk or soy formula in the first 2 years, compared with 24.5% of those with peanut allergy and 34.8% of those with a positive peanut challenge. They also found that creams containing peanut oil applied to the infant's skin to treat rashes during the first 6 months of life increased the risk of peanut allergies. No association was found with the mother's diet during pregnancy or lactation. Peanut-specific IgE was not detectable in the cord blood, indicating that sensitization had not occurred in utero, and mothers of children with peanut allergy did not eat more peanuts during breast-feeding than mothers in the control group.

There is no way to predict when a child will outgrow a food allergy, but 75% to 90% of milk-allergic children can tolerate cow's milk by 4 years of age. Some infants lose their milk allergy in as little as a few months, whereas others may remain symptomatic for as long as 8 to 10 years (Wood, 2003). Many also become tolerant to egg, soy, and wheat, although fish, tree nut, and peanut allergies may persist throughout the lifetime (Nowak-Wegrzyn, 2003). Other foods that may cause allergic reactions in infants and young children include berries, tomatoes, citrus, and apples. Children with non–IgE-mediated cow's milk allergy often outgrow their allergies by 5 years of age without the development of additional allergic complications. Children with IgE-mediated allergies often have persistent allergic symptoms at 8 years of age. They also more frequently have asthma, rhinoconjunctivitis, atopic eczema, and sensitization to other allergens and are at increased risk for sensitization to in-

halant allergens (Saarinen, Pelkonen, Makela, & Savilahti, 2005). Read more about food allergies in Chapter 7.

DIABETES AND CELIAC DISEASE

Two studies by Norris et al. (2005a, 2005b) looked at the association between the development of type 1 diabetes and celiac disease and early introduction of gluten-ontaining foods. The Diabetes Autoimmunity Study in the Young is a prospective study of triggers for diabetes and celiac disease in genetically predisposed children with a parent or sibling with type 1 diabetes or celiac disease. The timing of introduction of gluten-containing cereals was found to be associated with the risk of developing diabetes or celiac disease in children at increased risk for the disease. Children initially exposed to wheat, barley, or rye between birth and 3 months or later than 7 months were at increased risk of developing diabetes and celiac disease than children first exposed to cereal between 4 and 6 months.

In Sweden, where the prevalence of celiac disease is 1% to 2% of Swedish children, introducing gluten-containing foods at 4 to 6 months is recommended during the time of exclusive breast-feeding. Enacted in 1996, this policy was a change from previous recommendations to introduce gluten after 6 months. New evidence showed that the risk of childhood celiac disease could be reduced with concurrent breast-feeding during the time that gluten is introduced into the infant's diet. Despite public health programs to inform families of the recommendations, a survey in 2004 showed that only 45% were compliant with the recommendation to introduce gluten earlier than 6 months while breast-feeding. As many as 45% continued to avoid gluten until after 6 months and another 10% introduced gluten without breast-feeding (Odijk, Hulthen, Ahlstedt, & Borres, 2004). Read more about celiac disease and diabetes in Chapters 7 and 8, respectively.

Issues to Debate

1. Discuss the nutritional impact of pregnancy and lactation on teens.
2. Should more be done to promote breast-feeding?
3. Should there be more food labeling because of the prospect of infant food allergies?
4. What are some of the cultural aspects that affect the transitioning from an all-milk infant diet to a diet of family foods?

Normal Infant Nutrition Case Study

Caleb was born by standard vaginal delivery to a healthy 30-year-old mother. Caleb's mother decided while she was pregnant to exclusively breast-feed him for the first 6 months of life because she was familiar with the advantages associated with exclusive breast-feeding, such as reduction of illness and allergies, enhanced intelligence, convenience of feedings, and cost savings. Caleb weighed 7 pounds at birth (25% percentile) and gained weight appropriately for the first 6 months of life. At his 6-month checkup he weighed 18 pounds and was at the 50th to 75% percentile for weight.

Caleb's mother chose to introduce pureed foods she prepared herself when Caleb was 6 months old. At this time he exhibited an interest in what his parents were eating and had developed good head and neck control. She

prepared sweet potatoes, carrots, squash, and peas and pureed them in a food processor until they were a smooth consistency. She froze them in single serving portions in an ice cube tray. She introduced one food at a time and waited 3 to 5 days between foods while observing Caleb for signs of food allergy. Gradually, she added more foods to his diet, including chicken, turkey, beef, cereal, pears, peaches, and bananas. When Caleb was 7 months old he was offered a sippy cup with water at meals.

Caleb was developing fine motor control and was able to grasp foods and attempt self-feeding. His mother offered him small pieces of toast, Cheerios, cut-up fresh melon, soft-cooked carrots, French toast, and pieces of cheese and turkey. He also began to eat cottage cheese and yogurt and a greater variety of foods from the family meal. Caleb continued to breast-feed, but the number of feedings per day began to decrease as he increased his intake of complementary foods. Caleb was breast-fed without any supplemental formula until he was 13 months old, when he was offered whole cow's milk by cup. By 1 year of age he had gradually transitioned from an all-milk diet in the first 6 months to a mixed diet of breast milk and pureed foods and finally to a diet of family foods including a variety of fruits and vegetables, grains, meats, and dairy.

What did Caleb's mother do correctly?

References

Pregnancy and Lactation

American Dietetic Association. (2005). Position of the American Dietetic Association:

Promoting and supporting breastfeeding. *Journal of the American Dietetic Association, 105*, 810–818.

Barker, D. J. (1991). The foetal and infant origins of inequalities in health in Britain. *Journal of Public Health Medicine, 13*, 64–68.

Brost, B. C., Goldenberg, R. L., Mercer, B. M., Iams, J. D., Meis, P. J., Moawad, A. H., et al. (1997). The Preterm Prediction Study: Association of cesarean delivery with increases in maternal weight and body mass index. *American Journal of Obstetrics and Gynecology, 179*, 333.

Fairweather-Tait, S. J. (1995). Iron–zinc and calcium–iron interactions in relation to zinc and iron absorption. *Proceedings of the Nutrition Society, 54*, 465.

Institute of Medicine (IOM), National Academies of Science. (1990). *Nutrition During Pregnancy.* Washington, DC: National Academy Press.

Institute of Medicine (IOM), Food and Nutrition Board. (2002). *Dietary Reference Intakes for Energy and the Macronutrients, Carbohydrate, Fiber, Fat, and Fatty Acids.* Washington, DC: National Academy Press.

Rasmussen, K. M. (2000). The "fetal origins" hypothesis: Challenges and opportunities for maternal and child nutrition. *Annual Review of Nutrition, 21*, 73–95.

U.S. Department of Agriculture and U.S. Department of Health and Human Services. (2005). *Nutrition and Your Health: Dietary Guidelines for Americans* (6th ed.). Washington DC: U.S. Government Printing Office.

Villar, J., Merialdi, M., Gulmezoglu, A. M., Abalos, E., Carroli, G., Kulier, R., et al. (2003). Characteristics of randomized controlled trials included in systematic review of nutritional interventions reporting maternal morbidity, mortality, preterm delivery, intrauterine growth restriction and small for gestational age and birth weight outcomes. *Journal of Nutrition, 133*, 1632S–1639S.

Infant Nutrition

Altucher, K., Rasmussen, K., Barden, E., & Habicht, J. (2005). Predictors of improvement in hemoglobin concentration among toddlers enrolled in the Massachusetts WIC program. *Journal of the American Dietetic Association, 105*, 709–715.

American Academy of Pediatrics (AAP). (2004). *Pediatric Nutrition Handbook* (5th ed.). Elk Grove Village, IL: American Academy of Pediatrics.

American Academy of Pediatrics (AAP), Committee on Nutrition. (2000). Hypoallergenic infant formulas. *Pediatrics, 106*, 346–349.

American Academy of Pediatrics (AAP), Committee on Nutrition. (2003). Prevention of pediatric overweight and obesity. *Pediatrics, 112*, 424–430.

American Academy of Pediatrics (AAP), Section on Breastfeeding. (2005). Breastfeeding and the use of human milk. *Pediatrics, 115*, 496–506.

American Dietetic Association. (2003). Position of the American Dietetic Association and Dietitians of Canada: Vegetarian diets. *Journal of the American Dietetic Association, 103*, 748–765.

Auestad, N., Halter, R., Hall, R., Blatter, M., Bogle, M., Burks, W., et al. (2001). Growth and development in term infants fed long-chain polyunsaturated fatty acids: A double-masked, randomized, parallel, prospective, multivariate study. *Pediatrics, 108*, 372–381.

Baker, R. D. (2002). Infant formula safety. *Pediatrics, 110*, 833–835.

Bergmann, K. E., Bergmann, R. L., Kries, R. von, Böhm, O., Richter, R., Dudenhausen, J. W., et al. (2003). Early determinants of childhood overweight and adiposity in a birth cohort study: Role of breast-feeding. *International Journal of Obesity, 27*, 162–172.

Birch, L., Orlet Fisher, J., & Krahnstoever Davison, K. (2003). Learning to overeat: Maternal use of restrictive feeding practices promotes girls' eating in the absence of hunger. *American Journal of Clinical Nutrition, 78*, 215–220.

Bogen, D. L., Hanusa, B. H., & Whitaker, R. C. (2004). The effect of breast-feeding with and without formula use on the risk of obesity at 4 years of age. *Obesity Research, 12*, 1527–1535.

Briefel, R., Reidy, K., Karwe, V., & Devaney, B. (2004a). Feeding Infants and Toddlers Study: Improvements needed in meeting infant feeding recommendations. *Journal of the American Dietetic Association, 104*, S31–S37.

Briefel, R., Reidy, K., Karwe, V., Jankowski, L., & Hendricks, K. (2004b). Toddlers' transition to table foods: Impact on nutrient intakes and food patterns. *Journal of the American Dietetic Association, 104*, S38–S44.

Butte, N., Cobb, K., Dwyer, J., Graney, L., Heird, W., & Rickard, K. (2004). The Start Healthy Feeding Guidelines for infants and toddlers. *Journal of the American Dietetic Association, 104*, 442–454.

Butte, N., Wong, W., Hopkinson, J., Heinz, C., Mehta, N., & Smith, E. O. (2000a). Energy requirements derived from total energy expenditure and energy deposition during the first 2 y of life. *American Journal of Clinical Nutrition, 72*, 1558–1569.

Butte, N., Wong, W., Hopkinson, J., Smith, E. O., & Ellis, K. (2000b). Infant feeding mode affects early growth and body composition. *Pediatrics, 106*, 1355–1366.

Canadian Paediatric Society. (2003). Dietary manipulations for infantile colic. *Paediatrics & Child Health, 8*, 449–452.

Carruth, B. R., Skinner, J., Houck, K., & Moran, J. D. (2000). Addition of supplementary foods and infant growth. *Journal of the American College of Nutrition, 19*, 405–412.

Carruth, B. R., Ziegler, P., Gordon, A., & Hendricks, K. (2004). Developmental milestones and self-feeding behaviors in infants and toddlers. *Journal of the American Dietetic Association, 104*, S51–S56.

Centers for Disease Control Enterobacter sakazakii infections associated with the use of powdered infant formula—Tennesse, 2001. *Morbidity and Mortality Weekly Report*, 51, 297–300.

Clifford, T., Campbell, K., Speechley, K., & Gorodzinsky, F. (2002). Infant colic: Empirical evidence of the absence of an association with source of early infant nutrition. *Archives of Pediatric and Adolescent Medicine, 156*, 1123–1128.

Dawodu, A., Adarwal, M., Hossain, M., Kochiyil, J., & Zayed, R. (2003). Hypovitaminosis D and vitamin D deficiency in exclusively breastfeeding infants and their mothers in summer: A justification for vitamin D supplementation of breastfeeding infants. *Journal of Pediatrics, 142*, 169–173.

de Onis, G., Garza, C., Onyango, A. W., & Borghi, E. (2007). Comparison of the WHO Child Growth Standards and the CDC 2000 Growth Charts. *Journal of Nutrition, 137*, 144–148.

Devaney, B., Kalb, L., Briefel, R., Zavitsky-Novak, T., Clusen, N., & Ziegler, P. (2004a). Feeding Infants and Toddlers Study: Overview of the study design. *Journal of the American Dietetic Association, 104*, S8–S13.

Devaney, B., Ziegler, P., Pac, S., Karwe, V., & Barr, S. (2004b). Nutrient intakes of infants and toddlers. *Journal of the American Dietetic Association, 104*, S14–S21.

Dewey, K. G. (2000a). Protein and amino acids. *Pediatrics, 106*, 1292.

Dewey, K. G. (2000b). Complementary feeding and breastfeeding. *Pediatrics,* 106, 1301–1302.

Dewey, K. G. (2001). Nutrition, growth, and complementary feeding of the breastfed infant. *Pediatric Clinics of North America, 48*, 87–104.

Dewey, K. G., Beaton, G., Fjeld, C., Lonnerdal, B., & Reeds, P. (1996a). Protein requirements of infants and children. *European Journal of Clinical Nutrition, 50*, S119–S150.

Dewey, K. G., Cohen, R. J., Rivera, L. L., Canahuati, J., & Brown, K. H. (1996b). Do exclusively breast-fed infants require extra protein? *Pediatric Research, 39*, 303–307.

Dewey, K. G., Domellof, M., Cohen, R., Rivera, L. L., Hernell, O., & Lonnerdal, B. (2002). Iron supplementation affects growth and morbidity of breast-fed infants: Results of a randomized trial in Sweden and Honduras. *Journal of Nutrition, 132*, 3249–3255.

Dewey, K. G., Peerson, J. M., & Brown, K. H. (1998). Effects of age of introduction of complementary foods on iron status of breastfed infants in Honduras. *American Journal of Clinical Nutrition, 67*, 878–884.

Dietz, W. H. (2001). Breastfeeding may help prevent childhood overweight. *Journal of the American Medical Association, 285*, 2506–2507.

Domellof, M., Lonnerdal, B., Abrams, S., & Hernall, O. (2002). Iron absorption in breast-fed infants: Effects of age, iron status, iron supplements, and complementary foods. *American Journal of Clinical Nutrition, 76*, 198–204.

DuPont, C. (2003). Protein requirements during the first year of life. *American Journal of Clinical Nutrition, 77*(Suppl.), 1544S–1549S.

Dwyer, J., Suitor, C., & Hendricks, K. (2004). FITS: New insights and lessons learned. *Journal of the American Dietetic Association, 104*, S5–S7.

Eichenberger Gilmore, J., Hong, L., Broffitt, B., & Levy, S. (2005). Longitudinal patterns of vitamin and mineral supplement use in young white children. *Journal of the American Dietetic Association, 105*, 763–772.

Engelmann, M. D. M., Sandstrom, B., & Michaelsen, K. (1996). Meat intake and iron status in late infancy: An intervention study. *Journal of Pediatric Gastroenterology and Nutrition, 26*, 26–33.

Ermis, B., Demirel, F., Demircan, N., & Gurel, A. (2002). Effects of three different iron supplementations in term healthy infants after 5 months of life. *Journal of Tropical Pediatrics, 48*, 280–284.

European Food Safety Authority. (2004). EFSA Panel advises on how to avoid microbiological risks in infant formulae—at home and in hospital. Retrieved January 8, 2005, from http://www.efsa.eu.int/press_room/press_release/696/pr_biohaz03_microrisk_en1pdf

FDA Talk Paper. (2002). FDA warns about possible *Enterobacter sakazakii* infections in hospitalized newborns fed powdered infant formulas. Retrieved January 7, 2005, from http://www.cfsan.fda.gov/~lrd/tpinf.html

Fomon, S. (2001). Feeding normal infants: Rationale for recommendations. *Journal of the American Dietetic Association, 101*, 1002–1005.

Fox, M. K., Devaney, B., Reidy, K., Razafindrakoto, C., & Ziegler, P. (2006a). Relationship between portion size and energy intake among infants and toddlers: Evidence of self-regulation. *Journal of the American Dietetic Association, 106*, S77–S83.

Fox, M. K., Pac, S., Devaney, B., & Jankowski, L. (2004). Feeding infants and toddlers study: What foods are infants and toddlers eating? *Journal of the American Dietetic Association, 104*, S22–S30.

Fox, M. K., Reidy, K., Karwe, V., & Ziegler, P. (2006b). Average portions of foods commonly eaten by infants and toddlers in the United States. *Journal of the American Dietetic Association, 106*, S66–S76.

Fox, M. K., Reidy, K., Novak, T., & Ziegler, P. (2006c). Sources of energy and nutrients in the diets of infants and toddlers. *Journal of the American Dietetic Association, 106*, S28–S42.

Gartner, L., Greer, F., and the Section on Breastfeeding and Committee on Nutrition. (2003). Prevention of rickets and vitamin D deficiency: New guidelines for vitamin D intake. *Pediatrics, 111*, 908–910.

Gibson, R., & Holtz, C. (2000). The adequacy of micronutrients in complementary foods. *Pediatrics, 106*, 1298–1300.

Gillman, M. W., Rifas-Shiman, S. L., Camargo, C. A., Berkey, C. S., Frazier, A. L., Rockett, H. R. H., et al. (2001). Risk of overweight among adolescents who were breastfed as infants. *Journal of the American Medical Association, 285*, 2461–2467.

Greer, F., Shannon, M., the Committee of Nutrition, & the Committee on Environmental Health. (2005). Infant methemoglobinemia: The role of dietary nitrate in food and water. *Pediatrics, 116*, 784–786.

Heath, A. M., Tuttle, C. R., Simons, M. S. L., Cleghorn, C., & Parnell, W. (2002). Longitudinal study of diet and iron deficiency anaemia in infants during the first two years of life. *Asia Pacific Journal of Clinical Nutrition, 11*, 251–257.

Hediger, M., Overpeck, M., Kuczmarski, R., & Ruan, W. J. (2001). Association between infant breastfeeding and overweight in young children. *Journal of the American Medical Association, 285*, 2453–2460.

Heine, R., Hill, D., & Hosking, C. (2004). Primary prevention of atopic dermatitis in breastfed infants: What is the evidence? *Journal of Pediatrics, 44*, 564–567.

Henderson, A. (2005). Vitamin D and the breastfed infant. Journal of Obstetric, Gynecologic, and Neonatal Nursing. *34*, 367–372.

Hill, D., Roy, N., Heine, R., Hosking, C., Francis, D., Brown, J., et al. (2005). Effect of a low-allergen maternal diet on colic among breastfed infants: A randomized, controlled trial. *Pediatrics, 116*, e709–e715.

Institute of Medicine (IOM). (2001). *Dietary Reference Intake for Vitamin A, Vitamin K, Arsenic, Boron, Chromium, Copper, Iodine, Iron, Manganese, Molybdenum, Nickel, Silicon, Vanadium, and Zinc.* Washington, DC: National Academy Press.

Institute of Medicine (IOM). (2002). *Dietary Reference Intake for Energy, Carbohydrate, Fiber, Fat, Fatty Acids, Cholesterol, Protein, and Amino Acids. Part I.* Prepublication copy. Washington, DC: National Academy Press.

Institute of Medicine (IOM). (2005). Report brief. WIC Food Packages: Time for a Change. Retrieved October 4, 2007, from www.iom.edu/report.asp?id=26667

Jensen, C., Voigt, R., Prager, T., Zou, Y., Fraley, J. K., Rozelle, J., et al. (2005). Effects of maternal docosahexaenoic acid intake on visual function and neurodevelopment in breastfed term infants. *American Journal of Clinical Nutrition, 8*, 125–132.

Joppu, U., Kalliomaki, M., & Isolauri, E. (2000). Maternal diet rich in saturated fat during breastfeeding is associated with atopic sensitization of the infant. *European Journal of Clinical Nutrition, 54*, 702–705.

Kalliomaki, M., Salminen, S., Arvilommi, H., Kero, P., Koskinene, P., & Isolauri, E. (2001). Probiotics in primary prevention of atopic disease; a randomised placebo-controlled trial. *Lancet, 357*, 1076–1079.

Kattelmann, K. K., Ho, M., & Specker, B. L. (2001). Effect of timing of introduction of complementary foods on iron and zinc status of formula fed infants at 12, 24, and 36 months of age. *Journal of the American Dietetic Association, 101*, 443–447.

Kazal, L. (2002). Prevention of iron deficiency in infants and toddlers. *American Family Physician, 66*, 1217–1224.

Khedr, E. M., Farghaly, W. M., Amry Sel, D., & Osman, A. A. (2004). Neural maturation of breastfed and formula-fed infants. *Acta Paediatrics*, 93, 734–738.

Kill, I., Wickman, M., Lilja, G., Nordvall, S. L., & Pershagen, G. (2002). Breast feeding and allergic diseases in infants—a prospective birth cohort study. *Archives of Diseases in Children, 87*, 478–481.

Kleinman, R. (2000a). American Academy of Pediatrics recommendations for complementary feeding. *Pediatrics, 106*, 1274.

Kleinman, R. (2000b). Complementary feeding and later health. *Pediatrics, 106*, 1287–1288.

Kleinman, R. (2000c). Complementary feeding and neuromuscular development. *Pediatrics, 106*, 1279.

Koletzko, B. (2000). Complementary foods and the development of food allergy. *Pediatrics, 106*, 1285.

Koo, W. (2003). Efficacy and safety of docosahexaenoic acid and arachidonic acid addition to infant formulas: Can one buy better vision and intelligence? *Journal of the American College of Nutrition, 22*, 101–107.

Kramer, M., Guo, T., Platt, R., Shapiro, S., Collet, J. P., Chlamers, B., et al. (2002). Breastfeeding and infant growth: Biology or bias? *Pediatrics, 110*, 343–347.

Krebs, N. (2000). Dietary zinc and iron sources, physical growth and cognitive development of breastfed infants. *Journal of Nutrition, 130*, 358S–360S.

Krebs, N. F., Reidinger, C. J., Robertson, A. D., & Hambridge, K. M. (1994). Growth and intakes of energy and zinc in infants fed human milk. *Journal of Pediatrics, 124*, 32–39.

Kreiter, S., Schwartz, R., Kirkman, H., Charlton, P., Calikoglu, A., & Davenport, M. (2000). Nutritional rickets in African-American breast-fed infants. *Journal of Pediatric, 137*, 153–157.

Kries, R. von, Koletzko, B., Sauerwald, T., Mutius, E. von, Barnert, K., Grunert, V., et al. (1999). Breast feeding and obesity: Cross sectional study. *British Medical Journal, 319*, 147–150.

Lack, G., Fox, D., Northstone, K., & Golding, J. (2003). Factors associated with the development of peanut allergy in childhood. *New England Journal of Medicine, 348*, 977–985.

Lawrence, R. (1999). *Breastfeeding: A Guide for the Medical Profession* (5th ed.). St. Louis: Mosby.

Lucas, A., & St. James-Robert, I. (1998). Crying, fussing and colic behavior in breast and bottle-fed infants. *Early Human Development, 53*, 9–18.

Lust, K., Brown, J., & Thomas, W. (1996). Maternal intake of cruciferous vegetables and other foods and colic symptoms in exclusively breastfed infants. *Journal of the American Dietetic Association, 96*, 47–48.

Martorell, R., Stein, A. D., & Schroeder, D. G. (2001). Early nutrition and later adiposity. *Journal of Nutrition, 131*, 874S–880S.

Meeks Gardner, J. M., Powell, C. A., Baker-Henningham, H., Walker, S. P., Cole, T. J., & Grantham-McGregor, S. M.

(2005). Zinc supplementation and psychosocial stimulation: Effects on the development of undernourished Jamaican children. *American Journal of Clinical Nutrition, 2005, 82,* 399–405.

Michaelsen, K. F. (2000). Cow's milk in complementary feeding. *Pediatrics, 106,* 1302–1303.

Milner, J., Stein, D., McCarter, R., & Moon, R. (2004). Early infant multivitamin supplementation is associated with increased risk for food allergy and asthma. *Pediatrics, 114,* 27–32.

Morale, S., Hoffman, D., Castañeda, Y., Wheaton, D., Burns, R., & Birch, E. (2005). Duration of long-chain polyunsaturated fatty acids availability in the diet and visual acuity. *Early Human Development, 81,* 197–203.

Motarjemi, Y. (2000). Research priorities on safety of complementary feeding. *Pediatrics, 106,* 1304–1305.

Muraro, A., Dreborg, S., Halken, S., Høst, A., Niggemann, B., Aalberse, R., et al. (2004). Dietary prevention of allergic diseases in infants and small children. Part III. Critical review of published peer-reviewed observational and interventional studies and final recommendations. Pediatric Allergy and Immunology, 15, 291–307.

National Center for Health Statistics. (2000). Vital and health statistics of the Centers for Disease Control and Prevention. *Advance Data, 314.*

National WIC Association Position Paper. (2004). *Breastfeeding Promotion and Support in the WIC Program.* Washington, DC: Author.

Norris, J., Barriga, K., Hoffenber, E., Taki, I., Miao, D., Haas, J., et al. (2005a). Risk of celiac disease autoimmunity and timing of gluten introduction in the diet of infants at increased risk of disease. *Journal of the American Medical Association, 293,* 2343–2351.

Norris, J., Barriga, K., Klingensmith, G., Hoffman, M., Eisenbarth, G., Erlich, H., et al. (2005b). Timing of initial cereal exposure in infancy and risk of islet autoimmunity. *Journal of the American Medical Association, 290,* 1713–1720.

Nowak-Wegrzyn, A. (2003). Future approaches to food allergy. *Pediatrics,* 111, 1672–1680.

Odijk, J. van, Hulthen, L., Ahlstedt, S., & Borres, M. P. (2004). Introduction of food during the infant's first year: A study with emphasis on introduction of gluten and of egg, fish, and peanut in allergy-risk families. *Acta Paediatrics, 93,* 464–470.

Orlet Fisher, J., Birch, L., Smiciklas-Wright, H., & Picciano, M. F. (2000). Breast-feeding through the first year predicts maternal control in feeding and subsequent toddler energy intakes. *Journal of the American Dietetic Association, 100,* 641–646.

Owen, C. G., Martin, R. M., Whincup, P. H., Davey Smith, G., & Cook, D. G. (2005). Effect of infant feeding on the risk of obesity across the life course: A quantitative review of the published evidence. *Pediatrics, 115,* 1367–1377.

Pelto, G. (2000). Improving complementary feeding practices and responsive parenting as a primary component of interventions to prevent malnutrition in infancy and early childhood. *Pediatrics, 106,* 1300–1301.

Ponza, M., Devaney, B., Ziegler, P., Reidy, K., & Squatrito, C. (2004). Nutrient intakes and food choices of infants and toddlers participating in WIC. *Journal of the American Dietetic Association, 104,* S71–S79.

Rajakumar, K., & Thomas, S. (2005). Reemerging nutritional rickets: A historical perspective. *Archives of Pediatric and Adolescent Medicine, 159,* 335–341.

Rossander-Hulten, L., Brune, M., Sandstrom, B., Lonnerdal, B., & Hallberg, L. (1991). Comparative inhibition of iron absorption by manganese and zinc in humans. *American Journal of Clinical Nutrition, 54,* 152–156.

Ryan, A. S., Wenjun, Z., & Acosta, A. (2002). Breastfeeding continues to increase into the new millennium. *Pediatrics, 110,* 1103–1109.

Saarinen, K. M., Pelkonen, A. S., Makela, M. G., & Savilahti, E. (2005). Clinical course and prognosis of cow's milk allergy are dependent on milk-specific IgE status. *Journal of Allergy and Clinical Immunology, 116,* 869–875.

Sakashita, R., Inoue, N., & Kamegai, T. (2004). From milk to solids: A reference standard for the transitional eating process in infants and preschool children in Japan. *European Journal of Clinical Nutrition, 58,* 643–653.

Sakashita, R., Inoue, N., & Tatsuki, T. (2003). Selection of reference foods for a scale of standards for use in assessing the transitional process from milk to solid foods in infants and pre-school children. *European Journal of Clinical Nutrition, 57,* 803–809.

Savino, F., Costamagna, M., Prino, A., Oggero, R., & Silvestro, L. (2002). Leptin levels in breast-fed and formula-fed infants. *Acta Paediatrics, 91,* 897–902.

Schach, B., & Haight, M. (2002). Colic and food allergy in the breastfed infant: Is it possible for an exclusively breastfed infant to suffer from food allergy? *Journal of Human Lactation, 18,* 50–52.

Schmitz, J. (2000). Complementary feeding and enteropathies. *Pediatrics, 106,* 1286.

Sicherer, S. (2003). Clinical aspects of gastrointestinal food allergy in childhood. *Pediatrics, 111,* 1609–1616.

Skinner, J., Ziegler, P., Pac, S., & Devaney, B. (2004a). Meal and snack patterns of infants and toddlers. *Journal of the American Dietetic Association, 104,* S65–S70.

Skinner, J., Ziegler, P., & Ponza, M. (2004b). Transitions in infants' and toddlers' beverage patterns. *Journal of the American Dietetic Association, 104,* S45–S50.

Slaughter, C., & Bryant, A. H. (2004). Hungry for love: The feeding relationship in the psychological development of young children. *Permanente Journal, 8,* 23–29.

Stang, J. (2006). Improving the eating patterns of infants and toddlers. *Journal of the American Dietetic Association, 106,* S7–S9.

Stettler, N., Stallings, V. A., Troxel, A., Zhou, J., Schinnar, R., Nelson, S. E., et al. (2005). Weight gain in the first week of life and overweight in adulthood. *Circulation, 111,* 1897–1903.

Stettler, N., Zemel, B. S., Kumanyika, S., & Stallings, V. A. (2002). Infant weight gain and childhood overweight status in a multicenter, cohort study. *Pediatrics, 109*, 194–199.

Taveras, E., Scanlon, K., Birch, L., Rifas-Shiman, S., Rich-Edwards, J., & Gillman, M. (2004). Association of breastfeeding with maternal control of infant feeding at age 1 year. *Pediatrics, 114*, e577–e583.

Upham, J., & Holt, P. (2005). Environment and development of atopy. *Current Opinion in Allergy and Clinical Immunology, 5*, 167–172.

Vadas, P., Wai, Y., Burks, W., & Perelman, B. (2001). Detection of peanut allergens in breast milk of lactating women. *Journal of the American Medical Association, 285*, 1746–1748.

Villalpando, S. (2000). Feeding mode, infections, and anthropometric status in early childhood. *Pediatrics, 106*, 1282–1283.

Wagner, C. L., Hulsey, T. C., Fanning, D., Ebeling, M., & Hollis, B. W. (2006). High-dose vitamin D3 supplementation in a cohort of breastfeeding mothers and their infants; a 6-month follow-up pilot study. *Breastfeeding Medicine, 1*, 59–70.

Weaver, L. (2000). Gastrointestinal digestive and absorptive function. *Pediatrics, 106*, 1280–1281.

Weisberg, P., Scablon, K., Li, R., & Cogswell, M. (2004). Nutritional rickets among children in the United States: Review of cases reported between 1986 and 2003. *American Journal of Clinical Nutrition, 80*(Suppl.), 1697S–16705S.

Wharton, B. (2000). Patterns of complementary feeding (weaning) in countries of the European Union: Topics for research. *Pediatrics, 106*, 1273–1274.

WHO Working Group on the Growth Reference Protocol and the WHO Task Force on Methods for the Natural Regulation of Fertility. (2002). Growth of healthy infants and the timing, type and frequency of complementary foods. *American Journal of Clinical Nutrition, 76*, 620–627.

World Health Organization (WHO). (2003). *Global Strategy for Infant and Young Child Feeding* [pamphlet]. Geneva: Author.

Wood, R. A. (2003). The natural history of food allergy. *Pediatrics, 111*, 1631–1637.

Zeiger, R. (2003). Food allergen avoidance in the prevention of food allergy in infants and children. *Pediatrics, 11*, 1662–1671.

Zutavern, A., Mutius, E. von, Harris, J., Mills, P., Moffatt, S., White, C., et al. (2004). The introduction of solids in relation to asthma and eczema. *Archives of Diseases in Children, 89*, 303–308.

Special Section: Social and Cultural Aspects of Breast-Feeding

Yeemay Su Miller, M.S., R.D. and Virginia L. Marchant

> *"It's like making a choice between a car that runs perfectly and is free, or a lower quality car that's expensive . . . seems like a no-brainer to me."*

Statement from a man regarding the decision to breast-feed or formula feed a baby

---

A Brief History of Breast-Feeding

Deciding whether or not to breast-feed and for how long is not as simple as deciding what car to buy. Many complex social and cultural factors play interrelated roles in a woman's decision to breast-feed. Until the mid-18th century, aristocrat families, and later the urban middle class, employed wet nurses to feed their infants as the social norm until the age of weaning, usually at 2 years of age. The ability to hire a wet nurse was regarded as a status symbol, and the mothers who hired wet nurses could then carry out upper class social obligations and civic duties. One could draw parallels between these women and today's mothers who choose to bottle feed, free from being the only one who can perform the frequent and sometimes taxing task of feeding their infants. In an ironic twist of modern times, breast-feeding rates are higher among more educated and higher-income older mothers, whereas less educated lower-income mothers are more likely to bottle feed their infants (CDC, 2004).

Current Trends Affecting Breast-Feeding

Throughout history men have dictated the significance of the female breast, from sacred and life giving to a sensual erotic object. Not until the later half of the 20th century did women begin to repossess their breasts, with increasing numbers of women seeking breast augmentation surgeries, which place second only to liposuction for the most common cosmetic surgery. Sociologist Barbara Behrmann notes in her book, *The Breast-Feeding Café* (2005), "Women in the U.S. nurse [their babies] in a culture in which our breasts are used to sell everything from cars to beer; in which deep cleavage dominates the checkout aisle...and in which the number of women who artificially enhance their breasts has increased 533% from 1992 to 2002."

Surveys conducted by the American Society of Plastic Surgeons in 2001 reveal that 206,354 women underwent breast augmentation (i.e., breast implants) in the United States. The actual risk of impeding future breast-feeding varies, depending on the type of procedure, the skill and techniques of the surgeon, and physiology of the individual woman's breasts. Some women who receive breast implants may have the ability to do some breast-feeding as long as the surgery is done skillfully with proper technique (Hefter, Lindholm, & Elvenes, 2003).

Reduction mammoplasty (breast reduction surgery) procedures have tripled from 47,874 performed in 1997 to 126,614 in 2002 (Plastic Surgery Information Service, n.d.). Unfortunately, women who undergo this particular surgery are likely unable to breast-feed exclusively or successfully for very long (Souto, Giugliani, Giugliani, & Schneider, 2003). The research of Souto et al. with a cohort of Brazilian women who had undergone reduction mammoplasty revealed that most of them expressed a strong wish and intention to breast-feed and were told over-optimistically by their surgeons that lactation would be preserved. However, the women who had undergone reduction mammoplasty were not as successful with any or exclusive breast-feeding when compared with control subjects. These women expressed that they would have undergone the surgery even if told lactation may not be preserved (Souto et al., 2003).

Who Breast-Feeds?

Thirty percent of all women who give birth in the United States choose not to breast-feed at all, according to the most recent CDC National Immunization Survey. Although slightly more than 70% of women do initiate breast-feeding at birth or soon thereafter, significantly fewer woman continue to breast-feed their infants to 6 months, with 14% exclusively breast-feeding and 36% partially breast-feeding. Only 18% of women breast-feed their infants to 1 year of age, the duration recommended by the AAP (CDC, 2004). These rates fall short of the U.S. Department of Health and Human Services' *Healthy People 2010* public health initiative, which sets a national goal of 75% of all women breast-feeding their infants starting at birth or in the early postpartum period, 50% continuing to breast-feed at 6 months, and 25% at 1 year (U.S. Department of Health and Human Services and CDC, n.d.).

Women who choose to initiate breast-feeding at the highest rates tend to be white, over 25 years of age, college educated, and of middle to high socio-economic status (CDC, 2004). Although the breast-feeding rates for Hispanic or Latino women in the United States closely match or even exceed those of their white peers, the greatest disparity from the national overall rate occurs among African-American women, 50% of whom breast-feed at birth, with only 23% continuing to breast-feed to 6 months, and less than 10% to 1 year (CDC, 2004). Worldwide, the WHO (2005) estimates that only 35% of infants are breast-fed to 4 months of age.

A report by the CDC showed that children were more likely to have ever been breast-fed if they were ineligible for or did not receive WIC assistance (CDC Report, 2004). Another study showed that women who participated in the WIC program were significantly less likely to breast-feed to 6 months of age and that this factor was stronger than other demographic characteristics (Ryan & Zhou, 2006). Research also showed that overweight and obese mothers are less likely to breast-feed and for shorter duration than mothers of normal weight and body mass index (Kugyelka, Rasmussen, & Frongillo, 2004; Rasmussen & Kjolhede, 2004; Lovelady, 2005).

Breast-feeding rates also vary widely by region and state, with the lowest initiation rates (ranging from less than 55% to 64%) in the southern and midwestern states and the highest (75% or greater) in 14 western states, including Alaska, Idaho, Oregon, Washington, Utah, and California. At 6 months of life the percentage of breast-fed infants drops to below 30% in the south and below 40% in most other states, with a handful of western states maintaining 50% or better. The percentage of infants still breast-fed at 1 year dips below 20% in most states and into the single digits in at least five southern states, most notably Alabama, Mississippi, and Louisiana (CDC, 2004).

Barriers to Breast-Feeding

It is important to educate new mothers, their partners, family members, and healthcare professionals. The HHS Blueprint for Action on Breastfeeding (U.S. Department of Health and Human Services, 2000) lists the importance of educating the father or mother's partner, other family members, and healthcare pro-

viders, who all can greatly influence a woman's decision to breast-feed (Freed, Fraley, & Schanler, 1992; Ekulona, 1996). Within the U.S. medical system all healthcare providers, including obstetricians, pediatricians, and nurses, need more education on the physiology of lactation and the mechanics of breast-feeding to best support their breast-feeding patients. Yet the breadth of knowledge on these topics taught by most medical schools is likely limited. Providers inadvertently sabotage a mother's efforts to exclusively breast-feed by recommending supplementation with formula when he or she fail to recognize that breast-fed infants gain weight differently from formula-fed peers or recommend complete weaning when a mother reports a lactation problem rather than a referring her to a qualified lactation consultant. National surveys reveal that health care professionals who are educated on how best to support lactation in their patients play an important role in influencing the mother's decision to breast-feed and for longer duration (Lu, Lange, Slusser, Hamilton, & Halfon, 2001).

When the method a mother chooses to feed her baby can be viewed as a life-style decision, it can be determined by the mother's and other family members' attitudes and beliefs about breast-feeding as well as healthcare professionals' views, employment, stress levels, and amount of social support (Donath, Amir, & ALSPAC Study Team, 2003). A mother's perception of the father's attitude or preferences on how the baby should be fed is one top determinant of the mother's decision to initiate bottle feeding over breast-feeding (Freed et al., 1992; Arora, McJunkin, Wehrer, & Kuhn, 2000). Studies have also reported that the maternal grandmother's attitude also influences the type of feeding method by the mother and positively correlates with longer duration of breast-feeding if she supports her daughter's decision to breast-feed (Donath et al., 2003; Swanson & Power, 2005). The perceived influence of other people's views (subjective norms), including the views of the women's partners, other family members, and healthcare providers, is an important predictor of infant feeding behavior (Swanson & Power, 2005). Therefore promoting breast-feeding as a positive norm and as the ideal method to feed an infant within a mother's broad social context increases initiation and continuation of breast-feeding.

Routine Maternity Care Practices

Research has identified specific hospital nursery and maternity ward practices that interfere with breast-feeding, especially in the critical first week. Separating the mother and newborn without medical necessity can prevent the establishment of breast-feeding during the first hour of life when newborns are most alert. Introducing pacifiers and bottles to newborns too early often causes "nipple confusion," because the method of sucking artificial replacements is completely different from the type of suck needed to extract milk from a breast. As a result, an infant may suck improperly or inadequately at the breast.

Supplementation with formula or "sugar water" and pacifier use can also depress the infant's instinct to breast-feed frequently, which helps establish the mother's milk supply. The most recent research correlates early pacifier use with a significant decline in exclusive breast-feeding. In addition, "across all types of breastfeeding (exclusive, full, and overall), the most significant predictor of duration was the receipt of supplemental feedings while in the hospital" (Howard et al., 2003).

The WHO outlines a number of maternity care practices for the birthplace, whether it is hospital, clinic, or birth center, that facilitate and support breast-feeding; if these practices are fully implemented, the hospital earns the designation of "baby-friendly." Currently, fewer than 50 hospitals and maternity care facilities in the United States have earned the "baby-friendly" designation (Shealy, Li, Benton-Davis, & Grummer-Strawn, 2005). A recently published study of baby-friendly hospitals and birth centers in the United States showed that women who gave birth in a baby-friendly setting initiated breast-feeding and exclusively breast-fed their infants in the early postpartum period at significantly higher rates than state, regional, and national rates, and these rates were consistently elevated in a variety of settings (Merewood, Mehta, Chamberlain, Philipp, & Bauchner, 2005).

In addition to the UNICEF and WHO Baby Friendly Hospital Initiative, the U.S. Department of Health and Human Services and the CDC advocate that every facility providing maternity services and care for newborn infants should

- Have a written breast-feeding policy that is routinely communicated to all healthcare staff
- Train all healthcare staff in skills necessary to implement this policy
- Inform all pregnant women about the benefits and management of breast-feeding
- Help mothers initiate breast-feeding within a half-hour of birth

- Show mothers how to breast-feed and how to maintain lactation even if they should be separated from their infants
- Give newborn infants no food or drink other than breast milk, unless *medically* indicated and under no circumstances provide breast milk substitutes, feeding bottles, or pacifiers free of charge or at low cost
- Practice rooming-in (allow mothers and infants to remain together) 24 hours a day
- Encourage breast-feeding on demand
- Give no artificial teats or pacifiers to breast-feeding infants
- Foster the establishment of breast-feeding support groups and refer mothers to them on discharge from the hospital or clinic

Physiologic and Psychological Factors

One of the most common reasons reported by women who introduce formula to their babies and thereby begin to decrease breast-feeding is "lack of confidence in the sufficiency of their breast milk" (Donath et al., 2003; Swanson & Power, 2005), which is a self-efficacy issue. Confidence in one's body to nourish an infant adequately from the breast is not necessarily a physiologic issue of adequate production or supply of milk. Unlike bottle feeding, in which one can actually see how many ounces an infant is drinking, other measures, such as the number of wet diapers per day and proper weight gain over time, determine the adequacy of a breast-fed infant's intake. Increasing a mother's self-efficacy and confidence with breast-feeding appears to be important in helping women breast-feed successfully and for longer duration (Mitra, Khoury, Hinton, & Carothers, 2004; Kools, Thijs, & de Vries, 2005; Noel-Weiss, Bassett, & Cragg, 2006). Therefore helping women combat their lack of self-confidence, providing reassurance, and reinforcing that the more she breast-feeds the more milk she will produce assist mothers in their breast-feeding goals.

Breast-feeding can be painful initially for many women even when done correctly (i.e., correct positioning and hold of the infant, proper latch-on). Flat or inverted nipples, scar tissue, bacterial or yeast infection, changes in hormone levels, plugged ducts, an infant with a vigorous suck, or other underlying causes may not be immediately diagnosed, leading a mother to believe that breast-feeding will always cause pain and to wean her infant prematurely. However, often these problems can be addressed by knowledgeable healthcare professionals or may even resolve themselves within a few weeks. A study of breast-feeding discontinuation reported that 14% of women who initiated breast-feeding discontinued between the first and third week because of breast pain or soreness, whereas only 4% discontinued between the fourth and sixth week, and none after the seventh week (Taveras et al., 2003).

In addition, women with more symptoms of maternal depression had greater odds of discontinuing breast-feeding by 12 weeks. A woman's predelivery perception of breast-feeding and the strength of her intention to breast-feed also determine whether or not she will initiate breast-feeding and continue to do so "through the vulnerable post delivery period when women may experience the most discomfort" (Ahluwalia, Morrow, & Hsia, 2005). Healthcare providers interested in promoting breast-feeding should provide women with the tools and support to overcome potential difficulties, including pain and soreness.

Social Support and Acculturation

In some industrialized societies, but not all, breast-feeding has been intertwined with sexuality, making it difficult for some people to separate the two distinctly different functions of the breast. Some ignore the biological role of the breast as a mammary gland to produce milk ideally suited for the nutritional needs of a human child. Other individuals misconstrue breast-feeding in public as a form of indecent exposure. As author Gabrielle Palmer states in *The Politics of Breastfeeding*, "The very reason it [breast-feeding] is frowned upon in public is that breasts are perceived exclusively as objects of sexual attention (1988, p. 119)."

To increase the proportion of women who breast-feed and continue exclusively for at least 6 months, the U.S. Department of Health and Human Services in conjunction with the Ad Council launched the first-ever nationwide breast-feeding awareness campaign in 2004. Rather than just promoting the benefits of breast-feeding, the campaign featured television, radio, and print ads that emphasized the risks of not breast-feeding and its impact on infant and child health. The 2005 postsurvey results revealed that awareness of messages about breast-feeding rose from 28% to 38% and significantly more women surveyed had breast-fed a child in the 2004/2005 study (73%) than in the 2004 study (63%). In regard to breast-feeding in public, 42% of respondents surveyed in

2005 reported being somewhat comfortable or very comfortable with breast-feeding their infant in public, a 3% increase from the 2004 study, whereas 48% of women surveyed in 2005 reported being somewhat uncomfortable or very uncomfortable with breast-feeding their infant in a public place, which is a 1% increase from 2004 survey results. Clearly, much more needs to be done to enable women to feel more comfortable with breast-feeding in public and to make it a social norm.

Not only is American society often unsupportive of breast-feeding women, it can be outright hostile to women who breast-feed in public. Women from various regions of the country and different walks of life have reported incidents of discrimination and harassment while breast-feeding their children in public places such as restaurants, public pools, shopping malls, and supermarkets. Many times these stories appear in the local media, accompanied by editorials or letters to the editor, and some even make it into the national news. These media controversies and the public debate over public breast-feeding lead many women to view breast-feeding negatively when deciding on how to feed their infants.

The same factors that influence whether a mother initiates breast-feeding, as previously mentioned, also determine the *duration* of breast-feeding. Based on the AAP recommendation that a mother breast-feed her infant for at least 12 months, breast-feeding beyond this age has been reported in U.S. literature as "extended breastfeeding." However, the average age of weaning throughout the world, historically and currently, falls between ages 2 and 4 years (Stuart-Macadam & Dettwyler, 1995).

In addition, an analysis of data from NHANES indicates that the more highly acculturated a Hispanic woman becomes in the United States, the less likely she will breast-feed. Conversely, the less acculturated a Hispanic woman is in the United States, the more likely she will breast-feed in keeping with the rate of her country of origin (Gibson, 2005).

Marketing of Breast Milk Substitutes

Expectant mothers are heavily influenced by the plethora of advertisements in parenting magazines, marketing materials in their doctors' offices, coupons for free or steeply discounted breast milk substitutes (formula) that arrive in the mail, and the free samples distributed by the hospital where they give birth. Research suggests that this advertising during pregnancy seriously undermines a future breast-feeding relationship (Howard, Howard, Lawrence, Andresen, & DeBlieck, 2000). Formula companies also target their marketing to women who remain undecided or intend to just "give breast-feeding a try." This deluge of marketing material affects the feeding decisions of mothers to such an extent that the manufacture and sale of breast milk substitutes has grown into an 8 billion dollar industry.

Nearly all hospitals distribute discharge packs or "gift bags" provided by major pharmaceutical companies that contain cans or bottles of formula, with marketing materials including coupons for more formula and sometimes packaged with "breast-feeding success" brochures or books on infant care. Research has shown that the distribution of the bags reduces the number of women who exclusively breast-feed for any length of time (Donnelly, Snowden, Renfew, & Woolridge, 2004).

To curtail the inappropriate marketing of formula that interferes with lactation, the WHO set forth an International Code of Marketing of Breast Milk Substitutes in 1981 (WHO/UNICEF, 1981), which the United States also adopted in 1994. The main goal of the WHO Code is "to contribute to the provision of safe and adequate nutrition for infants, by the protection and promotion of breast-feeding and by the proper use of breast milk substitutes, when these are necessary, on the basis of adequate information and through appropriate marketing and distribution" (WHO/UNICEF, 1981). The Code specifically prohibits

- Advertising of breast milk substitutes
- Distributing free samples of breast milk substitutes to mothers
- Promoting breast milk substitutes through healthcare facilities
- Using company-appointed "nurses" to "advise" mothers on bottle feeding
- Giving gifts or personal samples to health workers
- Placing words or pictures idealizing artificial feeding, including pictures of infants, on the labels of the products
- Promoting unsuitable products for infants, such as sweetened condensed milk

In addition, the Code states that

- Information to health workers should be scientific and factual
- All information on artificial feeding, including the labels, should explain the benefits of breast-

feeding and the costs and hazards associated with artificial feeding
- All products should be of high quality and take into account the climatic and storage conditions of the country where they are used

Returning to Work

The most recent available statistics from the U.S. Department of Labor (2004) show that 57% of female employees are women with infants and children under the age of 3, and they are the fastest growing segment of today's labor force. At least 50% of women who are employed when they become pregnant return to the labor force by the time their child reaches 3 months of age. Research indicates that the timing of the mother's resumption of employment is a key factor that influences the duration of exclusive breast-feeding, and workplace policies and practices, particularly maternity/parental leave provisions, have considerable potential to positively influence breast-feeding practices (Galtry, 2003). Because there is a positive association between length of maternity leave and duration of breast-feeding, some contend that a country's breast-feeding rates are influenced by and reflected in its maternity leave programs (U.S. Department of Labor, 1996). In Norway and Sweden, which have the highest breast-feeding rates in the world, women are entitled to 12 months and 18 months, respectively, of job-protected maternity and child care leave and compensation at 80% to 100% of normal earnings (Organization for Economic Cooperation and Development, 2001). A 1997 report of the International Labor Organization found that for most industrialized countries, 75% to 100% of pay is guaranteed for up to 16 weeks of maternity leave. In stark contrast, the United States mandates only up to a 12-week maternity leave with no entitled pay and has relatively low breast-feeding rates in comparison with other industrialized countries. In addition, a 2000 report to the U.S. Congress on family and medical leave policies found that 77% of those surveyed who were eligible for Family Medical Leave did not take it, stating they could not afford to do so (Waldfogel, 2001).

The earlier a mother returns to work, the more likely her duration of breast-feeding will decrease (Piper & Parks, 1996; Visness & Kennedy, 1997; Vogel, Hutchison, & Mitchell, 1999), and the odds of a woman being able to continue breast-feeding after returning to work increase when her work hours are part-time as opposed to full-time. "Improved maternity leave provisions and more flexible working conditions may help women to remain at home with their infants longer and/or to combine successfully breastfeeding with employment outside the home (Scott, Binns, Oddy, & Graham, 2006)." Fortunately, more and more states are either encouraging or mandating that employers accommodate breast-feeding mothers when they return to work:

> After initiating lactation programs, many employers have seen positive results in the workplace, such as lower absenteeism, high productivity, high company loyalty, high employee morale, and lower healthcare costs. Because an ill child is a frequent cause of absenteeism among employed mothers and fathers, worksite programs that aim to improve child health may also bring about a reduction in absenteeism. Mothers with a formula-fed child are more prone to miss work because formula-fed children have been found to be ill three times more often than breast-fed children (Oregon Department of Health Services, n.d.).

The HHS Blueprint for Action in Breastfeeding (U.S. Department of Health and Human Services, 2000) lists specific aspects of worksite programs that support the continuation of breast-feeding once mothers return to the workplace:

- Prenatal lactation education specifically tailored to working women
- Corporate policies providing information to all employees on the benefits of breast-feeding and services to support breast-feeding women
- Education for personnel about why their breast-feeding coworkers need their support
- Adequate breaks, flexible work hours, job sharing, and part-time work
- Private "mother's rooms" for expressing milk in a secure, sanitary, and relaxing environment
- Access to hospital-grade autocycling breast pumps at the workplace
- Small refrigerators for the safe storage of breast milk
- Subsidization or purchase of individually owned portable breast pumps for employees
- Access to a lactation professional on-site or by phone to give breast-feeding education, counsel-

ing, and support during pregnancy, after delivery, and when the mother returns to work
- Coordination with on-site or near-site child care programs so that the infant can be breast-fed during the day
- Support groups for working mothers with children

Legislation: Protecting a Woman's Right to Breast-Feed

Florida and New York enacted the first state laws concerning breast-feeding in 1993 and 1994, and since then many state legislatures have added breast-feeding to their general statutes as a matter of public health policy. This legislation ranges from the protection of a mother's right to breast-feed in public, to requirements that an employer should accommodate a nursing mother's need to express her milk, to exemptions from jury duty for nursing mothers. The past 5 years have shown an upward trend in comprehensive breast-feeding legislation on the state level that addresses public breast-feeding, workplace issues, and exemption from jury duty. According to La Leche League International (n.d.), which tracks breast-feeding legislation, during the 2005–2006 legislative session 13 states considered bills to protect the right of nursing mothers to breast-feed their children wherever they have the legal right to be.

The provisions of breast-feeding laws can vary widely, as can their interpretations. Currently, 36 states clearly protect a woman's right to breast-feed in public, whereas 20 other states merely exempt nursing mothers from indecent exposure laws. At least eight states have legislation specifically maintaining that a woman may breast-feed wherever she is authorized to be, "irrespective of whether or not the nipple of the mother's breast is covered during or incidental to the breast-feeding."

Legislation that addresses discrimination against nursing mothers in the workplace can also vary. Six states require employers to provide adequate and sanitary facilities for mothers to express and safely store their milk during their lunch or break time. Other states permit but do not require employers to accommodate nursing mothers or designate a workplace as "mother friendly" by providing a flexible work schedule, a private location with an electrical outlet (other than a restroom), a sink with clean running water, and a hygienic refrigerator in the workplace.

References

Social and Cultural Aspects of Breast-Feeding

Ahluwalia, I. B., Morrow, B., & Hsia, J. (2005). Why do women stop breastfeeding? Findings from the pregnancy risk assessment and monitoring system. *Pediatrics, 116,* 1408–1412.

American Academy of Pediatrics. (2005). Breastfeeding and the Use of Human Milk Policy Statement. Breastfeeding and the use of human milk, section on breastfeeding. *Pediatrics, 115,* 496–506.

Arora, S., McJunkin, C., Wehrer, J., & Kuhn, P. (2000). Major factors influencing breastfeeding rates: Mother's perception of father's attitude and milk supply. *Pediatrics, 106,* E67.

Baby Milk Action. (n.d.). Cambridge, England: Center for Breastfeeding Information, Schaumburg, IL. Retrieved May 20, 2006, from http://www.babymilkaction.org

Behrmann, B. (2005). *The Breastfeeding Café.* Ann Arbor, MI: University of Michigan Press.

Bulk-Bunschoten, A. M., van Bodegom, S., Reerink, J. D., Pasker-de Jong, P. C., & de Groot, C. J. (2001). Reluctance to continue breastfeeding in The Netherlands. *Acta Paediatrics, 90,* 1047–1053.

Celi, A. C., Rich-Edwards, J. W., Richardson, M. K., Kleinman, K. P., & Gillman, M. W. (2005). Immigration, race/ethnicity, and social and economic factors as predictors of breastfeeding initiation. *Archives of Pediatrics & Adolescent Medicine, 159,* 255–260.

Centers for Disease Control and Prevention. (2005). Breastfeeding: Data and statistics. Breastfeeding practices—Results from the 2004 National Immunization Study. Retrieved October 4, 2007, from http://www.cdc.gov/breastfeeding/data/NIS data/data 2004.htm

Connecticut General Assembly, Office of Legislative Research. Retrieved May 30, 2006, from http://www.cga.ct.gov/ps99/rpt/olr/99-r-0760.doc

Donath, S. M., Amir, L. H., & ALSPAC Study Team. (2003). Relationship between prenatal infant feeding intention and initiation and duration of breastfeeding: A cohort study. *Acta Paediatrics, 92,* 352–356.

Donnelly, A., Snowden, H. M., Renfew, M. J., & Woolridge, M. W. (2004). Commercial hospital discharge packs for breastfeeding women (Cochrane review). *The Cochrane Library,* Issue 2.

Ekulona, E. (1996). Family health: Taking responsibility/making the difference. *Healthy Start Father's Journal,* 1–18.

Freed, G. I., Fraley, J. K., & Schanler, R. J. (1992). Attitudes of expectant fathers regarding breastfeeding. *Pediatrics, 90,* 224–227.

Galtry, J. (2003). The impact on breastfeeding of labour market policy and practice in Ireland, Sweden, and the USA. *Social Science and Medicine, 57,* 167–177.

Gibson-Davis, C. M., & Brooks-Gunn, J. (2006). Couples' immigration status and ethnicity as determinants of breastfeeding. *American Journal of Public Health, 96,* 641–646.

Giles, F. (2003). *Fresh Milk: The Secret Lives of Breasts.* New York: Simon and Schuster.

Giovannini, M., Riva, E., Banderali, G., Scaglioni, S., Veehof, S. H., Sala, M., et al. (2004). Feeding practices of infants through the first year of life in Italy. *Acta Paediatrica, 93,* 492–497.

Haynes, S. G. (2005). National Breastfeeding Awareness Campaign Results. U.S. Department of Health and Human Services Office on Women's Health (OWH).

Heath, A. L., Tuttle, C. R., Simons, M. S., Cleghorn, C. L., and Parnell, W. R. (2002). A longitudinal study of breastfeeding and weaning practices during the first year of life in Dunedin, New Zealand. *Journal of the American Dietetic Association, 102,* 937–943.

Hefter, W., Lindholm, P., & Elvenes, O. P. (2003). Lactation and breast-feeding ability following lateral pedicle mammaplasty. *British Journal of Plastic Surgery, 56,* 746–751.

Howard, C. R., Howard, F. M., Lanphear, B., Eberly, S., deBlieck, E. A., Oakes, D., et al. (2003). Randomized clinical trial of pacifier use and bottle-feeding or cupfeeding and their effect on breastfeeding. *Pediatrics, 111,* 511–518.

Howard, C. R., Howard, F., Lawrence, R., Andresen, E., & DeBlieck, E. (2000). Office prenatal formula advertising and its effects on breastfeeding patterns. *Obstetrics and Gynecology, 95,* 296–303.

Hurst, N. (2003). Breastfeeding after breast augmentation. *Journal of Human Lactation, 19,* 7–8.

International Labour Organization. (1998). Retrieved May 31, 2006, from http://www.ilo.org/public/english/bureau/inf/pr/1998/7.htm

Johnson, J. O., & Downs, B. (2005). Maternity leave and employment patterns of first time mothers. Current population reports. Retrieved June 5, 2006, from http://www.census.gov/prod/2005pubs/p70–103.pdf

Kools, E. J., Thijs, C., & de Vries, H. (2005). The behavioral determinants of breast-feeding in The Netherlands: Predictors for the initiation of breast-feeding. *Health Education Behaviors, 32,* 809–824.

Kronborg, H., & Vaeth, M. (2004). The influence of psychosocial factors on the duration of breastfeeding. *Scandinavian Journal of Public Health, 32,* 210–206.

Kugyelka, J. G., Rasmussen, K. M., & Frongillo, E. A. (2004). Maternal obesity is negatively associated with breastfeeding success among Hispanic but not Black women. *Journal of Nutrition, 134,* 1746–1753.

Le Leche League International. (n.d.). Breastfeeding and the law: A current summary of breastfeeding legislation in the US. Retrieved June 4, 2006, from http://www.lelecheleague/lawMain.com

Lewin, A. M. (2005). Breast-feeding moms take action: "lactivists" and lawmakers push to allow public nursing. *ABC News,* December 20, 2005.

Lovelady, C. A. (2005). Is maternal obesity a cause of poor lactation performance? *Nutrition Reviews, 63,* 352–355.

Lu, M. C., Lange, L., Slusser, W., Hamilton, J., & Halfon, N. (2001). Provider encouragement of breast-feeding: Evidence from a national survey. *Obstetrics and Gynecology, 97,* 290–295.

McIntyre, E., Hiller, J. E., & Turnbull, D. (2001). Attitudes towards infant feeding among adults in a low socioeconomic community: What social support is there for breastfeeding? *Breastfeeding Reviews, 9,* 13–24.

Merewood, A., Mehta, S. D., Chamberlain, L. B., Philipp, B. L., & Bauchner, H. (2005). Breastfeeding rates in US baby-friendly hospitals: Results of a national survey. *Pediatrics, 116,* 628–634.

Meyerink, R. O., & Marquis, G. S. (2002). Breastfeeding initiation and duration among low-income women in Alabama: The importance of personal and familial experiences in making infant-feeding choices. *Journal of Human Lactation, 8,* 38–45.

Mitra, A. K., Khoury, A. J., Hinton, A. W., & Carothers, C. (2004). Predictors of breastfeeding intention among low-income women. *Maternal and Child Health Journal, 8,* 65–70.

National Conference of State Legislatures. 50 State Summaries of Breastfeeding Laws. Retrieved April 20, 2006, from http://www.ncsl.org/programs/health/breast50.htm

Noel-Weiss, J., Bassett, V., & Cragg, B. (2006). Developing a prenatal breastfeeding workshop to support maternal breastfeeding self-efficacy. *Journal of Obstetric, Gynecologic, and Neonatal Nursing, 35,* 349–357.

Nommsen-Rivers, L. (2003). Cosmetic breast surgery—is breastfeeding at risk? *Journal of Human Lactation, 19,* 7–8.

Oregon Department of Human Services. (n.d.). Retrieved June 5, 2006, from http://www.dhs.state.or.us/policy/admin/safety/breastfeeding.htm

Organization for Economic Cooperation and Development. (2001). Balancing work and family life: Helping parents into paid employment. In *Employment Outlook* (pp. 129–166). Paris, France: Organization for Economic Cooperation and Development.

Palmer, G. (1988). *The Politics of Breastfeeding.* London: Pandora Press.

Piper, S., & Parks, P. L. (1996). Predicting the duration of lactation: Evidence from a national survey. *Birth, 23,* 7–12.

Plastic Surgery Information Service. (n.d.). Retrieved June 3, 2006, from http://www.plasticsurgery.org

Rasmussen, K. M., & Kjolhede, C. L. (2004). Prepregnant overweight and obesity diminish the prolactin response to suckling in the first week postpartum. *Pediatrics, 113,* e465–e471.

Rea, M. F., & Morrow, A. L. (2004). Protecting, promoting, and supporting breastfeeding among women in the labor force. *Advances in Experimental Medical Biology, 554,* 121–132.

Ryan, A. S., & Zhou, W. (2006). Lower breastfeeding rates persist among the special supplemental nutrition program for women, infants, and children participants, 1978–2003. *Pediatrics, 117,* 1136–1146.

Ryan, A. S., Zhou, W., & Acosta, A. (2002). Breastfeeding continues to increase into the new millennium. *Pediatrics, 110,* 1103–1109.

Shealy, K. R., Li, R., Benton-Davis, S., & Grummer-Strawn, L. M. (2005). *The CDC Guide to Breastfeeding Interventions.* Washington, DC: U.S. Department of Health and Human Services and the Centers for Disease Control and Prevention.

Stuart-Macadam, P., & Dettwyler, K. A. (1995). *Breastfeeding: Biocultural Perspectives.* Hawthorne, NY: Aldine De Gruyter.

Scott, J. A., Binns, C. W., & Aroni, R. A. (1995). Infant feeding practices in Perth and Melbourne: Report 1, p. 72 (breastfeeding rates in Australia).

Scott, J. A., Binns, C. W., Oddy, W. H., & Graham, K. I. (2006). Predictors of breastfeeding duration: Evidence from a cohort study. *Pediatrics, 117,* e646–e655.

Souto, G. C., Giugliani, E. R., Giugliani, C., & Schneider, M. A. (2003). The impact of breast reduction surgery on breastfeeding performance. *Journal of Human Lactation, 19,* 43–49; quiz 66–69, 120.

Swanson, V., & Power, K. G. (2005). Initiation and continuation of breastfeeding: Theory of planned behaviour. *Journal of Advanced Nursing, 50,* 272–282.

Sweden's Statistics in Health and Diseases. (1998). Retrieved June 3, 2006, from http://www.sos.se/FULLTEXT/0042-007/0042-007.pdf

Taveras, E. M., Capra, A. M., Braveman, P. A., Jensvold, N. G., Escobar, G. J., & Lieu, T. A. (2003). Clinician support and psychosocial risk factors associated with breastfeeding discontinuation. *Pediatrics, 112,* 108–115.

U.S. Department of Health and Human Services. (2000). *HHS Blueprint for Action on Breastfeeding.* Washington, DC: U.S. Department of Health and Human Services, Office on Women's Health.

U.S. Department of Health and Human Services and the Centers for Disease Control and Prevention. (n.d.). Healthy People 2010: Maternal, Infant, and Child Health. Retrieved July 1, 2007, from http://www.healthypeople.gov/Document/HTML/Volume2/16MICH.htm

U.S. Department of Labor. (1996). *A Workable Balance. Report to Congress on Family and Medical Leave Policies.*

U.S. Food and Drug Administration. Breast implants: An information update—2000. Retrieved July 1, 2007, from http://www.fda.gov/cdrh/breastimplants/index.html

van der Wal, M. F., de Jonge, G. A., & Pauw-Plomp, H. (2001). Increased percentages of breastfed infants in Amsterdam. *Ned Tijdschr Geneeskd, 18,* 1597–1601. In Dutch.

Vance, M. R. A current summary of breastfeeding legislation in the U.S. Retrieved July 1, 2007, from http://www.lalecheleague.org/LawBills.html. Also A current summary of proposed breastfeeding legislation in the U.S. Retrieved July 1, 2007, from http://www.lalecheleague.org/Law/proposedsummary.html

Visness, C., & Kennedy, K. (1997). Maternal employment and breast-feeding: Findings from the 1988 National Maternal and Infant Health Survey. *American Journal of Public Health, 87*, 945–950.

Vogel, A., Hutchison, B., & Mitchell, E. (1999). Factors associated with the duration of breastfeeding. *Acta Paediatrica, 88*, 1320–1326.

Waldfogel, J. (2001). Family and medical leave: Evidence from the 2000 surveys. *Monthly Labor Review*, 124. Retrieved October 4, 2007, from http://www.bls.gov/opub/mlr/2001/09/art2full.pdf

Walker, M. (2002). Breastfeeding after breast augmentation. *Journal of Human Lactation, 19*, 70–71.

WHO/UNICEF International Code of Marketing of Breast Milk Substitutes. (1981). Geneva, Switzerland.

Yalom, M. (1997). *A History of the Breast*. New York: Ballantine.

Special Section: Postpartum Depression and Maternal Nutrition

Rachelle Lessen, MS, RD, IBCLC

During fetal development the growth of the brain depends on the accumulation of large amounts of omega-3 fatty acids. DHA and AA are incorporated into the neural cell membranes during the period of rapid fetal brain development in the third trimester of gestation. A portion of this fatty acid can be endogenously synthesized by the fetus or newborn from its precursor alpha-linolenic acid; however, it is likely that most is provided directly from the mother through the placenta or in breast milk. Although the needs of the growing fetus and infant have been extensively studied, less is known about the needs of the mother, who is the primary source of DHA for her fetus or breast-fed child. Makrides and Gibson (2000) reported that there does not appear to be a detectable reduction of omega-3 fatty acids during pregnancy but there is a clear decrease of approximately 30% in the postpartum period. This decline occurs gradually from birth to 6 weeks and persists until 12 weeks or beyond. The decrease is largely independent of whether or not the mother is breast-feeding, suggesting that lactation is not contributing to this postpartum depletion. This decline is preventable and reversible with DHA supplementation.

Literature reports that an AI of omega-3 fatty acids is associated with major depression and other affective disorders, and there are reports of decreased levels of omega-3 fatty acids in depressed patients. DHA supplementation has been reported to be effective in treatment of bipolar disorder and schizophrenia. DHA is thought to modulate synaptic function directly through its effect on membrane structure. Because of the evidence supporting a relationship between DHA and brain function and the knowledge that DHA levels decrease in late pregnancy and lactation, researchers have proposed a relationship between DHA and postpartum depression.

Seafood is a major source of DHA, and studies have shown that women who regularly consume fish have higher levels of DHA in their breast milk than women who rarely or never eat fish. Also reported is an association between increased seafood consumption and decreased depression. Hibbeln (2002) proposed that the DHA content of mother's milk and seafood consumption would predict the prevalence rates of postpartum depression. Hibbeln hypothesized that because seafood consumption protects women from omega-3 fatty acid depletion during pregnancy, rates of postpartum depression would be lower in countries with greater rates of seafood consumption. Because the DHA content of breast milk serves as a marker of maternal DHA status postpartum, they also hypothesized that higher concentrations of DHA in breast milk would predict lower rates of postpartum depression. Their findings did indeed support the conclusion that lower DHA content in mothers' milk and lower seafood consumption were both associated with higher rates of postpartum depression. Because data on confounding variables were not available for all countries in the study, it could not be proved that higher levels of DHA caused a lower prevalence of rates of postpartum depression.

Llorente and colleagues (2003) found that DHA supplementation of 200 mg/day for 4 months after delivery prevented a decrease in plasma DHA that is often seen in postpartum women. In a randomly assigned, double-masked, interventional study they found that the mothers who received DHA supplementation increased their DHA levels by 8% compared with the placebo group, which had a 31% decrease in DHA. After 4 months of supplementation the supplemented group had a 50% higher DHA level than the unsupplemented group. However, these changes were not found to be associated with rates of depression. Repeated measurements of depression at 3 weeks, 2 months, and 4 months showed no difference between the groups at any time. Rates of depression were equally low in both groups. The authors conceded that perhaps a higher dose of DHA, or a combination of DHA and AA, or initiating supplementation during pregnancy may have more beneficial effects on postpartum depression.

References

Postpartum Depression and Maternal Nutrition

Hibbeln, J. R. (2002). Seafood consumption, the DHA content of mothers' milk and prevalence rates of postpartum depression: A cross-national, ecological analysis. *Journal of Affective Disorders, 69*, 15–29.

Llorente, A., Jensen, C. L., Voigt, R. G., Fraley, J. K., Berretta, M. C., & Heird, W. C. (2003). Effect of maternal docosahexaenoic acid supplementation on postpartum depression and information processing. *American Journal of Obstetrics and Gynecology, 188*, 1348–1353.

Makrides, M., & Gibson, R. (2000). Long-chain polyunsaturated fatty acid requirements during pregnancy and lactation. *American Journal of Clinical Nutrition, 71*, 307S–311S.

CHAPTER

3

Normal Nutrition for Toddler Through School-Aged Children and the Role of Parents in Promoting Healthy Nutrition in Early Childhood

Jennifer Sabo, RD, LDN, CNSD, and Barbara Robinson, MPH, RD, CNSD

CHAPTER OUTLINE

Reader Objectives

After studying this chapter and reflecting on the contents, you should be able to

1. Understand the different nutritional factors that may affect growth and development in a toddler.

2. Understand the use of vitamins and minerals in a toddler and how to provide them naturally.

3. Identify the differences in portion sizes that are appropriate for toddlers versus adults.

4. Understand the importance of "mealtime" with toddlers.

5. Identify reasons for excess weight gain in toddlers and how this can be prevented.

6. Use the information obtained in the chapter to assess three problems common to toddlers and determine the solution.

7. Identify the antecedents to eating behaviors that occur in the early childhood.

8. Discuss components of the mealtime feeding environment (structure, exposure, modeling, and repetition).

After infancy, nutrition continues to be vital to the growth and development of children. As the child becomes less dependent on breast milk and/or formula, a more comprehensive form of nutrition becomes essential to provide an appropriate variety of foods. This will ensure that the growing child is obtaining the necessary macro- and micronutrients for growth. This goal is made difficult by the emerging independence of the child. Strategies designed to incorporate, understand, and compensate for particular behaviors centered on mealtime and eating may be just as vital as providing healthy choices.

Normal Nutrition for Toddler Through School-Aged Children

Jennifer Sabo, RD, LDN, CNSD

Growth Expectations

Growth is measured and plotted on standard Centers for Disease Control and Prevention (CDC) growth charts based on age and sex. Head circumference and weight for height is measured and plotted until 36 months of age. After age 2 body mass index (BMI) is used to assess appropriate weight for height (National Institutes of Health, n.d.). The use of BMI after the age of 2 is appropriate because of a correlation between height and adiposity before age 12 (Freedman et al., 2004).

Growth rates may vary considerably for each individual child. This is thought to be associated with a variety of factors, including parents' growth history and patterns. It is essential for clinicians to note that approximately 25% of normal infants and toddlers in the first 2 years of life drop to a lower growth percentile and subsequently remain on this new growth track (Krugman & Dubowitz, 2003). Tables 3.1 and 3.2 demonstrate average weight and height growth, respectively, for the 1st through 10th years of life. It is helpful for healthcare professionals to be aware of these growth trends to assess each child's growth.

Energy and Nutrient Needs

As growth rates differ for each child, so do their energy needs. The energy requirements of toddlers and children vary greatly based on differences in both growth rate and level of activity (Zlotkin, 1996). As demonstrated in Tables 3.1 and 3.2, the growth rate for ages 1 to 3 years and 7 to 10 years are more rapid, thus necessitating greater energy needs. The chrono-

TABLE 3.1 Weight Growth

Age (yr)	Average Daily Growth (g/day)
1–3	4–10
4–6	5–8
7–10	5–12

Based on growth velocity of the 50th percentile weight for age and height for age from the National Center for Health Statistics growth charts (2000).

TABLE 3.2 Height Growth

Age (yr)	Average Daily Growth (g/day)
1–3	0.7–1.1
4–6	0.5–0.8
7–10	0.4–0.6

Based on growth velocity of the 50th percentile weight for age and height for age from the National Center for Health Statistics growth charts (2000).

logic age and the current stage of **development** of the child also relate to and influence energy needs. Current energy need recommendations from the Food and Agriculture Organization, World Health Organization, and United Nations University (1985) for growing children ages 1 to 10 years are based on the actual observed intakes of healthy children and can aid clinicians in establishing norms.

Development: A process in which something passes by degrees to a different more advanced stage.

Current weight and height, as well as trends in growth velocity, can also be used to assess a particular child's needs. It is essential to note that throughout childhood there appears to be no difference in energy requirements for boys and girls. A study by Butte et al. (2000) used the total energy expenditure and energy deposition data of a group of healthy children to demonstrate that current recommendations for energy intake in the first 2 years of life may exceed modern energy expenditures and perhaps need to be revised.

● **Learning Point** As a general rule, energy requirements are designed to promote an optimal rate of growth and adequate body composition (Butte et al., 2000). However, the overall energy requirements can be adjusted based on need for weight loss or gain, weight maintenance, or catch-up growth.

Protein

Protein is the primary factor in many body tissues. Proteins build, maintain, and restore tissues in the body, such as muscles and organs. As a child grows and develops, protein is a crucial nutrient needed to provide optimal growth. Current recommendations state that protein intake should comprise approximately 10% to 20% of the child's daily intake. This recommendation is designed to ensure that enough energy is provided to the body from all nutrients so that protein is spared for growth and development of tissues. Table 3.3 provides the current dietary reference intake for protein for growing toddlers and

TABLE 3.3	Protein Requirements

Age (yr)	Dietary Reference Intake for Protein (g/day)
1–3	0.7–1.1
4–6	0.5–0.8
7–10	0.4–0.6

Based on growth velocity of the 50th percentile weight for age and height for age from the National Center for Health Statistics growth charts (2000).

children (Institute of Medicine [IOM], Food and Nutrition Board, 2000–2005).

Learning Point Protein deficiencies are uncommon in the United States because most children exceed the daily recommended intake for protein. Children at risk for protein deficiency include those from low-income homes, those with multiple diet restrictions due to food allergies, and those who are provided a strict vegetarian diet that excludes most or all animal products (referred to as a vegan diet).

Fat

Until age 3 dietary fat plays a role in brain development. Fat comprises approximately 60% of the central and peripheral nervous systems that essentially control, regulate, and integrate every body system; thus it is essential that growing toddlers obtain adequate fat from their diet. Furthermore, the fat content of the diet is known to be the crucial element in providing satiety. Therefore low fat meals or snacks for children can lead to hunger and subsequent overeating between meals. After infancy most children are able to meet their daily calorie and nutrient requirements for growth with a diet consisting of 30% of total calories from fat (American Academy of Pediatrics [AAP] Committee on Nutrition, 1992; Butte, 2000). If excess weight gain is a concern, often only minor changes in dietary choices are needed to help keep fat intake at or below 30% of daily calories to promote optimal growth (Fisher, Van Horn, & McGill, 1997).

Learning Point The AAP recommends that children over age 2 receive at least 20% of calories from fat. Because children do not benefit from a restriction below this level (AAP, Committee on Nutrition, 1998), parents on low-fat diets should make certain to provide adequate fat to their growing child.

It should be noted that all fats are not equal in their benefits to one's health. Most fat intake should be derived from poly- and monounsaturated fat, such as fish, most nuts, and vegetable oils (American Heart Association [AHA], n.d.). These fats help to keep total cholesterol low and "good" cholesterol, or **high-density lipoproteins**, high. Foods high in saturated fat, such as butter, cheese, and beef, should be offered in moderation, because these can contribute to high total cholesterol and high **low-density lipoproteins**. Though hypercholesterolemia has not traditionally been a concern for this age group, recent trends in obesity coincide with a rise in cholesterol levels, therefore mandating that clinicians become more cognizant of fat intake.

High-density lipoprotein: A blood constituent involved in the transport of cholesterol and associated with a decreased risk of heart attack.

Low-density lipoprotein: A lipoprotein that transports cholesterol in the blood, composed of a moderate amount of protein and a large amount of cholesterol. High levels are associated with increased risk of heart disease.

Vitamins and Minerals

Calcium

Calcium is the principal mineral required by the body for the process of bone mineralization. Toddlers and young children have an increased need for calcium to promote the rapid bone growth and skeletal development that takes place during these early years of life. Despite the essential nature of this mineral, studies demonstrate only about 50% of children aged 1 to 5 years meet the Dietary Reference Intake for calcium (Dennison, 1996). Table 3.4 provides the current Dietary Reference Intake for calcium in growing children (IOM, 2000–2005).

Storey, Forchee, and Anderson (2004) demonstrated that soft drink and juice consumption begin to increase at 4 to 8 years of age, often replacing milk at meals and snacks. This study found that intake of milk and milk products decreased more significantly with age for girls as compared with boys. These authors suggest discouraging and/or restricting juice

TABLE 3.4	Calcium Requirements

Age (yr)	Dietary Reference Intake for Calcium (mg/day)
1–3	500
4–8	800
9–13	1,300

Based on current Dietary Reference Intake for calcium (IOM, 2000–2005).

and soft drink intake to avoid the displacement of milk with these largely unhealthy beverages (Storey et al., 2004).

If it is determined that the recommended daily calcium intake is not being met, by using diet histories and food frequencies, health professionals should consider recommendation of a daily calcium supplement. Many studies have shown that males demonstrate a superior result in building peak bone mass with calcium supplementation (Carter et al., 2001). It is essential to recognize that milk and milk products contain additional necessary nutrients for health, including protein and vitamin D, which continues to make these the superior means of meeting calcium needs. Thus healthcare professionals should continue to find means of increasing intake of milk and milk products (Storey et al., 2004). Because vitamin D is needed for the best utilization of calcium, many calcium supplements are now including vitamin D to aid in the efficiency of the product. As demonstrated by Johnston et al. (1992), daily calcium supplementation lasting greater than 12 months may result in great gains in bone mass as compared with control groups.

Recent studies indicate that calcium intake of about 800 mg/day is associated with adequate bone mineralization in preadolescent children (AAP, 1999). The importance of providing adequate calcium to growing children is becoming more apparent. Storey et al. (2004) found that adequate calcium intake in preadolescent and adolescent girls is necessary to help decrease the incidence of osteoporosis in adulthood. Therefore good prevention efforts for osteoporosis should focus on "young people in their growing years" (Carter et al., 2001).

Dairy products are typically the main source of calcium in the diet, including milk, yogurt, cheese, and ice cream. However, more recently and perhaps reflecting trends of inadequate calcium intake, many foods are being fortified with calcium, such as waffles, juice, and cereals. Calcium is often represented as a percent daily value on food labels, using 1,000 mg/day as 100% daily value (AAP, 1999). **Table 3.5** provides ways to increase calcium in a child's diet.

CRITICAL **Thinking**

Though controversial, flavored milk can be a good source of calcium and may increase compliance in young children. It may be helpful to choose lower fat milk and add flavoring with sugar-free syrups as a way to keep fat and added sugar intake low for toddlers over age 2 but still receive the benefits of calcium.

Vitamin D

Vitamin D is available to humans through the photochemical action of sunlight or ultraviolet light on 7-dehydrocholesterol in skin and through dietary sources such as fish oils, fatty fish, and foods fortified with vitamin D, including cow's milk and infant or supplemental formulas (Holick, Shils, Olsen, Shike, & Ross, 1999). The amount of vitamin D synthesized through sunlight exposure is affected by time spent outside, the amount of skin exposed, air pollution, cloud cover, time of day, latitude, time of year, and skin pigmentation (Tomashek et al., 2001).

Specker and colleagues (1985) estimated that white infants require approximately 30 minutes of sunlight per week to obtain adequate vitamin D if wearing only a diaper but require 2 hours per week if fully clothed without a hat. The melanin in our skin decreases the amount of

TABLE	
3.5	Easy Ways to Increase Calcium in the Diet

- Drink milk. Two 8-ounce glasses of milk each day can provide over 600 mg of calcium. Lactose-reduced milk is a good source of calcium if regular milk is not tolerated.
- Use heated milk in place of hot water to make hot cereals, such as oatmeal or hot chocolate.
- Add cheese to sandwiches, casseroles, meat loaf, salads, and snacks.
- Add broccoli and cheese to a baked potato.
- Choose desserts made with milk such as pudding, custard, frozen yogurt, and ice cream.
- Substitute milk and yogurt in recipes instead of cream or sour cream.
- Add dried powdered milk or evaporated milk when preparing soups, mashed potatoes, sauces, and hot cereals.
- Drink a glass of calcium-fortified juice, such as orange juice.
- Add almonds to muffin and bread recipes.
- Remember to read labels for percentage of calcium. If it has greater than 30% of your calcium requirement for the day, then it would be a high calcium choice. Many foods are fortified with calcium, such as orange juice, rice, cereals, waffles, and pasta.
- Choosing one high calcium food at each meal will help you to meet your goal every day!

Note: Low-fat products contain the same amount of calcium as whole milk products.

vitamin D synthesized from sunlight. Therefore children with darker skin need to spend more time outside than those with lighter skin to obtain sufficient vitamin D (Weisberg, Scanlon, Li, & Cogswell, 2004).

Adequate vitamin D intake is important for optimal calcium absorption. Dietary products such as yogurts and orange juice are now fortified with vitamin D. As toddlers are advanced off of infant formula and onto table foods, parents should be educated to offer a diet adequate in both nutrients (Weisberg et al., 2004). National data as to the prevalence of hypovitaminosis D among children are not yet available (Weisberg et al., 2004). Therefore more extensive study is needed to determine the extent of vitamin D deficiency in the United States.

Iron

Daily requirements for iron intake are based on age and iron stores. During periods of rapid growth the body's need for iron increases, as shown in **Table 3.6** (IOM, 2000–2005).

Iron can be classified as being derived from heme or nonheme sources. Heme sources include animal meats and products, such as beef and chicken, whereas nonheme sources include fortified grains, fruits, and vegetables (IOM, 2000–2005). Though iron can be obtained from either source, absorption of this essential nutrient is found to be higher from heme sources than from nonheme. Of note, consuming foods with vitamin C while eating an iron containing food can promote better absorption of iron into the body. Conversely, taking antacids during the meal may inhibit iron absorption. **Table 3.7** provides ways to increase iron the diet.

Iron deficiency **anemia** is the most common nutritional deficiency in the world and remains relatively common among at-risk groups in the United States (Schneider et al.,

Anemia: A quantitative deficiency of hemoglobin, often accompanied by a reduced number of red blood cells and causing pallor, weakness, and breathlessness. May be related to inadequate dietary consumption of iron or blood loss.

TABLE 3.7	Increasing Iron in the Diet

- Include a protein source at meals, such as fish, beef, or poultry.
- Look for iron enriched or fortified grains, such as cereals, breads, and pasta.
- Offer oatmeal or cream of wheat at breakfast.
- Add foods high in vitamin C to the meal, including citrus fruit, melon, and dark green leafy vegetables, for improved iron absorption.
- Add pureed meats to pasta sauce or casseroles for toddlers with difficulty advancing to chewing meats.
- Encourage children with advanced chewing skills to eat the skin of the baked potato for added dietary iron.

2005). Risk factors for iron deficiency include low household income, lack of consistent medical care, poor diet quality, and parents with minimal education. Identification of deficiency is crucial, because side effects for infants and children with iron deficiency may include impaired neurodevelopment, leading to decreased attention span and lower scores on standardized tests (Grantham-McGregor & Ani, 2001).

Deficiency often occurs as a secondary development to insufficient dietary iron intake. It should also be noted that increased calcium intake may lead to anemia. This is due to calcium and iron competing for absorption at the same receptor sites within the body. Therefore drinking large amounts of high calcium milk is a common cause of iron deficiency in children. Refusal of meats is also a common cause of low iron intake in developing children. The increased availability of iron fortified foods and formulas have helped to decrease the incidence of iron deficiency.

An objective of Healthy People 2010 is to reduce iron deficiency in 1- to 2-year-olds by 5% and in 3- to 4-year-olds by 1% (U.S. Department of Health and Human Services, 2000). The goal to reduce anemia and iron deficiency in high-risk populations, such as toddlers, has been addressed through programs such as the Special Supplemental Nutrition Program for Women, Infants, and Children (WIC) of the U.S. Department of Agriculture by enrolling families at the highest risk for anemia and iron deficiency and providing them with vouchers for iron fortified formulas and cereals. WIC also screens children for low hemoglobin with the goal of identifying at-risk children, educating families, and reducing the incidence of anemia (Schneider et al., 2005).

TABLE 3.6	Iron Requirements	
Age (yr)		Dietary Reference Intake for Iron (mg/day)
1–3		7
4–8		10
9–13		8

Based on current Dietary Reference Intake for iron (IOM, 2000–2005).

Vitamin Supplements

After infancy supplemental vitamin use decreases, but it is still relatively common. Typically, a general multivitamin is not routinely recommended for toddlers and young children unless the diet history demonstrates the child's intake to be inadequate.

Supplementation is recommended for children without the means to eat a balanced diet and for those with chronic medical conditions or treatments who may lose necessary vitamins, including dialysis, cystic fibrosis, gastrointestinal conditions, and food allergies. Megadoses of vitamins and minerals should be discouraged unless prescribed by a doctor for a specific medical condition.

Many everyday foods are being fortified with multiple vitamins and minerals; therefore vitamin and mineral deficiencies are rare in the United States (Dietz & Stern, 1999). Consuming the recommended daily servings of the many food groups typically provides adequate nutrients. A diet evaluation by a healthcare professional is recommended for those who are questioning their child's need for multivitamin intake. Many pediatricians believe minimal risk is involved if a child is given the daily standard multiple vitamin. However, although vitamin and mineral toxicities are rare, possible excess intakes of these nutrients due to supplements and high intake of fortified foods should be considered (Briefel, Hanson, Fox, Novak, & Ziegler, 2006).

> **● Learning Point** Many vitamins often look and taste like candy; therefore special care should be taken to keep them out of reach of children and under no circumstances should they be referred to as a treat by parents or caregivers.

If a child has an inadequate diet, simply providing a daily vitamin only addresses the problem in the short term. Working on improving the diet is the best way to ensure a child is receiving optimal nutrition. Healthcare professionals should stress the importance of whole foods rather than individual nutrients (Fox, Reidy, Novak, & Ziegler, 2006) to ensure the diet is complete with all nutrients, including fiber.

Fluoride

Fluorosis: An abnormal condition caused by excessive intake of fluorides, characterized in children by discoloration and pitting (mottling) of the teeth.

Fluoride has been demonstrated to promote tooth formation and also to inhibit the progression of dental caries (IOM, 2000–2005). However, children who begin to use fluoride toothpaste before age 2 are at higher risk for enamel **fluorosis**. This is due to a poorly controlled swallowing reflex, thereby leading to increased ingestion of fluoride. To avoid excess ingestion, child-strength toothpaste (which contains a decreased quantity of fluoride) may be used in children aged 2 to 6 years. After age 6 regular fluoridated toothpaste is approved in children (CDC, 2001).

Deficiencies in fluoride are not common but may occur in areas with nonfluoridated water or in children who receive nonfluoridated bottled water. Fluoride supplementation may be prescribed by a healthcare professional for infants over age 6 months who are at risk for dental caries and primarily drink water with minimal fluoride content (CDC, 2001).

Water

Water helps the body to maintain **homeostasis**, allows for the transport of nutrients into cells, and also functions in the removal of the waste products of metabolism (IOM, 2000–2005). Therefore water is a very important, though often overlooked, component of the daily diet. All beverages contain water, as do high moisture foods, such as fruit, soups, and ice cream. Water can be offered to the growing child for hydration, but care should be taken not to replace adequate milk or formula intake to prevent displacing vital nutrients in the diet.

Homeostasis: The tendency of the body to seek and maintain a condition of balance or internal stability.

Whole Milk

The use of whole milk should typically stop after age 2, unless otherwise directed by a healthcare professional. To promote adherence, families should take care to drink skim or 1% milk together.

Foods at 1 Year

After 1 year of age toddlers begin to eat more like their caregivers. An important aspect to feeding toddlers is the knowledge that portion sizes should be kept appropriate for their age. Toddlers often eat six small meals each day verses three larger meals. Dietz and Stern (1999) suggested that toddler serving sizes be one-fourth to one-half that of adults. Some examples follow:

- Grains: bread, one-fourth to one-half slice; cereal, rice, or pasta, cooked, 4 tablespoons; dry cereal, ¼ cup

- Cooked vegetables: 1 tablespoon per year of age
- Fruit: cooked or canned, ½ cup; fresh, one-half piece; 100% juice, ¼ to ½ cup
- Dairy: milk, ½ cup; cheese, ½ ounce; yogurt, ⅓ cup
- Protein: chicken, turkey, beef, or fish, 1 ounce; ground meat, 2 tablespoons

Mealtime With Toddlers

As toddlers continue to advance in their feeding skills, it is crucial to provide a healthy feeding and eating environment. Structure at meals can have a significant influence on a child's eating patterns (Patrick & Nicklas, 2005). Suggestions to provide such a structured environment include the complete absence of television and other distractions of a similar ilk. As often as possible the family should sit at the dining room or kitchen table together and enjoy the meal as a unit. In addition to providing structure and promoting family bonding, eating together as a family has been shown to be associated with increased intakes of fruits and vegetables at a meal (Patrick & Nicklas, 2005).

As with most behaviors, the child's stage of development can influence food choices. A toddler may prefer finger foods that encourage them to demonstrate their new independence. Table 3.8 provides examples of finger foods that are typically safe to offer. To avoid conflict at meals, parents should be educated that the child may also decide mealtime is over before a large amount of food is consumed because of their comparatively small stomach size. The AHA recommends that infants and young children should not be forced to finish a meal, because calorie intake is likely to vary at each mealtime (AHA, n.d.). In fact, Fisher et al. found that children forced to eat everything on their plates became less sensitive to their body's signs of satiety (Fisher & Birch, 1999).

TABLE 3.8	Finger Foods

- Foods should be easily dissolved.
- Serve cheese sticks, rice puffs, wagon wheels, cheese puffs, meat sticks, soft vegetable pieces, peeled apple or pear sticks, and soft fruit pieces.

Note: Types of foods offered *must* match developmental abilities.

Introducing New Foods

As toddlers and young children develop new feeding skills, there is potential for greater dietary variety. To the frustration of many caregivers, children often initially refuse a new food simply because it is unfamiliar. However, multiple exposures to a new food have been found to ultimately achieve food acceptance. It has been found that up to 10 exposures to the new food promote clear changes in acceptance of the food (Sullivan & Birch, 1993). However, Carruth et al. (1998) found that most caregivers tried a new food an average of 2.5 times before deciding the child disliked that particular food, falling well below the recommended number of experiences needed to truly determine an actual dislike for the food. This demonstrates that parents and caregivers can greatly benefit from consistent education regarding presentation of new foods.

It is important to introduce one food at a time to avoid confusion or overwhelming the child. Consistency with each new food, offering at least once per day, helps the child to develop a familiarity. Offering vegetables more frequently throughout the day has been shown to help increase a child's daily intake (Dennison, Rockwell, & Baker, 1998). Similar appearing foods may be more readily received once one type of food has previously been accepted. Conversely, limited exposure to a variety of foods could lead to rejection of other products that have a similar visual appearance to the initially rejected food (Carruth et al., 1998). Many parents state their child does not like vegetables, but vegetables are rarely available in the home for the child to become familiar with. Therefore not only exposure but also the *opportunity* to taste a food increases food acceptance (Birch & Fisher, 1998).

Caregivers should be educated on providing a healthy variety of new foods to their child. Foods without overall nutritional value should not be introduced merely to provide calories (AHA, n.d.). Table 3.9 provides tips on promoting increased fruit and vegetable intake.

Planning Children's Meals

When planning meals for the growing toddler or child it is important to keep in mind the different food groups and nutrient needs. It can be difficult to meet daily recommendations for fruit and vegetable

TABLE	
3.9	How To Promote Increased Fruit and Vegetable Intake

- Add fruit purees into mixes, such as pancakes, waffles, and muffins. Apples, pears, bananas, and blueberries are great fruits to try. Using purees avoids the child finding chunks of the fruit, which may prevent the child from eating the food. Sometimes starting with a very small amount of fruit and increasing the amount as the child becomes familiar with flavor is the best way for more sensitive children.
- Pureed fruits can also be mixed into yogurt, milk shakes, and pudding to add flavor.
- Adding dried fruits to cereal or trail mixes is a good way to increase fruit intake. Serving sizes are smaller for dried fruit, so the child does not have to eat as much. Note: This should be used for children over age 3 to prevent a choking risk.
- Mix vegetable purees into soups and sauces, such as spaghetti sauce or chicken noodle soup. Carrots, green beans, and sweet potatoes are good vegetables to start out with. You can also mix these purees into homemade meat loaf, meatballs, or hamburgers.
- Bring the child along to the store to select a new fruit or vegetable he or she would like to try. Have the child help prepare the new food. If the child feels more involved with the selection of the food, he or she is more likely to try it.

intake if one only offers these foods at the three main meals. Low intake of fruits and vegetables is correlated with suboptimal intake of many nutrients, including fiber and vitamins A and C, and also appears to be linked with higher fat intakes (Dennison et al., 1998). Fruits and vegetables are a good choice at snack time, thereby helping to meet optimal intake.

It is important to plan balanced meals, demonstrating healthy eating early while the child is developing feeding behaviors. Starting a heart healthy diet before reaching adulthood can help to reduce the prevalence of obesity (Fisher et al., 1997).

It is essential for healthcare providers to be aware that preparing and providing healthy meals can be expensive. The high cost of fruits and vegetables is often reported as the main reason a parent or caregiver does not frequently purchase these foods (Dennison et al., 1998). Parents should be educated on creative ways to provide fruits and vegetables. For example, shopping for produce at local farmers' markets provides a more affordable opportunity. Furthermore, canned fruits and vegetables are often less expensive and remain an excellent source of nutrients. It is important, however, to let caregivers know to purchase fruit canned in its own juice and vegetables without added salt to avoid providing extra sugar or sodium to the child.

Children tend to eat more of foods they are familiar with, so it is important for healthy foods to always be available in the home. Patrick and Nicklas (2005) reported that "children are more likely to eat foods that are available and easily accessible." This should always be considered when planning and shopping for a meal.

Hunger and Behavior

Children gain knowledge of dietary behaviors from watching others (Hayman, 2003; Patrick & Nicklas, 2005). As children age they begin to spend more time outside of the home, acquiring feeding behaviors from those around them. By age 3 or 4 eating becomes influenced by environmental cues more than the previous "deprivation-driven response" during infancy (Patrick & Nicklas, 2005).

However, regardless of behaviors developed the child should not control meal planning. Satter suggested caregivers develop a "division of labor" between caregivers and the child. In this model the caregiver's role is to provide healthy foods that are accessible. It is the child's responsibility to decide when to eat and how much food they will eat at a particular meal (Satter, 1986, 1996).

Food behaviors can also be related to the availability of certain foods and how easy they are to consume for the developing child. Baranowski, Cullen, and Baranowski (1999) found that children tend to choose foods more often that are in an accessible location and also of an appropriate size for their developmental capacity. Fruits and vegetables that are cut into sticks or bite size pieces are more likely to be chosen than whole fruits and vegetables simply because the child is able to handle them independently.

Growing toddlers and children should typically not be restricted at meals. Restriction of foods that are high in fat and sugar often lead to the child "fixating on the forbidden food" and consuming more of these foods outside of the home or when full (Fisher & Birch, 2000). If seconds are requested it is beneficial to develop a habit of offering an additional serving of vegetables or fruits, though not forcing the child to take what or *only* what is offered.

Picky Eating

Picky eating can be common in toddlers and may continue throughout childhood. Often, picky eating may represent an attempt at acquiring independence rather than a declaration of actual likes and dislikes. A caregiver may try to accommodate a picky eater or to develop techniques that may help increase amount and quality of foods eaten. However, using rewards, prodding, or punishment to encourage eating may only enforce the "picky eater phenomenon" (Pelcaht & Pliner, 1986). Caregivers should continue to provide healthy food options and not make special foods or entire meals for the picky child.

Working with a child who is exhibiting picky behaviors can certainly be challenging. Parents and caregivers may need information and strategies from their healthcare professional to increase the number of foods acceptable to their toddlers and children and to develop a sound eating plan (Carruth et al., 1998).

Grazing

The growing toddler and child may not be hungry on a schedule, and they often do not want to stop for a meal or snack that may interrupt their playtime. If a child asks for food or liquids more frequently than every 2 to 3 hours, it is important to encourage him or her to wait until the next meal or snack time to eat.

Grazing may produce a constant feeling of fullness and cause the child to avoid eating an appropriate amount at mealtime, therefore not expanding the stomach size. Constant snacking and early satiety may result in the child not receiving adequate calories each day, thereby ultimately leading to failure to thrive (Krugman & Dubowitz, 2003). It is important to have the child sit at a table away from distractions while eating to help them better understand the difference between mealtime and playtime.

Failure to Thrive

Failure to thrive is defined by "inadequate physical growth diagnosed by observation of growth over time using a standard growth chart" (Krugman & Dubowitz, 2003). This failure to maintain adequate growth can be caused by a multitude of factors. Most often, failure to thrive is classified as organic (inability to meet calorie needs due to medical conditions, malabsorption, or increased metabolism with specific disease states) or inorganic (food shortage, incorrect mixing of formula, or neglect) (Krugman & Dubowitz, 2003).

Healthcare professionals should be aware of any factors that may contribute to poor growth. Taking a full diet history, including formula mixing techniques, can help assess if adequate calories are in fact being provided to the child. If all possible inorganic etiologies are ruled out, then a medical workup for organic failure to thrive should be undertaken. Read more about failure to thrive in Chapter 5.

Lactose Intolerance

According to Vesa, Marteau, and Korpela (2000), lactose is the "most important source of energy during the first year of human life." Intolerance is uncommon in healthy infants but can present as a result of a gastrointestinal illness, ultimately resolving with improvement of the illness. Symptoms of intolerance are similar to other gastrointestinal dysfunctions (Vesa et al., 2000), causing stomach pain, flatulence, and loose stools.

Hypolactasia can present early in childhood in African-American and Asian children but seems to appear in late childhood or adolescence for white children (Scrimshaw & Murray, 1988). Many lactose maldigesters are able to tolerate small amounts of lactose without discomfort (Vesa et al., 2000). For example, children with lactose intolerance can often drink a small amount of regular milk. Alternatives exist, such as solid cheeses that are low in lactose, and yogurt may be better tolerated.

More recently, lactose-free and low-lactose milks and ice creams are readily available. Soy milk may also be a good substitute, but caregivers should be educated that whatever the variety of substituted milk, it must be fortified with calcium and vitamin D. Careful diagnosis is important to prevent unnecessary diet restrictions that may lead to deficiencies in the essential nutrients provided by dairy products (Vesa et al., 2000). Families should be instructed on ways to meet nutrient needs if a dairy restriction is ultimately recommended.

Television Watching and Media Influence on Food Cravings

Many children spend more time watching television than interacting with their families, creating a change in key influences. More than 50% of food advertisements on television target children (Story & French, 2004). Messages often show "junk" foods as fun, exciting, and glamorous. Young people often have difficulty discriminating between education provided in television programs and information in commercials, therefore misinterpreting advertising as life-style instruction. Furthermore, because commercials are brief and to the point, they target the child's short attention span, thereby conveying an efficient and powerful message.

It is suggested that television viewing contributes to obesity by one or more of three mechanisms: displacement of physical activity, an increase in calorie consumption while watching or as a direct result of the effects of advertising, and/or reducing resting metabolism (Robinson, 2001).

The AAP (2001) proposes that children should spend no more than 2 hours per day watching television or using other electronic forms of entertainment. (Note: The AAP recommends no television watching at all for children under age 2.) Making sure that meals and snacks are not eaten while watching television may help to reduce daily television viewing. Saelens et al. (2002) found that the frequency of meals eaten while watching television was the most important predictor of long-term increase in television viewing time among children. Creating rules about eating meals in front of the television was found to decrease the probability of the child watching television for greater than 2 hours per day (Saelens et al., 2002).

Simply restricting meals while watching television may not be an entirely adequate strategy for decreasing overall inactivity. The relationship between the family environment, television viewing, and low level of activity is complex. Restricting television viewing during mealtimes may be effective, but focusing on increasing physical activity is also a component not to be overlooked (Waller, Du, & Popkin, 2003; Salmon, Timperio, Telford, Carver, & Crawford, 2005).

In a study by Burdette and Whitaker (2005) on preschool children, it was found that television viewing and outdoor play minutes were not correlated to one another or to the child's BMI. However, in an article by Gortmaker, Must, and Sobol (1996), a dose-dependent relationship between television viewing and obesity was demonstrated. Given the conflicting evidence, more research is needed regarding any possible real-world correlation between daily television viewing, activity, and excessive weight gain.

Learning Through Participation

As children grow and mature, involving them in the preparation of the meal may help to increase variety in the diet. A child will often taste what he or she has participated in preparing. Time spent in the kitchen can also be used to talk about the different colors of fruit and vegetables, to help the child understand the healthy reasons behind eating a wider variety of foods, and to promote family bonding. Furthermore, offering a choice of fruits or vegetables at a meal may help the child feel a modicum of control and inclusion. Such a practice may also promote better intake of the chosen food during the meal.

Interestingly, many studies have shown that it can be beneficial to allow a child to be involved in portioning foods onto their own plate at meals. Orlet Fisher, Rolls, and Birch (2003) showed that allowing children to serve themselves at meals may decrease the incidence of exposure to excessive portion sizes.

Choking Prevention

Having an adult always present whenever a child is eating constitutes the ultimate in safe eating practices. Because many children do not develop the skill of chewing with a grinding motion until about 4 years of age (Dietz & Stern, 1999), foods with a firmer texture that need adequate chewing may not be appropriate for young children. To prevent choking, foods should be cut into small bite-size pieces and children should remain sitting at all times while eating. Choking is more likely to occur if the child is running or falling with food in the mouth. The child should be encouraged to take small bites and avoid stuffing his or her mouth full of food. **Table 3.10** provides foods that may present a choking risk.

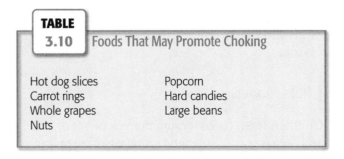

TABLE 3.10	**Foods That May Promote Choking**
Hot dog slices	Popcorn
Carrot rings	Hard candies
Whole grapes	Large beans
Nuts	

Snacks

Snacking among children is an important source of energy (Jahns, Siega-Riz, & Popkin, 2001). Toddlers and children have a comparatively small stomach size and cannot consume large amounts at meals; therefore snacks provide needed servings of healthy foods. However, Jahns et al. (2001) found that children obtain an inordinate percentage of their daily calories from snacks, so much so that at times children may snack to such an extent that they are not hungry at mealtime. On the other hand, many children continue to eat normal sized meals and simply consume excess calories during the day, leading to increased weight gain.

Instead of skipping snacks, caregivers should provide healthy snack choices. Nutritious snacks include, but are not limited to, cheese slices, carrot sticks, orange slices, yogurt, apple pieces, and peanut butter on wheat crackers. Snacks should be easy to prepare and on hand to reduce the need for quick, often unhealthy, snack choices.

Caregivers should be aware of what and how much their child is eating while watching television. Sometimes television viewing may condition a child who is not hungry to snack (Epstein, Coleman, & Myers, 1996). As stated previously, it can be helpful to prohibit meals or snacks in front of the television.

Dental Health

It is beneficial to start tooth care at a young age. Introducing a toothbrush during the toddler years can initiate a good oral hygiene routine that continues through life (Mahan & Escott-Stump, 2000). Children often snack on sugary sticky foods that may stay in the teeth and provide an ideal environment for growth of the bacteria that cause dental caries. Also, the continued exposure of the teeth to the sugary drinks, such as juice, contributes to dental caries in children (AAP, Committee on Nutrition, 2001). Teaching young children to brush their teeth after meals and snacks can help to reduce the incidence of cavities.

Role Models

Children learn by observing the behaviors of others and then incorporating and imitating these practices. Parents modeling healthy behaviors, accessibility to sedentary pursuits at home, sibling influences, and family television viewing habits may be important determinants of a child's activity level and healthy behaviors (Rachlin, Logue, Gibbon, & Frankel, 1986). Food choices and dietary quality in the early years of life are usually influenced by parents or other primary caregivers.

As children mature they tend to eat more meals outside the home. Therefore it is essential to model good habits while the child is at a young impressionable age. Modeling food behaviors is one of the most effective ways to promote increased consumption of healthy foods (Dennison et al., 1998). Parents who do not eat fruits and vegetables tend to raise children who refuse these foods as well.

Negatives thoughts regarding food can also begin at a young age. Preadolescent girls are becoming more at risk for picking up dieting habits from female caregivers. Girls who diet by adolescence tend to have mothers who are often overtly encouraging or unconsciously demonstrating the means to diet through their own restrictive habits (Birch & Fisher, 2000).

CRITICAL **Thinking**

Evidence suggests that more young girls are becoming concerned with gaining weight because of the influence by caregivers and the media. Can you give some examples of this? What can be done to prevent this?

Breakfast

As children enter school there becomes less time in the morning for simple things, such as eating a healthy breakfast. It is important to develop the habit of including breakfast in the daily morning routine. Eating breakfast has been shown to increase energy and concentration at school. It also allows for a balanced metabolism, thereby aiding in the child's ability to maintain a healthy weight. Studies have shown that skipping breakfast is related to increased BMI and risk of obesity (Cho, Dietrich, Brown, Clark, & Block, 2003).

Breakfast is an excellent time to consume a needed serving of fruit, whole grains, dairy, or protein. Many schools have a breakfast program, but it is important to be aware of what foods are being offered and how much the child is consuming during this time. At breakfast, schools provide 25% or more of the daily recommended levels of key nutrients that children need (School Breakfast Program Food and

Research Action Center, n.d.), but this is often not controlled to avoid excess. The child is usually able to make their own food choices, so education concerning appropriate portion sizes and healthy choices can be helpful.

Nutrition at School

Many schools participate in the government funded lunch program. The National School Lunch program is a federally assisted meal program. Regulations create a standard for school lunches in order to provide one-third of the Recommended Daily Allowance for protein, vitamins A and C, calcium, iron, and calories (U.S. Department of Agriculture, 2005). Meals must meet nutritional requirements, but individual schools are able to decide what foods to serve and how to prepare them.

The program guarantees that every child will meet at least 33% of his or her daily needs each day. It is true that many children rely on this program for needed nutrition. However, to meet the required 33% of calories, at times meal options do not contain particularly healthy choices. Less than nutritious options such as nachos, giant hoagies, and hot dogs are common at many schools. Also, many children receive a large portion of their daily calories from snacks, which often leads to excess daily calories when combined with school lunches and fast food consumption. Lunch is often provided at a discount or may be free to students, making it unrealistic to expect these children to pack lunches containing healthier options. Therefore it seems reasonable for schools to become more adept at offering well-balanced meals.

Peer influence also plays a roll in lunchtime nutrition. Food choices are often affected by what friends at school are eating. Children may be encouraged to try a new food if others around them are eating it. On the other hand, such influence may also contribute to requesting more "junk" foods that other children bring to school.

Parents and children may benefit from education on choosing healthier options at school. If available, reviewing the monthly menu with the child can prompt discussion on which foods are the healthier choice.

Physical Activity

Physical activity is an important part of a healthy life-style. It promotes muscle building, increased metabolism, and disease prevention. Among children, overweight, obesity, and low levels of physical activity have been shown to be associated with increased risk of disease later in life (Baranowski, 1992). Exercise is also a vital aspect of achieving maximal peak bone mass (AAP, 1999).

With age and increased independence, physical activity often decreases. The CDC demonstrated that 61% of 9- to 13-year-olds do not participate in organized after-school activities and 23% did not participate in any physical activity during their free time (CDC, 2003). Something as simple as parental encouragement may be all some children need to become more active. Studies have shown that parents who are supportive of their children's participation in physical activities are more likely to have an active child (Sallis, Prochaska, & Taylor, 2000).

Sedentary activities such as watching television and playing video games have become the preferred after-school pastime. Parents, caregivers, health educators, and teachers should promote enjoyable alternatives to sedentary behaviors to increase children's participation in physical activity and prevent unhealthy weight gain (Salmon et al., 2005). If the safety of the neighborhood is poor, then caregivers should work to create inside activities that keep the child active and away from sedentary pursuits.

The bottom line is that physical activity should be a part of everyday life. If children are cared for outside of the home after school, parents may need to discuss with day-care providers or other caregivers the stated preference that their child be active and not spend the afternoon involved in sedentary activities. Being active as a family can help everyone to stay healthy and provides an excellent means of spending quality time together.

Excessive Weight Gain

Obesity is becoming a more common problem with young children. Fifteen percent of children ages 6 to 11 years are estimated to be overweight in the United States (Ogden, Flegal, Carroll, & Johnson, 2002). Inactivity and larger portion sizes are contributors to this multifaceted and increasingly severe problem. Studies demonstrate that increased size of food portions offered can stimulate a young child's food intake, causing excess calorie consumption at meals (Orlet Fisher et al., 2003).

Obesity prevention programs focused on diet and exercise are becoming more and more available to young children. However, Etelson et al. (2003)

Juice Consumption

In the past fruit juice was consistently recommended by pediatricians as a good source of vitamin C for children and also an additional source of hydration (AAP, Committee on Nutrition, 2001). As mentioned previously, juices high in vitamin C have been shown to aid in the body's absorption of iron. However, the high carbohydrate content of juice often leads to malabsorption in children.

Over time juice has become the preferred beverage among many children. Children aged 1 to 12 years make up about 18% of the total population but are responsible for almost one-third of the average daily intake of juice and juice drinks (AAP, Committee on Nutrition, 2001).

In toddlers and children juice often inappropriately replaces formula, milk, and water intake and is also used as a replacement for whole fruit and vegetable servings. Fruit juice accounts for about 33% of all fruit and vegetable intake among preschoolers and 50% of fruit intake by children aged 2 to 18 (Dennison, 1996). When replacing formula and milk, the child often does not receive optimal calories and nutrients needed for growth. Excessive juice consumption has been shown to contribute to inorganic failure to thrive and decreased stature in some children. Juice provides empty carbohydrate calories and decreases the child's appetite at mealtime, causing overall decreased calorie intake (Smith & Lifshitz, 1994; Dennison, 1996). Conversely, it has also been shown to be associated with high caloric intake and obesity in some studies when consumed frequently throughout the day (Dennison, 1996).

Only pasteurized 100% fruit juice is recommended for growing children and is the specific type of juice provided by WIC. Juice should be watered down for the child and should not be available to be sipped throughout the day. Juice should be limited to no more than 4 to 6 ounces per day for children aged 1 to 6 years (AAP, Committee on Nutrition, 2001).

The IOM has recommended a change in the WIC package to decrease the juice content. Also, the AAP's Top Ten Resolutions for 2005 stated that their number 2 priority is to get the message out that juice is not a healthy choice for children.

reported that participation in obesity prevention programs and life-style changes are dependent on the parents' ability to recognize that their child is overweight. In their study it was determined that no parent of a child above the 75th percentile for BMI/age was able to correctly estimate how overweight their child was. These parents universally believed their children were less overweight than actually recorded. Therefore if a parent perceives a child to be at low risk for being overweight, the intervention is likely to be delayed. Read more about childhood obesity in Chapter 7.

Supplements for Increased Calories

Children who are not able to consume adequate calories each day may need a high calorie nutritional supplement. There are multiple supplements available designed specifically for growing children. Pediasure®, Nutren Jr®, Resource Just for Kids®, and Carnation Instant Breakfast Junior® are just a few supplements available for children ages 1 through 10 years. These supplements are often packaged in child friendly containers and come in a variety of popular flavors. After

age 10 most adult supplements, such as Ensure®, Boost®, and Nutren 1.0®, are acceptable. It is essential to note that supplements should be used under the care of a healthcare professional.

Role of Parents in Promoting Healthy Nutrition in Early Childhood
Barbara Robinson, MPH, RD, CNSD

Social science research contributes to our understanding of why young children consume particular foods and display specific eating behaviors. Historically, nutrition professionals have focused more on the science of nutrition in childhood rather than on why children eat what they eat. A comment to this effect by Lipsitt, Crook, and Booth (1985) is still true more than two decades later: "Research on the psychological aspects of feeding development has lagged behind the study of nutritional requirements for physiologic sustenance. . . ." Lipsitt et al. go on to state, ". . . the style and quality of caretaker–infant interactions are determinative of other (non-feeding) interactions and subsequent feeding behavior, including preferences and aversions."

The level of attention devoted to the influence of parenting in relationship to diet quality might be increasing. Recently, the burgeoning childhood obesity problem may have prompted medical and nutritional experts to focus more on the behavioral determinants of the nutritional content of children's diets. In 2004 The American Dietetic Association and the Gerber Products Company joined together to publish the "Start Healthy Feeding Guidelines for Infants and Toddlers" (Butte et al., 2004). These are comprehensive guidelines that advise feeding based on developmental readiness rather than on age and seek to help adult caregivers understand hunger and fullness cues in addition to nutritional requirements. In the Start Healthy Feeding Guidelines the value of repeated exposures to healthy foods and age-appropriate physical activity are addressed (Butte et al., 2004). In 2005 The American Heart Association published a scientific statement entitled "Dietary Recommendations for Children and Adolescents" (Gidding et al., 2005). As is typical in a statement such as this, specific nutrient goals are discussed and nutritional recommendations are provided. What makes this statement unique is the significant focus on the effects of parenting in relation to the nutritional content of children's diets.

The context in which complementary foods are offered can facilitate either acceptance or rejection of new flavors. There is a window of opportunity in the normal development of infant and child food preferences. To a large extent food preferences and eating behaviors are formed in the early years of a child's life and become the foundation for lifelong eating habits. "Parents are a child's first teachers" is often quoted in discussions on child development. Adult family members not only determine the content of a young child's diet, but they and older siblings are role models. There is another dimension to food acceptance: the emotional bond between the young child and the primary feeder. The influence of the family environment, including the type of foods to which a child is exposed, continues throughout childhood, but the impact of parenting on diet is greatest in the early years. The goal for this section is to discuss the relationship between the home environment and early childhood nutrition.

Eating Is a Learned Behavior: Acquisition of Flavor and Food Preferences

Children are not born with a preference for French fries rather than green beans. As demonstrated over and over again in behavioral research, eating is a behavior that is learned through exposure and repetition (Birch & Marlin, 1982; Sullivan & Birch, 1990; Skinner, Carruth, Bounds, & Zeigler, 2002). How early in a child's life does this learning begin to take place? What impact, if any, does exposure to flavor compounds in utero have on the developing fetus? Interestingly, researchers have found that the amnion, or the fetal environment, contains flavor compounds specific to the maternal food intake (Mennella, Johnson, & Beauchamp, 1995, 2001; Schall, Marlier, & Soussignan, 2000). Furthermore, it has been observed that the flavor compounds a fetus is exposed to from the maternal diet via amniotic fluid are recognized by the infant postnatally, as reflected by newborns' facial, mouthing, and orienting responses when exposed to the same flavors orally. Mennella, Jagnow, and Beauchamp (2001) demonstrated that intake of a specific food flavor (carrot) during either pregnancy or lactation influenced liking or disliking of carrot flavor in the mothers' infants at 5 to 6 months of age. One implication from the findings about breast-feeding and the maternal diet is that infants who are breast-fed are exposed to a wide variety of flavors that reflect the maternal diet. Conversely, formula-fed infants become accustomed to only one flavor, that of the formula.

Neonatal and Early Infant Weight Gain

The Infant Growth Study, conducted by the University of Pennsylvania and the Children's Hospital of Philadelphia, showed that infants who gained weight rapidly by 4 months of age tended to be heavier in later childhood. A higher weight at 24 months of age was observed in children who were also heavier at 3 months of age and who exhibited increased nutritive sucking and increased habitual food intake (Stettler, Zemel, & Kumanyika, 2002).

The potential for long-term consequences to very early nutritional experiences could have significant implications for guidance to pregnant women and new parents. Early childhood healthcare providers are appropriately concerned when an infant or young child is failing to grow at an acceptable rate. Newer research into the potential for negative health consequences of rapid weight gain should promote careful guidance for adequate but not excessive rate of weight gain. This has important implications, as discussed by Stettler et al. (2002), who found a strong association between early toddler weight gain and obesity at age 7.

Similar results were found in a study conducted in England on children who were infants in 1991 and 1992 (Ong et al., 2006). Parents reported intake at 4 months of age and children were weighed and measured up to 10 additional times up to the age of 5 years. Among infants who were bottle fed or who received a combination of formula and breast milk, a higher calorie intake as early as 4 months of age predicted more weight gain in early childhood and a higher BMI at ages 1, 2, 3, and 4 years.

Development of Food Preferences

Although there seems to be an association between consumption of certain foods during both pregnancy and breast-feeding and food preferences of the infant, there has been insufficient research to determine the degree of influence that maternal diet has on an infant's flavor preference. This remains an intriguing area for further investigation. There has been more exploration into the developmental nature of how children learn what to eat. Transitioning from the suckling and sucking that occurs with breast-feeding or bottle feeding to tasting, chewing, and selecting food flavors and textures is a developmental process that occurs in the context of the family environment. Eating is an activity that is repeated over and over again; feeding behaviors and preferences are shaped through this repetition. Because eating behaviors are shaped through repetition, parents will have the best chance of helping their children learn to like healthy foods if they continue to offer a food in spite of apparent expression of dislike the first few times a child tastes a new food.

Why is it typically necessary to provide several exposures before infants will accept new foods? Although infants are curious, they are also neophobic; that is, they are cautious about trying new foods and/or might not like them until they have tried them numerous times (Birch & Fisher, 1995; Addessi, Galloway, Visalberghi, & Birch, 2005). Parents should not become discouraged and should continue to offer healthy foods in the context of a pleasant feeding experience. Although there is no guarantee that a child will like a given food, early exposure to a variety of healthy foods appears to be a critical factor in fostering preferences for healthy foods. Birch and Marlin (1982) showed that a higher number of food exposures were necessary in children aged 4 to 5 years than in children aged 2 years, indicating that younger children are more likely to accept new flavors. Children aged 2 years accepted new foods after 10 exposures, but it took 11 to 15 exposures to a new food before children aged 4 to 5 years established a preference for that food. Skinner et al. (2002) showed that 8-year-old children preferred the same foods that they liked at the age of 4, demonstrating the durability of previously established food preferences. These findings suggest that food preferences are more difficult to change as children become older. There might be implications for confronting the increasing incidence of childhood obesity, which is becoming evident even in very young children. Changing established food preferences is very difficult for the family and is a challenge for healthcare providers.

The conventional approach to childhood obesity can be used to illustrate this point, as the emphasis has been on identification of existing childhood obesity by measuring BMI and then intervening if the BMI is over the 95th percentile. The BMI has become the standard by which practitioners screen for excessive weight status. Because BMI is not measured until 24 months of age, early excessive weight gain would not lead to a categorization of risk. It takes more training and skill to determine risk of becoming overweight based on food intake patterns, and physicians might not make a special effort to discuss an infant's or toddler's eating habits or opportunities for physical activity with parents. Therefore indicators of emerging childhood obesity might be missed (Salsberry & Reagan, 2005). Setting the stage for positive eating behaviors in early childhood as a vehicle for obesity prevention is just beginning to be considered by pediatric researchers and clinicians. Data from a descriptive survey (Feeding Infants and Toddlers Study [FITS]) conducted in 2003 by Dwyer, Sutor, and Hendricks (2004) highlights for child health professionals the benefit of shifting the focus from changing established eating habits when a weight problem is identified to promoting healthy eating behaviors to parents of all infants and toddlers whether they meet risk criteria for becoming overweight or not.

Feeding Infants and Toddlers Study

FITS explored the diet composition of infants and toddlers ages 4 to 24 months (Fox, Pac, Devaney, & Janowski, 2004). FITS data show that 18% to 23% of infants and toddlers consumed no vegetables and 23% to 33% consumed no fruits during a day. And by 1 year of age white potatoes were the most commonly consumed vegetables (often in the form of French fries), whereas the deep yellow/orange vegetables that were consumed in infancy were no longer a part of the diet. Foods high in added fats and sugars, including sweetened beverages, sweetened cereals, cookies, processed meats, cakes, and pies, provided approximately 19% of calories in toddlers. By the end of the second year more than 11% of children were consuming carbonated sodas. Such foods and beverages can be classified as **competitive foods**, which are those foods that are less nutritious, such as high-fat high-sugar snacks, soda, and other sweetened beverages. Easy access to these foods competes with healthier food choices for attention and consumption.

> **Competitive foods:** Those foods that are less nutritious, such as high-fat high-sugar snacks, soda, and other sweetened beverages. Easy access to these foods competes with healthier food choices for attention and consumption.

Parents

Parents and/or adult caregivers play a central role in the development of early childhood feeding behaviors. FITS describes poor quality dietary intakes of infants and toddlers, which are a direct reflection of the choices that parents are making for their young children. The proliferation of commercially available high-sugar high-fat food and beverages contributes to the poor diet quality, but there are other influences on parents as well. Carruth and Skinner (2000) performed multiple interviews of mothers of children aged 2 to 54 months to identify sources and types of information and advice mothers received about feeding their children and to determine whether these sources differed as infants grew into toddlers and preschoolers. Sources of nutrition and feeding included family, especially grandmothers; professionals; magazines; books; and videotapes. (Unfortunately, the interview process did not include questions about more insidious influences such as corporate food advertising geared toward children.) Other contemporary influences on mothers' food choices for children included family composition (e.g., single-parent families versus two-parent families) and lack of time due to employment outside of the home.

From 1970 to 1999 the percentage of women with young children (under age 6) who were working outside the home increased from 30% to 62%. Mothers have traditionally been more involved in preparing meals, offering foods, and feeding. Skinner et al. (2002) found that food preferences of 2- and 3-year-olds are related to mothers' food preferences, based on foods that were liked, disliked, or never tasted by both the mother and the child. If a mother never learned to like vegetables and fruits, for example, she is less likely to prepare and offer these foods.

Modeling

In addition to repeatedly exposing children to a variety of healthy foods, parents have another important role to play. Parents, other adults who are with a young child regularly, and older siblings all serve as models for young children in regard to eating. The effects of modeling on a child's food preferences are additive to the effects of repeated exposure. The social learning theory as described by Bandura (1972) became the foundation on which behavioral psychology experts conducted research on how children acquire food preferences. Bandura showed that in other areas of human interaction, modeling is a process that is a strong influence on behavior.

Eating is both a social experience and a repetitive experience. Other people in a young child's environment become the models for food choice, and children develop preferences for the foods they see others eating. Harper and Sanders (1975) contrasted the degree of modeling influence between mothers and strangers on young children. There were several pertinent findings. When mothers modeled eating a certain food, children were more willing to try the new food than when strangers modeled consumption of the same food. Older children were influenced by modeling but to a lesser degree than younger children. And finally, but perhaps most important, new foods were accepted more readily by children when the adult model ate the food with the child rather than just offering the food to the child. This has implications for the value of encouraging family meals, which have become less frequent as families become busier with work and extracurricular activities.

Birch (1980) investigated whether the effects of modeling on food preferences were sustained after the modeling event. She found that preschoolers who learned to like previously "nonpreferred foods" through modeling exposure continued to like the new food several weeks later. This was interpreted as learned behavior rather than just the conformity that would be expected when others at the table are eating the same foods. An additional finding found in other studies is that 3-year-old children are more readily influenced in their feeding behaviors than 4-year-old children. The greater magnitude of influence seems to indicate that earlier influences on food preferences have the greatest impact.

Research by Addessi et al. (2005) showed the importance of modeling on preference of a specific food. Three groups of 2- to 5-year-old children were offered pasta with very strong food flavors added. The added flavors were cumin, caper paste, and anchovy paste. These food flavors were considered to be new or "novel" to the children. The respective flavors of the semolina were colored yellow, green, and red. Familiar adults served as eating models. In one group the children were served the food and the model was present but was not eating. In the second group the children were served yellow pasta but the adult model was eating different colored pasta. Children and the adult model in the third group were both given the same color pasta served in clear containers. When each of the trials was over, the children switched groups after a "break period" of 1 week. The pasta for the adult models was flavored to be palatable so they would eat with enthusiasm. The result of this simple experiment was very informative. Children who were given the same food (children identified it by color) as the adult model ate the most, seemed to enjoy it the most, and had the least hesitation when first trying the food. The authors of this study suggested that children might learn to like more foods if day-care and preschool teachers routinely and enthusiastically ate with young children. However, a 2002 study found that preschool teachers typically eat very few of the foods that are offered to children (Hendy, 2002).

Historically, efforts at improving nutrition and activity behaviors have targeted school-aged children, and children have been regarded as the "agents of change." More recently, however, settings where young children are together have been targeted as well. Brocodile the Crocodile was a 9-month study of 307 children ages 3 to 5 (and their parents) in 18 day care/preschools to compare changes over the 9 months in BMI z-scores for appropriate weight gain in a control and intervention group. The intervention promoted healthier food intake, more activity, and less television and video viewing. The results were positive for all the intended behaviors and for no increase in the BMI z-score in the intervention group as opposed to a slight increase in the control group. Parents and daytime caregivers were considered to be the agents of change, that is, the people who intentionally changed their behaviors to achieve the desired outcome (Dennison, 2002).

Self-Regulation

Flavor and food preferences are learned and can be modified through repeated exposure and modeling. Conversely, the ability to regulate volume of food intake is believed to be a normal human newborn behavior. Based on social science research, many child development experts believe that infants are innate "self-regulators" and possess the ability to respond to their own internal cues of hunger and satiety and that they communicate these feelings to feeders (Shea, Basch, Contento, & Rand Zybert, 1992). In young infants, crying, excited arm and leg movements, and moving forward as the breast or bottle is offered with mouth open can be signs of hunger. Signs of satiety can include fussing during feeding, slowing down the pace of eating, falling asleep, or spitting out or refusing the nipple.

● Learning Point Some parents are not skilled at interpreting infant "cues" or signals, and without proper guidance parents' behaviors can disrupt this natural regulation and children can develop responses that manifest in disordered eating.

One of the many reasons breast-feeding is encouraged is because it allows infants to choose their own portion sizes. The infant guides the feeding because mothers typically nurse until the infant indicates he or she is satisfied. The quantity of breast milk consumed by the infant is primarily under the infant's control (Dewey, Heinig, Nommensen, & Lonnerdal, 1991). The mother does not teach over-consumption by expecting her infant to finish the bottle. After the first few months of an infant's life, because of the belief that their infant is not being satisfied by infant formula or for other reasons, some parents are eager to begin solid foods before an infant is ready.

The AAP supports exclusive breast-feeding for approximately 6 months but recognizes that infants are often developmentally ready to accept complementary (solid) foods between 4 and 6 months (Kleinman, 2004). Developmental readiness should be the guide for when to begin offering complementary foods. Control of the tongue, which is important for swallowing, chewing, and handling of foods, and the ability to hold the head up are two developmental indicators of readiness. Fomon and Bell (1993) advised that when an adult spoons food into the mouth of an infant who does not yet posses the skills to show that he or she is no longer hungry, this adult behavior might increase the likelihood that the infant will learn to overeat.

When feeding their infants, some parents react to fussing or crying by persisting in offering food when a child is not actually hungry and is expressing something entirely different from hunger. At other times parents do not respond to signs of fullness and continue to feed beyond a child's hunger. Starting at around the age of 6 months infants display more overt signs of interest or disinterest in eating. Children who are being spoon-fed will close their lips and turn away when offered food if they are not hungry. Quite simply, infants seem to eat when hungry and stop when full. Although it appears that infants possess the innate ability to self-regulate, childhood eating behaviors are formed in a social context, usually within a family. Many parents do not practice healthy eating themselves and/or may not understand the value of repeated exposures to healthy foods for young children or that their infants and young children know when they are hungry and full.

Parents' expectations that infants will immediately either accept or reject a new food can be a barrier to successful feeding. It has long been known that repeated exposures to new foods are typically necessary for acceptance (Birch & Marlin, 1990). Furthermore, when parents do not accurately interpret cues or messages from their infants and are also concerned that their children are eating too much or too little, they might resort to coercion of a child at mealtimes to respond to a meal or snack according to guidelines imposed by the parents. Parents often believe they have to motivate their infants to eat. However, children are naturally curious about trying new foods and will consume a varied diet if the foods are made available to them in the context of a pleasing and positive feeding experience. Children should be allowed to use their own hunger and satiety cues to initiate and terminate eating. Repeated opportunities to taste a new food are positively correlated with eventual preference, but coaxing, coaching, urging, or bribing, even when conducted in a pleasant fashion, interferes with the learning process of exploring and ultimately enjoying new foods, which comes from within the child.

Both coercing a child to eat a defined amount or limiting access to foods can promote disordered eating (i.e., lack of response to internal cues and overeating or under-eating). Some parents become overly controlling in regard to what foods their young children are expected to eat. This has the unintended effect of promoting disordered eating in children, which persists into adulthood. Many pediatric nutritionists are familiar with the work of Ellyn Satter, who has written extensively on the feeding relationship between parent and child. Satter (1999) advised that parents should offer healthy foods at regular times during the day but that children should be the ones to determine whether and how much they will eat. Carper, Fisher, and Birch (2000) developed the kids' child-feeding questionnaire and used it to assess the relationship between controlling parental behavior during feeding and diminished use of their own hunger and satiety cues by 5-year-old girls. These researchers found that girls who perceived they were pressured to eat (parents' urging) engaged in both restrained eating and disinhibited eating. Cutting and colleagues (2000) found an association between the overeating styles of mothers who engaged in disinhibited eating and their daughters, who exhibited the same tendencies in an experimental environment.

Some social scientists believe that children can relearn self-regulation of energy intake through training to focus on internal cues to hunger and satiety. In an intriguing study, Johnson (2000) used dolls with detachable stomachs of three sizes to correspond with an empty, in-between, and full stomach. Over the course of 6 weeks children learned to focus on feelings of hunger and fullness based on the three stomach sizes.

Although some individuals continue to self-regulate their calorie intake into adulthood, many people do not, as demonstrated by the work of Engell et al. (1995) and Booth, Fuller, and Lewis (1981). In general, when does the shift away from self-regulation occur? There is evidence that this process begins early. In a small study of 32 children, Rolls and coworkers (2000) demonstrated that children at the age of 3½ responded well to internal cues and ate only the amounts they were accustomed to eating, but 5-year-old children ate larger amounts when the portions served were larger than their usual portions. The larger portions responded to by the 5-year-old children were an "external" cue. The findings of a similar study were interesting in that when 3- to 5-year-old children were repeatedly given a larger portion, they consumed about 25% more calories. However, when the same children were allowed to serve themselves they did not eat a larger than usual portion even though more food was available. This study suggests that the difference in response to more available food is that although parents offered a particular food, the children chose how much to eat and were better able to self-regulate their energy intake.

The impact of parenting related to feeding can be seen in eating styles of the children; the strongest association has been seen between mothers and their daughters. Birch and Fisher (2000) examined the influence on daughters' eating habits of maternal–child feeding practices. Mothers who reported they tended to restrict their own food consumption also restricted their daughters' food consumption. This is an example of how the inborn ability to self-regulate can be disrupted. Birch and Fisher also looked at short-term energy regulation of 3- to 6-year-old children after a meal. Daughters of mothers who scored higher on a scale measuring **dietary disinhibition** ate more when they had free access to food after they had already eaten a meal than did the children of mothers who were able to self-regulate. Although fathers and sons were also evaluated in this study, no relationship was found between dietary disinhibition between fathers and

Dietary disinhibition: Unrestrained eating without regard to hunger or satiety.

daughters, fathers and sons, or mothers and sons. Both maternal excessive weight and maternal dietary disinhibition were correlated with excessive weight in 3- to 6-year-old daughters. "Emotional" eating is commonly used to represent the phenomenon of disinhibited eating.

Are there some specific parenting styles that might be more likely to foster disordered eating in children? Baumrind (1998) described four different parenting styles. Rhee et al. (2006) examined the relationship between each of four parenting styles and excessive weight status in first-graders. In this study, parenting style was classified when the children were 4½ years old and the children were weighed 2 years later. The results of the study showed that a strict environment coupled with a lack of emotional responsiveness (authoritarian style) is most strongly associated with excessive weight in children. The kind of parent who is insensitive to the child's emotional needs and development might, for example, create a structure that requires a child to finish his or her entire meal, regardless of hunger. In this scenario an external cue would be imposed, disturbing the child's innate self-regulation. In the study by Rhee et al. first-graders with authoritarian parents were found to have almost five times the odds of being overweight. The odds for children with permissive or neglectful parents were also higher than those with authoritative parents by almost twice as much. Children whose parents displayed an authoritative parenting style (firm but loving) had the lowest prevalence of excessive weight.

> **Parenting Styles**
>
> Parenting styles affect all areas of children's behavior and development, including eating behaviors. Baumrind (1998) defined four different parenting styles:
>
> 1. **Authoritative:** Parents exhibit consistent firm regulations and control; however, they give a clear explanation to their child for their standards. Authoritative parents are loving and supportive. In addition, these parents believe in autonomy for their children.
> 2. **Authoritarian:** Parents are very demanding of their child and are not strong believers of giving children a response and providing explanations. They discourage give-and-take feedback with their child. A parent who exhibits this style of parenting believes that it is "his/her way or no way." They tell their child what they should do and do not expect any feedback from the child.
> 3. **Permissive:** Parents demand very little of their children in regard to following rules, and they allow their children to do what they want. They provide minimal guidance. They are not neglectful, but they do not provide the structure of rules and consequences for behaviors.
> 4. **Rejecting-neglecting:** Parents do not monitor their child's behavior and tend to be disengaged from their child. They do not set limits for what the child does. Also, they are not responsive, so they do not provide any type of warmth to their child.

Anticipatory Guidance

Well-child visits to primary care providers (i.e., pediatricians, family practitioners, and pediatric nurse practitioners) represent a missed opportunity for helping parents to promote healthy eating behaviors in their very young children. Well-child visits are most frequent in the first 2 years of a child's life, coinciding with the time of establishment of food preferences and eating behaviors. The concept of anticipatory guidance, or the provision of accurate messages before a practice is established, is well known in pediatric primary care medicine. Conceptually, enhancing the nutrition information that is usually discussed with behavioral strategies for promoting healthy eating makes sense. The reality is that primary care physicians are concerned about the lack of time they have for each well-child visit and, also, parents might suffer from information overload if too many topics are discussed on visits (Barkin et al., 2005). Nevertheless, physician–parent encounters at well-child visits present a potential opportunity for primary care providers to use age-appropriate "talking points" as a way to discuss early childhood nutrition. Some key messages, such as fruit is a more healthy choice than juice, could be reiterated at several well-child visits at various ages. If supported by teaching of primary care physicians to make them more adept at providing anticipatory guidance counseling and age-appropriate handouts that parents can take home, such discussions with parents of all children might foster healthier eating habits and might have a secondary effect of reducing the incidence of new cases of childhood obesity.

To accompany the above discussion between healthcare providers and parents, the parents can be provided with a handout to take home such as the one seen here:

Helping Your Child Stay Healthy
at 12 to 15 months

What does your child drink?

Now is a good time to offer whole milk and water in a cup.

- Soda, fruit drinks, and Kool-Aid don't help your child's body. Why not?
- They are easy to drink and taste so sweet that your child might not learn to like flavors of other foods, like fruits and vegetables.
- They add extra calories but not many nutrients. Milk is more nutritious.

Your child is learning about her world, including what foods she likes.

- She will learn to eat healthy foods by watching you eat them.

Children learn to like foods they are given, especially before age 2.

- Now is the time to offer a wide variety of healthy foods, so that your child learns good eating habits for life.
- Did you know that children do best when they eat at a regular time and place?
- Make mealtimes pleasant. Turn off the television. Enjoy one another!

What are some healthy foods at this age?

- All fruits and vegetables (cut grapes in half and carrots lengthwise) are good choices.
- Soft beans, such as kidney beans, make good finger foods.
- Yogurt, cheese, and whole-wheat toast with jam are healthy snacks for your child.
- Sweet potato, broccoli, mango, oatmeal, beans, watermelon, cantaloupe, and milk are so nutritious that some experts call these "super foods."
- Do you know that children will learn to prefer less healthy foods such as French fries, doughnuts, candy, and other sweets if they are given them often?

Activity

- Have fun together inside and outside! Enjoy active playtime together such as walking, running, jumping, kicking and throwing a ball, or dancing.
- This is a great age for visiting zoos, beaches, and parks. Babies love swings.
- Your child will learn to be active if it is fun and if she sees that you enjoy being active.

Good Nutrition for Your 1-Year-Old Child

- Encourage your child to drink water during the day.
- Limit juice to 4 ounces a day.
- Serve milk with meals and snacks.

These foods are healthy and just right for your 1 year-old

Breakfast
½ cup of plain Cheerios
½ cup whole milk (red top)
½ banana, sliced

Snack
½ cup of yogurt
2 to 3 slices of fresh or canned peaches (drain juice from can)

Lunch
¼ cup rice
½ cup kidney beans cooked with tomatoes and a small amount of oil
¼ cup soft melon slices (no seeds)

Snack
½ cup whole milk
1 to 2 graham crackers
2 teaspoons peanut butter

Dinner
¼ cup meat loaf
¼ cup mashed potatoes
¼ cup cooked broccoli, cut up
1 small piece of corn bread
1 fresh orange, cut up, no seeds
½ cup whole milk

Used with permission from Shalon, L. S., Robinson, B. B., & DeLessio, D. (2003). Anticipatory Guidance in Early Childhood for Overweight Prevention.

Summary

It is undeniable that to provide essential nutrients for optimal growth and development, toddlers and young children must consume a wide variety of foods. This varied diet, coupled with physical fitness, is an excellent beginning for these young lives.

Growing toddlers and children rely on caregivers to provide them with adequate nutrition and guide them in the development of proper mealtime behaviors, ultimately resulting in healthy life-styles into the adult years and beyond. However, outside influences, including the media and the food and beverage industries, make this challenge ever more difficult. Healthcare professionals must provide support for each family, with the goal of fostering understanding regarding the importance of good nutrition and consistent physical activity, and they must help parents acquire the necessary parenting skills to put their beliefs into practice when raising their young children.

There are many influences on the diet quality of the young child. As detailed in this chapter, constructing an environment for promotion of healthy eating in early childhood includes authoritative parenting style, repeated and early exposure to healthy foods, family dining, keeping competitive foods out of the home, and provision of sound advice before childhood eating habits are established (anticipatory guidance).

These are guidelines for parents that encompass the domains of infant and toddler development, parent–child interaction, the feeding relationship, nutritional requirements, development of food preferences, and eating behaviors as well as television viewing and physical activity during infancy and the toddler years. Central to the recommendations is the concept put forth in the guidelines as follows: "Responsive parenting is at the core of a healthy infant–parent feeding relationship (Butte et al., 2004).

Case Study 1

Anna is a 2½ year old girl. Her mother considers her a picky eater. She loves milk, and sometimes will only drink at a meal and pick at the other foods. Her favorite foods are oatmeal, yogurt, dried cereal, macaroni and cheese, and pasta with tomato sauce. Her mom is concerned that she is not getting enough nutrients. Her growth has started to slowly fall off her normal curve, and she also seems pale and more tired during the day.

Questions: What are some nutritional concerns you may have for Anna? What suggestions could you make to her mother?

Case Study 2

Mark is a 5-year-old boy who loves snack foods. He doesn't really like to sit down for a meal. His mom leaves the snacks out so while he is playing he can grab a bite or two and then continue to play. He carries his sippy cup of juice around with him too in case he gets thirsty. He has not been growing well, but his mom says that once he grows out of this phase, he will catch up.

Questions: Why might Mark's growth be inadequate? What changes to Mark's current eating habits would you recommend?

Case Study 3

Tony is an 11-year-old boy whose favorite activity is his PlayStation system. He loves to come home from school and start playing right away. He usually grabs a large bag of potato chips and a soda from the fridge and snacks while he plays. He takes a break for dinner, but then he heads right back to the game. Tony has always plotted around the 50th percentile for weight and height for age, but lately he has been gaining weight and is now greater than the 95th percentile for weight. His father is not concerned, reporting that he was the same way at his age but "thinned out" as he got older.

Questions: Should Tony's weight gain be a concern, despite his family history? What recommendations could be made to the family?

Websites

For Families and Professionals

Bright Futures www.brightfutures.org
Food for Tots http://www.foodfortots.com
Kids Health http://websrv01.kidshealth.org/parent
Nutrition for Kids http://www.nutritionforkids.com
Satter, Ellyn www.ellynsatter.com
Tiny Tummies http://www.tinytummies.com

For Professionals

Pediatric Basics: *Journal of Pediatric (Early Childhood) Nutrition and Development* www.gerber.com/content/usa/html/pages/pediatricbasics
Zero to Three: a resource organization for the first 3 years of life www.zerotothree.org

For Parents, Professionals, and Children

www.celebratehealthyeating.org
www.smallsteps.gov

References

Normal Nutrition for Toddler Through School-Aged Children

American Academy of Pediatrics (AAP). (1999). Calcium requirements of infants, children, and adolescents. *Pediatrics, 104*, 1152–1157.

American Academy of Pediatrics (AAP). (2001). Children, adolescents, and television. *Pediatrics, 107*, 423–426.

American Academy of Pediatrics (AAP), Committee on Nutrition. (1992). Statement on Cholesterol. *Pediatrics, 90*, 469–473.

American Academy of Pediatrics (AAP), Committee on Nutrition. (1988). *Cholesterol in Childhood*. Elk Grove, IL: Author. Retrieved October 11, 2007, from http://aappolicy.aappublications.org/cgi/content/full/pediatrics;101/1/141

American Academy of Pediatrics (AAP), Committee on Nutrition. (2001). The use and misuse of fruit juice in pediatrics. *Pediatrics, 107*, 1210–1213.

American Heart Association (AHA). (n.d.). AHA scientific position. Dietary guidelines for healthy children. Retrieved February 10, 2007, from http://www.americanheart.org

Baranowski, T. (1992). Assessment, prevalence, and cardiovascular benefits of physical activity and fitness in youth. *Medicine and Science in Sports and Exercise, 24*, S237–S247.

Baranowski, T., Cullen, K. W., & Baranowski, J. (1999). Psychosocial correlates of dietary intake: Advancing dietary intervention. *Annual Review of Nutrition, 9*, 17–40.

Birch, L. L., & Fisher, J. O. (1998). Development of eating behaviors among children and adolescents. *Pediatrics, 101*, 539–549.

Birch, L. L., & Fisher, J. O. (2000). Mothers' child-feeding practices influence daughters' eating and weight. *American Journal of Clinical Nutrition, 71*, 1054–1061.

Briefel, R., Hanson, C., Fox, M. K., Novak, T., & Ziegler, P. (2006). Feeding infants and toddlers study: Do vitamin and mineral supplements contribute to nutrient adequacy or excess among US infants and toddlers? *Journal of the American Dietetic Association, 1*(Suppl.), S52–S65.

Burdette, H. L., & Whitaker, R. C. (2005). A national study of neighborhood safety, outdoor play, television viewing, and obesity in preschool children. *Pediatrics, 116*, 657–662.

Butte, N. (2000). Fat intake of children in relation to energy requirements. *American Journal of Clinical Nutrition, 72*(Suppl.), 1246S–1252S.

Butte, N. F., Wong, W. W., Hopkinson, J. M., Heinz, C. J., Mehta, N. R., & O'Brian Smith, E. (2000). Energy requirements derived from total energy expenditure and energy deposition during the first 2 y of life. *American Journal of Clinical Nutrition, 72*, 1558–1569.

Carruth, B. R., Skinner, J., Houck, K., Moran, J., Coletta, F., & Ott, D. (1998). The phenomenon of "picky eater": A behavioral marker in eating patterns of toddlers. *Journal of the American College of Nutrition, 17*, 180–186.

Carter, L. M., Whiting, S. J., Drinkwater, D. T., Zello, G. A., Faulkner, R. A., & Baily, D. A. (2001). Self-reported calcium intake and bone mineral content in children and adolescents. *Journal of the American College of Nutrition, 20*, 502–509.

Centers for Disease Control and Prevention (CDC). (2001). Recommendations for using fluoride to prevent and control dental caries in the United States. *Morbidity and Mortality Weekly Report, 50*(RR-14), 26–27.

Centers for Disease Control and Prevention (CDC). (2003). Physical activity levels among children aged 9-13 years: United States, 2002. *Morbidity and Mortality Weekly Report, 52*, 785–788.

Cho, S., Dietrich, M., Brown, C. J., Clark, C. A., & Block, G. (2003). The effect of breakfast type on total daily energy intake and body mass index: Results from the Third National Health and Nutrition Examination Survey (NHANES III). *Journal of the American College of Nutrition, 22*, 296–302.

Dennison, B. A. (1996). Fruit juice consumption by infants and children: A review. *Journal of the American College of Nutrition, 15* (Suppl. 5), 4S–11S.

Dennison, B. A. (2004). Site specific approaches prevention or management of pediatric obesity.

Dennison, B. A., Rockwell, H. L., & Baker, S. L. (1998). Fruit and vegetable intake in young children. *Journal of the American College of Nutrition, 17*, 371–378.

Dietz, W. H., & Stern, L. (1999). *American Academy of Pediatrics: Guide to Your Child's Nutrition* (pp. 41–60). New York: Random House.

Epstein, L. H., Coleman, K. J., & Myers, M. D. (1996). Exercise in treating obesity in children and adolescents. *Medicine and Science in Sports and Exercise, 28*, 428–435.

Etelson, D., Brand, D. A., Patrick, P. A., & Shirali, A. (2003). Childhood obesity: Do parents recognize this health risk? *Obesity Research, 11*, 1362–1368.

Food and Agricultural Organization, World Health Organization, and United Nations University Expert Consultation. (1985). Energy and protein requirements. *World Health Organization Technical Report Series, 724*, 1–206.

Fisher, E. A., Van Horn, L., & McGill, H. C. (1997). Nutrition and children: A statement for healthcare professionals from the Nutrition Committee, American Heart Association. *Circulation, 95*, 2332–2333.

Fisher, J. O., & Birch, L. L. (1999). Restricting access to palatable foods affects children's behavioral response, food selection, and intake. *American Journal of Clinical Nutrition, 69*, 1264–1272.

Fisher, J. O., & Birch, L. L. (2000). Parent's restrictive feeding practices are associated with young girls' negative self-evaluation of eating. *Journal of the American Dietetic Association, 100*, 1341–1346.

Fox, M. K., Reidy, K., Novak, T., & Ziegler, P. (2006). Sources of energy and nutrients in the diets of infants and toddlers. *Journal of the American Dietetic Association, 1*(Suppl.), S28–S42.

Freedman, D. S., Thornton, J. C., Mei, Z., Wang, J., Dietz, W. H., Pierson, R. N., et al. (2004). Height and adiposity among children. *Obesity Research, 12*, 846–853.

Gortmaker, S. L., Must, A., & Sobol, A. M. (1996). Television viewing as a cause of increasing obesity among children in the United States. *Archives of Pediatric and Adolescent Medicine, 150*, 356–362.

Grantham-McGregor, S., & Ani, C. (2001). A review of studies on the effect of iron deficiency on cognitive development in children. *Journal of Nutrition, 131*, 649S–668S.

Hayman, L. L. (2003). The Dietary Intervention Study in Children (DISC): Progress and prospects for primary prevention. *Progress in Cardiovascular Nursing, 18*, 4–5.

Holick, M. F., Shils, M. E., Olsen, J., Shike, M., & Ross, C.A. (Eds.). (1999). *Modern Nutrition in Health and Disease* (9th ed., p. 329). Baltimore, MD: Williams & Wilkins.

Institute of Medicine (IOM), Food and Nutrition Board. (2000–2005). Dietary reference intakes. Retrieved February 10, 2007, from http://www.nal.usda.gov/fnic/etext/000105.html

Jahns, L., Siega-Riz, A. M., & Popkin, B. M. (2001). The increasing prevalence of snacking among U.S. children from 1977 to 1996. *Journal of Pediatrics, 138*, 493–498.

Johnston, C. C., Miller, J. Z., Slemenda, C. W., Reister, T. K., Hui, S., Christian, J. C., et al. (1992). Calcium supplementation and increases in bone mineral density in children. *New England Journal of Medicine, 327*, 82–87.

Kaiser, L. (2004). What are infants and toddlers eating? Maternal and Infant Briefs: Jan/Feb edition. Retrieved February 10, 2007, from http://nutrition.ucdavis.edu/briefs/Issues/JanFeb04.htm

Krugman, S., & Dubowitz, H. (2003). Failure to thrive. *American Family Physician, 68*, 879–884.

Mahan, L. K., & Escott-Stump, S. (2000). *Krause's Food, Nutrition, and Diet Therapy* (10th ed.). Philadelphia: W. B. Saunders.

National Center for Health Statistics in collaboration with the National Center for Chronic Disease Prevention and Health Promotion. (2000). Retrieved February 1, 2007, from http://www.cdc.gov/growthcharts

National Institutes of Health. (n.d.). BMI Chart. Retrieved October 11, 2007, from www.nhlbi.nih.gov/guidelines/obesity/bmi_tbl.pdf

Ogden, C. L., Flegal, K. M., Carroll, M. D., & Johnson, C. L. (2002). Prevalence and trends in overweight among US children and adolescents, 1999–2000. *Journal of the American Medical Association, 288*, 1728–1732.

Orlet Fisher, J., Rolls, B. J., & Birch, L. L. (2003). Children's bite size and intake of an entrée are greater with large portions than with age-appropriate or self selected portions. *American Journal of Clinical Nutrition, 77*, 1164–1170.

Patrick, H., & Nicklas, T. A. (2005). A review of family and social determinants of children's eating patterns and diet quality. *Journal of the American College of Nutrition, 24,* 83–92.

Pelcaht, M. L., & Pliner, P. (1986). Antecedents and correlates of feeding problems in young children. *Journal of Nutrition Education, 18,* 23–29.

Rachlin, H., Logue, A. W., Gibbon, J., & Frankel, M. (1986). Cognition and behavior in studies of choice. *Psychology Review, 93,* 33–45.

Robinson, T. N. (2001). Television viewing and childhood obesity. *Pediatric Clinics of North America, 48,* 1017–1025.

Saelens, B. E., Sallis, J. F., Nader, P. R., Broyles, S. L., Berry, C. C., & Taras, H. L. (2002). Home environment influences on children's television watching from early to middle childhood. *Journal of Developmental and Behavioral Pediatrics, 23,* 127–132.

Sallis, J. F., Prochaska, J. J., & Taylor, W. C. (2000). A review of correlates of physical activity of children and adolescents. *Medicine and Science in Sports and Exercise, 32,* 963–975.

Salmon, J. O., Timperio, A., Telford, A., Carver, A., & Crawford, D. (2005). Association of family environment with children's television viewing and with low level of physical activity. *Obesity Research, 13,* 1939–1951.

Satter, E. M. (1986). The feeding relationship. *Journal of the American Dietetic Association, 86,* 352–356.

Satter, E. M. (1996). Internal regulation and the evolution of normal growth as the basis for prevention of obesity in children. *Journal of the American Dietetic Association, 96,* 860–864.

Schneider, J. M., Fujii, M. L., Lamp, C. L., Lonnerdal, B., Dewey, K. G., & Zidenberg-Cherr, S. (2005). Anemia, iron deficiency, and iron deficiency anemia in 12-36-mo-old children from low-income families. *American Journal of Clinical Nutrition, 82,* 1269–1275.

School Breakfast Program and Food and Research Action Center. (n.d.). Child nutrition fact sheet. Retrieved January 15, 2007, from www.frac.org/pdf/cnsbp.PDF

Scrimshaw, N. S., & Murray, E. B. (1988). Prevalence of lactose maldigestion. *American Journal of Clinical Nutrition, 48*(Suppl.), 1086–1098.

Smith, M. M., & Lifshitz, F. (1994). Excess fruit juice consumption as a contributing factor in nonorganic failure to thrive. *Pediatrics, 93,* 438–443.

Specker, B. L., Valanis, B., Hertzberg, V., Edwards, N., & Tsang, R. (1985). Sunshine exposure and serum 25-hydroxyvitamin D concentrations in exclusively breast-fed infants. *Journal of Pediatrics, 107,* 372–376.

Storey, M. L., Forchee, R.A., & Anderson, P. A. (2004). Associations of adequate intake of calcium with diet, beverage consumption, and demographic characteristics among children and adolescents. *Journal of the American College of Nutrition, 23,* 18–33.

Story, M., & French, S. (2004). Food advertising and marketing directed at children and adolescents in the US. *International Journal of Behavioral Nutrition and Physical Activity, 1,* 1–17.

Sullivan, S. A., & Birch, L. L. (1993). Infant dietary experience and acceptance of solid foods. *Pediatrics, 93,* 271–278.

Tomashek, K. M., Nesby, S., Scanlon, K. S., Cogswell, M. E., Powell, K. E., Parashar, U. D., et al. (2001). Nutritional rickets in Georgia. *Pediatrics, 107,* e45.

U.S. Department of Agriculture, Food and Nutrition Service. (n.d.). Women, Infants, and Children (WIC). Retrieved February 2, 2007, from www.fns.usda.gov/wic/aboutwic/default.htm

U.S. Department of Agriculture. (2005). Nutrition program facts. National school lunch program. Retrieved February 10, 2007, from www.fns.usda.gov/cnd/Lunch/AboutLunch/NSLPFactSheet.pdf

U.S. Department of Health and Human Services. (2000). Tracking Healthy People 2010. Retrieved February 21, 2007, from http://www.healthypeople.gov/document/html/tracking/THP_Intro.htm

Vesa, T. H., Marteau, P., & Korpela, R. (2000). Lactose intolerance. *Journal of the American College of Nutrition, 19,* 165S–175S.

Waller, C. E., Du, S., & Popkin, B. M. (2003). Patterns of overweight, inactivity, and snacking in Chinese children. *Obesity Research, 11,* 957–961.

Weisberg, P., Scanlon, K. S., Li, R., & Cogswell, M. E. (2004). Nutritional rickets among children in the United Stated: Review of cases reported between 1986 and 2003. *American Journal of Clinical Nutrition, 80*(Suppl.), 1697S–1705S.

Zlotkin, S. H. (1996). A review of the Canadian nutrition recommendations update: Dietary fat and children. *Journal of Nutrition, 126*(Suppl.), 1022S–1027S.

Role of Parents in Promoting Healthy Nutrition in Early Childhood

Addessi, E., Galloway, A. T., Visalberghi, E., & Birch, L. L. (2005). Specific social influences on the acceptance of novel foods in 2-5 year-old children. *Appetite, 45,* 264–271.

Bandura, A. (1972). Modeling theory: Some traditions, trends, and disputes. In R. D. Parke (Ed.), *Recent Trends in Social Learning Theory.* New York: Academic Press.

Barkin, S. L., Scheindlin, B., Brown, C., Ip, E., Finch, S., & Wasserman, R. C. (2005). *Ambulatory Pediatrics, 5,* 372–356.

Baumrind, D. (1998). Rearing competent children. In W. Damon (Ed.), *Child Development Today and Tomorrow.* San Francisco: Jossey-Bass Publishers.

Birch, L. L. (1980). Effects of peer models' food choices and eating behaviors on preschoolers' food preferences. *Child Development, 5,* 489–496.

Birch, L. L., & Fisher, J. A. (1995). Appetite and eating behavior in children. *Pediatric Clinics of North America, 42,* 931–935.

Birch, L. L., & Fisher, J. O. (2000). Mothers' child-feeding practices influence daughters' eating and weight. *American Journal of Clinical Nutrition, 71,* 1054–1061.

Birch, L. L., & Marlin. D. W. (1982). "I don't like it; I never tried it": Effects of exposure on two-year-old children's food preferences. *Appetite, 3,* 353–360.

Booth, D., Fuller, J., & Lewis, V. (1981). Human control of body weight: Cognitive or physiological? Some energy-related perceptions and misperceptions. In L. Cioffi, W. James, & T. van Italie (Eds.), *The Body Weight Regulatory System: Normal and Disturbed Mechanisms* (pp. 305–314). New York: Raven Press.

Butte, N., Cobb, K., Dwyer, J., Graney, L., Heird, W., Richard, K., et al. (2004). The Start Healthy Feeding Guidelines for Infants and Toddlers. *Journal of the American Dietetic Association, 104*, 443–454.

Carper, J. L., Fisher, J. O., & Birch, L. L. (2000). Young girls' emerging dietary restrain and disinhibition are related to parental control in child feeding. *Appetite, 35*, 121–129.

Carruth, B. R., & Skinner, J. (2000). Preschoolers food product choices at a simulated point of purchase and mothers' consumer practices. *Journal of Nutrition Education, 33*, 143–147.

Cutting, T. M., Fisher, J. O., Grimm-Thomas, K., & Birch, L. L. (1999). Like mother, like daughter: Familial patterns of overweight are mediated by mothers' dietary disinhibition. *American Journal of Clinical Nutrition, 69*, 608–613.

Dewey, K. G., Heinig, J., Nommensen, L. A., & Lonnerdal, B. (1991). Maternal versus infant factors related to breast milk intake and residual milk volume. *Pediatrics, 87*, 829–837.

Dwyer, J. T., Sutor, C. W., & Hendricks, K. (2004). FITS: New insights and lessons learned. *Journal of the American Dietetic Association, 104*(Suppl. 1), s25–s27.

Engell, D., Kramer, M., Zaring, D., Birch, L. L., & Rolls, B. J. (1995). Effects of serving size on food intake in children and adults. *Obesity Research, 3*(Suppl. 3), 381s.

Fomon, S. J., & Bell, E. F. (1993). *Nutrition of Normal Infants: Energy* (pp. 443–454). St. Louis, MO: Mosby-Year Book.

Fox, M. K., Pac, S., Devaney, B., & Janowski, L. (2004). Feeding Infants and Toddlers Study. What are infants and toddlers eating? *Journal of the American Dietetic Association, 104*(Suppl. 1), S22–S30.

Gidding, S., Dennison, B., Birch, L. L., Daniels, S., Gilman, M. W., Lichtenstein, A. H., et al. (2005). Dietary recommendations for children and adolescents: A guide for practitioners. Consensus Statement from the American Heart Association. *Circulation, 112*, 2061–2075.

Harper, L. V., & Sanders, K. M. (1975). The effect of adults' eating on young children's acceptance of unfamiliar foods. *Journal of Experimental Child Psychology, 20*, 206–214.

Hendy, H. M. (2002). Effectiveness of trained peer models to encourage food acceptance in preschool children. *Appetite, 39*, 217–225.

Johnson, S. L. (2000). Improving preschoolers' self-regulation of energy intake. *Pediatrics, 106*, 1429–1435.

Kleinman, R. E. (Ed.). (2004). *Pediatric Nutrition Handbook* (p. 105). Elk Grove, IL: American Academy of Pediatrics.

Lipsitt, L. P., Crook, C., & Booth, C. (1985). The transitional infant: Behavioral development and feeding. *American Journal of Clinical Nutrition, 41*, 485–496.

Mennella, J. A., Jagnow, C. J., & Beauchamp, G. K. (2001). Pre- and postnatal flavor learning by human infants. *Pediatrics, 107*, 88–93.

Mennella, J. A., Johnson, A., & Beauchamp, G. K. (1995). Garlic ingestion by pregnant women alters the odor of amniotic fluid. *Chemical Senses, 20*, 207–209.

Ong, K. K., Emmett, P. M., Noble, S., Ness, A., Dunger, D. B., & The ALSPAC Study Team (2006). Dietary energy intake at the age of 4 months predicts postnatal weight gain and childhood body mass index. *Pediatrics, 117*, 503–508.

Rhee, K. E., Lumeng, J. C., Appugliese, D. P., Kaciroti, N., & Bradley, R. H. (2006). Parenting styles and overweight status in first grade. *Pediatrics, 117*, 2047–2054.

Salsberry, P. J., & Reagan, P. B. (2005). Dynamics of early childhood overweight. *Pediatrics, 116*, 1329–1338.

Satter, E. (1999). *Secrets of Feeding a Healthy Family* (p. 2). Madison, WI: Kelcy Press.

Schall, G., Marlier, L., & Soussignan, R. (2000). Human fetuses learn odours from their pregnant mothers' diet. *Chemical Senses, 25*, 729–737.

Shea, S., Basch, C. E., Contento, I., & Rand Zybert, P. (1992). Variability and self-regulation of energy intake in young children in their everyday environment. *Pediatrics, 90*, 542–546.

Skinner, J. D., Carruth, B. R., Bounds, W., & Zeigler, P. J. (2002). Children's food preferences: A longitudinal analysis. *Journal of the American Dietetic Association, 102*, 1638–1647.

Stein, K. (2000). Children with feeding disorders: An emerging issue. *Journal of the American Dietetic Association, 100*, 1000–1001.

Stettler, N., Zemel, B. S., & Kumanyika, S. (2002). Infant weight gain and childhood overweight status in a multicenter, cohort study. *Pediatrics, 109*, 194–199.

Sullivan, S. A., & Birch, L. L. (1990). Pass the sugar, pass the salt: Experience dictates preference. *Developmental Psychology, 26*, 546–555.

Sullivan, S. A., & Birch, L. L. (1994). Infant dietary experience and acceptance of solid foods. *Pediatrics, 93*, 271–277.

CHAPTER 4

Normal Adolescent Nutrition

Pamela S. Hinton, PhD

With a Special Section: Public Health Nutrition Programs for Children
Rachel Colchamiro, MPH, RD, LDN, and Jan Kallio, MS, RD, LDN

CHAPTER OUTLINE

Reader Objectives

After studying this chapter and reflecting on the contents, you should be able to

1. Understand nutritional regulation of the hormones that moderate growth and sexual maturation.
2. Describe gender differences in growth and development and in nutrient requirements.
3. Appreciate how psychosocial development during adolescence affects health-related behaviors, including dietary patterns.
4. Identify and describe sociodemographic factors affecting dietary patterns.
5. Describe trends in chronic disease incidence among adolescents.

Normal Adolescent Nutrition

Pamela S. Hinton, PhD

Adolescence is a period of rapid linear growth, altered body composition, reproductive maturation, and psychosocial development. Nutrient requirements are increased to meet the demands of growth and development. There are significant gender differences in the timing and rate of peak linear growth, puberty, and sexual development, resulting in divergent nutrient needs. Normal growth and development are influenced by nutritional status because the hormones responsible for linear growth, alteration in body composition, and sexual development are nutritionally regulated. Food intake during adolescence is influenced by psychosocial factors; peers and popular culture, including the mass media and advertising, significantly affect dietary patterns.

Growth and Development

Physical Growth

Peak Height Velocity

The adolescent growth spurt takes 2 to 4 years to complete and is generally longer in boys than in girls. The average height velocity is 5 to 6 cm/yr during adolescence; peak height velocity is 8 to 10 cm/yr. Girls, on average, begin their pubertal growth spurt at age 9 years (Veldhuis et al., 2005) and achieve their maximal rate of linear growth (i.e., peak height velocity) at an average chronologic age of 11.5 years, corresponding to Tanner breast stages 2 and 3. The onset of the pubertal growth spurt occurs at age 11 years in boys, and peak height velocity occurs at age 13.5 years, normally Tanner genital stages 3 and 4. The onset of the adolescent growth spurt is more closely associated with bone age than with chronologic age. Boys, because their peak height velocity is greater than that of girls, 9.5 cm/yr versus 8.3 cm/yr, and because peak height velocity occurs later in boys than in girls, are on average 13 cm taller than girls. Interindividual variation in the onset and rate of pubertal growth and development is significant because of interaction between a child's genetic potential and his or her environment.

Body Composition

Normative body composition data from prospective population-based samples are lacking in adolescent populations, especially ethnic and gender specific data. During adolescence girls gain fat mass at an average rate of 1.14 kg/yr. In contrast, boys do not experience a significant increase in absolute fat mass. Boys also gain fat-free mass at a greater rate and for a longer period of time than girls; as a result, boys are relatively leaner than girls after puberty. At ages 8 to 10 boys, on average, have 15% body fat and 24 kg fat free mass. At the end of puberty, ages 18 to 20 years, young men have 13% body fat and 60 kg fat free mass. In contrast, girls have 20% body fat and 24 kg fat-free mass at ages 8 to 10 years. By ages 18 to 20 years young women have 26% body fat and 44 kg fat-free mass (Guo, Chunlea, Roche, & Siervogel, 1997).

Bone Growth and Mineralization

In the immature skeleton the ends of the long bones (**epiphyses**) are separated from the shafts of the long bones (**diaphyses**) by the growth plate. After puberty the growth plate becomes mineralized and the epiphyses fuse. Thus the mature skeleton is incapable of additional growth in height or length.

> **Epiphyses:** Ends of long bones.
>
> **Diaphyses:** Shafts of long bones.

CRITICAL **Thinking**

After reading the statement, "Thus the mature skeleton is incapable of additional growth in height or length," how does nutrition in childhood affect skeletal growth?

Bone mass doubles between the onset of puberty and young adulthood. Bone growth is greatest approximately 6 months after peak height velocity (Whiting et al., 2004); approximately 25% of peak adult bone mass is acquired during the 2 years of peak adolescent skeletal growth. Growth of the skeleton occurs via modeling, which changes both the size and shape of the bones. Bones increase in length by ossification of the growth plates and in diameter by **periosteal apposition** and **endosteal resorption**. When the growth plates fuse after puberty, bone mass density (BMD) is 90% to 95% of peak BMD (Riggs, Khosla, & Melton, 2002). Boys are, on average, 10% taller and have 25% greater peak bone mass than girls because of their later pubertal onset and longer growth spurt (Riggs et al., 2002).

> **Periosteal apposition:** Deposition of bone on the outer surface.
>
> **Endosteal resorption:** Removal of bone from the inner surface.

> ● **Learning Point**   There are ethnic differences in BMD; African-American teenagers have higher BMD than white teenagers.

Calcium Absorption and Retention

The maximal rate of calcium accretion in the skeleton occurs at ages 11 to 14 years in girls and 16 to

18 years in boys. During the 2 years of peak bone growth, boys gain approximately 400 g of bone mineral and girls deposit approximately 325 g). Fractional calcium absorption is increased to approximately 40% during peak bone mineral deposition (Molgaard, Thomsen, & Michaelsen, 1999). In adolescents there is a linear relationship between dietary calcium intake and calcium retention. During adulthood, fractional absorption decreases with increasing dietary calcium. In contrast, increasing calcium consumption to 47.4 mmol/day did not reduce fractional calcium absorption compared with 21.2 mmol/day in adolescent girls (Wastney et al., 2000; Weaver, 2000). Because the additional calcium suppressed bone resorption, calcium retention was significantly increased by the higher calcium intake (Weaver, 2000). In a calcium balance study of adolescent girls, African-Americans were found to have increased calcium retention, bone formation relative to bone resorption, fractional calcium absorption, and decreased urinary excretion compared with whites (Bryant et al., 2003).

Bone Turnover Markers

Biochemical markers of bone formation and resorption also are increased during puberty and generally parallel the rate of linear growth (Federico, Baroncelli, Vanacore, Fiore, & Saggese, 2003). Bone turnover during puberty is up to 10-fold higher than during adulthood (Eastell, 2005): The rate of remodeling is increased, linear growth occurs at the epiphyseal growth plates, and there is modeling of bone, which changes the shape of the bones by periosteal or endosteal apposition. Longitudinal studies demonstrate that bone turnover markers are greatest early in puberty, whereas maximal mineral deposition occurs late in puberty when bone turnover markers in serum are decreasing (Eastell, 2005). Mechanical stress on the skeleton is critical to all these processes; the growing skeleton is more sensitive to loading than the mature skeleton. Thus physical activity during adolescence is necessary to maximize peak bone mass.

Peak Bone Mass and Prevention of Osteoporosis

Loss of bone mass during adulthood is inevitable; thus prevention of osteoporosis depends, in part, on maximizing peak bone mass, which is achieved in young adulthood. Because a large fraction of adult bone mass is acquired during adolescence, it is important to optimize skeletal growth during this stage in the life cycle. Strategies to maximize peak bone mass include adequate nutrition, regular weight-bearing exercise, and normal endocrine function to retain calcium and stimulate bone growth (Weaver, 2000).

Fracture Risks

Although 75% to 85% of the variance in bone strength can be attributed to bone mass, the fragility of a bone also is determined by the shape of the bone, remodeling rates, and chemical properties of the bone. Most fractures occur later in life; thus fracture risk depends not only on bone mass but on bone geometry, bone turnover, and risk of falling. Furthermore, the rate of bone loss during adulthood is accelerated by poor nutrient intake and lack of regular weight-bearing exercise. Therefore acquisition of peak bone mass during adolescence does not guarantee that an individual will be protected against fractures during late adulthood (Schonau, 2004).

Hormonal Mediators of the Adolescent Growth Spurt

Pattern of Hormone Secretion

Normal physical growth and development during puberty depends on the integration of the growth hormone–(GH) insulin-like growth factor (IGF) and gonadotropin axes. Nutritional and metabolic signals, in part, control these hormonal systems by acting on the hypothalamus and pituitary gland. During childhood, the activity of the hypothalamic–pituitary–gonadal axis is suppressed by the central nervous system. Animal data suggest that in females gamma-aminobutyric acid is responsible for the juvenile pause; in males **neuropeptide Y** prevents the onset of puberty. At puberty, excitatory neurotransmitters stimulate the release of gonadotropin-releasing hormone in the hypothalamus. As a result the pulse amplitude of the **gonadotropins**, luteinizing hormone (LH) and follicle-stimulating hormone (FSH), increases and the nocturnal rise in LH secretion is amplified. Pulse frequency, however, is unchanged during puberty. This nocturnal rhythm is specific to puberty and disappears in adulthood. Increased circulating concentrations of LH and FSH stimulate development of the gonads and production of sex steroid hormones. Androgens are synthesized in the Leydig cells of the testes, to a lesser degree the ovaries, and are secreted in response to LH. Testosterone stimulates sperm protein synthesis and development of secondary sex characteristics. FSH stimulates release of estrogens from the ovaries. Progesterones are synthesized in the **corpus luteum** and secreted in response to LH. Estrogen and progesterone control the menstrual cycle and the development of the female secondary sex characteristics.

An increase in spontaneous GH secretion precedes the onset of puberty. GH peak amplitude per

Neuropeptide Y: A 36 amino acid peptide neurotransmitter found in the brain and autonomic nervous system; it augments the vasoconstrictor effects of noradrenergic neurons.

Gonadotropin: Hormones secreted by the pituitary gland that affect the function of the male or female gonads.

Corpus luteum: A yellow glandular mass in the ovary formed by an ovarian follicle that has matured and released its egg; secrets progesterone.

pulse is elevated, and integrated 24-hour GH secretion (Styne, 2003) is increased 1.5- to 3-fold (Leung, Johannsson, Leong, & Ho, 2004). GH release stimulated by insulin, arginine, and other secretagogues also is elevated during puberty. Serum levels of IGF-I increase in parallel with increased GH secretion and are elevated threefold above prepubertal levels (Leung et al., 2004). Because the secretion of the acid-labile subunit and IGF binding protein 3 (IGFBP-3) do not match the increased production of IGF-I, free IGF-I concentrations also are elevated. GH deficiency diseases illustrate the importance of the somatotropic axis in pubertal growth. Children with GH deficiency are of short stature and have reduced growth velocity and delayed pubertal onset. Thus normal function of the GH–IGF axis is needed for onset and maintenance of puberty and male sexual development.

Sex Hormones

The sex steroids, estrogen and testosterone, increase spontaneous and stimulated GH secretion. Estrogen appears to be primarily responsible for increased GH secretion associated with the pubertal growth spurt. The effects of testosterone are likely mediated through conversion to estradiol by the enzyme aromatase. Sex steroids also modulate IGF-I bioactivity via regulation of IGFBPs and proteases. IGF-I enhances gonadotropin-releasing hormone secretion in some species and augments the effects of LH and FSH on sex steroid production in the ovaries and testes both in vitro and in vivo (Veldhuis et al., 2005).

Leptin, a peptide hormone secreted by adipocytes, plays a role in pubertal development, although its role in the onset of puberty is not clear. Leptin levels parallel the changes observed in fat mass during puberty, suggesting that leptin does not initiate puberty. However, administration of recombinant human leptin to postmenarcheal women with hypothalamic amenorrhea increases secretion of LH, FSH, and estradiol and stimulates follicular development independent of changes in body weight (Welt et al., 2004). In addition, individuals who are deficient in leptin or who have leptin receptor defects fail to go through puberty. Boys have lower serum leptin concentrations than girls, and this gender difference increases throughout puberty. The lower leptin concentrations in males compared with females at a given body mass index (BMI) may be due to the suppressive effects of androgens on leptin expression (Federico et al., 2003).

Hormone Actions on Muscle

GH, IGF-I, and testosterone apparently have synergistic effects on anabolism in skeletal muscle, although the cellular mechanisms are not completely understood. Administration of GH or IGF-I to individuals with GH deficiency increases lean body mass by inhibition of protein breakdown and stimulation of amino acid uptake and protein synthesis. Testosterone replacement therapy at physiologic doses in hypogonadal boys and men causes an increase in lean tissue mass due to enhanced rates of protein synthesis and suppression of proteolysis. Testosterone reduces **myocyte** apoptosis via induction of **myostatin**. Some of the anabolic effects of testosterone are due to induction of IGF-I and inhibition of IGFBP-4 expression in skeletal muscle. IGF-I promotes myoblast differentiation from satellite cells and causes hypertrophy of existing myocytes. Endogenous androgens likely drive muscle anabolism in pubertal girls, as well as in pubertal boys.

Myocyte: A single muscle cell.

Myostatin: A growth factor that limits muscle tissue growth.

Hormone Actions on Adipose

Total fat mass is under control of multiple hormones and neurotransmitters, including the sex steroids, GH, insulin, glucocorticoids, and **adrenergic agonists**. Testosterone, GH, and adrenergic agonists stimulate lipolysis; estrogen and insulin cause lipogenesis. Regional fat distribution is determined by tissue distribution of the sex steroid receptors. Adipocytes in the mammary gland and gluteofemoral region have estradiol receptors; intraabdominal fat cells have androgen receptors. Testosterone has many lipolytic effects that may contribute to the changes in regional fat distribution that occur during puberty. Testosterone enhances the actions of GH and adrenergic agonists, stimulates androgen receptor expression, and reduces the lipogenic effects of insulin and lipoprotein lipase. In contrast, estrogen increases expression of insulin receptors in adipose tissue and may attenuate the lipolytic effects of GH.

Adrenergic agonists: Bind to and activate adrenergic receptors.

Exogenous female reproductive hormones administered orally or as intramuscular injections affect body composition in adolescent girls. Oral contraceptive agents and depot **medroxyprogesterone acetate** promote excessive adiposity in adolescent girls. In a longitudinal study of adolescents, depot medroxyprogesterone acetate use resulted in significantly greater weight gain after 18 months compared with oral contraceptives and no hormonal contraception in obese girls. Among nonobese teens, either form of hormonal contraception resulted in a greater incidence of obesity compared with control subjects (Eastell, 2005; Bonny et al., 2006).

Medroxyprogesterone acetate: A synthetic progestin.

Hormone Actions on Bone

The sex steroids have opposing actions on bone. Androgens and estrogens stimulate both bone growth and fusion of the epiphysis. Individuals with subnormal levels of estrogen or testosterone at puberty have reduced peak bone mass, resulting in osteopenia or osteoporosis and increased fracture risk during adulthood. Some of the osteogenic effects of testosterone and estrogen are likely due to increased pulsatile GH secretion, which is the primary stimulus of longitudinal bone growth; IGF-I synthesis in bone; increased intestinal absorption of calcium and magnesium; and increased osteoblast activity. Androgen receptors are present on osteoblasts and osteocytes. In vitro studies demonstrated that testosterone inhibits apoptosis of osteoblasts and osteocytes, suppresses osteoclastogenesis, and causes deposition of mineral on periosteal surfaces of cortical bone. The effects of testosterone may be partially mediated by estradiol via conversion of testosterone via aromatase. Aromatase deficiency in humans and animals causes osteoporosis, and aromatase antagonists increase bone resorption and impair pubertal bone mineralization.

Estrogen, like testosterone, promotes bone growth by suppressing bone resorption and enhancing bone deposition. Estrogen stimulates proliferation and differentiation of osteoblasts as well as osteoblast secretion of osteoprotegerin. Osteoprotegerin is a glycoprotein that inhibits osteoclastogenesis. Estrogen also increases intestinal absorption of calcium, thereby indirectly enhancing bone mineralization. Estrogen is responsible for the sexual dimorphism of bone, explaining why females have smaller skeletons relative to males. Age at menarche is associated with BMD and fracture risk. Delayed menarche is associated with low adult BMD and fracture risk. The relative risk of hip fracture was 2.1 in women who experienced menarche after age 17 years (Fujiwara, Kasagi, Yamada, & Kodama, 1997); the relative risk of vertebral fractures was 1.8 in women who began menstruating after age 16 years (Roy et al., 2003). There are two possible explanations for this finding (Eastell, 2005). The first hypothesis is that lower lifetime exposure to estrogen reduces BMD. The second explanation is that both early menarche and BMD result from greater body weight per height, and body weight is a strong predictor of BMD.

Menarche: First menstrual period.

GH, IGF-I, IGF-II, and IGFBPs also regulate bone modeling and growth. GH stimulates IGF-I synthesis in bone, proliferation of prechondrocytes, and hypertrophy of osteoblasts. In vitro experiments demonstrated that GH reduces production of IGFBP-4 in bone and increases synthesis of IGFBP-2, -3, and -5. IGFBP-4 antagonizes the actions of IGF-I in bone, whereas IGFBP-2, -3, and -5 augment the effects of IGF-I.

Assessment of Growth and Development

Growth

Serial measurements of height and weight plotted on height for age, weight for age, and weight for height growth charts from the National Center for Health Statistics (2000) are used to evaluate growth statistics (see Appendix 1). Height growth potential is calculated from parental height. Skeletal age is assessed using radiography of the left hand and wrist. An open epiphysis indicates skeletal immaturity and potential for additional growth. Stature of pregnant adolescents should be assessed using a knee height measuring device to determine the length of the lower leg. Vertebral compression during pregnancy due to changes in posture (increased **lordosis**) and gestational weight gain makes stature an invalid measure of growth.

Lordosis: An abnormal forward curvature of the lumbar spine.

Height and weight are used to calculate BMI (kg/m^2); BMI for age growth charts also are available. Excessive weight in adolescents is defined as BMI greater than or equal to the 95th percentile; adolescents with the 85th percentile less than or equal to BMI less than or equal to the 95th percentile are classified as "at risk for overweight." Underweight is defined as BMI less than the 5th percentile.

Reproductive Development

Reproductive development is assessed using Tanner stages that characterize pubic hair and breast (female) and genital (male) maturation. Progression from Tanner stages 2 to 5 typically takes 2.5 to 5 years. In girls Tanner staging of breasts and pubic hair usually occurs in parallel; for boys genital staging precedes pubic hair staging. Menarche typically occurs at Tanner stage 4. Pubertal onset, including age at menarche, is in part genetically determined. The normal age of pubertal onset is ages 8 to 16 years in girls and ages 9 to 17 years in boys.

Adolescent Growth Disorders

Identification of Normal Short Stature

It is important to differentiate between an adolescent who is small relative to his or her peers and a teenager who is growing poorly. To make this distinction and to evaluate growth, serial determinations of height and weight are required. Two benign conditions that result in short stature are familial short stature and constitutional/maturational delay. Parental stature is used to assess growth potential. A child with constitutional delay experiences retarded growth at ages 3 and 11 to 12 years; this condition is often familial. Bone age, height age, and growth velocity can be used to differentiate familial short stature and constitutional delay. Adolescents with constitutional delay have delayed bone and height age and slowed growth, whereas those with familial short stature have normal bone age, height age less than bone age, and normal growth (Simm & Werther, 2005). Chronologic age and bone age may differ by as much as 2 years and still be within the normal range. Puberty can be induced in boys older than 14 years by testosterone administration without compromising linear growth. Girls with extreme constitutional delay may be treated with low dose estrogen. Because estrogen causes fusion of the growth plates, adult height may be compromised.

Pathologic Causes of Short Stature

Changes in weight trajectories also can be used to determine the cause of short stature, because weight gain is affected before linear growth. A teenager whose weight percentile is declining may be suffering from chronic illness or poor dietary intake, possibly of psychosocial etiology. Other pathologic causes of short stature include endocrine disorders such hypothyroidism and GH deficiency; intrauterine growth retardation; chromosomal defects, Turner, Down, and Prader-Willi syndromes; and skeletal dysplasia. Diagnosis of these disorders requires thyroid function, bone age, karyotype, and provocative GH testing. Some catch-up growth usually occurs after the underlying pathology is resolved. GH deficiency and Turner syndrome can be treated with GH.

Pathologic Causes of Tall Stature

Tall stature in adolescents is rare compared with short stature; most cases of tall stature are benign familial tall stature (Simm & Werther, 2005). Pathologic tall stature must be diagnosed with thyroid function tests, bone age, karyotyping, and determination of serum IGF-I concentrations. Endocrine causes of tall stature include hyperthyroidism, precocious puberty, and GH secreting tumors. Adolescents with precocious puberty end up with compromised adult height because estrogen and androgen levels peak early, causing premature fusion of the growth plates. Klinefelter, Marfan, Sotos, and Beckwith-Widermann syndromes are rare genetic disorders that result in tall stature. Most adolescents with tall stature do not require medical intervention. Sex steroid treatment can be used to induce premature fusion of the epiphyseal growth plates, thereby reducing final height. However, estrogen treatment of tall stature may impair fertility; thus it rarely is used (Simm & Werther, 2005).

Cognitive and Psychosocial Development During Adolescence

Cognitive and Affective Development

The brain develops during puberty; in particular, areas involved in regulation of behavior and emotion and in perception and evaluation of risk and reward undergo considerable change (Steinberg, 2005). Cognitive development during adolescence results in increased self-awareness, self-direction, and self-regulation. However, the changes in arousal and motivation that take place during puberty occur before acquisition of the ability to regulate affect (Steinberg, 2005). The limbic areas of the brain associated with emotion increase in volume during puberty. The cortical gray area is reduced in volume, and there is localized synaptic pruning that increases the efficiency of information processing. Frontal brain activity, the location of abstract thought, planning, and attention, is increased (Waylen & Wolke, 2004). There is increased connectivity among brain regions via myelination of nerve fibers; in particular, increased connections between the cortex and the **limbic systems** augment the ability to evaluate and make decisions regarding risk and reward.

> **Affect:** Emotion.

> **Limbic system:** A group of brain structures and their connections with each other as well as their connections with the hypothalamus and other areas; largely associated with emotions.

During early adolescence, teenagers improve their deductive reasoning, information processing, and specialized knowledge. The capacity for abstract, multidimensional, planned, and hypothetical thought increases into middle adolescence. Although adults and adolescents have similar reasoning capacities, adolescents and adults differ in social and emotional factors, leading to divergent behaviors with age. For example, adolescents are more susceptible to peer influences than adults, and their reasoning about real-life situations or personal choices is not as sound as their reasoning about hypothetical or ethical questions.

Age and life experience are associated with most aspects of cognitive development during adolescence; however, maturation in arousal, motivation, and emotion are more closely linked with the onset of puberty. Emotional intensity and reactivity and reward-seeking and risk-taking behaviors also are influenced by puberty and not by chronologic age. Vulnerability to social status appears to increase at pubertal onset, coinciding with increased risk-taking behaviors. Cognitive development enhances the ability to regulate affect; conversely, emotion alters decision-making thought processes and behavior. Because teenagers are more likely to engage in high-risk behaviors (e.g., drug use and unprotected sex), it previously was thought that their ability to accurately evaluate risk was lacking. However, there is evidence that adolescents are able to understand risk but make poor decisions, regardless. Thus decision-making behaviors that affect health, including diet and exercise, are highly influenced by emotion and social influences, despite understanding of associated risks and benefits.

Psychosocial Development

Adolescence is the transition from childhood to adulthood, requiring maturation of psychosocial functioning. During the teenage years, individuals move from same- to mixed-sex peer groups, develop romantic relationships, and transfer relational dependence and modeling of behaviors from parents to peers (Waylen & Wolke, 2004). Adolescence also is a time of increased independence with regard to academic performance and economic self-sufficiency. In the United States and other Western societies physical maturity precedes achievement of these developmental tasks; this period of prolonged adolescence has been termed the "maturity gap." The length of the maturity gap differs significantly between genders and among individuals; the maturity gap is larger for boys than for girls.

The cognitive and affective development that occurs during adolescence changes a teenager's self-concept and self-esteem. Adolescents are concerned with the identity they project to others (Waylen & Wolke, 2004). The discrepancy between an adolescent's self-identity and the expectations of others may be problematic. Rapid pubertal development or pubertal onset that deviates from one's peers also may result in maladaptive behaviors. In females early maturation is associated with increased affective disorders, delinquency and drop-out rates, and pregnancy.

In boys early physical maturation has mostly positive consequences, namely increased social status and high self-esteem. In contrast, males with late pubertal onset are more likely to engage in status-seeking antisocial behaviors. Thus biological and social factors interact to affect behaviors, including those with long-term effects on health.

Drug use is one maladaptive coping mechanism that adolescents may adopt to deal with stress. Puberty is associated with the onset of mental health disorders in girls; in particular, the incidence of anxiety and depressive disorders, eating disorders, and smoking is increased in female adolescents. Among U.S. girls participating in the National Longitudinal Study of Adolescent Health (Harris, Gordon-Larsen, Chantala, & Udry, 2006), 10% to 15% reported feelings of depression and 13% to 33% had suicidal thoughts. In contrast, boys were less likely to feel depressed (6% to 9%) or to report suicidal ideation (8% to 14%). Girls also are more likely to attempt to suicide (Grunbaum et al., 2002). This gender difference may be attributed to hormonal changes and to the female ruminative response style.

> **● Learning Point** Tobacco use, poor diet/inactivity, alcohol abuse, and illicit drug use are among the leading modifiable causes of death in the United States (McGinnis, 1993; Mokdad et al., 2000). Unfortunately, the prevalence of these risk factors is high among adolescents.

In the Youth Risk Behavior Surveillance nearly one-half of high school students use alcohol, 30% binge drink, and approximately one-fourth report current marijuana use (Grunbaum et al., 2002). The prevalence of cocaine, inhalant, heroin, and methamphetamine use is lower; lifetime rates of use range from 3% to 15% (Grunbaum et al., 2002). Five percent of high school students reported using illegal steroids during their lifetime (Grunbaum et al., 2002). Among girls 13% to 33% binge drink, 7% to 21% use marijuana, and 2% to 8% use hard drugs (Harris et al., 2006). Adolescent boys are more likely than girls to binge drink (17% to 32%), use marijuana (14% to 28%), or use hard drugs (3% to 8%) (Grunbaum et al., 2002; Harris et al., 2006). In a national sample of U.S. youth 49.3% consumed at least one drink in the previous month. On average, adolescents aged 15 to 21 years consumed 14.3 drinks per month (Snyder, Milici, Slater, Sun, & Strizhakova, 2006).

Alcohol use, smoking, marijuana use, and truancy are co-occurring behaviors; teens who use marijuana are more likely to also use tobacco than nonusers (Weden & Zabin, 2005). Regular or excessive alcohol consumption is positively associated with marijuana use (Boys et al., 2003; Rey, Martin, & Krabman, 2004). These behaviors are less likely to persist into adulthood if the onset occurs during adolescence, if the frequency of the behaviors is occasional, and if the behaviors occur within the peer group (Waylen & Wolke, 2004).

Tobacco use, particularly cigarette smoking, also is common among adolescents. In 2004 about 12% of middle school students and 28% of high school students smoked at least one cigarette in the past 30 days (Centers for Disease Control and Prevention [CDC], 2005). Each day approximately 4,000 children and adolescents younger than 18 years of age smoke their first tobacco cigarette. One-half of these teens become regular smokers (U.S. Department of Health and Human Services, Office of Applied Studies, 2003). Teenagers perceive increased social status from cigarette smoking. Girls often smoke cigarettes to control their body weight. Adolescents also believe cigarette smoking is harmless during the first few years of smoking (Waylen & Wolke, 2004). Advertising increases risk of cigarette smoking by glamorizing smoking and by fostering brand recognition and desirability (CDC, 2005).

Nutrient Requirements and Temporal Consumption Trends

Absolute nutrient requirements are increased in adolescence compared with childhood due to increased growth and body size. Adolescent boys have greater requirements for most nutrients compared with girls due to differences in growth and development. The exception is iron; postmenarcheal adolescent girls need more iron than boys due to menstrual blood losses (Institute of Medicine [IOM], Food and Nutrition Board, 2001).

Macronutrients

Average daily energy consumption assessed in National Health and Nutrition Examination Survey (NHANES) I (1971–1974) and III (1988–1994) has remained relatively constant, except for adolescent girls, whose energy intake increased from 1,735 to 1,996 kcal/day (Troiano, Briefel, Carroll, & Bialostosky, 2000; Briefel & Johnson, 2004). The proportion of energy derived from fat and saturated fat decreased over time but remains above the recommendations in the Dietary Guidelines at 33.5% for total fat and 12.5% for saturated fat (Troiano et al., 2000). In children over 6 years of age 10% to 18% of saturated fat and 5% to 10% of total fat was consumed in 2% fat and whole milk products.

Minerals

Calcium

The Food and Nutrition Board of the IOM established the adequate intake (AI) for calcium based on maximal calcium retention using data from epidemiologic studies, randomized controlled trials, and balance studies (IOM, Food and Nutrition Board, 1997). Calcium balance studies in adolescents determined that retention increased with dietary intake up to 1,300 mg/day. Recent longitudinal data of bone mineral deposition suggest that calcium requirements may be higher—1,500 mg for girls and 1,700 mg for boys—during peak calcium accretion (Whiting et al., 2004). Dairy foods supply 75% of the calcium in the American diet (Weaver, 2000). Some vegetables contain calcium, but the bioavailability is poor: 5 servings of broccoli and 15 servings of spinach provide as much absorbable calcium as 1 cup of milk (Weaver, 2000).

Adolescent boys aged 9 to 13 years consume, on average, 79% of the AI for calcium (1,022 mg/day) and girls 65% of the AI for calcium (842 mg/day) (Storey, Forshee, & Anderson, 2004). Older adolescent boys aged 14 to 18 years consume 1,156 mg calcium per day (89% of AI per day). However, calcium consumption is reduced among older adolescent girls aged 14 to 18 years; average daily calcium intake among these girls is only 750 mg/day or 57% of the AI (Storey et al., 2004). There also are significant ethnic differences in calcium consumption; African-American and Hispanic-American teenagers have lower daily calcium intakes than whites (Storey et al., 2004).

CRITICAL Thinking

Milk consumption has declined 36% among teenaged girls from the late 1970s to the mid-1990s. Teenaged girls may avoid dairy products because they believe dairy products promote weight gain. Lactose intolerance is another reason that teenagers, especially nonwhites, do not consume dairy products. Consumption of soft drinks has been associated with reduced bone mineral deposition in adolescent girls with average calcium intakes less than 900 mg/day but not in boys, whose calcium intakes averaged more than 1,000 mg (Whiting et al., 2004). Noncaffeinated carbonated soft drinks do not increase urinary calcium losses (Heaney & Rafferty, 2001). Because soft drinks often replace milk, reduced calcium consumption likely explains the relationship between soft drinks and bone mineral. What effects will this have in the aging process?

Iron

Iron requirements increase during adolescence to meet the demands of growth and inevitable losses. Iron is lost from the gastrointestinal tract, skin, and urine and from menstrual blood in females. The requirements for absorbed iron for adolescent boys and girls are estimated to be 1.47 and 1.15 mg/day, respectively (Fomon et al., 2003). The mean iron intake of adolescent boys aged 14 to 16 years is approximately 15 mg/day (Egan, Tao, Pennington, & Bolger, 2002). Thus most boys probably meet the absorbed iron requirement. In contrast, female adolescents average a daily intake of 11 mg (Egan et al., 2002) and thus are at risk for iron deficiency.

Sodium

Average daily sodium consumption has increased by approximately 1,000 mg for adolescent boys and girls between NHANES I (1971–1974) and NHANES (1999–2000). The average daily sodium intake for teenaged boys was about 4,000 mg and for girls, 3,000 mg.

Vitamins

Vitamin D

The AI for vitamin D is 5 µg (200 IU) per day for individuals aged 1 to 50 years (IOM, Food and Nutrition Board, 1997). Synthesis of vitamin D in the skin is adequate to meet the requirement with sufficient exposure to ultraviolet light. Skin vitamin D synthesis is reduced by use of sunscreen and by dark skin pigmentation. Recently, there have been increased reports of vitamin D insufficiency and deficiency, including reports of rickets among African-American children and vitamin D deficiency in adolescents. Individuals with darkly pigmented skin have reduced ability to synthesize vitamin D and therefore are at greater risk for insufficiency when dietary intakes are marginal.

Dietary intake of vitamin D among adolescents varies by ethnicity; non-Hispanic-American whites had the highest intakes of vitamin D and African-Americans the lowest (Moore, Murphy, & Holick, 2005). As a group adolescent boys are more likely to have adequate vitamin D intakes than girls and older males. However, there are significant ethnic differences; approximately 75% of non-Hispanic-American whites meet or exceed the AI, compared with 45% of non-Hispanic African-Americans and 58% of Mexican-Americans (Moore et al., 2005). Approximately one-half of adolescent girls meet or exceed the AI for vitamin D; only 38% of non-Hispanic African-Americans met the AI compared with 59% of whites and 60% of Mexican-Americans (Moore et al., 2005).

Fortified foods, mainly fortified milk, are the primary dietary sources of vitamin D. Because the prevalence of lactose intolerance is higher among African-Americans (75%) than among Hispanic-Americans (53%) and whites (6% to 22%), avoidance of dairy products may explain the reduced vitamin D intakes among African-American adolescents (Jackson & Savaiano, 2001). In 2003 the U.S. Food and Drug Administration approved vitamin D fortification of calcium-fortified juices and juice drinks. African-Americans and Mexican-Americans who avoid dairy products may benefit from these fortified products; for example, 8 ounces of fortified orange juice provides up to 2.5 µg (100 IU) vitamin D.

The current recommended intakes for vitamin D are probably too low, based on optimal calcium absorption. Without ultraviolet synthesis of vitamin D, 20 to 25 µg (800 to 1,000 IU) dietary vitamin D a day are needed to maintain serum vitamin D concentrations within the desired range (Dawson-Hughes, 2004). During peak pubertal growth, low serum concentrations of 25-hydroxyvitamin D increase serum **parathyroid hormone** and 1,25-dihydroxyvitamin D and, consequently, fractional calcium absorption (Abrams et al., 2005). In contrast to the relationship observed in adults, 25-hydroxyvitamin D was not correlated with fractional calcium absorption in adolescents. These findings suggest that adolescents adapt to suboptimal vitamin D status better than adults. Possible mechanisms include enhanced responsiveness of calcium absorption to 1,25-dihydroxyvitamin D, increased conversion of 25-hydroxy to 1,25-dihydroxyvitamin D, or increased vitamin D–independent calcium absorption (Abrams et al., 2005).

> **Parathyroid hormone:** Peptide hormone secreted by the parathyroid gland; it increases blood calcium by acting on the bone, intestine, and kidneys.

CRITICAL **Thinking**

Individuals who live at northern latitudes above the 35th parallel do not receive enough ultraviolet radiation to support adequate synthesis of vitamin D; between November and March vitamin D synthesis is dramatically reduced in the Northern Hemisphere (Moore et al., 2005). What effect does global warming have on this issue?

Dietary Patterns

Serving Size

Average serving sizes for foods eaten at home and away from home have increased during the past 30 years. The average serving sizes for foods frequently consumed by adolescents—salty snacks, French fries, ready to eat cereals, and soft drinks—have significantly increased. The volume of soft drinks consumed per occasion increased more than 50% among female adolescents. Foods with low nutrient density, such as soft drinks, candy, desserts, and salty and snacks, added sugar and fats, account for 30% of daily energy intake in children aged 8 to 18 years (Briefel & Johnson, 2004). Consumption of these low nutrient density foods is associated with higher energy intakes and lower consumption of vitamin A, folate, calcium, magnesium, iron, and zinc.

Food Groups

Adolescents do not consume the recommended number of servings of fruits, vegetables, and dairy products, and they consume excessive amounts of added sugar (Xie, Gilliland, Li, & Rockett, 2003), fat, and saturated fat (Briefel & Johnson, 2004). In a study of 18,000 adolescents who participated in the National Longitudinal Study of Adolescent Health, many did not eat the minimum recommended number of servings of vegetables (71%), fruits (55%), and dairy products (47%) (Videon & Manning, 2003). Teenagers who did not consume milk had inadequate intakes of vitamin A, folate, calcium, phosphorous, and magnesium (Briefel & Johnson, 2004).

Skipping Breakfast

One-fifth of adolescents report skipping·breakfast (Videon & Manning, 2003). Children who skip breakfast have lower daily intakes of vitamins A, E, D, and B_6; calcium; phosphorous; and magnesium compared with breakfast eaters (Nicklas, Bao, Webber, & Berenson, 1993). Eating breakfast also is associated with increased school attendance and academic performance (Pollitt, 1995).

Added Sugars

Adolescents have the highest intake of added sugars than any other age group; approximately 40% of added sugars are consumed in carbonated soft drinks (Briefel & Johnson, 2004). Soft drinks supply approximately 8% of total energy intake among adolescents. Overweight adolescents derive more of their daily energy intake from soft drinks than normal weight teens (Troiano et al., 2000). Teenagers consume more carbonated soft drinks than they do fruit juices, fruit ades, or milk. Consumption of soda and fruit drinks among adolescent girls doubled and milk consumption decreased between NHANES I (1971–1974) and

NHANES III (1988–1994). Based on the U.S. Department of Agriculture (USDA) Continuing Survey of Food Intakes by Individuals for adolescents age 12 to 17 years, consumption of sweetened breakfast cereals is positively associated with dietary intakes of calcium, folate, and iron and sweetened dairy products increase calcium intakes. However, consumption of other foods and beverages that are high in sugar was associated with poor diet quality, including reduced intakes of calcium, iron, and folate (Frary, Johnson, & Wang, 2004). Displacement of milk by high sugar beverages reduces consumption of protein, calcium, and vitamins B_2, B_{12}, and D (St. Onge, Keller, & Heymsfield, 2003).

Fast Food Consumption

Most adolescents frequently eat meals and snacks away from home. In one study 26% of all meals and snacks were consumed away from home, accounting for 32% of total energy (Lin, Guthrie, & Frazao, 1999). In another survey 75% of adolescents reported eating at a fast food restaurant in the previous week (French, Story, Neumark-Sztainer, Fulkerson, & Hannan, 2001). Teens who ate at a fast food restaurant at least three times in the past week had energy intakes about 40% higher than adolescents who did not eat fast food. Frequency of fast food consumption also is inversely related to daily servings of vegetables, fruit, and dairy products (French et al., 2001). Adolescents who described themselves as overweight were more likely to have poor dietary consumption patterns (Videon & Manning, 2003) but did not differ in frequency of fast food consumption compared with normal weight teens (French et al., 2001). Adolescent boys are more likely than girls to eat away from home (Briefel & Johnson, 2004). Teenagers who were employed ate fast food more frequently than those who did not work (French et al., 2001).

Sociodemographic Moderators of Dietary Intake

Gender, ethnicity, parental income, and education affect diet quality in adolescents. Non-Hispanic-American whites have the lowest intakes of fruit; African-Americans and Asian-Americans have significantly higher consumption of vegetables (Xie et al., 2003). Degree of acculturation affects nutrient intake among Hispanic-American youths. Adolescents whose families were less acculturated had lower intakes of energy, protein, sodium, and percent of energy from fat and saturated fat and greater intakes of folate compared with acculturated families (Mazur,

Marquis, & Jensen, 2003). Higher parental education level was associated with better diet quality, and the presence of a parent at the evening meal was positively associated with consumption of fruits, vegetables, and dairy products. Another study of 3,200 adolescents reported higher intakes of polyunsaturated fat, protein, calcium, and folate in teenagers from families with higher incomes and lower intakes of total fat, saturated fat, and cholesterol with higher parental education (Xie et al., 2003). Snacking is more common among families with higher incomes, and income modifies the selection of snack foods. Family income at or below 130% of the poverty line reported higher intakes of fried potatoes, potato chips, whole milk, and fruit drinks and ades than those with incomes at or above 300% of the poverty line (Briefel & Johnson, 2004).

As children make the transition from dependence on their parents to autonomy, normative family development includes increased frequency and intensity of parent–child conflicts. During this time peer influence on values and behavior becomes stronger as peers replace parents as the primary source of social support. Teenagers may use diet as a means of expressing their self-identity and autonomy. Peers may exert either positive or negative influences on food intake.

Advertising and marketing of foods and beverages influences the food preferences, purchase requests, purchase, and consumption of children and youth (IOM, Food and Nutrition Board, 2006). Television is the primary source of advertising, but other forms of marketing such as radio, print, billboards, and the Internet also are used to influence purchases by adolescents. Most products marketed to children and teenagers are high in energy, sugars, fat, and salt and low in micronutrients. Children are more vulnerable to advertising than teenagers because they are not able to differentiate between informative and commercial programming. There is strong evidence that advertising influences food preferences, purchase requests, and short-term food consumption of children 2 to 11 years of age. There are insufficient data to determine the effect of advertising on teenagers. However, television advertising is positively

Effect of Advertising

Advertising influences the consumption of alcoholic beverages by adolescents. Exposure to alcohol advertising on television, radio, magazines, and billboards increased alcohol consumption in a dose-dependent manner in individuals aged 15 to 20 years. Each additional advertisement seen increased the number of drinks consumed by 1% (Snyder et al., 2006).

correlated with body fat in children and adolescents (IOM, Food and Nutrition Board, 2006). Television and video viewing are associated with reduced consumption of fruits and vegetables in adolescents (Boynton-Jarrett et al., 2003).

School Food Environment

The recent increase in excessive weight and obesity in adolescents has brought the food environment in schools under increasing scrutiny. Most schools have "competitive" foods for sale in addition to the USDA National School Breakfast and Lunch Programs that provide free and reduced cost meals to students from low-income families. The USDA meals programs are subject to federal regulations, including nutrient standards (USDA, 2005). Despite these regulations, the meals offered by these programs have been reported to exceed the USDA's recommendations for fat (38% versus <30% of total energy), saturated fat (15% versus <10% of total energy), and sodium (~1,500 mg per meal versus <2,400 mg/day).

Competitive foods include those that are sold a la carte, in vending machines, from school stores, or by school fundraisers. The only federal regulation regarding competitive foods is restriction of the sale of "foods of minimal nutritional value" (e.g., carbonated beverages, water ices, chewing gum, and some candy) in the lunch rooms during meals (French, 2005). Fruits, fruit juices, and vegetables are rarely offered for sale in school stores or in vending machines (St. Onge et al., 2003). Concern about the increasing incidence of excessive weight in children has caused some states and local school districts to regulate competitive foods through legislation and policy. Sales of a la carte foods and vending machine purchases are significant in middle and high schools, and many of the available selections are high in fat and/or added sugar (Kann, Grunbaum, McKenna, Wechsler, & Galuska, 2005). The School Health Profiles assessment of schools from 27 states and 11 large urban school districts found that nearly 90% of districts offered competitive foods. The most prevalent types of less nutritious foods were chocolate candy (65% of schools); other candy (68%); salty snacks, not low in fat (75%); soft drinks, sports drinks, or fruit drinks. Low-fat salty snacks (80%) and 100% fruit juice (84%) were the most common choices with higher nutritional value; fruits and vegetables were offered by 45% of schools surveyed (Kann et al., 2005). In a survey of public high schools in Pennsylvania the top-selling items were pizza, hamburgers, or sandwiches; baked goods not low in fat; French-fried potatoes; salty snacks not low in fat; carbonated beverages, sports drinks, and fruit drinks; and bottled water (Probart et al., 2005).

Availability of competitive foods reduces diet quality (French & Stables, 2003a). Interventions to the school food environment designed to promote consumption of fruits and vegetables significantly increase fruit intake with a negligible effect on vegetable consumption (French & Stables, 2003a). Increased availability of fruit and fruit juices effectively increase intake. Reducing the cost of healthy food items offered in school snack bars and vending machines increases the purchases of these items. Alternatively, increasing the cost of higher fat "junk" foods reduces purchase and consumption of these foods (French, 2005). Other innovative strategies include school gardening programs, use of produce from local farmers' markets in school salad bars, and free fruit and vegetables.

Health Status of U.S. Adolescents

Excessive Weight and Obesity

The prevalence of excessive weight (i.e., ≥ 95th percentile for BMI on 2000 CDC growth charts) among adolescents has increased from 6.1% in NHANES I (1974–1976) to 15.5% in NHANES (1999–2000). The increase in excessive weight was greatest in African-American and Mexican-American teens; the prevalence of excessive weight approaches 25% in these ethnic groups (Moore, 2004). Adolescents from lower income households are twice as likely to be overweight or obese compared with those from higher income families.

The increase in excessive weight and obesity in adolescents has been attributed to a dietary shift away from fruits and vegetables toward fats and simple carbohydrates and to decreased energy expenditure in physical activity. Among children aged 12 to 19 years, only 50% report regular vigorous physical activity and 25% do not get any vigorous exercise (Moore, 2004). The time spent in sedentary activities also is increasing among adolescents. In 1997 parents reported that their children (aged 2 to 17 years) watched an averaged of 2.1 hours of television per day; by 2000 the average time spent watching television increased to 2.45 hours per day, and a total of 382 minutes were spent watching television, playing video games, using a computer, talking on the telephone, or reading (Ford, Mokdad, & Ajani, 2004).

Excess adiposity during adolescence increases the risk of adult obesity and chronic diseases. In the National Longitudinal Study of Adolescent Health of 9,795 adolescents, baseline prevalence of obesity was 12.5%, and only 1.6% of adolescents who were obese between ages 13 and 20 years were not obese 5 years later (Ford et al., 2004). Non-Hispanic African-American females were more likely to become and remain obese than non-Hispanic-American whites; Asian women were less likely to become and remain obese (Ford et al., 2004). The risk of hypertension is increased 10-fold, dyslipidemias 3- to 8-fold, and diabetes mellitus 2-fold by excess adiposity. Surprisingly, only 39.6% of adolescents aged 12 to 15 years and 51.6% of older teens aged 16 to 19 years were ever informed of their overweight status by a physician or healthcare provider (Ogden, 2005). Read more about childhood obesity in Chapter 7.

Metabolic Syndrome

The comorbidities of diabetes, hypertension, and hyperlipidemia in patients with cardiovascular disease have been described as the metabolic syndrome. Using the guidelines from NHANES III, the metabolic syndrome is defined as having three or more of the following risk factors: abdominal obesity (i.e., waist circumference 90th percentile for age and gender), triglycerides at least 110 mg/dL, fasting glucose at least 110 mg/dL, systolic or diastolic blood pressure at least in the 90th percentile (age, height, gender specific), and no more than 40 mg/dL high-density lipoprotein for males and no more than 50 mg/dL for females.

Data from NHANES III of 1,366 adolescents aged 12 to 17 years found the prevalence of the metabolic syndrome to be 6.3% among boys and 4.1% among girls. Abdominal obesity, assessed by waist circumference, was identified in 17.9%, hypertriglyceridemia was present in 21.0%, and 18.0% had low high-density lipoprotein and 7.1% had hypertension. Furthermore, the prevalence of elevated C-reactive protein was nearly four times greater in adolescents with the metabolic syndrome compared with those without it (Ford, Ajani, Mokdad, & National Health and National Examination, 2005). Using slightly different criteria for the metabolic syndrome (i.e., waist circumference ≥ 75th percentile and high-density lipoprotein ≤ 45 mg/dL for adolescent boys), the prevalence of the metabolic syndrome was 9.2% in 1,960 adolescents aged 12 to 19 years and was comparable among boys and girls (de Ferranti et al., 2004).

There were small changes in risk factors for the metabolic syndrome in children and adolescents between NHANES III and NHANES (1999–2000): Waist circumference increased by 2.0 cm in children aged 2 to 17 years, systolic blood pressure increased 2.2 mm Hg in children aged 8 to 17 years, and triglycerides decreased by 8.8 mg/dL and glucose by 2.5 mg/dL in teens aged 12 to 17 years. Total cholesterol, high-density lipoprotein and low-density lipoprotein cholesterol, and glycosylated hemoglobin were unchanged (Ford et al., 2004).

Iron Deficiency

Approximately 9% of girls aged 12 to 15 years and 16% of adolescent girls aged 16 to 19 years are iron deficient (Looker, 2002). Iron deficiency anemia affects 2% of girls aged 12 to 19 years. The prevalence of iron deficiency among males 12–15 years is 5%. Iron deficiency causes reduced exercise capacity, immune function, and cognitive performance. Adolescent girls who were iron deficient scored lower in verbal learning and memory (Ford et al., 2004) and in math (Halterman, Kaczorowski, Aligne, Auinger, & Szilagyi, 2001) compared with those with normal iron status. Iron deficiency also may contribute to attention deficit hyperactivity disorder. Children with attention deficit hyperactivity disorder have significantly lower concentrations of ferritin than control subjects (Konofal, Lecendreux, Arnulf, & Mouren, 2004).

Tobacco Use and Nutritional Status

Although the prevalence of smoking among adults in the United States has decreased in the 40 years after the Surgeon General's report describing the adverse consequences of cigarette smoking, more adolescents are smoking now than in the past. In 2004 30% of adolescents smoked. In addition, children are starting to smoke at a younger age. Rates of regular tobacco use increase significantly at age 11 years (DuRant & Smith, 1999; Winkleby, Robinson, Sundquist, & Kraemer, 1999). Non-Hispanic-American white adolescents are more likely to smoke cigarettes than African-American, Mexican-American, and Native American teens (CDC, Division of Adolescent and School Health and Office on Smoking and Health, 1999). Most adolescents smoke to control their weight, and some substitute smoking a cigarette for eating (Dowdell & Santucci, 2004).

Adult smokers have significantly higher intakes of energy, total fat, saturated fat, cholesterol, and alcohol and lower intakes of polyunsaturated fat, fiber, vitamin C, vitamin E, and beta-carotene than nonsmokers (Dallongeville, Marécaux, Fruchart, & Amouyel, 1998). Similarly, adolescent smokers consume less fiber, vitamins, and minerals than nonsmokers (Hampl & Betts, 1999). The more a teenager smokes, the less likely they are to exercise at least three times per week and consume at least one serving per day of vegetables or milk/dairy products (Wilson et al., 2005). Adolescents who smoke consume more alcohol than nonsmokers (Crawley & While, 1996). For some teens who smoke, their poor diet may reflect the poor diet quality of their parents, who also smoke. Nonsmoking children of parents who smoke had lower intakes of folate and vitamins C and E than children whose parents do not smoke (Crawley & While, 1996). Among young women passive and active smokers had lower intakes of folate and concentration of folate in serum compared with nonsmokers and values reported in 1999–2000 NHANES (Ortega et al., 2004).

Data from NHANES III show that environmental tobacco smoke exposure and active cigarette smoking increase the risk of the metabolic syndrome among adolescents. Teens exposed to environmental tobacco smoke were 4.7 times as likely to develop the metabolic syndrome compared with nonexposed adolescents; the odds ratio for active smokers was 6.1 (Weitzman et al., 2005). Among overweight adolescents 19.6% of those exposed to environmental tobacco smoke and 23.6% of smokers had the metabolic syndrome compared with 5.6% of nonexposed teens (Weitzman et al., 2005). Unfortunately, 43% of children in the United States live in a household with at least one smoker. Alcohol and marijuana users eat more snack foods and less fruit, vegetables, and milk than nonusers (Farrow, Rees, & Worthington-Roberts, 1987).

Adolescent Pregnancy

There are approximately 0.9 million adolescent pregnancies in the United States per year; more than 40% of adolescent girls have been pregnant at least once before 20 years of age (Kirby, Coyle, & Gould, 2001). About 51% of these pregnancies end in live births. Pregnant adolescents are more likely to have nutritional and medical complications than adult women; the risk is greatest for the youngest teenagers.

Teenagers are twice as likely to deliver a low birth weight infant and the rate of neonatal death is increased nearly threefold compared with adult women. Premature delivery is more common in teenagers. Inadequate and excessive maternal weight gain (Howie, Parker, & Schoendorf, 2003), pregnancy-induced hypertension, and anemia are common nutrition-related problems among pregnant adolescents (Klein, 2005). Low prepregnancy body weight and **gynecologic age**, parity, and poor nutritional status negatively affect pregnancy outcome (Klein, 2005). Smoking tobacco or marijuana, behaviors that are relatively common among adolescents, reduces birth weight (Fergusson & Woodward, 2000).

Gynecologic age: Years since menarche.

To optimize infant birth weight the IOM (1990) recommended that pregnant adolescents gain weight at the upper end of the recommended rates for each prepregnancy BMI category. However, the recommendation for greater weight gain in adolescents is controversial because it may increase the risk of maternal obesity (McAnarney & Stevens-Simon , 1993). Early and continuous weight gain is also important (American Dietetic Association, 1994). Inadequate weight gain in the first 24 weeks increases the risk of having a small for gestational age infant; low rates of weight gain late in gestation increase the risk of premature delivery (Hediger, Scholl, Belsky, Ances, & Salmon, 1989).

In addition to gestational weight gain, maternal growth is an important determinant of birth weight. Among teens who are still growing, gestational weight gain is positively associated with increased maternal subcutaneous adiposity and not with birth weight (Scholl, Hediger, Schall, Khoo, & Fischer, 1994). Growing adolescents give birth to infants that weigh 150 to 200 g less than nongrowing teens or adult women. Reduced placental perfusion and transfer of micronutrients to the fetus explain, at least in part, the lower birth weight.

> **● Learning Point** An increase in leptin during gestation may mediate the increased maternal adiposity and fetal growth restriction in growing adolescents (Scholl, Stein, & Smith, 2000). Leptin also may mediate the increased postpartum weight retention observed in growing adolescents compared with nongrowing teens (Scholl et al., 2000).

Nutrition is one of the most important modifiable factors that alters pregnancy outcome. Adolescents may improve their diet quality during pregnancy, but total energy and iron intake often are inadequate (American Dietetic Association, 1994). Suboptimal intakes of magnesium, zinc, folate, and vitamin B$_6$ also have been reported among pregnant adolescents (Pope, Skinner, & Carruth, 1992). Calcium, vitamin B$_6$, vitamin C, and folate supplements are recommended for teens at risk for poor dietary intakes (American Dietetic Association, 1994). Food cravings and aversions to previously preferred foods are common among adolescents. Cravings for sweet foods increase the consumption of sugar, and craving salty snacks is associated with increased consumption of sodium and fat (Pope et al., 1992).

Body Dissatisfaction, Dieting, and Eating Disorders

Nearly 30% of high school students believe they are overweight; girls are more likely to believe they are overweight (35%) than boys (23%). More than one-half of female students (62%) were trying to lose weight compared with 29% of males. Exercise is the most common weight control behavior (60% of all students), followed by dieting (44%), fasting (14%), diet pills (9%), and vomiting or laxative use (5%). All weight control behaviors are more prevalent among female adolescents than males (Grunbaum et al., 2002).

Eating disorders are psychiatric disorders with significant medical and psychosocial complications that affect about 5 million Americans, primarily adolescent girls and young women. Three eating disorders have been identified by the American Psychiatric Association, anorexia nervosa, bulimia nervosa, and eating disorder not otherwise specified; the diagnostic criteria are outlined in the *Diagnostic and Statistical Manual of Mental Disorders,* 4th edition (American Psychiatric Association, 2000). The eating disorders share an excessive importance of body weight and shape to self-concept and self-esteem.

The estimated combined prevalence of anorexia nervosa and bulimia nervosa in the United States is 3% among young women and an additional 3% have eating disorder not otherwise specified, affecting about 5 million Americans (Becker, Grinspoon, Klibanski, & Herzog, 1999). The incidence of anorexia nervosa is 19 females and 2 males per 100,000 per year compared with 29 females and 1 male for bulimia nervosa (Fairburn & Harrison, 2003). It is thought that the incidence of both anorexia nervosa and bulimia nervosa has increased in the recent past. It is very difficult to accurately determine the frequency of eating disorders in the general population (Agras et al., 2004).

Because of the reluctance to seek treatment, many eating disorders go undiagnosed in the community. In addition, there is bias in access to treatment, which in turn biases the reported prevalence of eating disorders among different ethnic and racial groups and between the genders. There is very little epidemiologic data regarding eating disorder not otherwise specified, although these atypical eating disorders seem to primarily affect adolescents and young adult women (Fairburn & Bohn, 2005). Read more about eating disorders in Chapter 8.

Issues to Debate

1. If girls experience peer pressure to eat like other teens, including boys, what might be the result?
2. Discuss how psychosocial development during adolescence affects health-related behaviors, including dietary patterns.
3. What are the sociodemographic factors affecting dietary patterns? How does this affect a pregnant teen?
4. What are the dietary implications to chronic disease incidence among adolescents?

Case Study

Anne is 5'8" tall and from her sophomore year in high school until she began her freshman year at MU she weighed 145 pounds. After arriving on campus she began to restrict her food intake by skipping breakfast and lunch. At the end of the first semester Anne now weighs 110 pounds but is not satisfied with her weight or the shape of her body. Anne has been amenorrheic for 4 months. Occasionally (about once a month) she becomes so hungry that she finds herself consuming large amounts of food and feels out of control while eating. Afterward, Anne is so consumed with guilt she does not eat anything for the next 24 hours and increases her exercise to "make up" for the extra calories.

What diagnosis would you give Anne? What subtype diagnosis would you give Anne?

What diagnosis would you give Anne if the frequency of her bingeing increased to everyday, she began to purge by vomiting, and these behaviors lasted for 6 months?

References

Abrams, S. A., Griffin, I. J., Hawthorne, K. M., Gunn, S. K., Gundberg, C. M., & Carpenter, T. O. (2005). Relationships among vitamin D levels, parathyroid hormone, and calcium absorption in young adolescents. *Journal of Clinical Endocrinology and Metabolism, 90,* 5576–5581.

Agras, W. S., Brandt, H. A., Bulik, C. M., Dolan-Sewell, R., Fairburn, C. G., Halmi, K. A., et al. (2004). Report of the National Institutes of Health workshop on overcoming barriers to treatment research in anorexia nervosa. *International Journal of Eating Disorders, 35,* 509–521.

American Dietetic Association. (1994). Position of the American Dietetic Association: Nutrition care for pregnant adolescents. *Journal of the American Dietetic Association, 94,* 449–450.

American Psychiatric Association. (2000). *Diagnostic and Statistical Manual of Mental Disorders* (4th ed., text revision). Washington, DC: Author.

Becker, A. E., Grinspoon, S. K., Klibanski, A., & Herzog, D. B. (1999). Eating disorders. *New England Journal of Medicine, 340,* 1092–1098.

Bonny, A. E., Ziegler, J., Harvey, R., Debanne, S. M., Secic, M., & Cromer, B. (2006). Weight gain in obese and non-obese adolescent girls initiating depot medroxyprogesterone, oral contraceptive pills, or no hormonal contraceptive method. *Archives of Pediatric and Adolescent Medicine, 160,* 40–45.

Boynton-Jarrett, R., Thomas, T. N., Peterson, K. E., Wiecha, J., Sobol, A. M., & Gortmaker, S. L. (2003). Impact of television viewing patterns on fruit and vegetable consumption among adolescents. *Pediatrics, 112,* 1321–1326.

Boys, A., Farrell, M., Taylor, C., Marsden, J., Goodman, R., Brugha, T., et al. (2003). Psychiatric morbidity and substance use in young people aged 13–15 years: Results from the Child and Adolescent Survey of Mental Health. *British Journal of Psychiatry, 182,* 509–517.

Briefel, R. R., & Johnson, C. L. (2004). Secular trends in dietary intake in the United States. *Annual Review of Nutrition, 24,* 401–431.

Bryant, R. J., Wastney, M. E., Martin, B. R., Wood, O., McCabe, G. P., Morshidi, M., et al. (2003). Racial differences in bone turnover and calcium metabolism in adolescent females. *Journal of Clinical Endocrinology and Metabolism, 88,* 1043–1047.

Centers for Disease Control and Prevention. (2005). Tobacco use, access, and exposure to tobacco in media among middle and high school students—United States, 2004. *Morbidity and Mortality Weekly Report, 54,* 297–301.

Centers for Disease Control and Prevention, Division of Adolescent and School Health and Office on Smoking and Health. (1999). Cigarette smoking among high school students—11 states, 1991–1997. *The Journal of School Health, 69*(8), 303–306.

Crawley, H. F., & While, D. (1996). Parental smoking and the nutrient intake and food choice of British teenagers aged 16–17 years. *Journal of Epidemiology and Community Health, 50,* 306–312.

Dallongeville, J., Marécaux, N., Fruchart, J. C., & Amouyel, P. (1998). Cigarette smoking is associated with unhealthy patterns of nutrient intake: A meta-analysis. *Journal of Nutrition, 128,* 1450–1457.

Dawson-Hughes, B. (2004). Racial/ethnic considerations in making recommendations for vitamin D for adult and elderly men and women. *American Journal of Clinical Nutrition, 80,* 1763S–1766S.

de Ferranti, S. D., Gauvreau, K., Ludwig, D. S., Neufeld, E. J., Newburger, J. W., & Rifai, N. (2004). Prevalence of the metabolic syndrome in American adolescents: Findings from the Third National Health and Nutrition Examination Survey. *Circulation, 110*, 2494–2497.

Dowdell, E. B., & Santucci, M. E. (2004). Health risk behavior assessment: Nutrition, weight, and tobacco use in one urban seventh-grade class. *Public Health Nursing, 21*, 128–136.

DuRant, R. H., & Smith, J. A. (1999). Adolescent tobacco use and cessation. *Primary Care, 26*, 553–575.

Eastell, R. (2005). Role of oestrogen in the regulation of bone turnover at the menarche. *Journal of Endocrinology, 185*, 223–234.

Egan, S. K., Tao, S. S. H., Pennington, J. A. H., & Bolger, P. M. (2002). US Food and Drug Administration's Total Diet Study: Intake of nutritional and toxic elements, 1991–96. *Food Additives and Contaminants, 19*, 103–125.

Fairburn, C. G., & Harrison, P. J. (2003). Eating disorders. *Lancet, 361*, 407–416.

Fairburn, C. G., & Bohn, K. (2005). Eating disorder NOS (EDNOS): An example of the troublesome "not otherwise specified" (NOS) category in DSM-IV. *Behavioral Research Therapy, 43*, 691–701.

Farrow, J. A., Rees, J. M., & Worthington-Roberts, B. S. (1987). Health, developmental, and nutritional status of adolescent alcohol and marijuana abusers. *Pediatrics, 79*, 218–223.

Federico, G., Baroncelli, G. I., Vanacore, T., Fiore, L., & Saggese, G. (2003). Pubertal changes in biochemical markers of growth. *Hormone Research, 60*, 46–51.

Fergusson, D. M., & Woodward, L. J. (2000). Educational, psychosocial, and sexual outcomes of girls with conduct problems in early adolescence. *Journal of Child Psychology and Psychiatry, 41*, 779–792.

Fomon, S. J., Drulis, J. M., Nelson, S. E., Serfass, R. E., Woodhead, J. C., & Ziegler, E. E. (2003). Inevitable iron loss by human adolescents, with calculations of the requirement for absorbed iron. *Journal of Nutrition, 133*, 167–172.

Ford, E. S., Mokdad, A. H., & Ajani, U. A. (2004). Trends in risk factors for cardiovascular disease among children and adolescents in the United States. *Pediatrics, 114*, 1534–1544.

Ford, E. S., Ajani, U. A., Mokdad, A. H., & National Health and National Examination. (2005). The metabolic syndrome and concentrations of C-reactive protein among U.S. youth. *Diabetes Care, 28*, 878–881.

Frary, C. D., Johnson, R. K., & Wang, M. Q. (2004). Children and adolescents' choices of foods and beverages high in added sugars are associated with intakes of key nutrients and food groups. *Journal of Adolescent Health, 34*, 56–63.

French, S. A. (2005). Public health strategies for dietary change: Schools and workplaces. *Journal of Nutrition, 135*, 910–912.

French, S. A., Story, M., Neumark-Sztainer, D., Fulkerson, J. A., & Hannan, P. (2001). Fast food restaurant use among adolescents: Associations with nutrient intake, food choices and behavioral and psychosocial variables. *International Journal of Obesity and Related Metabolic Disorders, 25*, 1823–1833.

French, S. A., & Stables, G. (2003a). Environmental interventions to promote vegetable and fruit consumption among youth in school settings. *Preventive Medicine, 37*, 593–610.

French, S. A., Story, M., Fulkerson, J. A., & Gerlack, A. F. (2003b). Food environment in secondary schools: À la carte, vending machines, and food policies and practices. *American Journal of Public Health, 93*, 1161–1167.

Fujiwara, S., Kasagi, F., Yamada, M., & Kodama, K. (1997). Risk factors for hip fracture in a Japanese cohort. *Journal of Bone and Mineral Research, 12*, 998–1004.

Grunbaum, J. A., Kann, L., Kinchen, S. A., Williams, B., Ross, J. G., Lowry, R., et al. (2002). Youth risk behavior surveillance—United States, 2001. *Journal of School Health, 72*, 313–328.

Guo, S. S., Chunlea, W. C., Roche, A. F., & Siervogel, R. M. (1997). Age- and maturity-related changes in body composition during adolescence into adulthood: The Fels Longitudinal Study. *International Journal of Obesity and Related Metabolic Disorders, 21*, 1167–1175.

Halterman, J. S., Kaczorowski, J. M., Aligne, C. A., Auinger, P., & Szilagyi, P. G. (2001). Iron deficiency and cognitive achievement among school-aged children and adolescents in the United States. *Pediatrics, 107*, 1381–1386.

Hampl, J. S., & Betts, N. M. (1999). Cigarette use during adolescence: Effects on nutritional status. *Nutrition Reviews, 57*, 215–221.

Harris, K. M., Gordon-Larsen, P., Chantala, K., & Udry, J. R. (2006). Longitudinal trends in race/ethnic disparities in leading health indicators from adolescence to young adulthood. *Archives of Pediatric and Adolescent Medicine, 160*, 74–81.

Heaney, R. P., & Rafferty, K. (2001). Carbonated beverages and urinary calcium excretion. *American Journal of Clinical Nutrition, 74*, 343–347.

Hediger, M. L., Scholl, T. O., Belsky, D. H., Ances, I. G., & Salmon, R. W. (1989). Patterns of weight gain in adolescent pregnancy: Effects on birth weight and preterm delivery. *Obstetrics and Gynecology, 74*, 6–12.

Howie, L. D., Parker, J. D., & Schoendorf, K. C. (2003). Excessive maternal weight gain patterns in adolescents. *Journal of the American Dietetic Association, 103*, 1653–1657.

Institute of Medicine (IOM). (1990). *Nutrition During Pregnancy. Part I. Weight Gain. Part II. Supplements.* Washington, DC: National Academy Press.

Institute of Medicine (IOM), Food and Nutrition Board. (1997). *Dietary Reference Intakes for Calcium, Magnesium, Phosphorous, Vitamin D.* Washington, DC: National Academy of Sciences.

Institute of Medicine (IOM), Food and Nutrition Board. (2001). *Dietary Reference Intakes for Vitamin A, Vitamin K, Arsenic, Boron, Chromium, Copper, Iodine, Iron,*

Manganese, Nickel, Silicon, Vanadium, and Zinc. Washington, DC: National Academy Press.

Institute of Medicine (IOM), Food and Nutrition Board. (2006). *Food Marketing to Children and Youth: Threat or Opportunity.* Washington, DC: National Academy Press.

Jackson, K. A., & Savaiano, D. A. (2001). Lactose maldigestion, calcium intake and osteoporosis in African-, Asian-, and Hispanic-Americans. *Journal of the American College of Nutrition, 20*, 198S–207S.

Kann, L., Grunbaum, J., McKenna, M. L., Wechsler, H., & Galuska, D. A. (2005). Competitive foods and beverages available for purchase in secondary schools—selected sites, United States, 2004. *Morbidity and Mortality Weekly Report, 54*, 917–921.

Kirby, D., Coyle, K., & Gould, J. B. (2001). Manifestations of poverty and birthrates among young teenagers in California zip code areas. *Family Planning Perspectives, 33*, 63–69.

Klein, J. D. (2005). Adolescent pregnancy: Current trends and issues. *Pediatrics, 116*, 281–286.

Konofal, E., Lecendreux, M., Arnulf, I., & Mouren, M. C. (2004). Iron deficiency in children with attention-deficit/hyperactivity disorder. *Archives of Pediatric and Adolescent Medicine, 158*, 1113–1115.

Leung, K. C., Johannsson, G., Leong, G. M., & Ho, K. K. (2004). Estrogen regulation of growth hormone action. *Endocrine Reviews, 25*, 693–721.

Lin B-H., Guthrie, J., & Frazao, E. (1999). Nutrient contribution of food away from home. In Frazao, E. (Ed.), *America's Eating Habits: Changes and Consequences.* USDA, ERS Agriculture Information Bulletin 750.

Looker, A. C. (2002). Iron deficiency—United States, 1999–2000. *Mortality and Morbidity Weekly Report, 51*, 897–899.

Mazur, R. E., Marquis, G. S., & Jensen, H. H. (2003). Diet and food insufficiency among Hispanic-American youths: Acculturation and socioeconomic factors in the third National Health and Nutrition Examination Survey. *American Journal of Clinical Nutrition, 78*, 1120–1127.

McAnarney, E. R., & Stevens-Simon, C. (1993). First, do no harm. Low birth weight and adolescent obesity. *American Journal of Diseases of Children, 147*, 983–985.

McGinnis, J. M. (1993). Actual causes of death in the United States. *Journal of the American Medical Association, 270*, 2207–2212.

Mokdad, A. H., Serdula, M. K., Dietz, W. H., Bowman, B. A., Marks, J. S., & Koplan, J. P. (2000). The continuing epidemic of obesity in the United States. *Journal of the American Medical Association, 284*, 1650–1651.

Molgaard, C., Thomsen, B. L., & Michaelsen, K. F. (1999). Whole body bone mineral accretion in healthy children and adolescents. *Archives of Disease in Childhood, 81*, 10–15.

Moore, C. E., Murphy, M. M., & Holick, M. F. (2005). Vitamin D intakes by children and adults in the United States differ among ethnic groups. *Journal of Nutrition, 135*, 2478–2485.

Moore, T. R. (2004). Adolescent and adult obesity in women: A tidal wave just beginning. *Clinical Obstetrics and Gynecology, 47*, 884–889.

National Center for Health Statistics. (2000). CDC growth charts: United States. U.S. Department of Health and Human Services, Centers for Disease Control and Prevention.

Nicklas, T. A., Bao, W., Webber, L. S., & Berenson, G. S. (1993). Breakfast consumption affects adequacy of total daily intake in children. *Journal of the American Dietetic Association, 93*, 886–891.

Ogden, C. (2005). Children and teens told by doctors that they are overweight—United States, 1999–2002. *Mortality and Morbidity Weekly Report, 54*, 848–849.

Ortega, R. M., Requejo, A. M., López-Sobaler, A. M., Navia, B., Mena, M. C., Basabe, B., et al. (2004). Smoking and passive smoking as conditioners of folate status in young women. *Journal of the American College of Nutrition, 23*, 365–371.

Pollitt, E. (1995). Does breakfast make a difference in school? *Journal of the American Dietetic Association, 95*, 1134–1139.

Pope, J. F., Skinner, J. D., & Carruth, B. R. (1992). Cravings and aversions of pregnant adolescents. *Journal of the American Dietetic Association, 92*, 1479–1482.

Probart, C., McDonnell, E., Weirich, J. E., Hartman, T., Bailey-Davis, L., & Prabhakher, V. (2005). Competitive foods available in Pennsylvania public high schools. *Journal of the American Dietetic Association, 105*, 1243–1249.

Rey, J. M., Martin, A., & Krabman, P. (2004). Is the party over? Cannabis and juvenile psychiatric disorder: The past 10 years. *Journal of the American Academy of Child and Adolescent Psychiatry, 43*, 1194–1205.

Riggs, B. L., Khosla, S., & Melton, L. J. 3rd. (2002). Sex steroids and the construction and conservation of the adult skeleton. *Endocrine Reviews, 23*, 279–302.

Roy, D. K., O'Neill, T. W., Finn, J. D., Lunt, M., Silman, A. J., Felsenberg, D., et al. (2003). Determinants of incident vertebral fracture in men and women: Results from the European Prospective Osteoporosis Study (EPOS). *Osteoporosis International, 14*, 19–26.

Scholl, T. O., Hediger, M. L., Schall, J. L., Khoo, C. S., & Fischer, R. L. (1994). Maternal growth during pregnancy and the competition for nutrients. *American Journal of Clinical Nutrition, 60*, 183–188.

Scholl, T. O., Stein, T. P., & Smith, W. K. (2000). Leptin and maternal growth during adolescent pregnancy. *American Journal of Clinical Nutrition, 72*, 1542–1547.

Schonau, E. (2004). The peak bone mass concept: Is it still relevant? *Pediatric Nephrology, 19*, 825–831.

Simm, P. J., & Werther, G. A. (2005). Child and adolescent growth disorders—An overview. *Australian Family Physician, 34*, 731–737.

Snyder, L. B., Milici, F. F., Slater, M., Sun, H., & Strizhakova, Y. (2006). Effects of alcohol advertising exposure on drinking among youth. *Archives of Pediatric and Adolescent Medicine, 160*, 18–24.

St. Onge, M. P., Keller, K. L., & Heymsfield, S. B. (2003). Changes in childhood food consumption patterns: A cause for concern in light of increasing body weights. *American Journal of Clinical Nutrition, 78*, 1068–1073.

Steinberg, L. (2005). Cognitive and affective development in adolescence. *Trends in Cognitive Science, 9*, 69–74.

Storey, M. L., Forshee, R. A., & Anderson, P. A. (2004). Associations of adequate intake of calcium with diet, beverage consumption, and demographic characteristics among children and adolescents. *Journal of the American College of Nutrition, 23*, 18–33.

Styne, D. M. (2003). The regulation of pubertal growth. *Hormone Research, 60*, 22–26.

Troiano, R. P., Briefel, R. R., Carroll, M. D., & Bialostosky, K. (2000). Energy and fat intakes of children and adolescents in the United States: Data from the national health and nutrition examination surveys. *American Journal of Clinical Nutrition, 72*, 1343S–1353S.

U.S. Department of Agriculture (USDA). (2005). National School Lunch Program: Nutrition program facts. Retrieved October 11, 2007, from http://wwwfnsusdagov/cnd/lunch/AboutLunch/NSLPFactSheetpdf

U.S. Department of Health and Human Services, Office of Applied Studies. (2003). Results from the 2002 National Survey on Drug Use and Health: National findings. Retrieved October 11, 2007, from http://oassamhsagov/nhsda/

Veldhuis, J. D., Roemmich, J. N., Richmond, E. J., Rogol, A. D., Lovejoy, J. C., Sheffield-Moore, M., et al. (2005). Endocrine control of body composition in infancy, childhood, and puberty. *Endocrine Reviews, 26*, 114–146.

Videon, T. M., & Manning, C. K. (2003). Influences on adolescent eating patterns: The importance of family meals. *Journal of Adolescent Health, 32*, 365–373.

Wastney, M. E., Martin, B. R., Peacock, M., Smith, D., Jiang, X. Y., Jackman, L. A., et al. (2000). Changes in calcium kinetics in adolescent girls induced by high calcium intake. *Journal of Clinical Endocrinology and Metabolism, 85*, 4470–4475.

Waylen, A., & Wolke, D. (2004). Sex 'n' drugs 'n' rock 'n' roll: The meaning and social consequences of pubertal timing. *European Journal of Endocrinology, 151*, S151–S159.

Weaver, C. M. (2000). The growing years and prevention of osteoporosis in later life. *Proceedings of the Nutrition Society, 59*, 303–306.

Weden, M. M., & Zabin, L. S. (2005). Gender and ethnic differences in the co-occurrence of adolescent risk behaviors. *Ethnic Health, 10*, 213–234.

Weitzman, M., Cook, S., Auinfer, P., Florin, T. A., Daniels, S., Nguyen, M., et al. (2005). Tobacco smoke exposure is associated with the metabolic syndrome in adolescents. *Circulation, 112*, 862–869.

Welt, C. K., Chan, J. L., Bullen, J., Murphy, R., Smith, P., DePaoli, A. M., et al. (2004). Recombinant human leptin in women with hypothalamic amenorrhea. *New England Journal of Medicine, 351*, 987–997.

Whiting, S. J., Vatanparast, H., Baxter-Jones, A., Faulkner, R. A., Mirwald, R., & Bailey, D. A. (2004). Factors that affect bone mineral accrual in the adolescent growth spurt. *Journal of Nutrition, 134*, 696S–700S.

Wilson, D. B., Smith, B. N., Speizer, I. S., Bean, M. K., Mitchell, K. S., Uguy, L. S., et al. (2005). Differences in food intake and exercise by smoking status in adolescents. *Preventive Medicine, 40*, 872–879.

Winkleby, M. A., Robinson, T. N., Sundquist, J., & Kraemer, H. C. (1999). Ethnic variation in cardiovascular disease risk factors among children and young adults: Findings from the Third National Health and Nutrition Examination Survey, 1988–1994. *Journal of the American Medical Association, 281*, 1006–1013.

Xie, B., Gilliland, F. D., Li, Y. F., & Rockett, H. R. (2003). Effects of ethnicity, family income, and education on dietary intake among adolescents. *Preventive Medicine, 36*, 30–40.

Adequate nutrition during infancy, childhood, and adolescence is critical to promote optimal growth and development and is essential for realizing good health in adulthood. It is recognized that healthy dietary patterns established in the early childhood years tend to be carried into adulthood and set the stage for lifelong good health. Conversely, it is well known that poor health conditions and negative nutritional behaviors observed in childhood have a significant deleterious impact on the incidence of disease later in life.

Many families in the United States struggle to provide their children with the foods needed to achieve optimal growth and prevent disease. The federal government established numerous public health nutrition programs to provide access to resources and services to guide and assist these families in meeting the needs of their growing children. These public health nutrition programs evaluate and document nutritional status and need, provide food and financial support to prevent hunger, deliver nutrition-related services to those with special health and developmental needs, and offer nutrition education and counseling that supports the development of healthy behaviors that can be carried into adulthood.

This special section identifies priority nutrition issues to be addressed in a public health setting and explores the federal public health nutrition programs serving the nutritional needs of infants, children, and adolescents. In addition, this special section presents federal nutrition monitoring systems that provide programs with data for planning and evaluation.

Critical Need for Pediatric Public Health Nutrition Services

The U.S. Department of Health and Human Services established national goals for improving public health and, together with the USDA, developed the Healthy People 2010 initiative and policy document. Healthy People 2010 includes a number of goals targeted to the nutritional health of infants, children, and adolescents. These Healthy People 2010 objectives provide a framework for public health nutrition programs to understand national priority areas for health promotion and disease prevention. These objectives provide benchmarks and can be used to build administrative support for public health nutrition initiatives. Collecting and reviewing nutrition-related data elements in a community can justify and support the implementation of nutrition programs within public health settings. The list below features the Healthy People 2010 objectives that relate to nutrition issues of infants, children, and adolescents:

16-1 Reduce fetal and infant deaths

16-10 Reduce low birth weight and very low birth weight

16-19 Increase the proportion of mothers who breast-feed their babies

19-3 Reduce the proportion of children and adolescents who are overweight or obese

19-4 Reduce growth retardation among low-income children under age 5 years

19-5 Increase the proportion of persons aged 2 years and older who consume at least two daily servings of fruit

19-6 Increase the proportion of persons aged 2 years and older who consume at least three daily servings of vegetables, with at least one-third of those being dark green or orange vegetables

19-7 Increase the proportion of persons aged 2 years and older who consume at least six daily servings of grain products, with at least three being whole grains

19-8 Increase the proportion of persons aged 2 years and older who consume less than 10% of calories from saturated fat

19-9 Increase the proportion of persons aged 2 years and older who consume no more than 30% of calories from total fat

19-10 Increase the proportion of persons aged 2 years and older who consume 2,400 mg or less of sodium daily

19-11 Increase the proportion of persons aged 2 years and older who meet dietary recommendations for calcium

19-12 Reduce iron deficiency among young children and females of childbearing age

19-15 Increase the proportion of children and adolescents aged 6 to 19 years whose intake of meals and snacks at school contributes to good overall dietary quality

19-18 Increase food security among U.S. households and in so doing reduce hunger

These objectives outline the priority nutrition needs of infants, children, and adolescents, creating a critical need for public health nutrition programs to establish initiatives and programming to address these issues. A brief discussion of the importance of addressing these issues follows.

Prematurity

Prematurity, defined as less than 37 weeks of completed pregnancy, and subsequent low birth weight (a birth weight less than 5 pounds 8 ounces) are the leading causes of death in the first month of life. Rates of prematurity have grown steadily over the past decade. Premature infants are at higher risk for general illness and disability, including developmental delays, chronic respiratory problems, and vision and hearing impairment, all of which have a critical impact on the nutritional needs and dietary intake of these high-risk infants.

In 2003 there were nearly 500,000 infants born premature in the United States, representing 12.3% of live births. Disparities in prematurity exist between ethnic groups. Between 2001 and 2003 the highest rates of prematurity were experienced by African-American infants (17.7%), followed by Native Americans (13.2%), Hispanic-Americans (11.6%), whites (11%), and Asians (10.4%) (March of Dimes Birth Defects Foundation, 2006).

Overweight Status

Pediatric overweight status is defined as a BMI at or about the 95th percentile for age and sex. Nationally representative data from NHANES conducted between 1999 and 2002 indicate that an estimated 16% of children and adolescents ages 6 to 19 years were overweight. This represents an alarming 45% increase from those estimates of 11% obtained in an earlier survey between 1988 and 1994. An additional 15% of children and adolescents were found to be at risk for excessive weight, defined as a BMI for age between the 85th and 95th percentiles (CDC, National Center for Health Statistics, 2004).

Even among the youngest children, being overweight (>95% BMI for age) is a significant problem—and is even more evident among the low-income toddlers and preschoolers enrolled in federal food programs. Pediatric Nutrition Surveillance System (PedNSS) data report that nearly 15% of 2- to 5-year-olds enrolled in the Special Supplemental Nutrition Program for Women, Infants, and Children (WIC) or other federally funded maternal and child health programs are overweight compared with 10% nationally. An additional 16% of 2- to 5-year-olds assessed by PedNSS were found to be at risk for excessive weight (Hedley et al., 2004). This particular trend in overweight status is of great concern. As the prevalence of being overweight in young children increases, so does the incidence of diseases that in the past were primarily associated with adults, such as heart disease and type 2 diabetes. Being overweight in young children impacts their ability to be physically active and participate in age-appropriate play. It also affects a child's social health and has been linked to difficulties with low self-esteem and depression. Excessive weight in childhood significantly increases the likelihood of adult obesity and the consequent reduction in quality of life and risk of serious chronic disease (Krebs & Jacobson, 2003).

Anemia

Iron-deficiency is a common, yet preventable, nutritional condition that has serious lifelong health consequences. Although it is often thought that iron deficiency anemia—the most severe form of iron deficiency—is necessary for adverse effects to be evident, it has been established that negative impacts on cognitive development in children and adolescents are evident without the full expression of anemia. Iron deficiency is associated with motor and mental development in children and impacts the ability to learn by influencing attention span and memory; it also puts children at higher risk of lead poisoning (Brown, 1998; Center on Hunger and Poverty, 2002).

Rates of iron deficiency remain higher than Healthy People 2010 goals. The prevalence of iron deficiency is greatest among certain categories of individuals; 5% to 7% of children under age 5 are iron deficient, as are 16% of adolescent girls and 12% of women. Non-Hispanic African-American and Mexican-American females experience iron deficiency at twice the rate of non-Hispanic-American white females (CDC, 2002).

Breast-Feeding

Breast-feeding is one of the most important contributors to the optimal health and development of infants. All major medical and public health organizations in the United States recommend exclusive breast-feeding for the first 6 months of life, followed by the addition of complementary foods for the second 6 months of life, as the preferred method of infant nutrition.

Human milk contains an ideal balance of nutrients that matches an infant's needs for growth and development. Because a mother's antibodies are passed to her infant through breast milk, breast-fed infants are significantly less likely to suffer from a number of common infant illnesses—including ear infections, upper respiratory infections, and gastrointestinal infections—than infants who are fed formula. Numerous studies have also shown links between breast-feeding and a reduction in risk for many chronic pediatric conditions such as diabetes, celiac disease, childhood cancers, and obesity. Some studies suggest that infants who are exclusively breast-fed for the first year of life or longer may be protected from chronic diseases such as diabetes, lymphoma, leukemia, obesity, high cholesterol, and asthma (Gartner et al., 2005).

Despite the overwhelming evidence of the superiority of breast-feeding over formula feeding, breast-feeding rates in the United States lag behind the Healthy People 2010 goals. National breast-feeding initiation, duration, and exclusivity data are collected on a periodic basis as part of the CDC's National Immunization Survey. The most recent data available from 2004 indicate that 70% of infants were breast-fed at least once after delivery, compared with the 75% goal set by Healthy People 2010. Thirty-six percent of infants continue to breast-feed at 6 months, well below the goal of 50%, and 18% of infants are breast-feeding at their first birthdays, compared with the goal of 25%. The need for increased breast-feeding promotion and support initiatives in the United States becomes clearer when rates of exclusive breast-feeding are examined. Only 39% of infants are exclusively breast-feeding at 3 months, and this rate drops to 14% at 6 months (CDC, National Center for Health Statistics, 2004).

Hunger and Food Insecurity

Food insecurity and hunger continue to be problems of significance to infants, children, and adolescents. Food security is the ensured access to enough food for an active healthy life as well as access to enough food that is safe, nutritious, and acquired in socially acceptable ways. There are different levels of food insecurity, both with and without hunger. Hunger is the outcome of limited or uncertain access to food.

Both food insecurity and hunger have significant detrimental effects on the health and well-being of children because of the critical need of adequate energy and nutrients to promote growth and cognitive development. Children who experience inadequate food intake have poorer health status, are sick more often, are more likely to have ear infections, and are more likely to experience impaired growth. In addition, children who experience food insecurity have more missed days of school and learning difficulties and have more frequent hospitalizations. These children also experience higher rates of iron deficiency anemia and higher risk of lead poisoning (Brown, 1998; Center on Hunger and Poverty, 2002). Excessive weight and obesity are also a consequence of hunger and food insecurity resulting from an adaptive response to episodic food insufficiency or the result of consuming low-cost, low-nutrient, high-fat foods to prevent hunger when households lack money to buy more nutrient-dense food (Center on Hunger and Poverty and the Food Research and Action Center, 2003).

It 2004 over 13 million households (11.9% of all U.S. households) were food insecure. This figure represents 38.2 million Americans, 13.9 million of whom were children. Households with children had nearly twice the rate of food insecurity than those without children. More than 7 million adults and 3 million children lived in households where someone experienced hunger during the year. Data show that in most households children themselves appear to be protected from hunger unless the hunger among adults in the household becomes severe. Only 0.7% of children in the United States were classified as having experienced hunger (USDA, Economic Research Service, 2006). Current public health nutrition programs that provide interventions and programs that promote achieving healthy dietary habits and target the prevention and treatment of these critical nutrition issues are warranted to reduce the incidence and prevalence of these conditions in infants, children, and adolescents.

Federal Public Health Nutrition Programs

The federal government administers several public health nutrition programs that exclusively or primarily address the nutritional needs of infants, children, and adolescents. These programs work individually or in partnership with community programs to provide a food availability safety net and promote the development of sound nutrition patterns to promote lifelong nutritional health for its recipients.

Federal spending on food assistance programs is classified as either mandatory or discretionary. Mandatory programs, often referred to as entitlement programs, use eligibility guidelines that are written into law. All eligible individuals are entitled to the benefits offered. Discretionary programs are funded annually based on budgets determined in federal appropriations acts. Although the eligibility guidelines for discretionary programs may be broad, higher-need individuals may be prioritized to receive benefits in times of fiscal shortfall.

Special Supplemental Nutrition Program for Women, Infants, and Children (WIC)

The three primary goals of the WIC program are to provide supplemental nutrient-dense foods, to offer nutrition education, and to supply health and social service referrals to pregnant, postpartum, and breast-feeding women, infants, and children to 5 years of age who are at nutritional risk and meet specific income guidelines. (Refer to the USDA's WIC website at http://www.fns.usda.gov/wic for current eligibility criteria for and information on the WIC program.) WIC is a discretionary program funded by the USDA and administered by state agencies and Indian Tribal Organizations; some states also provide funding to broaden their program's ability to serve participants.

Nutritional eligibility of WIC applicants is determined by a thorough health and dietary assessment completed during the certification process. Nutrition staff use assessment outcomes to provide personalized nutrition education and counseling to meet the participant's needs and interests. Anticipatory guidance tailored to the stage of development of infants and children is also provided.

A key objective of WIC nutrition services is to promote and support breast-feeding as the ideal method of infant nutrition, unless contraindicated. WIC offers a range of breast-feeding education and support services, including peer counseling services. Many WIC programs offer breast pump loan programs to their participants. Breast-feeding mothers enrolled in WIC receive more food benefits and a longer eligibility period than women who formula feed their infants.

WIC participants receive checks for monthly food benefits that are individually tailored to meet dietary preferences and needs. Foods available from WIC were chosen to provide key nutrients, such as iron, calcium, protein, and vitamin C, commonly deficient in the diets of low-income families. In 2005 an expert panel from the IOM recommended revisions to the WIC food package to be consistent with current national dietary recommendations. The panel's recommendations strive to make the WIC food package more culturally appropriate and provide families with a framework to establish lifelong healthy dietary patterns.

WIC participants may also receive coupons to purchase fresh fruits and vegetables during the summer months at authorized farmers' markets through the WIC Farmers' Market Nutrition Program (FMNP). This program—administered through a federal and state partnership with USDA's Food and Nutrition Service—provides seasonal unprepared produce to WIC families and expands the awareness, use of, and sales at farmers' markets. The federal food benefit for Farmers' Market Nutrition Program recipients may be no less than $10 and no more than $30 per recipient per year. States may supplement the federal funds with state, local, or private dollars (USDA of Agriculture, 2006).

In 2005 the WIC program served more than 8 million participants, of whom roughly one-half are children ages 1 to 5; one-fourth are pregnant, postpartum, or breast-feeding women; and one-fourth are infants under 12 months (USDA, 2005a). The WIC program has significant potential impact on the health and nutritional status of the pediatric population, as almost half of all infants and one-fourth of all children ages 1 to 4 years in the United States are program participants (Oliveira, Racine, Olmsted, & Ghelfi, 2002).

The WIC program is the most studied of all the federal nutrition programs in terms of its influence on health and nutrition status. The bulk of the research has focused on the impact of WIC participation during pregnancy on birth outcomes. The General Accounting Office in 1992 studied and concluded that prenatal WIC participation reduced the incidence of low birth weight (less than 2,500 g) by 25% and the incidence of very low birth weight (less than 1,500 g) by 44%. In a later General Accounting Office study, researchers calculated that the provision of WIC services saves more than $1 billion in costs for federal, state, local, and private payers (Oliveira et al., 2002). Although some analysts believe this figure overestimates the cost savings associated with WIC participation, the body of WIC research in general is strongly suggestive of WIC's positive impact on birth weight and several other key birth outcomes and that these positive effects lead to savings in healthcare costs (Fox, Hamilton, & Lin, 2004).

The WIC program's impact on breast-feeding outcomes is an important area for evaluation. Although breast-feeding rates for women enrolled in WIC are improving, these rates lag behind non-WIC participants and behind the Healthy People 2010 objectives.

According to data collected in the Ross Mothers' Survey, more than twice as many non-WIC mothers than WIC participants breast-fed their infants at 6 months of age (Ryan & Zhou, 2006). Because poverty and low education levels are negatively correlated with breast-feeding incidence and low-income and poorly educated women are more likely to participate in WIC, participants tend to be of a demographic less likely to breast-feed (Oliveira, 2003). WIC strives to offer culturally appropriate services to combat this disparity and has added a significant focus on breast-feeding peer counseling in recent years. Some researchers have questioned whether the provision of infant formula by the program acts as a disincentive to breast-feeding. Reducing the impact of this element is one of the key components of the IOM recommendations for the revision of the WIC food package.

Based on a number of studies, data show that children who participate in WIC have significantly higher intakes of folate, vitamin B_6, and iron than WIC eligible children who are not enrolled in the program. Rose, Habicht, & Devaney (1998) reported that WIC participation also increased children's iron and zinc intake and was found to be significantly and positively associated with the intake of 10 of 15 key nutrients studied. Recent data suggest that WIC participation decreases children's consumption of added sugar (Fox et al., 2004) and that WIC children were found to be significantly less likely than income eligible nonparticipant children to be iron deficient (Cole & Fox, 2004). It has also been found that children who participate in the WIC program are significantly more likely to be fully immunized by 24 months than nonparticipating children of similar socioeconomic background (Luman, McCauley, Shefer, & Chu, 2003) and that WIC participation has a significant positive effect on the utilization of health and dental care services (Fox et al., 2004).

The Children's Sentinel Nutrition Assessment Program (C-SNAP), a national network of pediatric health experts aimed at combating hunger and promoting children's health, studied the impact of WIC participation on growth and health in young children. A 2004 study found that infants who did not enroll in the WIC program because of access problems were more likely to be underweight, undersized, and perceived by their caregivers to be in fair or poor health compared with those infants who did receive WIC services (Black et al., 2004). C-SNAP findings released in 2006 detail the impact of WIC, as well as the other major federal public assistance programs,

on the health of young children of color. Compared with African-American infants who received WIC benefits, those who were eligible but did not receive services were 56% more likely to be at nutritional risk for growth problems, more than twice as likely to be underweight, and more likely to be shorter in height. The C-SNAP report also concluded that compared with Hispanic-American infants enrolled in WIC, those infants who were eligible but did not participate in the program were more likely to have a lower weight and shorter height (Joint Center for Political and Economic Studies, 2006).

Because the rates of young overweight children are climbing, and the rise is even more significant among low-income and minority children, some critics have blamed the WIC program for these negative trends. These attacks, however, remain unfounded. In research published in 2006, the receipt of WIC services was not linked to increased rates of excessive weight in young children (Joint Center for Political and Economic Studies, 2006). Another recent study found a positive impact of WIC participation on weight status—at the age of 4, children enrolled in WIC were significantly less likely to be "at risk" for excessive weight (defined as BMI above the 85th percentile for sex and age). Thus WIC participation may result in a significant positive reduction of future risk of obesity-related diseases (Institute for Research on Poverty, 2004).

Food Stamp Program

The intention of the Food Stamp Program is to be the nation's first line of defense against hunger. The program provides low-income households with coupons and electronic benefit transfer cards to purchase eligible foods for a nutritionally adequate diet at authorized food stores. The Food Stamp Program is a mandatory program funded by the USDA Food and Nutrition Service and is administered by state welfare, social service, or human service agencies. Local welfare, social service, or human service offices provide the actual services.

Eligibility and allotments for the Food Stamp Program are based on household size, income, assets, and other factors. (For specific information on income eligibility criteria, refer to the USDA's Food Stamp Program website at http://www.fns.usda.gov/fsp.) Legal immigrants who are children or disabled are eligible for food stamps, as well as legal immigrants who have legally resided in the United States for at least 5 years. Able-bodied, childless, unemployed adults may have time limits on their receipt of food stamp benefits.

States have the option of providing nutrition education to food stamp recipients as a part of their program services. The goal of Food Stamp Nutrition Education is to improve the likelihood that individuals and families will make healthy food choices within a limited budget. State Cooperative Extension Systems are the primary agencies contracted to provide Food Stamp Nutrition Education services; however, state nutrition education networks, public health departments, welfare agencies, and other university academic centers can also be sponsoring agencies.

In 2005 the Food Stamp Program served nearly 26 million individuals who each received an average of $93 per month in benefits. The average monthly household benefit for each of the 11 million households enrolled in the program that year was approximately $213. Total costs for the year, including both the direct cost of program benefits and the administrative expenses, exceeded $31 billion (USDA, 2005b).

Most food stamp recipients are either children or elderly. More than half of program participants are children, one-third of whom are under the age of 5. Eight percent of recipients are age 60 or older. Working age women represent 28% of the caseload, whereas working age men represent 13%. Food stamp participants tend to have very little income: A recent review found that just 12% of program participants were living above the poverty line (Poikolainen, 2005). Food stamp benefits are based on the "Thrifty Food Plan," the national governmental standard for a minimally nutritionally adequate diet at a low cost. The Food Stamp Program allocation formula assumes that households will be able to purchase sufficient foods to reach Thrifty Food Plan levels using their benefits in addition to 30% of any income they receive (Food Research and Action Center, 2004).

In addition to providing the instruments to purchase foods, states have the option—and are actively encouraged—to provide nutrition education to food stamp recipients as part of their program operations. The goal of Food Stamp Nutrition Education is to provide educational programs that increase the ability of food stamp recipients to make healthy food choices and choose active life-styles that are consistent with national nutrition and health guidance.

Studies have found a positive correlation between Food Stamp Program participation and food security in the household in which a preschooler lives if the food stamp benefits last throughout the entire month (Perez-Escamilla et al., 2000). The Food Stamp Program has been shown to significantly attenuate the negative impact of food insecurity on a child's health status (Cook et al., 2004).

Recently, researchers have found food stamps to be effective in reducing hunger among children of color. Compared with African-American children whose food stamp benefits were not reduced in the previous year, African-American infants and toddlers whose family benefits were reduced were 33% more likely to be food insecure and those whose benefits were sanctioned were 84% more likely to be food insecure. Those who experienced a reduction in food stamp benefits were also 38% more likely to be reported as being in fair or poor health. Hispanic-American children whose family food stamp benefits were reduced were more than twice as likely as those receiving their full benefits to be food insecure (Joint Center for Political and Economic Studies, 2006).

Food stamp households buy more food on average than other low-income households that do not participate in the program. Food stamp recipients have been shown to obtain more nutrients for every dollar they spend on food than shoppers who do not utilize food stamps (www.frac.org). In particular, food stamp participation has been shown to significantly increase preschoolers' intake of iron, zinc, folate, and vitamin B_6 (Rose et al., 1998; Perez-Escamilla et al., 2000).

National School Lunch Program

The National School Lunch Program (NSLP) provides nutritious low-cost lunch at full or reduced prices—or free—to children enrolled in school or residential child care institutions. Any child attending school may participate; free meals are available to children from families with incomes at or below 130% of poverty level; reduced price meals are available to children from families with incomes between 131% and 185% of poverty level. The NSLP is a mandatory program funded by the USDA and administered by each state's Department of Education and local school districts. NSLP services are provided by all public schools; they are voluntary in private schools. The total cost of administering the NSLP in 2003 was $7.1 billion (USDA, 2005c).

NSLP also includes reimbursement for snacks for students enrolled in after-school programs. These snacks are provided to children on the same income eligibility basis as school meals; however, programs may serve all their snacks for free if they operate in schools where at least 50% of students are eligible for free or reduced price meals.

In the 2003–2004 school year over 28.4 million children in 98,000 schools and residential child care institutions participated in the NSLP, serving 16.5 million children with free or reduced priced lunches. This represents 58% of this nation's school children (Food Research and Action Center, 2006a). African-American children are almost five times more likely to participate in the NSLP than other children (Dunifon & Kowaleski-Jones, 2003).

School lunches offered under the NSLP must conform to the Dietary Guidelines for Americans, which recommend that no more than 30% of an individual's calories come from fat and less than 10% from saturated fat. School lunches must meet specific standards for key nutrients necessary for growth and development; NSLP requirements state that lunches must provide one-third of the Recommended Dietary Allowances of protein, vitamin A, vitamin C, iron, calcium, and calories. Although school lunches must meet these federal nutrition requirements, the decisions about what specific foods to serve and how foods are prepared are made by local school food authorities (USDA, 2005c).

Participation in the NSLP appears to reduce hunger among families with children ages 5 to 18 (Kabbani & Yazbeck, 2004). Researchers have identified seasonal differences in food security between spring and summer for school-aged children, thereby reducing the prevalence of hunger during the school year (Nord & Romig, 2003).

NSLP has also been found to improve the growth of children less than 10 years of age. Children who participate in the NSLP are less likely to fall below the 25th percentile of weight for height (Hanes, Vermeersch, & Gale, 1984). Another study confirmed that participation in the NSLP was protective of the BMI of children from families living below the poverty line—nonparticipating poor students had below average BMIs compared with similar income students who did utilize the school lunch program (Hofferth & Curtin, 2005).

Many of the available evaluations of the NSLP document the relationship between participating in the program and increased nutrient intake, particularly noting increases in intakes at lunch of vitamin A, calcium, and zinc. However, NSLP participants' lunches also provide a higher percentage of food energy from fat and saturated fat and a lower percentage from carbohydrate than do nonparticipants' lunches (Burghardt, Devaney, & Gordon, 1995). A study published in 2003 found that NSLP participants had significantly higher intakes of dietary fiber and 11 key nutrients (vitamin A, vitamin B$_6$, vitamin B$_{12}$, thiamin, riboflavin, folate, calcium, magnesium, phosphorus, iron, and zinc) and significantly lower intakes of added sugars than children not consuming school lunch. This study also confirmed that children utilizing the NSLP consumed more total fat and saturated fat than nonparticipants (Gleason & Suitor, 2003).

While some may be concerned with these findings—providing nutrients that assist children in meeting the Recommended Daily Allowance goals, yet higher in fat and saturated fat than recommended by The Dietary Guidelines for Americans, studies do show that participating in NSLP can lead to improvements in test scores of children and did not have a negative effect on a child's weight (Dunifon & Kowaleski-Jones, 2004; Hofferth & Curtin, 2005).

USDA research indicates that children who participate in the NSLP have superior nutritional intakes compared with those who bring lunch from home or otherwise do not participate (Food Research and Action Center, 2006b). Finally, a study noted a positive impact on behavior of children in families experiencing hunger (Dunifon & Kowaleski-Jones, 2002).

School Breakfast Program

The School Breakfast Program provides nutritious low-cost breakfast at full or reduced prices or free to children in participating schools or institutions. The goal of the School Breakfast Program is to promote learning readiness and improve healthy eating behaviors. All children attending schools where the breakfast program operates may participate: Free breakfast is available to children from families with incomes at or below 130% of poverty level, and reduced priced breakfast is available to children from families with incomes between 131% and 185% of poverty level. The School Breakfast Program is a mandatory program funded by the USDA and administered by each state's Department of Education and local school districts. Services are provided by both public and private schools as well as residential child care facilities.

On average, 9.2 million children in more than 80,000 schools and institutions participated in the School Breakfast Program on a typical day during the 2004–2005 school year. Of these children 7.5 million, or 82%, received free or reduced price breakfasts (Food Research and Action Center, 2006c). Like school lunch, the School Breakfast Program must follow the Dietary Guidelines for Americans and limit fat to 30% of the calories in the meal; saturated fat is limited to 10% of calories. School breakfasts must provide one-fourth of the Recommended Daily Allowance for protein, calcium, iron, vitamin A, vitamin C, and calories.

Research shows that children who have school breakfast eat more fruits, drink more milk, and consume less saturated fat than those who do not eat breakfast or have breakfast at home (Food Research and Action Center, 2006c). Children who have the School Breakfast Program available consume a better overall diet as measured by the Healthy Eating Index (Bhattacharya, Currie, & Haider, 2004).

Studies have concluded that students who eat school breakfast have increased intakes of food energy, protein, and calcium. In addition, students experience increased math and reading scores and improve their speed and memory in cognitive tests. Research shows that children who eat breakfast at school—closer to class and test-taking time—perform better on standardized tests than those who skip breakfast or eat breakfast at home (Food Research Action Center, 2001).

Summer Food Service for Children

The Summer Food Service Program provides free meals and/or snacks to children as a substitute for the National School Lunch and School Breakfast Programs during summer vacation. Children under 18 years of age who come to an approved site will be served. People over age 18 who are enrolled in school programs for persons with disabilities may also participate in the Summer Food Service Program. The Summer Food Service Program is funded by the USDA and administered generally by each state's Department of Education, but state health or social service department or a Food and Nutrition Service regional office may be designated.

Summer Food Service Program sites are hosted by local governments and agencies at such places as schools, parks, recreation centers, housing projects, migrant centers, houses of worship, and summer camps. Most Summer Food Service Program sites are considered "open sites," that is, they are open to all the children in the community provided they are located in an area in which at least 50% of the children are from households that would be eligible for free or reduced price school meals.

In 2004 the Summer Food Service Program served over 1.6 million children in 30,000 sites operated by over 3,500 sponsoring organizations and 1.3 million children received school lunch through summer school. These numbers, however, represent less than one in five of the children served school lunch during the school year (Food Research and Action Center, 2005). Improving participation in the Summer Food Service Program is key to ensuring that low income school-aged children receive the nutrition they need during the summer months so they are better able to learn when they return to school.

Most studies evaluating the Summer Food Service Program focus on participation and service delivery. However, one study did report that the meals served by the Summer Food Service Program supplied at least 33% of the Recommended Daily Allowance for most nutrients (USDA, Food and Nutrition Service, 1998).

Special Milk Program

The Special Milk Program provides milk to children in schools, summer camps, and child care institutions that have no federally supported meal program. Milk is free to children from families that would be income eligible for free meals through the NSLP. The Special Milk Program is funded by the USDA and administered by the each state's Department of Education. Program services are provided by public or nonprofit private schools of high school grade and under, eligible camps, and public or nonprofit private child care institutions not participating in other federally supported meal programs. In 2003 more than 6,000 schools and residential child care institutions, 1,000 summer camps, and 550 nonresidential child care institutions participated in the Special Milk Program (USDA, 2005d). This program helps to supply important nutrients to growing children in the absence of the availability of other programs.

Child and Adult Care Food Program

The Child and Adult Care Food Program (CACFP) provides cash reimbursements and commodity foods for meals served in child and adult day-care centers, Head Start programs, family and group day-care homes, homeless shelters, and approved after-school care programs. The program provides reimbursement for food and meal preparation costs, ongoing training in the nutritional needs of children, and on-site assistance in meeting the program's strong nutritional requirements.

CACFP is funded by the USDA and administered by each state's Department of Education or alternate state agency (state health or social service department). CACFP services are provided by public and nonprofit private licensed child and adult day-care centers and homes, outside after-school-hours care centers, Head Start, other licensed/approved day-care centers, and homeless shelters. Any child up to age 12 or adult attending a participating adult day-care facility is entitled to meals.

Research has found that children in sites receiving CACFP funds consume meals that are nutritionally superior to those served to children in child care settings without CACFP. They have higher intakes of key nutrients and fewer servings of fats and sweets than children not receiving CACFP-funded meals. Studies have documented that participation in CACFP is one of the major factors influencing quality child care; in one review the vast majority of family child care homes considered to be providing quality child care had participated in CACFP (Food Research and Action Center, 2006c).

Commodity Supplemental Food Program

The Commodity Supplemental Food Program (CSFP) provides commodity foods to low-income pregnant, postpartum, and breast-feeding women; infants; children to 6 years of age; and the elderly. Pregnant, postpartum, and breast-feeding women; infants; and children (up to 6 years) with household income determined to be at or below 185% of poverty level are eligible. Elderly participants must be at least 60 years of age and be living at or below 130% of poverty. Some states have residency and nutrition risk criteria. Individuals cannot participate in both WIC and CSFP at the same time.

USDA uses CSFP funds to purchase commodity foods, which are then stored by state health, social service, education, or agriculture agencies. The foods are distributed to local public and nonprofit agencies for provision to eligible individuals. CSFP foods are not intended to constitute a complete diet but rather provide good sources of the nutrients typically lacking in the diets of the target population. Available foods are generally canned or packaged and include fruits, vegetables, meats, infant formula, cereals, rice, pasta, beans, cheese, and peanut butter.

There is very limited research on CSFP. An evaluation completed by the USDA in 1982 reported positive findings related to pregnancy outcomes; however, for children the findings were inconclusive to positive health outcomes associated with program participation (Fox et al., 2004).

Emergency Food Assistance Program

The Emergency Food Assistance Program provides commodity foods to low-income persons, food banks,

food pantries, and soup kitchens. Each state sets criteria for household income eligibility. Households may participate in another federal, state, or local food health or welfare program for which eligibility is based on income and still receive foods funded by the Emergency Food Assistance Program. Recipients of prepared meals funded by the Emergency Food Assistance Program, such as participants in congregate meal programs for the elderly or homeless, are considered to be the most needy and do not need to prove income eligibility. Funded by the USDA, foods are purchased and sent to state agencies for distribution to food banks, food pantries, soup kitchens, and other public and private nonprofit organizations that distribute food to needy individuals and families.

Expanded Food and Nutrition Education Program

The Expanded Food and Nutrition Education Program (EFNEP) aims to provide low-income individuals with the skills and education necessary to engage in behaviors that lead to nutritious diets and to provide overall nutritional well-being for their families. EFNEP services are provided in all 50 states and are funded through the Cooperative State Research, Education, and Extension Service, an agency within the USDA. Programs are administered on a state level through the Cooperative Extension Service at the state universities.

EFNEP designates a major portion of its resources to services targeted at adults, largely consisting of a series of lessons in food preparation, purchasing, and safety taught by paraprofessional staff and volunteers. Lessons are generally provided in a group format. In 2005, EFNEP reached nearly 151,000 adults, most of whom had extensive contact with EFNEP staff over a period of many months.

EFNEP has had great success connecting school-aged youth with nutrition education. EFNEP services for youth are provided as an addition to the regular curriculum in a variety of settings, including after-school programs, 4-H clubs, camps, and community centers. In 2005, 412,000 youth nationwide received an EFNEP educational contact. Data from EFNEP's evaluation and reporting system show that EFNEP education has a significant impact on youths' nutrition knowledge and behavior. After receiving EFNEP services 73% of youth ate a greater variety of foods, 70% increased their knowledge of basic human nutrition, 65% increased their ability to select low-cost nutritious foods, and 65% improved their food handling and preparation practices (Montgomery & Willis, 2006).

Team Nutrition

Although not a separate public health nutrition program, the USDA funds the Team Nutrition initiative in an effort to support its Child Nutrition Programs. Team Nutrition's goal is to improve children's lifelong nutrition and physical activity behaviors using the principles of the Dietary Guidelines for Americans and the Food Guide Pyramid. Team Nutrition activities fall into one of three key strategies: (1) to provide training and technical assistance to Child Nutrition Program food service staff to assist them in serving meals that taste good and meet nutrition standards, (2) to provide nutrition education for children and their parents through the school system and with community programs, and (3) to provide support for healthy eating and physical activity by facilitating communication between school administrators and other community partners.

Team Nutrition activities benefit 50 million school children in more than 96,000 schools nationwide. The bulk of these dollars are focused on supporting the school meal programs, the CACFP, and the Summer Food Service Program. Schools are encouraged to enroll themselves as "Team Nutrition schools" and to affirm their commitment to prioritize the nutritional health and education of their students. State agencies recruit Team Nutrition schools and assist them with the training and support necessary to sustain the local implementation of the initiative. Team Nutrition also makes efforts to provide reinforcing nutrition education messages to children and their parents through partnerships with the WIC Program and the Food Stamp Program (USDA, 2006b).

Other Federal Programs That Respond to the Nutritional Needs of Infants, Children, and Adolescents

The following programs' goals are not primarily targeted to respond to the nutritional health of infants and children. However, their services are comprehensive and include nutritional components that contribute to the nutritional health and well-being of program participants. Evaluations of the programs' services indicate a range of positive outcomes related to program participation, but generally nutritional outcomes are not specifically identified.

Head Start and Early Head Start

The Head Start Program provides comprehensive medical, educational, nutrition, social, and dental services; referrals to social services; and other related assessment and early intervention services in a preschool setting to low-income children between the ages of 3 and 5 and their families. Early Head Start offers early education both in and out of the home, parenting education, comprehensive health and mental health services, nutrition education, and family support services to women before, during, and after pregnancy and to young children up to age 3. Both Head Start and Early Head Start provide nutritious meals and snacks to children in its care.

Low-income families receiving public assistance (i.e., Temporary Assistance for Needy Families or Supplemental Security Income) or who have a total annual income less than 100% of the federal poverty level are eligible to receive Head Start services, as are children in foster care. Head Start reserves at least 10% of total enrollment for children with physical disabilities. Head Start is funded by the Federal Department of Health and Human Services' Administration for Children & Families and is administered by U.S. Department of Health and Human Services regional offices. Services are provided by local public agencies, private nonprofit and for-profit organizations, American Indian Tribes, and school systems.

More than 905,000 children and pregnant women were enrolled in Head Start in 2004. Children under age 3 and pregnant women receiving Early Head Start services accounted for approximately 8% of program enrollment (Hamm & Ewen, 2006).

Early Intervention

The early intervention program for infants and toddlers with disabilities is funded under Part C of the Individuals with Disabilities Education Act. Federal grants are provided to states to offer children under the age of 3 and their families a comprehensive multidisciplinary system of services. In most states the Department of Health and Human Services or Department of Education administers the program. Early intervention services include audiology, health and medical services, nutrition services, occupational therapy, physical therapy, psychological and social work services, speech and language services, and vision care.

Program eligibility is based on state-determined evaluation and assessment systems that identify children who have or who are at risk for a developmental delay. States receiving Part C funds must ensure that all children birth to age 3 who are eligible for program services are identified, located, and evaluated for need. Once need is determined, services are either provided free of charge to families or fees are determined on a sliding scale basis. Health insurance plans often cover the cost of services (American Academy of Pediatrics, n.d.).

Nutrition Surveillance Systems in the United States

Policymakers, program administrators, and program evaluators rely on the comprehensive collection of health statistics to set public health priorities, strategically design public health and nutrition programs, and determine the impact of program components on the health status of those served. The CDC administers the three largest federal monitoring systems that regularly collect, analyze, interpret, and disseminate data on key indicators of nutritional status among infants, children, and adolescents.

The Pregnancy Nutrition Surveillance System annually monitors risk factors associated with infant morbidity and mortality as well as poor birth outcomes among low-income pregnant women who participate in federally funded public health programs such as WIC and Title V Maternal and Child Health Programs. Although most of the data elements reported are related to maternal conditions, the Pregnancy Nutrition Surveillance System does collect data on prematurity, low birth weight, and breast-feeding initiation—indicators significantly associated with the growth and nutritional status of infants and young children. More than three-fourths of a million women were represented in the 2004 Pregnancy Nutrition Surveillance System reporting (www.cdc.gov/pednss/what_is/pnss/).

The PedNSS collects data each year on birth weight, breast-feeding duration, anemia, short stature, and underweight and overweight status among children birth to 5 years of age. Although the vast majority (86%) of the PedNSS data come from children who participate in the WIC program, PedNSS also monitors children enrolled in the Early and Periodic Screening, Diagnosis, and Treatment Program and the Title V Maternal and Child Health Program. In 2004 the PedNSS data set included records for approximately 7 million children (2004 PedNSS Summary Report, 2006).

The Youth Risk Behavior Surveillance System monitors six categories of high-risk behaviors among 9th to 12th grade youth (i.e., behaviors that contribute to unintentional injuries and violence, tobacco use, alcohol and other drug use, sexual behaviors that contribute to unintended pregnancy and sexually transmitted diseases, unhealthy dietary behaviors, and physical inactivity) as well as indicators of weight status. Youth Risk Behavior Surveillance System data represent a national school-based survey conducted by the CDC as well as state and local school-based surveys conducted by education and health agencies. Youth Risk Behavior Surveillance System data are used to measure progress toward achieving national health objectives and to monitor leading health indicators for youth. In addition, education and health officials at national, state, and local levels use Youth Risk Behavior Surveillance System data to improve policies and programs that reduce high-risk, health-related behaviors among young people (CDC, 2004c).

The CDC also conducts NHANES on an ongoing basis. The survey assesses the health and nutritional status of all age segments of the population and monitors changes over time. A major objective of the survey's nutrition component is to provide data for nutrition monitoring purposes, including tracking nutrition, identifying risk factors related to food insecurity, and estimating the prevalence of compromised nutritional status. A second major objective is to provide information for studying the relationships among diet, nutritional status, and health. A dietary 24-hour recall is used to obtain dietary data. The survey is unique because it combines data from both interviews and physical examinations.

Summary

It is well established that achieving optimal nutritional status during infancy, childhood, and adolescence is critical to proper growth and development and for setting the stage for good health in adulthood. Federal nutrition programs provide a range of services that strive to target the nutritional needs of this population. These programs provide a food availability safety net and promote sound nutritional patterns for program participants and their families. These programs have demonstrated long-term success in delivering services that improve the nutritional well-being of infants, children, and adolescents. With the Healthy People 2010 goals as nutritional benchmarks and the available nutrition monitoring systems, these federal nutrition programs can enhance and adapt their services to meet the nutritional needs of infants, children, and adolescents in this population.

Issues for Debate

1. What are the advantages and disadvantages of being designated and funded as a mandatory program versus a discretionary program? What are the consequences to program services and participation?

2. Federal nutrition programs were originally developed to combat hunger and nutrient insufficiencies. In today's environment, what is the role of these programs to provide preventive services to provide long-term health and well-being? How can this preventive component be promoted and evaluated to ensure adequate funding?

3. What are the differences in eligibility criteria between the different federal nutrition programs? What groups are included and what groups are missed? What are the consequences to society by excluding identified groups?

4. What could a family living at the federal poverty line purchase with 1 week of food stamps? How could these families meet their nutritional requirements? Consider the expense and availability of utilities and equipment as well.

5. Examine the contents of the current WIC food package and the food stamp benefit. How do these food benefits ensure adequate nutrition and contribute to good health?

References

American Academy of Pediatrics. (n.d.). The Medical Home and Early Intervention program. Retrieved July 17, 2006, from http://www.medicalhomeinfo.org/health/Downloads/EIBrochureF.pdf

Bhattacharya, J., Currie, J., & Haider, S. J. (2004). *Evaluating the Impact of School Nutrition Programs Final Report.* Washington, DC: U.S. Department of Agriculture, Economic Research Service.

Black, M. M., Cutts, D. B., Frank, D. A., Geppert, J., Skalicky, A., Levenson, S., et al. (2004). Special Supplemental Nutrition Program for Women, Infants, and Children participation and infants' growth and health: A multisite surveillance study. *Pediatrics, 114*, 169–176.

Brown, J. (1998). *Statement on the Link Between Nutrition and Cognitive Development in Children.* Center on Hunger, Poverty and Nutrition Policy, Tufts University.

Burghardt, J. A., Devaney, B. L., & Gordon, A. R. (1995). The School Nutrition Dietary Assessment Study: Summary and discussion. *American Journal of Clinical Nutrition, 61*, 252S–257S.

Center on Hunger and Poverty. (2002). *Consequences of Hunger and Food Insecurity for Children, Evidence From Recent Scientific Studies.* Brandeis University. Con Agra Foods. Retrieved October 11, 2007, from http://centeron hunger. brandeis.edu/pdf/ConsequencesofHunger. pdf

Center on Hunger and Poverty and the Food Research and Action Center. (2003). *Paradox of Hunger and Obesity in America.*

Centers for Disease Control and Prevention (CDC). (2002). Iron deficiency—United States, 1999. *Morbidity and Mortality Weekly Review, 51*, 897–899.

Centers for Disease Control and Prevention (CDC), National Center for Health Statistics. (2004a). Prevalence of overweight among children and adolescents: United States, 1999–2002. Retrieved May 28, 2006, from http://www. cdc.gov/nchs/products/pubs/pubd/hestats/overwght 99.htm

Centers for Disease Control and Prevention (CDC), National Center for Health Statistics. (2004b). National Immunization Survey, 2004. Retrieved July 26, 2006, from http:// www.cdc.gov/breastfeeding/data/NIS_data/data_2004.htm

Centers for Disease Control (CDC). (2004c).Youth Risk Behavior Surveillance—United States, 2000. MMWR Surveill Summary. Retrieved [DATE] from www.cdc.gov/mmwr/ preview/mmwrhtml/mm5620a2.htm—Vol 56, No 20; 4972007-05-25.

Cole, N., & Fox, M. K. (2004). *Nutrition and Health Characteristics of Low-Income Populations: Volume II, WIC Program Participants and Nonparticipants.* E-FAN Report No. 04014-2. Washington, DC: U.S. Department of Agriculture, Economic Research Service.

Cook, J. T., Frank, D. A., Berkowitz, C., Black, M. M., Casey, P. H., Cutts, D. B., et al. (2004). Food insecurity is associated with adverse health outcomes among human infants and toddlers. *Journal of Nutrition, 134*, 1432–1438.

Dunifon, R., & Kowaleski-Jones, L. (2002). *Associations Between Participation in the National School Lunch Program, Food Insecurity, and Child Well-Being.* Discussion Paper No. 1249-02. Madison, WI: Institute for Research on Poverty.

Dunifon, R., & Kowaleski-Jones, L. (2003). The influences of participation in the National School Lunch Program and food insecurity on child well-being. *Social Service Review, 72*–92.

Dunifon, R., & Kowaleski-Jones, L. (2004). *Exploring the Influence of the National School Lunch Program on Children.* Discussion Paper No. 1277-04. Madison, WI: Institute for Research on Poverty.

Food Research and Action Center. (2001). Breakfast for learning. Retrieved June 8, 2006, from http://www.frac. org/pdf/breakfastforlearning.pdf

Food Research and Action Center. (2004). Federal food programs: Food Stamp Program. Retrieved June 8, 2006, from http://www.frac.org/html/federal_food_programs/ programs/fsp.html

Food Research and Action Center. (2005). Federal food programs: Summer Food Service Program for Children. Retrieved June 8, 2006, from http://www.frac.org/html/ federal_food_programs/programs/sfsp.html

Food Research and Action Center. (2006a). Federal food programs: National School Lunch Program. Retrieved June 8, 2006, from http://www.frac.org/html/federal_food_programs/programs/nslp.html

Food Research and Action Center. (2006b). Federal food programs: School Breakfast Program. Retrieved June 8, 2006, from http://www.frac.org/html/federal_food_programs/programs/sbp.html

Food Research and Action Center. (2006c). Child and Adult Care Food Program. Retrieved July 26, 2006, from http://www.frac.org/html/federal_food_programs/programs/cacfp.html

Fox, M., Hamilton, W., & Lin, B. (2004). *Effects of Food Assistance and Nutrition Programs on Nutrition and Health.* Food Assistance and Nutrition Report No. FANRR-19-3. Washington, DC: U.S. Department of Agriculture, Food and Rural Economic Division, Economic Research Service.

Gartner, L. M., Morton, J., Lawrence, R. A., Naylor, A. J., O'Hare, D., Schanler, R. J., et al. (2005). Breastfeeding and the use of human milk. *Pediatrics, 115*, 496–506.

Gleason, P. M., & Suitor, C. W. (2003). Eating at school: How the National School Lunch Program affects children's diets. *American Journal of Agricultural Economics, 85*, 1047–1061.

Hamm, K., & Ewen, D. (2006). *From the Beginning: Early Head Start Children, Families, Staff, and Programs in 2004.* Washington, DC: Center for Law and Social Policy.

Hanes, S., Vermeersch, J., & Gale, S. (1984). The national evaluation of school nutrition programs: Program impact on dietary intake. *American Journal of Clinical Nutrition, 40*, 390–413.

Hedley, A., Ogden, C., Johnson, C., Carroll, M., Curtin, L., & Flegal, K. (2004). Overweight and obesity among US children, adolescents, and adults, 1999–2002. *Journal of the American Medical Association, 291*, 2847–2850.

Hofferth, S. L., & Curtin, S. (2005). Poverty, food programs and obesity. *Journal of Policy Analysis and Management, 24*, 703–726.

Institute for Research on Poverty. (2004). *Medicaid at Birth, WIC Take-Up, and Children's Outcomes.* Discussion Paper no. 1286-04.

Joint Center for Political and Economic Studies Health Policy Institute. (2006). *Protecting the Health and Nutrition of Young Children of Color: The Impact of Nutrition Assistance and Income Support Programs.* Washington, DC: Author.

Kabbani, N. S., & Yazbeck, M. (2004). *The Role of Food Assistance Programs and Employment Circumstances in Helping Households With Children Avoid Hunger.* Discussion Paper No. 1280-04. Madison, WI: Institute for Research on Poverty.

Krebs, N., & Jacobson, M. (2003). American Academy of Pediatrics policy statement: Prevention of pediatric overweight and obesity. *Pediatrics, 112*, 424–430.

Luman, E. T., McCauley, M. M., Shefer, A., & Chu, S. (2003). Maternal characteristics associated with vaccination of young children. *Pediatrics, 111*, 1215–1218.

March of Dimes Birth Defects Foundation. (2006). Born too small and too soon. Retrieved July 11, 2006, from http://www.marchofdimes.com/peristats

Montgomery, S., & Willis, W. (2006). Fiscal year 2005 impact and review of the Expanded Food and Nutrition Education Program. Retrieved July 24, 2006, from http://www.csrees.usda.gov/nea/food/efnep/pdf/2005_impact.pdf

Nord, M., & Romig, K. (2003). Hunger in the summer: Seasonal food insecurity and the National School Lunch and Summer Food Service Programs. Presented at the Association for Public Policy Analysis and Management Annual Research Conference, Washington, DC.

Oliveira, V. (2003). *Food Assistance Research Brief—WIC and Breastfeeding Rates.* Food Assistance and Nutrition Report No. FANRR-34-2. Washington, DC: U.S. Department of Agriculture, Economic Research Service.

Oliveira, V., Racine, E., Olmsted, J., & Ghelfi, L. (2002). *The WIC Program: Background, Trends, and Issues.* Food Assistance and Nutrition Report No. FANRR27. Washington, DC: U.S. Department of Agriculture, Food and Rural Economic Division, Economic Research Service.

Perez-Escamilla, R., Ferris, A. M., Drake, L., Haldeman, L., Peranick, J., Campbell, M., et al. (2000). Food stamps are associated with food security and dietary intake of inner-city preschoolers from Hartford, Connecticut. *Journal of Nutrition, 130*, 2711–2717.

Poikolainen, A. (2005). *Characteristics of Food Stamp Households: Fiscal Year 2004.* Report No. FSP-05-CHAR. Alexandria, VA: U.S. Department of Agriculture, Food and Nutrition Service, Office of Analysis, Nutrition and Evaluation.

Rose, D., Habicht, J., & Devaney, B. (1998). Household participation in the food stamp and WIC programs increases the nutrient intakes of preschool children. *Journal of Nutrition, 128*, 548–555.

Ryan, A. S., & Zhou, W. (2006). Lower breastfeeding rates persist among the Special Supplemental Nutrition Program for Women, Infants and Children participants, 1978–2003. *Pediatrics, 117*, 1136–1146.

U.S. Department of Agriculture, Economic Research Service. (2006). Food security in the United States: Conditions and trends. Retrieved July 12, 2006, from www.ers.usda.gov/briefing/foodsecurity/trends.htm

U.S. Department of Agriculture, Food and Nutrition Service. (1998). Evaluation of the Summer Food Service Program, Final Report. Washington, DC: Author.

U.S. Department of Agriculture. (2005a). Women, Infants and Children. Retrieved May 28, 2006, from http://www.fns.usda.gov/wic/

U.S. Department of Agriculture. (2005b). Program data: Food Stamp Program. Retrieved June 8, 2006, from http://www.fns.usda.gov/pd/fspmain.htm

U.S. Department of Agriculture. (2005c). Nutrition program facts, Food and Nutrition Service: National School Lunch Program. Retrieved May 8, 2006, from http://www.fns.usda.gov/cnd/Lunch/AboutLunch/NSLPFactSheet.pdf

U.S. Department of Agriculture. (2005d). Special Milk Program. Retrieved July 26, 2006, from http://www.fns.usda.gov/cnd/milk/AboutMilk/SMP.05.pdf

U.S. Department of Agriculture. (2006a). WIC farmers' market nutrition program. Retrieved July 17, 2006, from http://www.fns.usda.gov/WIC/WIC-FMNP-Fact-Sheet.pdf

U.S. Department of Agriculture. (2006b). Team Nutrition policy statement. Retrieved July 24, 2006, from http://www.fns.usda.gov/tn/TN_PolicyStatement.pdf

CHAPTER

5

Special Topics in Prenatal and Infant Nutrition: Genetics and Inborn Errors of Metabolism and Failure to Thrive

Laura Harkness, PhD, RD, Sara Snow, MS, RD, and Claire Blais, RD, LDN, CNSD

With a Special Section: Neonatal Intensive Care Nutrition: Prematurity and Complications
Liesje Nieman, RD, CNSD, LDN

CHAPTER OUTLINE

Reader Objectives

After studying this chapter and reflecting on the contents, you should be able to

1. Define and describe the biochemistry of some of the more prevalent inborn errors of metabolism.
2. Describe the prevalence, diagnosis, clinical symptoms, and long-term complications of inborn errors of metabolism.
3. Discuss medical nutrition therapy for inborn errors of metabolism.
4. Identify and classify failure to thrive.
5. Evaluate the diet of the patient with failure to thrive and describe techniques to treat failure to thrive in the outpatient and inpatient settings.

Genetics and Inborn Errors of Metabolism

Laura Harkness, PhD, RD, and Sara Snow, MS, RD

The inheritance of a genetic disease is determined by whether the gene is dominant or recessive as well as the type of chromosome that carries the gene (autosomal or sex chromosome). **Autosomal recessive** describes a form of inheritance of genetic traits located on the autosomes (the non-sex chromosomes 1–22). Sex-linked diseases are inherited through the X chromosome (because diseases cannot be inherited through the Y chromosome).

A *recessive gene* is an allele that causes a phenotype (a detectable or visible characteristic) that is only seen on a homozygous genotype (having two copies of the same allele). Each of us has two copies of every gene on an autosomal chromosome, one from the mother and one from the father.

For a child to inherit a recessive disease, both parents must carry at least one gene for the disease and the child must inherit two abnormal alleles; in other words, the individual is homozygous for the trait. If only one gene is inherited, the child will not have the disease but will be a carrier and can pass the gene on to future generations.

If both parents are carriers (heterozygous for the trait), there is a 25% chance a child will inherit two abnormal genes and inherit the disease and a 50% chance a child will inherit one abnormal gene and be a carrier for the disease. If only one parent is a carrier, the trait will only occur if the other parent is also a carrier of the trait.

The number and complexity of **inborn errors of metabolism** present a notable challenge to health care providers. More than 300 genetic disorders are associated with adverse production, either deficiency, excess, or altered metabolism, of normally occurring cellular compounds (Burton, 1998). Because early diagnosis and treatment are vitally important to prevent poor outcomes in infants born with inherited metabolic disorders, newborn screening programs are common nationwide to diagnose many of these genetic disorders. In many cases early treatment has been shown to be effective in reducing long-term risks in such disorders as phenylketonuria (PKU), maple syrup urine disease (MSUD), isovaleric academia, and galactosemia. For some inborn errors of metabolism, medical nutrition therapy is the primary treatment modality and will prevent manifestation of toxic substances. Unfortunately, diagnosis of genetic disorders often takes place after irreversible damage has occurred. Early diagnosis and appropriate medical nutrition therapy are paramount to optimal patient outcome.

For nutritional management of inborn errors of metabolism, use of restricted diets and medical nutritional foods are principle components of disease treatment. Medical nutrition therapy must be maximized to maintain normal growth and development. Frequently, energy needs are higher in individuals with inborn errors of metabolism, because protein, carbohydrate, or fat is restricted. Children can require supplemental feedings in the form of enteral or parenteral support to promote growth and to prevent protein catabolism. For inborn errors of metabolism of essential amino acids, it is not possible to completely eliminate the amino acids from the diet for a long period of time without causing adverse outcomes, so careful and continuous monitoring of biochemical measures is crucial. In addition, identifying and managing all key metabolic pathways and compounds that are affected by the inborn error are essential for adequate medical nutritional therapy. The adverse consequences that can result from inborn errors of metabolism include accumulation of toxic substances both locally and remotely, loss of production of key intermediates and products, increased production of intermediates or products that are normally produced in small amounts, lack of substrates for formation of biological compounds, and loss of normal feedback compounds that normally inhibit or stimulate other pathways (Elsas & Acosta, 2006). Therefore the purpose of this chapter is to review the more prevalent inborn errors of metabolism and to discuss key aspects of medical nutrition therapy management.

Branched Chain Amino Acids and Inborn Errors of Metabolism

The **branched chain amino acids** (BCAAs) (leucine, valine, and isoleucine) comprise most of the essential amino acids in healthy individuals, accounting for 40% of essential amino acids. The primary role of BCAAs is incorporation into body proteins. In newborns 75% of BCAAs are used for the synthesis of protein. BCAAs are an important source of nitrogen for the synthesis of nonessential amino acids. Those

Autosomal recessive: Both parents must be carriers of a gene on one of the autosomal (non-sex) chromosomes for a child to inherit the disease. If both parents are carriers, there is a 25% chance that a child will inherit the disease and a 50% chance the child will be a carrier.

Inborn errors of metabolism: Traits arising from a variation in the structure of enzymes or protein molecules.

Branched chain amino acids: Leucine, isoleucine, and valine; present in and help maintain skeletal muscle tissue; important in gluconeogenesis.

not used in protein metabolism are catabolized to provide intermediates (acetyl-coenzyme A [CoA], succinyl-CoA, and acetoacetate) for energy metabolism. The BCAAs share common first steps in catabolism with tricarboxylic acid cycle intermediates. This irreversible oxidative decarboxylation of the keto acids yields intermediates for energy metabolism.

Branched Chain Amino Acid Metabolism

The first step in the metabolism of the BCAAs is a reversible transamination of leucine, isoleucine, and valine by branched chain amino transferase to the resultant keto acid (alpha-ketoisocaproate, alpha-keto-beta-methylvalerate, and alpha-ketoisovalerate). The second step involves the irreversible oxidative decarboxylation by branched chain alpha-keto acid dehydrogenase complex to alpha-ketoacyl-CoA (isovaleryl-CoA, alpha-methylbutyryl-CoA, and isobutyryl-CoA) (Chuang, Chuang, & Wynn, 2006). Branched chain alpha-keto acid dehydrogenase is located in the inner mitochondrial membrane and requires thiamin pyrophosphate, lipoic acid, CoA, and Nicotinamide adenine dinucleotide (NAD) (Figure 5.1).

Maple Syrup Urine Disease (Branched Chain Alpha-Ketoaciduria)

Maple syrup urine disease is a defect in the metabolism of the BCAAs (isoleucine, leucine, and valine). This autosomal recessive disorder is caused by a deficiency of branched chain α-ketoacid dehydrogenase, which is needed for the oxidative decarboxylation of the keto acids that are produced from the BCAAs. The result is accumulation of the BCAAs in the plasma (Harris et al., 1990).

MSUD is rare in the general population (1/100,000 to 1/300,000 births) but has a high incidence (1/200 to 1/700 births) in the Mennonite population. In 1954 Menkes and colleagues at Boston Children's Hospital first described MSUD. Menkes, Hurst, and Craig (1954) documented the deaths of four children from the same family. All the children displayed severe ketoacidosis in the first week of life, and their urine had a strong smell of maple syrup.

Maple syrup urine disease (MSUD): An autosomal recessive disorder characterized by a defect in the metabolism of the branched chain amino acids isoleucine, leucine, and valine caused by a deficiency of branched chain α-ketoacid dehydrogenase resulting in the accumulation of the branched chain amino acids in the plasma.

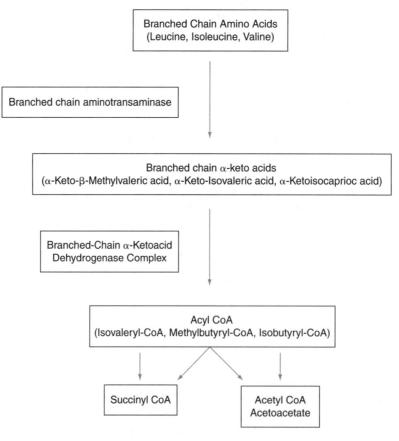

Figure 5.1 Branched Chain Amino Acid Metabolism.

Clinical Features of MSUD

The clinical symptoms that occur in MSUD are the result of neurotoxicity from the accumulation of leucine, valine, and isoleucine and their alpha-keto acids (alpha-ketoisocaproate, alpha-keto-beta-methylvalerate, and alpha-ketoisovalerate) (Riazi et al., 2004). MSUD has a heterogenous clinical phenotypic expression, such that the disease can range from mild to severe. There are presently five known clinical phenotypes for MSUD: classic, intermediate, intermittent, thiamin responsive, and dihydrolipoamide dehydrogenase (E3) deficient (Chuang et al., 2006). Approximately 100 mutations have been identified in four (branched chain alpha-keto acid decarboxylase/dehydrogenase-alpha [E1alpha], E1beta, dihydrolipoyl transacylase [E2], and E3) of the six genes that encode branched chain alpha-keto acid dehydrogenase (Chuang et al., 2006). Accumulation of the branched chain alpha-keto acids in the brain leads to reduced glutamate, glutamine, and gamma-aminobutyrate concentrations. This is considered to be the cause of MSUD encephalopathies. Symptoms of MSUD appear after the infant is fed a protein-containing food. The most severe symptoms can include seizures, apnea, and death within 2 weeks of birth. Additional characteristics of the disorder are elevated blood and urine levels of alpha-ketoisocaproate, alpha-keto-beta-methylvalerate, alpha-ketoisovalerate, leucine, isoleucine, and valine. Elevated urine concentrations result in a maple syrup odor. Infants exhibit a sharp cry, lethargy, vomiting, loss of normal tendon reflexes, poor sucking ability, respiratory failure, metabolic acidosis, and alternating flaccidity and rigidity, leading to spasms of the body with the back fully arched and the heels and head bent back and seizures (Riviello, Rezvani, DiGeorge, & Foley, 1991; Morton, Strauss, Robinson, Puffenberger, & Kelley, 2002).

In both children and adults severe episodes can occur after infections, exercise, injuries, surgery, or some other kind of physiologic stressor. Muscle fatigue, vomiting, sleep disturbances, hallucinations, anorexia, hyperactivity, decreased cognitive function, and dystonia characterize these episodes. Prolonged deficiencies of BCAAs can result from excessive dietary restriction, so careful monitoring of nutrition therapy is important to prevent growth failure, anemia, immunodeficiency, and developmental delay.

Clinical Assessment of MSUD

Clinical symptoms include elevated leucine, isoleucine, and valine levels; ketonuria; poor sucking; irritability; lethargy; seizures; and focal cerebral edema. Laboratory findings in MSUD include metabolic acidosis with anion gap, elevated urine and plasma ketones, and high blood concentrations of BCAAs. Most notably, leucine levels greater than 4 mg/dL (305 µmol/L) should be evaluated for MSUD.

Nutrition Therapy for MSUD

Long-term nutrition therapy is required to provide appropriate dietary BCAA intake to support optimal growth and development while maintaining plasma concentrations of BCAA at nontoxic levels. Timely initiation of nutrition therapy is key to preventing impaired physical and mental development. The aim of the therapeutic regime in MSUD is to keep the concentration of toxic metabolites within individual tolerance limits. BCAAs are essential amino acids and therefore cannot be eliminated from the diet. BCAA requirement in patients with MSUD is mainly determined using indirect markers such as growth and elimination of symptoms. Direct measurement of BCAA requirements in patients with MSUD has been done using indicator amino acid oxidation technique (Riazi et al., 2004). Total mean BCAA requirement was found to be 45 mg/kg/day with an upper limit of 62 mg/kg/day (Raizi et al., 2004). Nutritionally complete protein substitutes, free from leucine, isoleucine, and valine, are used to provide protein and calories for patients with MSUD (Hallam, Lilburn, & Lee, 2005)

The long-term restriction of BCAA intake in diets has proven effective in controlling plasma BCAA levels and mitigating some of the neurologic manifestations. Individualized nutrition therapy must be carefully planned to provide for adequate growth and development while maintaining BCAA concentrations at nontoxic levels. Nutrition therapy that is frequently modified is necessary using laboratory analysis of plasma BCAA concentrations. Long-term plasma leucine levels are associated with impaired cognitive outcome in patients with classic MSUD. To achieve the best possible intellectual outcome for affected individuals, the target range for plasma leucine should not exceed 200 µmol/L in children (Hoffman, Helbling, Schadewaldt, & Wendel, 2006). All patients with MSUD should be evaluated for thiamin responsiveness, because some forms of MSUD respond to thiamin therapy. Thiamin-responsive MSUD is due to a reduced affinity of the mutant branched chain alpha-keto acid dehydrogenase for thiamin pyrophosphate (Chuang, Ku, & Cox, 1982). For these patients, 100 to 500 mg of oral thiamin should be provided for up to 3 months (Fernhoff, 1985).

Disorders of Leucine Catabolism: Isovaleric Acidemia

Isovaleric academia: A disorder of leucine metabolism caused by a deficiency of isovaleryl-CoA characterized by the excessive production of isovaleric acid upon ingestion of protein or during infectious episodes resulting in severe metabolic acidosis.

Isovaleric acidemia is the result of impairment of isovaleryl-CoA dehydrogenase, which leads to toxic accumulation of free isovaleric acid and its precursors (Fries, Rinaldo, Schmidt-Sommerfeld, Jurecki, & Packman, 1996). Isovaleryl-CoA dehydrogenase is required for the conversion of isovaleryl-CoA to β-methylcrotonyl-CoA. To reduce accumulation of free isovaleric acid and toxic precursors, two alternative metabolic routes take place. Free isovaleric acid is detoxified with the addition of carnitine, and toxic precursors are converted to isovaleryl glycine (Naglak, Salvo, Madsen, Dembure, & Elsas, 1988; Fries et al., 1996).

Clinical Diagnosis and Symptoms of Isovaleric Acidemia

There are two forms of isovaleric acidemia, acute or chronic intermittent. The acute form typically occurs in normal full-term infants, who with the start of feeding develop severe symptoms. These can include vomiting, diarrhea, tachypnea, poor feeding, lethargy, hypotonia, tremors, and a "sweaty feet" odor of the urine and blood (Elsas & Acosta, 2006). If infants are not treated or do not respond to treatment, death can occur from metabolic acidosis, cardiac arrest, or central nervous system hemorrhage. Chronic intermittent isovaleric academia is characterized by periods of vomiting, acidosis, and coma during late infancy. The telltale "sweaty feet" odor in urine and blood is present. In some patients hematologic abnormalities have been reported, including low hemoglobin, neutropenia, leukopenia, and thrombocytopenia (Gilbert-Barness & Barness, 1999)

Diagnosis of isovaleric academia is measured by urinary isovaleryl glycine and the presence of metabolic acidosis and elevated plasma and urine ketones (Burton, 1998). In addition, isovaleric acidemia is associated with marked reduction of free carnitine in both plasma and urine (Roe, Millington, Maltby, Kahler, & Bohan, 1984).

Medical Nutrition Therapy for Isovaleric Acidemia

The aim of treatment is to reduce the isovaleric acid burden to a minimum. Therapy, consisting of leucine restriction with supplemental glycine and carnitine, should be started as soon as possible after birth. During acute ketosis, metabolic acidosis must be corrected immediately with glycine and L-carnitine therapy to prevent serious complications, such as mental re-

tardation and intraventricular hemorrhage (Naglak et al., 1988). For long-term therapy dietary restriction of leucine, combined with supplemental glycine and L-carnitine, are used as the cornerstones of treatment. Control of endogenous protein turnover, via supplemental glycine and carnitine, is recommended to limit production of toxic metabolites (Millington, Roe, Matlby, & Inoue, 1991). This is the preferred choice of medical nutrition therapy when compared with protein restriction. The dose of 150 mg glycine/kg/day combined with L-carnitine for two patients was an optimum glycine supplement under stable condition when leucine was restricted (Naglak et al., 1988). When supplemental glycine and L-carnitine were combined in therapy in an 8-year-old patient with isovaleric academia, isovalerylglycine excretion increased compared with providing glycine or L-carnitine alone (Fries et al., 1996). In this case the patient was given a 3-week course of supplementation with glycine alone (250 mg/kg/day), L-carnitine alone (100 mg/kg/day), and both agents combined. The combined therapy leads to increased excretion of isovalerylglycine and isovalerylcarnitine. Moreover, Roe et al. (1984) found that when L-carnitine was given alone, excretion of isovalerylglycine decreased in preference to enhanced excretion of isovalerylcarnitine and hippurate. Treatment with L-carnitine alone has proven effective in preventing further hospitalizations in one patient tested (Roe et al., 1984).

Protein restriction (1.2 to 2.0 g/kg/day), combined with glycine and carnitine supplementation, has been used to improve clinical symptoms; however, careful attention to growth and development are necessary when protein is restricted. With modest protein restriction and monitoring, normal growth is possible. Nine patients with isovaleric acidemia treated with a lower protein diet (1.5 to 2.0 g/kg) and supplemental glycine (250 mg/kg/day) for up to 10 years exhibited no significant side effects and experienced normal growth velocity (Berry, Yudkoff, & Segal, 1988). Of these nine children, four were provided with sup-

CRITICAL Thinking

Critical Thinking About Protein Restriction: Endogenous catabolism of protein and amino acids is a problem in inborn errors of metabolism. It is thought that the endogenous catabolism leads to worsening symptoms and disease progression. Frequently, endogenous catabolism of protein is caused by restrictive diets. It is suggested that therapy should be directed toward control of endogenous protein turnover rather than the restriction of dietary protein during treatment of inborn errors of protein metabolism.

plemental carnitine (50 mg/kg/day) to maintain serum carnitine levels within normal limits.

Aromatic Amino Acids and Inborn Errors of Metabolism

Phenylalanine Metabolism

Phenylalanine is an essential amino acid used for tissue protein synthesis and hydroxylation reactions that result in the formation of tyrosine. The reaction requires phenylalanine hydroxylase, tetrahydrobiopterin, and dihydropteridine reductase (Scriver, Kaufman, Eisensmith, & Woo, 2001) (Figure 5.2). Hyperphenylalaninemia is caused by a defect in phenylalanine hydroxylase activity. If phenylalanine hydroxylase or its cofactor tetrahydrobiopterin are absent or deficient, phenylalanine accumulates in body fluids and the central nervous system and tyrosine becomes an essential amino acid (Behrman, Kleigman, & Arvin, 1996; Scriver et al., 2001).

Hyperphenylalaninemia primarily affects the brain tissue. The high concentration of phenylalanine interferes with the transport of the amino acids tyrosine and tryptophan into the brain (Behram et al., 1996). Tyrosine is needed to provide energy and to synthesize protein, catecholamines, melanin, and thyroid hormones (Elsas & Acosta, 2006). Excess phenylalanine in the blood results in the accumulation of phenyl ketones that are excreted in the urine, thus the term *phenylketonuria*.

> **Phenylketonuria:** A form of hyperphenylalaninemia caused by the complete or near complete deficiency of the liver enzyme phenylalanine hydroxylase resulting in an accumulation of phenylalanine in body fluids and the central nervous system.

Phenylketonuria

PKU, first described in 1933, is a form of hyperphenylalaninemia, defined as plasma phenylalanine value above 120 µM (2 mg/dL) (Scriver et al., 2001). It is an autosomal recessive disorder caused by the complete or near complete deficiency of the liver enzyme phenylalanine hydroxylase. The most severe form is classic PKU. The observation that phenylpyruvic acid was excreted in the urine of patients with mental defects was the first identification of a specific chemical deficiency in a central nervous system disorder (Udenfriend, 1961). Untreated, PKU can result in severe to profound mental retardation and behavioral difficulties. The severity of the disease can vary with each affected person. Mild and moderate PKU are less severe forms and carry less risk for brain damage; however, most patients with the disorder need to follow a lifelong restricted diet.

At least 200 different mutations that cause the "PKU phenotype" have been identified. They involve deletions in coding frames, missense mutations, and intron splice mutations (Scriver et al., 2001). PKU is an autosomal recessive disorder (both parents must have and pass on the gene). A rare disorder, PKU occurs in approximately 1 in 13,500 to 19,000 newborns. The incidence of non-PKU hyperphenylalaninemia is 1 in 48,000. PKU is more common in whites and Native Americans and occurs less in African-Americans, Hispanics, and Asians (National Institutes of Health [NIH], Consensus Development Panel, 2006). It is also common in those of Irish descent (Acosta & Yannicelli, 2001; Elsas & Acosta, 2006).

Clinical Symptoms and Diagnosis of PKU

The infant with PKU is normal at birth. Mental retardation can develop over time and may not be evident for the first few months. Left untreated, mental retardation can become very severe. On physical examination, infants with PKU are lighter in complexion than their siblings and have blue eyes and fair skin because phenylalanine cannot be converted to melanin. Some appear with seborrheic or eczematoid rash that disappears as the child gets older. A musty odor caused by phenylacetic acid may be present in the child's breath, skin, and/or urine. Most infants with PKU are hypertonic with hyperactive deep tendon reflexes. Twenty-five percent of children have seizures, with more than 50% exhibiting electroencephalographic abnormalities. Other common findings include microencephaly, prominent maxilla with widely spread teeth, enamel hyperplasia, and growth retardation (Behrman et al., 1996).

Newborn screening and subsequent dietary treatment of PKU have significantly reduced the incidence of severe mental retardation (MacCready, 1974; Luder & Greene, 1989; Koch et al., 2003). Screening for PKU was initiated in the early 1960s after the

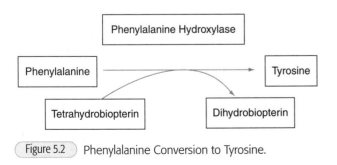

Figure 5.2 Phenylalanine Conversion to Tyrosine.

Guthrie bacterial inhibition assay was developed (Guthrie, 1961; Guthrie & Susi, 1963). All states require that newborns be screened for PKU. Blood is routinely collected from the infant's heel within the first 24 to 48 hours of life after protein ingestion (Behrman et al., 1996). Criteria for a positive PKU screen can vary state to state, and decision-making policies, funding, and availability of follow-up services can also vary. Because of this, not all newborns and families have the same level of care for PKU (NIH, 2006). In addition to newborn testing, prenatal screening can be done using chorionic villus sampling, DNA analysis, or enzyme assay (Scriver et al., 2001). Early screening coupled with early dietary treatment has lead to major improvements in the intellectual and behavioral outcomes for persons with PKU (Fishler, Azen, Henderson, Friedman, & Koch, 1987; Fishler, Azen, Friedman, & Koch, 1989).

Medical Nutrition Therapy for PKU

Treatment of PKU involves the immediate and life-long avoidance of excess dietary phenylalanine. It was once thought that the diet could be discontinued in adolescence, but today it is recommended the diet be followed for life (Scriver et al., 2001; Elsas & Acosta, 2006). The diet provides supplemental tyrosine and small amounts of phenylalanine for essential functions. Frequent laboratory testing and growth records are used to determine phenylalanine and tyrosine requirements. Requirements differ for each person depending on the extent of phenylalanine hydroxylase deficiency, age, health status, and, for pregnant women, the stage of pregnancy. The diet consists of phenylalanine-free medical foods that supply protein and essential nutrients and measured amounts of low-protein foods and free foods (foods with little or no phenylalanine). High-protein foods such as meat, fish, poultry, eggs, dairy products, nuts, dried beans, and peas are not allowed. Foods without PHE, such as sugar, oil, and pure starch, are added as needed to meet energy needs. Although expensive, low-protein specialty products such as bread, pasta, and baking mixes are available and can help to provide variety. A diet that is too low in phenylalanine may cause a phenylalanine deficiency, which could cause harm; thus small measured amounts of low-protein foods such as cereals, fruits, and vegetables are allowed (Acosta & Yannicelli, 2001; NIH, 2006). The amount of protein may be greater than the Dietary Reference Intake when an elemental formula is the primary source of protein equivalent (Acosta et al., 2003). Aspartame products should not be used because they contain 56% phenylalanine. Baby formulas and breast milk contain phenylalanine so infants must be fed phenylalanine-free formula; however, some infants can tolerate a measured amount of breast milk depending on the level of enzyme deficiency (Acosta & Yannicelli, 2001; Elsas & Acosta, 2006).

The strict limitations of the diet make compliance difficult and lead to noncompliance in 80% of patients (Walter et al., 2002). In addition, nutrient deficiencies, such as vitamin B_{12}, are associated with protein restriction (Hanley, Feigenbaum, Schoonheyt, & Austin, 1996; Robinson et al., 2000). As a result, researchers have been investigating alternatives to traditional diet therapy. The transport of phenylalanine across the blood–brain barrier has been shown to be completely inhibited by dietary supplementation of large neutral amino acids in adults who have been unable to follow the PKU diet (Pietz et al., 1999; Weglage et al., 2001; Moats, Moseley, Koch, & Nelson, 2003). Treatment using tetrahydrobiopterin, a cofactor of phenylalanine hydroxylase, has been shown to decrease blood phenylalanine in tetrahydrobiopterin-sensitive PKU, although more research needs to be done to find the optimal dose (Trefz, Scheible, Frauendienst-Egger, Korall, & Blau, 2005).

To determine the adequacy of phenylalanine and tyrosine in the diet, frequent blood testing for concentrations of these amino acids is necessary. The NIH consensus panel concluded that blood phenylalanine levels should be checked once a week during the first year of life, twice a month from ages 1 to 12 years, and monthly after age 12 (NIH, 2006). Because of the rapid growth that occurs in infancy, other practitioners have recommended that testing should be done twice a week during the first 3 months of life, along with measurements of height, weight, and head circumference (Elsas & Acosta, 2006). After the first 3 months, testing should be done weekly until age 1. If blood phenylalanine is greater than 300 µmol (5 mg/dL), then the frequency should be increased until the blood concentration reaches 30 to 60 µmol. Food records kept by the caregiver are necessary to determine what alterations need to be made in the diet (Elsas & Acosta, 2006; NIH, 2006). Especially in children, energy intake, physical activity, and weight should be monitored carefully (Fishler et al., 1989). Although the appropriate level of blood phenylalanine for children and adults has been an issue of debate, most practitioners recommend levels between 120 and 360 µmol/L (2 to 6 mg%)

(Waisbren, Schnell, & Levy, 1980; Fisch et al., 1995; Scriver et al., 2001; NIH, 2006).

Docosahexanoic acid and arachidonic acid play an important role in brain and retinal function. Moseley, Koch, and Moser (2002) found that docosahexanoic acid and arachidonic acid concentrations and red blood cell docosahexanoic acid concentration were slightly but significantly reduced. They recommended that blood lipid docosahexanoic acid and arachidonic acid be monitored in all PKU patients and supplemented if levels are significantly low.

Maternal Phenylketonuria

Women with PKU who have elevated levels of phenylalanine during pregnancy are at an increased risk of giving birth to offspring with intrauterine growth retardation, psychomotor retardation, microencephaly, and congenital heart defects (Koch et al., 1984; Michals-Matalon, Platt, Acosta, Azzen, & Walla, 2002). The Collaborative Study on Reproductive Outcome was initiated in 1984 in response to a lack of information about the management of PKU (Koch et al., 2003). The prospective study was convened to answer questions about diet and reproductive outcome and to evaluate the efficacy of dietary treatment in decreasing morbidity of offspring. Three hundred eighteen pregnancies were studied, with a total of 207 live births. The best fetal outcomes were seen when strict control of blood phenylalanine was obtained 10 weeks before pregnancy and maintained throughout the entire pregnancy. Blood phenylalanine levels in women with PKU should be maintained at 120 to 360 μmol/L. Blood levels greater than 600 μmol/L after 10 weeks gestation significantly increase the risk of congenital anomalies (Koch et al., 2003).

It is difficult for pregnant women to achieve desired blood phenylalanine levels (Lenke & Levy, 1980; NIH, 2006). Special populations are particularly vulnerable to dietary noncompliance. This is especially true for adolescents, who stop following their prescribed diet in late adolescence, leading to elevated levels of phenylalanine. To achieve the best outcomes, phenylalanine intake and all nutrients in the diet should be monitored (Acosta et al., 2001; Michals-Matalon et al., 2002; Matalon, Acosta, & Azen, 2003). Even when phenylalanine levels are elevated, adequate protein and vitamin intakes in the early stages of pregnancy may have a protective effect for congenital heart disease (Michals-Matalon et al., 2002; Matalon et al., 2003). Normal pregnancy weight gain may reduce microencephaly and should be encouraged and monitored (Michals-Matalon

et al., 2002; Matalon et al., 2003). Inadequate protein, fat, and energy intakes may contribute to elevated plasma phenylalanine concentrations and to poor outcomes (Acosta et al., 2001). Offspring of women who have a low protein intake during pregnancy combined with elevated blood phenylalanine levels appear to have an increased incidence of congenital heart defects (Michals-Matalon et al., 2002). Protein from medical foods, fat, and energy intakes should be increased to help prevent elevated PHE levels (Michaels-Matalon et al., 2003). The fact that only 36% of the women entering the maternal PKU study achieved blood PHE control by 8 weeks emphasizes the need for preconception education (Brown et al., 2002; Rouse & Azen, 2004). Tracking, education, and follow-up of pregnant women with PKU are essential to improve fetal outcomes (Acosta, 1995; Koch et al., 2003).

Tyrosinemias

Tyrosinemias are a group of inherited inborn errors of metabolism characterized by disordered tyrosine metabolism. Left untreated, tyrosine and its byproducts build up

> **Tyrosinemias:** A group of inherited inborn errors of metabolism characterized by disordered tyrosine metabolism.

in organs and tissues, resulting in serious medical problems. Tyrosine is used to synthesize protein and is a precursor for thyroxine, melanin, dopamine, norepinephrine, and epinephrine.

Seven types of tyrosinemia have been identified (Elsas & Acosta, 2006). Tyrosinemia type Ia is a result of a deficiency of fumarylacetoacetate hydrolyase, the last enzyme in the degradation pathway of tyrosine. Lack of this enzyme causes succinylacetone to accumulate in the liver and kidneys, resulting in a variety of symptoms such as severe liver disease that can lead to liver failure in infancy, cirrhosis, liver cancer, and renal Fanconi syndrome. Infants with tyrosinemia type Ia have increased blood concentrations of phenylalanine and tyrosine right after birth. The prevalence of tyrosinemia type Ia is 1 in 100,000 to 120,000 in the general population, with a higher incidence reported in the French-Canadian and Scandinavian population. In the Saguenay-Lac Saint Jean region of Quebec, Canada, the prevalence is estimated to be 1 in 1,846. (Behrman, Kleigman, & Arvin, 2004). Tyrosinemia type Ib, reported in only one infant, is believed to be caused by a deficiency of maleylacetoacetone isomerase (Mitchell, Grompe, Lambert, & Tanguay, 2001).

Type II tyrosinemia is a rare disorder caused by a deficiency of tyrosine aminotransferase. It is also known as oculocutaneous tyrosinemia, tyrosine aminotransferase deficiency, keratosis palmoplantaris with corneal dystrophy, and Richner-Hanhart syndrome. Mental retardation reportedly occurs in half of affected individuals with tyrosinemia type II. Restriction of dietary phenylalanine and tyrosine helps to alleviate skin and ophthalmic symptoms (Mitchell et al., 2001).

Type III tyrosinemia is a caused by a defect in the functioning of 4-hydroxyphenylpyruvate dioxygenase, the second enzyme in the catabolic pathway of tyrosine. Three different types have been identified: hereditary 4-hydroxyphenylpyruvate dioxygenase deficiency (type IIIa), hawkinsuria (type IIIb), and transient tyrosinemia of the newborn (type IIIc) (Mitchell et al., 2001). Transient tyrosinemia of the newborn can occur as a result of a high-protein diet, ascorbate deficiency, and immature function of 4-hydroxyphenylpyruvate dioxygenase. Normal plasma tyrosine is commonly achieved within weeks to months with treatment with oral ascorbate and/or protein restriction. The use of lower-protein commercial formulas and increased breast-feeding has decreased the incidence of transient tyrosinemia (Mitchell et al., 2001). Types IIIa and IIIb are extremely rare, with only 13 reported cases (Ellaway et al., 2001).

Clinical Features of Tyrosinemia Type Ia

The severe form of tyrosinemia type Ia is characterized by symptoms of acute liver failure, renal tubular dysfunction and coagulopathy, jaundice, vomiting, diarrhea, and hypoglycemia. A cabbage-like odor may be present, possibly due to methionine metabolites (Behrman et al., 2004). Children with the late onset or chronic form usually present after age 1, and symptoms are usually milder. Symptoms include hypophosphatemic rickets, hypertension, nervous system disorders, and liver and kidney dysfunction (Elsas, 1999; Scriver et al., 2001).

Diagnosis is made by measuring fumarylacetoacetate hydroxylase activity in liver biopsy specimens, lymphocytes, and erythrocytes (Behrman et al., 2004). Succinylacetate and succinylacetone are often present in the serum and urine, and blood phenylalanine and tyrosine are elevated.

Medical Nutrition Therapy for Tyrosinemias

The goals for medical nutrition therapy for tyrosinemias types Ia and Ib are to restrict dietary phenylalanine and tyrosine to amounts that maintain postprandial plasma amino acid concentration goals and support normal growth and development and

good health. To prevent deficiency, when plasma phenylalanine and tyrosine are at desired levels, plasma amino acids should be measured frequently (Acosta et al., 2001). Plasma phenylalanine should be maintained between 40 and 80 μmol and tyrosine between 50 and 15 μmol (Elsas & Acosta, 2006). Insufficient phenylalanine and tyrosine intake can result in anorexia, lethargy, hypotonia, inadequate growth, and decreased plasma fibrinogen (Cohn, Yudkoff, Yost, & Segal, 1977). Levels of protein should be supplied to support normal growth and development and prevent catabolism and rickets. Plasma bicarbonate, phosphate, and potassium should be maintained at normal levels, and plasma and urine should be free of or contain only trace amounts of succinylacetate and parahydroxyphenyl organic acids (Acosta et al., 2001). Phenylalanine and tyrosine need to be restricted more for type I than for types II and III. Adequate protein can be obtained with the addition of medical foods. A diet low in tyrosine and phenylalanine in addition to treatment with the enzyme 4-hydroxyphenylpyruvate dioxygenase by 2-(nitro-4-trifluoromethylbenzoyl)-1,2-cyclohexanedione has shown the most promising results (Crone et al., 2003).

Sulfur-Containing Amino Acids and Disorders of Sulfur-Containing Amino Acids

Methionine, a sulfur-containing essential amino acid present in dietary proteins, is to a small extent used for body protein synthesis, with most metabolized via the transsulfuration pathway to homocysteine Figure 5.3 . In the transsulfuration pathway, methionine is converted to S-adenosylmethionine, which is subsequently hydrolyzed to homocysteine. Homocysteine can be remethylated to form methionine (via two different pathways), metabolized to cystathionine, and oxidized to homocystine. Oxidation to homocysteine only happens when homocysteine accumulates to abnormal levels. Most homocysteine is metabolized to cystathionine via cystathionine beta-synthase (vitamin B_6 dependent enzyme).

Homocystinuria

The most common form of homocystinuria is caused by a lack of cystathionine beta-synthase. **Homocystinuria** caused by cystathionine beta-synthase deficiency affects at least 1 in 200,000 to 335,000 people (Mudd et al., 1985). The disorder appears to be

Homocystinuria: An inborn error of metabolism characterized by urinary excretion of homocysteine caused by a lack of cystathionine beta-synthase.

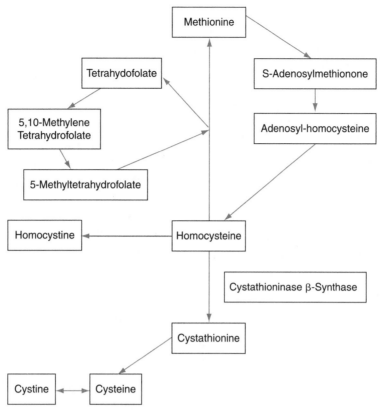

Metabolism of Methionine Homocysteine and Cystathionine.

more common in Ireland (Yap & Naughten, 1998). Approximately13% of cases of cystathionine beta-synthase deficient homocystinuria are responsive to vitamin B₆, which sometimes results in milder symptoms (Mudd et al., 1985). Other rarer forms of homocystinuria are caused by defects of the other enzymes responsible for metabolizing homocysteine.

Clinical Symptoms and Diagnosis of Homocystinuria

Cystathionine beta-synthase deficient homocystinuria is characterized by developmental delay and/or mental retardation, ectopia lentis (dislocation of the ocular lens) and/or severe myopia, skeletal abnormalities (excessive height and length of the limbs), osteoporosis, and thromboembolism (Mudd et al., 1985). Developmental delay is often the first abnormal sign in individuals with homocystinuria. Intelligence quotient in individuals with homocystinuria ranges from 10 to 138. The mean intelligence quotient of individuals with B₆ responsiveness is 79 versus 57 for those who are B₆ nonresponsive.

Thromboembolism, which can affect any vessel, is the major cause of early death and morbidity. Cerebrovascular accidents have been described in infants, although problems typically appear in young adults (Yap, Boers, et al., 2001).

Diagnosis of homocystinuria is evident by screening for increased methionine concentrations. Additional testing includes plasma and urine concentrations of methionine, homocysteine, and total homocysteine to confirm or exclude the diagnosis of homocystinuria. The cardinal biochemical features of classic homocystinuria are (1) markedly increased concentrations of plasma homocysteine, total homocysteine, homocysteine-cysteine mixed disulfide, and methionine and (2) increased concentration of urine homocysteine.

Medical Nutrition Therapy for Homocystinuria

Medical nutrition therapy should be closely managed to correct biochemical abnormalities, especially to control plasma homocysteine concentration, prevent thrombosis, and provide for optimal growth and development. Individuals identified by newborn screening should be treated shortly after birth to maintain plasma homocysteine concentration below 11 μmol/L (preferably no higher than 5 μmol/L) (Yap, Rushe, Howard, & Naughten, 2001). Treatment includes using vitamin B₆ therapy, protein-restricted and methionine-restricted diets, betaine treatment, and/or folate and vitamin B_{12} supplementation.

Dietary protein restriction reduces methionine intake, with additional use of methionine-free amino acid formulas and medical nutritional foods. It is important that cysteine is provided in the diet, because the normal conversion from methionine is not available. In those who are shown to be B_6 responsive, treatment with pyridoxine in a dose of approximately 100 to 200 mg/day, or the lowest dose that produces the maximum benefit, should be given. Betaine, given in two divided doses of 6 to 9 g/day, provides an alternative remethylation pathway to convert excess homocysteine to methionine (Yap, Rushe, et al., 2001; Lawson-Yuen & Levy, 2006). The optimal dose for betaine has not been determined, but betaine can become the treatment of choice in those individuals who are noncompliant with dietary restrictions or cannot be controlled through protein restriction alone (Schwahn et al., 2003; Singh, Kruger, Wang, Pasquali, & Elsas, 2004).

Betaine lowers homocysteine concentrations but increases methionine levels, so plasma methionine concentrations should be monitored in all persons receiving betaine. Side effects of betaine, although rare, have been reported, including body odor, resulting in reduced compliance, and cerebral edema when hypermethioninemia is greater than 1,000 μmol/L (Yaghmai et al., 2002; Devlin et al., 2004; Tada, Takanashi, Barkovich, Yamamoto, & Kohno, 2004; Braverman, Mudd, Marker, & Pomper, 2005). Omitting betaine results in rapid reduction of the hypermethioninemia and resolution of the cerebral edema (Lawson-Yuen & Levy, 2006). Thus plasma methionine as well as homocysteine must be monitored in patients receiving betaine.

Supplementation with folate and vitamin B_{12} can be used to optimize the conversion of homocysteine to methionine, because methionine synthase is a folate/vitamin B_{12} dependent enzyme. When red blood cell folate concentration and serum B_{12} concentration are reduced, folic acid (5 mg/day) and vitamin B_{12} (1 mg/mo intramuscularly) should be given (Fowler, Schutgens, Rosenblatt, Smit, & Lindemans, 1997).

Urea Cycle Disorders

Urea cycle disorders are caused by a deficiency of one of the enzymes (carbamyl phosphate synthetase, n-acetylglutamate synthetase, ornithine transcarbamylase, argininosuccinic acid synthetase, argininosuccinate lyase, arginase) in the urea cycle Figure 5.4 . There are six enzyme disorders of the urea cycle, collectively known as inborn errors of urea synthesis, or urea cycle enzyme defects. Urea, formed to remove nitrogen as ammonia during protein metabolism, is excreted in the urine. In urea cycle disorders ammonia accumulates, causing hyperammonemia. Ammonia can cross the blood–brain barrier and cause irreversible brain damage and death. The most common urea cycle disorder is ornithine transcarbamylase deficiency, which leads to decreased synthesis of citrulline from ornithine and carbamyl phosphate (Scaglia et al., 2003). Incidence of urea cycle disorders is estimated at 1 in 10,000 births (Bachman, 2003). Expression of urea cycle disorders can vary from complete to partial enzyme deficiency. Individuals with childhood or adult onset disease have partial enzyme deficiency. The percentage, or amount, of enzyme function varies widely between individuals with partial enzyme deficiencies. Patients with late onset forms may present at any age and carry a 28% mortality rate (Nassogne, Heron, Touati, Rabier, & Saudubray, 2005).

Urea cycle disorders: Inborn errors of urea synthesis caused by a deficiency of the enzymes in the urea cycle (carbonyl phosphate synthetase, n-acetylglutamate synthetase, ornithine transcarbamylase, arginosuccinic acid synthase, arginosuccinate lyase, arginase).

Clinical Symptoms and Diagnosis of Urea Cycle Disorders

Symptoms, including irritability, poor feeding, vomiting, and lethargy, usually occur after the first 24 hours of life. If untreated, symptoms progress to seizures, hypotonia, respiratory distress and alkalosis, coma, and death. Children with mild urea cycle enzyme deficiencies may not display noticeable symptoms until early childhood. These symptoms may develop as failure to thrive, vomiting, and behavior changes, including inconsolable crying, lethargy, agitation, infliction of self-injury, and refusal to eat high-protein foods. If the child is not diagnosed with a urea cycle disorder, hyperammonemic coma or death can occur.

Medical Nutrition Therapy for Urea Cycle Disorders

The primary objectives of medical nutrition therapy are to limit ammonia production and to maximize alternative pathways for removal of ammonia. Careful provision of dietary protein is needed to minimize am-

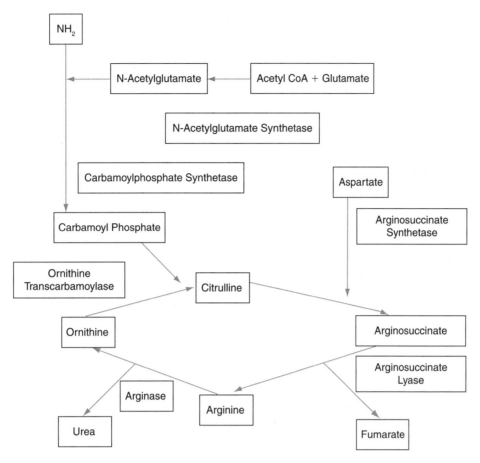

Figure 5.4   Urea Cycle.

monia production without adversely affecting growth and development. Optimization of calories from carbohydrate and fat are necessary to ensure that energy needs are met, because poor growth is often reported in patients who are prescribed lower protein diets. The protein restriction prescription requires careful calculations of need, which depend on many variables, including specific enzyme defect, age-related growth rate, current health status, physical activity, amount of free amino acids administered, energy intake, residual urea cycle function, family life-style, use of nitrogen-scavenging medications, and the patient's eating behaviors (Singh et al., 2005). Special formulas can be used to provide essential amino acids to help provide for anabolism and growth. In a 6-month clinical trial in which 17 infants and toddlers were provided amino acid medical food, significant increases in length and weight with nonsignificant gains in head circumference were seen (Acosta et al., 2005). In addition, albumin and transthyretin concentrations increased with provision of amino acid medical foods, with no increase in plasma ammonia levels. Additional nutrition therapy includes supplementation with branched chain amino

acids, L-citrulline, and multivitamins and minerals as needed based in clinical evaluation. Careful monitoring of a patient's appetite is important because frequent anorexia is present (Acosta et al., 2005).

Disorders of Carbohydrate Metabolism

Galactosemia

Most cases of **galactosemia** are categorized as classic, or type I, galactosemia and are caused by mutations in the *GALT* gene. This gene produces the enzyme galactose-1-phosphate uridyl-transferase, which is important in processing galactose. Mutations in the *GALT* gene cause two forms of type I galactosemia, classic and Duarte variant. Individuals with the classic type of galactosemia lack nearly all the enzyme activity necessary to metabolize galactose. Individuals with the Duarte variant have approximately 5% to 20% of the enzyme activity necessary to metabolize galactose and often do not

Galactosemia: An inborn error of carbohydrate metabolism caused by a deficiency of galactosyl-1-phosphate uridyl-transferase, which inhibits glycogen breakdown and glucose synthesis causing severe hypoglycemia after the ingestion of fructose.

have signs or symptoms of galactosemia (Podskarbi et al., 1996). Classic galactosemia is an inherited disorder that occurs in approximately 1 in 30,000 live births. The incidence of the Duarte variant, a mild type of galactosemia, is more common. This variant affects an estimated 1 in 16,000 live births (Tyfield et al., 1999).

Clinical Symptoms and Diagnosis of Galactosemia

Vomiting, liver enlargement, and jaundice are often the earliest signs of the disease, but bacterial infections (often severe), irritability, failure to gain weight, and diarrhea may also occur (Bosch, 2006). If unrecognized in the newborn period, the disease may produce liver, brain, eye, and kidney damage; thus galactosemia should be considered in any jaundiced infant (Bosch, 2006). Galactosemia is diagnosed by measuring levels of galactose-1-phosphate uridyl-transferase. In patients with galactosemia there is no enzyme activity. If infants are fed galactose-containing feedings, there will be large amounts of galactose excreted in urine (Bosch, 2006).

Medical Nutrition Therapy for Galactosemia

Nutrition therapy is to provide a galactose-free diet by using galactose-free foods. For infants with galactosemia, feeding special galactose- and lactose-free formula is required. Infants cannot be fed breast milk. With early therapy any liver damage that occurred in the first few days of life will nearly completely heal. Careful lifelong monitoring of dietary therapy must be maintained, including elimination of both lactose and galactose from the diet. Galactose is found mainly in milk and dairy products as part of lactose, but it is also contained in galactoproteins and galactolipids in others foods. The use of galactose-restricted diets must include attention to galactose contributions from all food sources, including bound galactose found in meat, dairy, and cereals as well as free galactose in peas, lentils, some legumes, organ meats, cereals, and some fruits and vegetables (Gropper, Weese, West, & Gross, 2000; Weese, Gosnell, West, &Groppper, 2003).

Careful monitoring of growth in children with galactosemia is important, because altered growth has been found with decreased height, less fat mass, and less lean body mass (Panis, Forgot, Nieman, Van Kroonenburgh, & Rubio-Gozalbo, 2005). Long-term complications usually develop in patients with galactosemia, despite a restricted diet. Complications, including mental retardation, motor abnormalities, hypergonadotropic hypogonadism, and speech disorders, are common (Bosch, 2006).

Fructose Intolerance

Fructose intolerance, also called fructosemia, hereditary fructose intolerance, and fructose aldolase B-deficiency, is caused by the lack of the enzyme fructose-1-phosphate aldolase (aldolase B). Aldolase B is the major aldolase isozyme in the liver and functions in both fructose metabolism, using fructose-1-phosphate as a substrate, and in gluconeogenesis, producing fructose-1,6-bisphosphate from the two triose phosphates, glyceraldehyde-3-phosphate and dihydroxyacetone phosphate (Figure 5.5). Fructoaldolase B deficiency leads to accumulation of fructose-1-phosphate, decreased ATP concentrations, and hypoglycemia (Van den Berghe, Bruntman, Vannestes, & Hers, 1977). The accumulated fructose-1-phosphate inhibits glycogen breakdown and glucose synthesis, thereby causing severe hypoglycemia after ingestion of fructose (Hommes, 1993). Incidence of fructose intolerance is estimated at 1 in 20,000 to 40,000 births.

> **Fructose intolerance:** An inborn error of metabolism caused by the lack of the enzyme fructose-1-phosphate aldolase (aldolase B).

Symptoms and Diagnosis of Fructose Intolerance

Consumption of fructose, sucrose, or sorbitol leads to severe symptoms of vomiting, poor feeding, irritability, jaundice, profound hypoglycemia, enlarged spleen and liver, and progressive liver damage (Ali, Rellos, & Cox, 1998). Continued ingestion of sucrose or fructose leads to hepatic and renal injury and growth retardation. Parenteral administration of fructose or sorbitol may be fatal (Ali et al., 1998). Diagnosis is confirmed by increased urine levels of glucose, lactate, bicarbonate, protein, and urate; increased blood levels of fructose, uric acid, bilirubin, and lactate; and reduced concentrations of glucose, bicarbonate, and proteins. Liver failure can occur with

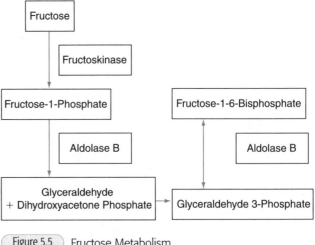

Figure 5.5 Fructose Metabolism.

resulting poor production of coagulation factors and increased enzyme concentrations of aspartate amino transferase and alanine amino transferase.

Medical Nutrition Therapy for Fructose Intolerance

Medical nutrition therapy includes removal of fructose, sorbitol, and sucrose from the diet (less than 40 mg/kg/day) and results in complete alleviation of most symptoms and a normal life span (Baerlocher, Baerlocher, Gitzelmann, Steinmann, & Gitzelmann-Cumarumsay, 1978; Odiévre, Gentil, Gautier, & Alagille, 1978). Complete exclusion of fructose is often difficult, however, and many patients develop a syndrome of chronic fructose intoxication characterized by retarded growth, chronic liver disease, and hepatomegaly (Baerlocher et al., 1978; Mock. Perman, Thaler, & Morris, 1983). Failure to comply with the dietary prescription can lead to progressive liver failure. Other side effects of fructose consumption include severe hypoglycemia, seizures, bleeding, gout, and death (Hommes, 1993). A noteworthy feature of fructose intolerance is the development of powerful aversions to fruit, nuts, and sweet-tasting foods and drinks (Cox, 1994). In fact, older subjects with fructose intolerance who adhere to a self-imposed fructose-restricted diet may continue to live undiagnosed and lead relatively normal lives.

Failure to Thrive

Claire Blais, RD, LDN, CNSD

The American Academy of Pediatrics (AAP) uses two criteria for diagnosing failure to thrive. The first of these is when weight (or weight for height) falls to less than two standard deviations below the mean (z-score less than –2.0) for sex- and age-matched peers (Kleinman, 2004). The second relates to weight for age having declined across more than two major percentile lines after having achieved a previously stable growth pattern. The latter definition highlights the importance of clinical judgment when diagnosing a child with failure to thrive. Up to 39% of infants cross two major percentile lines before stabilizing into a growth pattern (Mei, Grummer-Strawn, Thompson, & Dietz, 2004), so it is prudent not to use weight for age as a single measure for identifying failure to thrive.

A **z-score** is defined as the standard deviation from the mean. For example, in the National Center for Health Statistics (NCHS) growth

z-score: A numeric value assigned to the standard deviation from the mean of a data set. A z-score of 1.0 equates to one standard deviation above the mean.

charts the mean weight for age is defined by the 50th percentile. The fifth percentile expresses 1.75 standard deviations below the mean, or a z-score of −1.75. Categorizing growth according to z-scores is the most accurate technique for classifying growth failure. It is more precise than defining an infant's growth as "at or near" a percentile or "just below" a percentile (Kleinman, 2004). Nonetheless, this technique is less practical in the acute care setting, and growth charts tend to be the established norm.

It is important to distinguish children who are constitutionally small from those who are truly failing to thrive. Bone age can be useful in differentiating genetic short stature from abnormal growth (Corrales & Utter, 2004). If the bone age is less than the chronologic age, there exists potential for more growth, and the child is likely failing to thrive. If the bone age is consistent with the chronologic age, then the child is likely exhibiting genetic short stature.

CRITICAL **Thinking**

Critical Thinking About Clinical Judgment: Never let definitions outweigh your clinical judgment. These classifications are meant to help guide your practice, not replace it. If you have a child who was born at low birth weight and is plotting consistently below the third percentile on the weight for age chart, would you classify her with failure to thrive? Some previously accepted definitions would say yes—weight for age below the third percentile classifies as failure to thrive. But use your judgment; perhaps this patient is just following her own growth curve. Someone has to be in the bottom 3%!

Classification of Failure to Thrive

In 1972 Waterlow established criteria for comparing weight and height of a malnourished child with standards for age- and sex-matched peers. He described a weight for height deficit as wasting, indicating acute malnutrition, and a height for age deficit as stunting, indicating chronic malnutrition. No one method of classifying failure to thrive is infallible (Raynor & Rudolf, 2000), providing further evidence for the need to exercise clinical judgment when making the diagnosis of failure to thrive. The **Waterlow criteria** (Table 5.1) are still widely accepted today as among the primary classifications of pediatric malnutrition.

Waterlow criteria: A set of calculations used to classify the severity of malnutrition in children.

The three factors that lead to energy imbalance in the failure to thrive population are inadequate energy intake, inefficient energy utilization, and increased

TABLE 5.1	Waterlow Criteria		
Acute malnutrition (wasting) Actual weight (kg) × 100 ──────────────────── Expected weight (kg) for ht (cm) at 50th %ile	Grade 0 (normal)	>90%	
	Grade I (mild)	81–90%	
	Grade II (moderate)	70–80%	
	Grade III (severe)	<70%	
Chronic malnutrition (stunting) Actual height (cm) × 100 ──────────────────── Expected height (cm) for age at 50th %ile	Grade 0 (normal)	>95%	
	Grade I (mild)	90–95%	
	Grade II (moderate)	85–89%	
	Grade III (severe)	<85%	

Source: Reprinted with permission from Waterlow, C. (1972). Classification and definition of protein-calorie malnutrition. *British Medical Journal*, 3, 577–579.

energy expenditure (**Table 5.2**). Failure to thrive can be characterized by the presence of one or more of the above conditions.

There are a variety of causes for the three factors, which are broken up into two classes: organic and nonorganic. **Organic failure to thrive** is lack of growth associated with an identifiable disease or disorder. Almost all chronic illnesses in childhood can result in poor weight gain related to any of the factors described in Table 5.2. **Nonorganic failure to thrive** is present in most of all diagnosed cases of failure to thrive (Kleinman, 2004). Children have nonorganic failure to thrive

Organic failure to thrive: Lack of growth associated with an identifiable disease.

Nonorganic failure to thrive: Lack of growth that cannot be attributed to an identifiable disease or condition.

The Cultural Diversity of Poverty

Poverty is the most omnipresent of the social risk factors for failure to thrive. One study documented that 13% of their patients with poor growth are homeless, which makes access to the medical care needed to prevent and correct malnutrition difficult (Frank & Zeisel, 1998). It becomes crucial to proper treatment of your patients that you consider their socioeconomic status in designing an individualized care plan.

when their lack of growth cannot be attributed to an identifiable disease. The cause of nonorganic failure to thrive is psychosocial in origin. Risk factors for the development of nonorganic failure to thrive can be found in **Table 5.3**.

The development of failure to thrive is multifactorial and complex. It would be errant to assume that all cases of failure to thrive have a mutually exclusive presentation. In fact, many children present with features of both organic and nonorganic failure to thrive (Corrales & Utter, 2004).

Assessment of the Patient with Failure to Thrive

Assessment of the patient with failure to thrive should include a thorough medical, social, and nutritional evaluation. The medical evaluation should include a complete

TABLE 5.2	Energy Imbalance

Inadequate Energy Intake
   Anorexia
   Inappropriate formula preparation
   Poor nutritional quality of breast milk
   Poor nutritional quality of food offered
   Poor oral feeding (including dysphagia, uncoordinated
     suck/swallow)
Inefficient Energy Utilization
   Frequent emesis
Gastroesophageal Reflux
   Malabsorption/maldigestion (cystic fibrosis, inflammatory
     bowel disease, short gut syndrome, pancreatitis)
Increased Energy Expenditure
   Bronchopulmonary dysplasia
Cancer
Congential Heart Disease
Cystic Fibrosis

Source: Compiled from Corrales and Utter (2004) and Kleinman 2004).

TABLE 5.3	Risk Factors for the Development of OFTT and NOFTT	

Risk Factors for OFTT	Risk Factors for NOFTT
Bronchopulmonary dysplasia	Poverty
	Abuse
Cleft palate	Maternal/paternal
Cystic fibrosis	deficits in appropriate
Developmental delay	feeding practices
Fetal alcohol syndrome	Feeding difficulties
HIV/AIDS	Factors leading to poor
Intrauterine growth	bonding
restriction	Unwanted pregnancy
Prematurity	Mother of young age
Low birth weight	(<17 yr)
Very low birth weight	Depression
Extremely low birth weight	Psychopathology
Short gut syndrome	(including Munchausen
	syndrome by proxy)

Source: Compiled from Corrales and Utter (2004), Kleinman (2004), and Feldman et al. (2004).

history and physical, paying careful attention to pre- and perinatal history, clinical examinaiton, and family history, especially that of older siblings (Kleinman, 2004). The medical evaluation should also assess for lead toxicity, anemia, and zinc deficiency. A low serum alkaline phosphatase may indicate zinc deficiency. During the clinical examination the physician should observe for signs of neglect, which may include poor general hygiene, poor oral health, or diaper rash (Kleinman, 2004).

Given that the vast majority of cases of failure to thrive present with some form of inadequate caloric intake, nutritional rehabilitation should be attempted before extensive laboratory workup is commenced. A social evaluation should be conducted to assess the family dynamics and economic situation (Kleinman, 2004). During all evaluations careful attention should be paid to caregiver–child interaction, including eye contact, physical proximity, and verbalization.

The assessment performed by the nutrition professional is most essential. A thorough assessment of intake and output is necessary to evaluate truly the child's nutriture. If the infant is breast-feeding, the registered dietitian should ask if the child feeds at both breasts at each feeding, how long the child sucks at each breast, and how many times daily the child feeds. If the infant is formula feeding, careful attention must be paid to formula preparation. The most common error in formula feeding is improper dilution of the formula (Kleinman, 2004). The dietitian should determine how the formula is prepared, how much the child feeds, and how often. It is important here to be specific. Many parents are tempted to say, "2 to 3 ounces every 3 to 4 hours." This could be as little as 12 ounces of formula or as much as 24 ounces of formula. A detailed 3- to 5-day food record is the most accurate method, but it is not always possible, in which case a 24-hour recall can be very effective (Kleinman, 2004).

For the child who is also taking solid foods, it is important to ask what types and textures are being offered, how long the child takes to eat, what the portion size is and how much the child actually eats of it, and the timing of meals and snacks. The dietitian should also inquire into food allergies or intolerances, including the child's reaction to the food item. If possible, a direct observation of the feeding would be helpful. An in-home evaluation is ideal, but oftentimes an office or hospital setting must suffice. In addition to evaluating intake, the dietitian should also garner an understanding of the child's output. Number and consistency of stools and number of wet diapers (or strict measurement of urine

output in the acute care setting) can be helpful in determining the child's absorptive capacity. The dietitian should also ask about spits or emesis and, if at all possible, try to quantify the frequency and volume of such spits and emesis.

It is important to inquire about the child's activity level as well, because fidgety or very active children can be difficult to feed and could also be burning off more calories than they are consuming. It is also the responsibility of the dietitian to plot the growth curves carefully, correcting for prematurity where necessary. For a child who was born premature, the weight should be corrected until the child is 24 months old, the length until the child is 40 months old, and the head circumference until the child is 18 months old (Kleinman, 2004).

The nutrition evaluation should also include an assessment of kilocalorie and protein needs for catch-up growth. The equation for catch-up growth is as follows:

$$\frac{(\text{Ideal Body Weight for Height} \times \text{RDA for Weight Age})}{\text{Current Weight}}$$

where Ideal Body Weight for Height is the weight at the 50th percentile for the current height, RDA is the Recommended Daily Allowance, and the Weight Age is the age at which the current weight is at the 50th percentile (Corrales & Utter, 2004; Kleinman, 2004). This equation can be used for both kilocalorie needs and protein needs. For example, an 8-month-old male who weighs 7 kg and is 78 cm long has a weight age of 4.5 months and an ideal body weight for length of 8 kg. You would then multiply 8 kg 108 kcal/kg and divide by 7 kg. The result is 123 kcal/kg. If the RDA for weight age is equal to the RDA for current age, then it is generally acceptable to use 120 kcal/kg as the standard reference for this value. For example, a 5-month-old female who weighs 5 kg and measures 59 cm long has a weight age of 2.5 months and an ideal body weight for length of 5.7 kg. The RDA for her weight age is the same as the RDA for her chronologic age, so we would multiply 5.7 kg 120 kcal/kg and divide by 5 kg to get 134 kcal/kg.

Calculation of needs for catch-up growth is always an estimate. It is important to exercise clinical judgment. If a child's catch-up needs calculate out to be substantially more than his or her current level of intake, it is best to make small increases in the level of intake, following weight gain and adjusting as needed. Efforts to promote catch-up should continue until the child regains his or her previously established growth percentiles (Kleinman, 2004). The best measure of whether a child is meeting his or her needs for growth is by following the child's weight gain after interventions (Corrales & Utter, 2004). If the child is gaining weight at or above the expected rate for age, then the child is receiving adequate kilocalories. See Table 5.4 for expected rates of weight gain by age.

Nutritional Interventions

Weight gain or loss in the hospital may not be reproducible in the home environment, and it may not distinguish between organic and nonorganic failure to thrive, so it is best to avoid hospitalization if possible (Kleinman, 2004). Many failure to thrive cases are initially treated in the outpatient setting, with behavioral and nutritional interventions.

Regardless of the cause of the failure to thrive, the primary intervention is to increase intake of kilocalories. This presents a unique challenge for the breast-fed infant, because breast milk is only 20 kcal/oz. What will inevitably take place is that the mother will pump her breast milk, add infant formula powder or other modular kilocalorie supplements to the breast milk to fortify it, and feed this to the infant by bottle. In a case where malnutrition is present, the benefits of direct nursing are outweighed by the infant's need for adequate kilocalories. In the formula-fed infant the first intervention is to concentrate the formula to a higher caloric density. This can be done by concentration up to 24 kcal/oz and by modular kilocalorie supplements as needed up to 30 kcal/oz. The modular kilocalorie supplements typically used are in the form of fat or glucose polymers. It is not generally recognized as safe to concentrate beyond 24 kcal/oz strictly from powder, because the potential renal solute load becomes too high for the infant and vomiting and dehydration could occur (Corrales & Utter, 2004).

For the child who is taking additional solid foods, adding kilocalories to food without adding volume becomes imperative to maximize their intake. Parents should be taught label reading to offer their infants younger than 12 months old high-kilocalorie baby foods. These foods can also be fortified with small amounts of infant cereal, glucose polymer modular supplements, corn oil, or margarine. Children over 1 year of age can be offered drinks with added powdered skim milk, instant breakfast powder, glucose polymer modular supplements, table sugar, or corn oil. Cheese, gravy, margarine, peanut butter, and cream cheese can be added to solid foods, in addition to the supplements listed above for beverage addition. Juice should be limited to 4 ounces daily or eliminated completely from the diet (Corrales & Utter, 2004).

It is important to teach caregivers to develop a standard mealtime routine with their children. Some suggestions for what to tell caregivers are as follows (University of Iowa, 2002):

- Set definitive meal and snack times, and limit their duration to 30 minutes or less.
- Do not allow eating between scheduled meals and snacks, regardless of how much was eaten at the previous feeding.
- Always feed your child at the table in a high chair or a booster seat.
- Praise the positive behaviors.
- Ignore the negative behaviors.
- Allow your child to get messy while eating.
- Model good eating behavior.

Another less common approach to treatment includes the use of appetite stimulants. Homnick and coworkers (2004) found the use of appetite stimulants such as cyproheptadine to be effective in promoting weight gain among individuals aged 5 and older with organic failure to thrive; however, the AAP and U.S. Food and Drug Administration (FDA) believe the costs outweigh the benefits of the use of this appetite stimulant in infants with failure to thrive (Kleinman, 2004).

Occasionally, when behavioral management fails and the child continues to fail to take adequate amounts of nutrition by mouth, a nasogastric feeding tube must be placed. It is up to the health care

TABLE 5.4	Expected Rates of Growth by Age
Age	Expected growth (g/day)
Preterm infant	15–30
0–3 months	20–30
3–7 months	15–21
7–12 months	10–13
1–7 years	5–8

Source: Reproduced with permission from Fomon, S. J., Haschke, F., Zeigler, E. E., & Nelson, S. E. (1982). Body composition of reference children from birth to age 10 years. *American Journal of Clinical Nutrition, 35*, 1175.

team to determine how much of the child's nutrition will be administered through the tube at this point, but it generally depends on how much the child can reliably take by mouth. In most cases 77% to 75% of the child's nutritional needs should be provided through nasogastric feedings. For infants under age 1 year, standard infant formulas can be given. It is best to start with the standard dilution of 20 kcal/oz and advance by 2 kcal/oz daily as tolerated by the infant until the goal concentration is met. The same rules for concentrating infant formula and breast milk as for oral feedings apply for tube feedings as well. For children over 1 year of age, a standard 30 kcal/oz pediatric formula can be used, provided there is no cow's milk protein allergy present. If the child is allergic, there are a variety of hydrolyzed protein and hypoallergenic formulas available on the market. Full-strength feedings should be initiated at a low rate and advanced slowly as tolerated, monitoring for vomiting, diarrhea, or abdominal distension. If it becomes evident that the child will need aggressive nutrition supplementation for a period of several weeks to months, it would be wise to consider more permanent enteral access, typically in the form of a gastrostomy tube.

The prognosis of children with failure to thrive depends largely on the severity of the illness and the risk factors present. Evidence from studies on the effects on cognitive development in children with a history of failure to thrive in infancy has shown an adverse effect on intellectual outcomes in older childhood (Corbett & Drewett, 2004). A multidisciplinary team (a registered dietitian, a speech-language pathologist, and an occupational therapist, at a minimum) approach to the treatment of the patient with failure to thrive is the most effective method of intervention in these patients. In many cases prognosis can be excellent if the diagnosis is made early enough and intervention is commenced immediately (Corrales & Utter, 2004).

Summary

Individualized medical nutrition therapy must be initiated immediately upon diagnosis of an inborn error of metabolism. Nutrition therapy is necessary to prevent further adverse health outcomes and to optimize growth and development. Medical nutrition therapy must be continuously monitored to ensure that the individual needs for each patient are being met and that blood levels of key substances are being monitored. In addition, for some inborn errors of metabolism, consumption of foods may cause physical distress such as gastrointestinal (GI) pain, and the individual may be reluctant to eat foods or may develop anorexia. In planning nutrition support, a formal dietary prescription must be carefully written, including all macronutrients and key micronutrients as well as fluid. A plan for monitoring the nutrition support must also be enacted to ensure that both physical and biochemical status are monitored regularly. Last, compliance with the medical nutrition therapy is a very challenging area and must be constantly supported to enable parents and patients to maintain their diet.

Failure to thrive is a term used to describe children whose growth is significantly below that of their peers. This term has been used for centuries but remains controversial (Kleinman, 2004). There exists no one agreed-on definition for failure to thrive but rather several clinically acceptable diagnostic criteria. This section touched on some of these diagnostic criteria as well as accepted methods for classifying malnutrition in the pediatric population. It reviewed necessary components of the medical and nutritional evaluation of the patient with failure to thrive and described several techniques found to be effective in treatment of failure to thrive. Because there are so many factors that can contribute to the development of failure to thrive, outcomes are variable. Continued education and heightened awareness of clinicians is necessary to prevent and treat failure to thrive in at-risk populations.

Issues to Debate

The assessment and provision of adequate protein and optimal levels of essential amino acids are necessary for normal growth and development in children with inborn errors of metabolism. However, there is scant evidence regarding the amount of protein and amino acids needed to support normal development. In addition, there is little evidence to establish tolerance levels for amino acids levels in individuals with inborn errors of metabolism. Frequently, medical nutrition therapy is based on case studies with little research evidence to support the recommendations of the therapy. In addition, patient compliance with the medical nutrition therapy is problematic.

1. How does the health care provider ensure optimal growth and development for patients?
2. How does the health care provider write a prescription for medical nutrition therapy when little evidence is available to justify the prescription?

3. How does the health care provider work with patients and families to ensure compliance with medical nutrition therapy?

In failure to thrive:

1. When is it appropriate to feed an infant naso-gastrically? Moreover, when does it become imperative?

2. At what point should permanent enteral access be considered in a failure to thrive infant or toddler?

Case Study: Inborn Errors of Metabolism

A 5-day-old infant presented to the pediatrician with poor feeding, irritability, lethargy, and vomiting. Upon examination, there was poor tendon reflex.

Laboratory studies were obtained and included urinalysis, complete blood count, blood glucose, and serum electrolytes. Subsequent laboratory tests included blood gases. Key laboratory findings included

Blood pH	7.35
Potassium	5.5 mM
Glucose	160 mg/dL
Ketones	200 mg/dL
Chloride	94 mM
Bicarbonate	12 mEq/L
Urine pH	4.3
+ ketones in urine	

It was determined that this infant had 1) what kind of metabolic imbalance? Once the metabolic imbalance was diagnosed, what other laboratory findings would be useful?

Case Study: Failure to Thrive

MN is a 2-year, 2-month-old boy admitted to the hospital with failure to thrive. As the clinical dietitian you are consulted to evaluate this patient on his first day of admission. In your chart review you determine that he was a full-term infant and was strictly breast-fed until 6 months old, then began to take rice cereal and eventually added strained fruits and vegetables to his diet. During your interview mom reports that MN is difficult to feed. He throws food on the floor, plays with it, pushes the spoon away, laughs at his older brothers (ages 4 and 7), and generally does not seem interested in eating. It takes him over an hour to eat each meal and snack, and it is not a pleasant experience for the patient or his mother.

Birth Wt: 7 lb, 2 oz
Birth Lt: 20.5"
12-month check-up: 19 lb, 6 oz
Current Wt: 9.86 kg
Current Length: 90.5 cm
Labs: unremarkable, albumin WNL
Meds: none

24-hr Recall
Breakfast: 6–8 oz orange juice, ½ cup toasted oat o-shaped cereal, ½ banana, sliced. MN mostly throws the cereal on the floor and mashes the banana into his hair.
Morning snack: 4–6 oz apple juice, 2–3 wheat crackers, 1 string cheese.
Lunch: 8 oz whole milk, 1 cup spaghetti with tomato sauce. MN very much enjoys the milk, but most of the spaghetti ends up on his clothes and in the high chair.
Afternoon snack: 4oz water, ½ cup cooked carrot coins.
Dinner: 8 oz whole milk, 1 to 2 chicken nuggets, a few bites of corn.
Dessert: 8 oz whole milk, a few bites of chocolate brownie

Questions
1. Other than the information provided above, what other questions would you ask mom?
2. What other services do you believe should be consulted on this patient while in the hospital?
3. Plot MN's weights on a NCHS growth chart. Describe his weight trend.
4. Estimate MN's calorie and protein needs.
5. What suggestions can you give to this mom?

Websites

Genetic and Inborn Errors of Metabolism

www.ncbi.nlm.nih.gov/entree/dispomim.cgi?id=230400

http://rarediseases.info.nih.gov/html/resources/info_cntr.html

www.nlm.nih.gov/medlineplus/phenylketonuria/html/ency/article/00366.htm

www.nlm.nih.gov/medlineplus/ency/article/000359.htm

www.nlm.nih.gov/medlineplus/ency/article/000373.htm

www.nlm.nih.gov/medlineplus/ency/article/001199.htm

www.ghr.nlm.nih.gov/condition=argininosuccinicaciduria/show/PubMed

www.ghr.nlm.nih.gov/condition=isovalericacidemia

www.ghr.nlm.nih.gov/condition=tyrosinemia

Failure to Thrive

American Academy of Pediatrics (AAP) http://www.aap.org

American Dietetic Association (ADA) http://www.eatright.org

References

Genetics and Inborn Errors of Metabolism

Acosta, P. (1995). Nutrition support of maternal phenylketonuria. *Seminars in Perinatology, 19*, 182–190.

Acosta, P., Matalon, K., Castiglioni, L., Rohr, F. J., Wenz, E., Austin, V., et al. (2001). Intake of major nutrients by women in the Maternal Phenylketonuria (MPKU) Study and effects on plasma phenylalanine concentrations. *American Journal Clinical Nutrition, 73*, 792–796.

Acosta, P., & Yannicelli, S. (2001). *The Ross Metabolic Formula System: Nutrition Support Protocols* (4th ed.). Columbus, OH: Abbott Laboratories.

Acosta, P. B., Yannicelli, S., Ryan, A. S., Arnold, G., Marriage, B. J., Plewinska, M., et al. (2005). Nutritional therapy improves growth and protein status of children with a urea cycle enzyme defect. *Molecular Genetics and Metabolism, 86*, 448–455.

Acosta, P. B., Yannicelli, S., Singh, R., Modidi, S., Steiner, R., DeVincentis, E., et al. (2003). Nutrient intakes and physical growth of children with phenylketonuria undergoing nutritional therapy. *Journal of the American Dietetic Association, 103*, 1167–1173.

Ali, M., Rellos, P., & Cox, T. M. (1998). Hereditary fructose intolerance. *Journal of Medical Genetics, 35*, 353–365.

Bachman, C. (2003). Long-term outcome of patients with urea cycle disorders and the question of neonatal screening. *European Journal of Pediatrics, 162*, S29–S33.

Baerlocher, K., Gitzelmann, R., Steinmann, B., & Gitzelmann-Cumarumsay, N. (1978). Hereditary fructose intolerance in early childhood: A major diagnostic challenge. *Helvetica Paediatrica Acta, 33*, 465–487.

Behrman, R. E., Kleigman, R. M., & Arvin, A. A. (1996). *Nelson Textbook of Pediatrics* (15th ed.) Philadelphia: W. B. Saunders.

Behrman, R. E., Kleigman, R. M., & Arvin, A. A. (2004). *Nelson Textbook of Pediatrics* (17th ed.). Philadelphia: W. B. Saunders.

Berry, G. T., Yudkoff, M., & Segal, S. (1988). Isovaleric academia: Medical and neurodevelopmental effects of long-term therapy. *Pediatrics, 113*, 58–64.

Bosch, A. M. (2006). Classical galactosaemia revisited. *Journal of Inherited Metabolic Disease,* July 11 [epub]. Retrieved October 29, 2007, from http://www.springerlink.com/content/102938/

Braverman, N. E., Mudd, S. H., Barker, P. B., & Pomper, M. G. (2005). Characteristic MR imaging changes in severe hypermethioninemic states. *AJNR American Journal of Neuroradiology, 26*, 2705–2706.

Brown, A. S., Fernhoff, P. M., Waisbren, S. E., Frazier, D. M., Singh, R., Rohr, F., et al. (2002). Barriers to successful dietary control among pregnant women with PKU. *Genetic Medicine, 4*, 84–89.

Burton, B. K. (1998). Inborn errors of metabolism in infancy: A guide to diagnosis. *Pediatrics, 102*, 69–78.

Chuang, D. T., Chuang, J. L., & Wynn, R. M. (2006). Lessons from genetic disorders of branched-chain amino acid metabolism. *Journal of Nutrition, 136*, 243S–249S.

Chuang, D. T., Ku, L. S., & Cox, R. P. (1982). Thiamin-responsive maple-syrup-urine disease: Decreased affinity of the mutant branched-chain alpha-keto acid dehydrogenase for alpha-ketoisovalerate and thiamin pyrophosphate. *Proceedings of the National Academies of Science, 79*, 3300–3304.

Cohn, R. M., Yudkoff, M., Yost, B., & Segal, S. (1977). Phenylalanine–tyrosine deficiency syndrome as a complication of the management of hereditary tyrosinemia. *American Journal of Clinical Nutrition, 30*, 209–214.

Cox, T. M. (1994). Aldolase B and fructose intolerance. *FASEB Journal, 8*, 62–71.

Crone, J., Moslinger, D., Bodamer, Q. A., Schima, W., Huber, W. D., Holme, E., et al. (2003). Reversibility of cirrhotic regenerative live nodules upon NTBC treatment in a child with tyrosinaemia type I. *Acta Paediatrica, 92*, 625–628.

Devlin, A. M., Hajipour, L., Gholkar, A., Fernandes, H., Ramesh, V., & Morris, A. A. (2004). Cerebral edema associated with betaine treatment in classical homocystinuria. *Journal of Pediatrics, 144*, 545–548.

Ellaway, C. J., Holme, E., Standing, S., Preece, M. A., Green, A., Ploechl, E., et al. (2001). Outcome of tyrosinemia type III. *Journal of Inherited Metabolic Disease, 24*, 824–832.

Elsas, L. J., & Acosta, P. B. (2006). Inherited metabolic disease: Amino acids, organic acids, and galactose. In M. E. Shils, M. Shike, A. C. Ross, B. Caballero, & R. J. Cousins (Eds.), *Modern Nutrition in Health and Disease* (9th ed., pp. 909–959). Baltimore: Williams & Wilkins.

Fernhoff, P. M., Lubitz, D., Danner, D. J., Dembure, P. P., Schwartz, H. P., Hillman, R., et al. (1985). Thiamine response in maple syrup urine disease. *Pediatric Research, 19*, 1011–1016.

Fisch, R. O., Chang, P. N., Weisberg, S., Gulberg, P., Guttler, F., & Tsai, M. Y. (1995). Phenylketonuria patients decades after diet discontinuation. *Journal of Inherited Metabolic Disease, 18*, 347–353.

Fishler, K., Azen, C. G., Friedman, E. G., & Koch, R. (1989). School achievement in treated PKU children. *Journal of Mental Deficiency Research, 33*, 493–498.

Fishler, K., Azen, C. G., Henderson, R., Friedman, E. G., & Koch, R. (1987). Psychoeducational findings among children treated for phenylketonuria. *Journal of Mental Deficiency Research, 92*, 65–73.

Fowler, B., Schutgens, R. B., Rosenblatt, D. S., Smit, G. P., & Lindemans, J. (1997). Folate-responsive homocystinuria and megaloblastic anaemia in a female patient with functional methionine synthase deficiency (cbIE disease). *Journal of Inherited Metabolic Disease, 20*, 731–741.

Fries, M. H., Rinaldo, P., Schmidt-Sommerfeld, E., Jurecki, E., & Packman, S. (1996). Isovaleric acidemia: A response to a leucine load after three weeks of supplementation with glycine, L-carnitine, and combined glycine-carnitine therapy. *Journal of Pediatrics, 129*, 449–452.

Gilbert-Barness, E., & Barness, L. A. (1999). Isovaleric academia with promylecystic myeloproliferative syndrome. *Pediatric and Developmental Pathology, 2*, 286–291.

Gropper, S. S., Weese, S. J. O., West, P. A., & Gross, K. C. (2000). Free galactose content of fresh fruits and strained fruits and vegetable baby foods: More foods to consider for the galactose-restricted diet. *Journal of the American Dietetic Association, 100*, 573–575.

Guthrie, R. (1961). Blood screening for phenylketonuria. *Journal of the American Medical Association, 178*, 863.

Guthrie, R., & Susi, A. (1963). A simple phenylalanine method for detecting phenylketonuria in large populations of newborn infants. *Pediatrics, 32*, 338–343.

Hallam, P., Lilburn, M., & Lee, P. J. (2005). A new protein substitute for adolescents and adults with maple syrup urine disease (MSUD). *Journal of Inherited Metabolic Disease, 28*, 665–672.

Hanley, W. B., Feigenbaum, A. S., Clarke, J. T., Schoonheyt, W. E., & Austin, V. J. (1996). Vitamin B$_{12}$ deficiency in adolescents and young adults with phenylketonuria. *European Journal of Pediatrics, 155*, 145S–147S.

Harris, R. A., Zhang, B., Goodwin, G. W., Kuntz, M. J., Shimomura, Y., Rougraff, P., et al. (1990). Regulation of the branched-chain alpha-ketoacid dehydrogenase and elucidation of a molecular basis for maple syrup urine disease. *Advances in Enzyme Regulation, 30*, 245–263.

Hoffman, B., Helbling, C., Schadewaldt, P., & Wendel, U. (2006). Impact of longitudinal plasma leucine levels on the intellectual outcome in patients with classic MSUD. *Pediatric Research, 59*, 17–20.

Hommes, F. A. (1993). Inborn errors of fructose metabolism. *American Journal of Clinical Nutrition, 58*, 788S–795S.

Hutchinson, R. J., Bunnell, K., and Thoene, J. G. (1985). Suppression of granulopoietic progenitor cell proliferation by metabolites of branched-chain amino acids. *Journal of Pediatrics, 106*, 62–65.

Kaufman, U., and Froesch, E. R. (1973). Inhibition of phosphorylase-a by fructose 1-phosphate, alpha-glycerolphosphate and fructose1,6-diphosphate: explanation for fructose-induced hypoglycaemia in hereditary fructose intolerance and fructose 1,6-diphosphatase deficiency. *European Journal of Clinical Investigation, 3*, 407–413.

Koch, R., Hanley, W., Levy, H., Matalon, K., Matalon, R., Rouse, B., et al. (2003). The maternal phenylketonuria international study: 1984–2002. *Pediatrics, 112*, 1523–1529.

Lawson-Yuen, A., & Levy, H. L. (2006). The use of betaine in the treatment of elevated homocysteine. *Molecular Genetics and Metabolism, 88*, 201–207.

Lenke, R. R., & Levy, H. L. (1980). Maternal phenylketonuria and hyperphenylalaninemia: An international survey of the outcome of untreated and treated pregnancies. *New England Journal of Medicine, 303*, 1202–1208.

Luder, A. S., & Greene, C. L. (1989). Maternal phenylketonuria and hyperphenylalaninemia: Implications for medical practice in the United States. *American Journal of Obstetrics and Gynecology, 161*, 1102–1105.

MacCready, R. A. (1974). Admissions of phenylketonuric patients to residential institutions before and after screening programs of the newborn infant. *Journal of Pediatrics, 85*, 383–385.

Matalon, K. M., Acosta, P. B., & Azen, C. (2003). Role of nutrition in pregnancy with phenylketonuria and birth defects. *Pediatrics, 112*, 1534–1553.

Menkes, J. H., Hurst, P. L., & Craig, J. M. (1954). A new syndrome: Progressive familial infantile cerebral dysfunction associated with an unusual urinary substance. *Pediatrics, 14*, 462–467.

Michals-Matalon, K., Acosta, P., and Azen, C. (2003). Role of nutrition in pregnancy with phenylketonuria and birth defects. *Pediatrics, 112*, 1534–1536.

Michals-Matalon, K., Platt, L. D., Acosta, P. P., Azen, C., & Walla, C. A. (2002). Nutrient intake and congenital heart defects in maternal phenylketonuria. *American Journal of Obstetrics and Gynecology, 187*, 441–444.

Millington, D. S., Roe, C. R., Maltby, D. A., & Inoue, F. (1991). Endogenous catabolism is the major source of toxic metabolites in isovaleric acidemia. *Pediatric Neurology, 7*, 137–140.

Mitchell, G. A., Grompe, M., Lambert, M., & Tanguay, R. M. (2001). Hypertyrosinemia. In C. R. Scriver, A. L. Beaudet, W. S. Sly, & D. Valle (Eds.), *The Metabolic and Molecular Basis of Inherited Disease* (8th ed., pp. 1777–1806). New York: McGraw-Hill.

Moats, R. A., Moseley, K. D., Koch, R., & Nelson, M. (2003). Brain phenylalanine concentrations in phenylketonuria: Research and treatment of adults. *Pediatrics, 112*, 1575–1579.

Mock, D., Perman, J., Thaler, M., & Morris, R. C. (1983). Chronic fructose intoxication after infancy in children with hereditary fructose intolerance. *New England Journal of Medicine, 309*, 764–770.

Morton, D. H., Strauss, K. A., Robinson, D. L., Puffenberger, E. G., & Kelley, R. I. (2002). Diagnosis and treatment of maple syrup disease: A study of 36 patients. *Pediatrics, 109*, 999–1008.

Moseley, K., Koch, R., & Moser, A. B. (2002). Lipid status and lon-chain polyunsaturated fatty acid concentrations in adults and adolescents with phenylketonuria on a phenylalanine-restricted diet. *Journal of Inherited Metabolic Disease, 25*, 56–64.

Mudd, S. H., Skovby, F., Levy, H. L., Pettigrew, K. D., Wilcken, B., Pyeritz, R. E., et al. (1985). The natural history of homocystinuria due to cystathionine-β-synthase deficiency. *American Journal of Human Genetics, 37*, 1–31.

Naglak, M., Salvo, R., Madsen, K., Dembure, P., & Elsas, L. (1988). The treatment of isovaleric academia with glycine supplement. *Pediatric Research, 24*, 9–13.

Nassogne, M. C., Heron, B., Touati, G., Rabier, D., & Saudubray, J. M. (2005). Urea cycle defects: Management and outcome. *Journal of Inherited Metabolic Disease, 28*, 407–414.

National Institutes of Health (NIH), Consensus Development Panel. (2006). National Institutes of Health Consensus

Development Conference statement: Phenylketonuria: screening and management, October 16–18, 2000. *Pediatrics, 105*, 972–982.

Odiévre, M., Gentil, C., Gautier, M., & Alagille, D. (1978). Hereditary fructose intolerance in childhood: Diagnosis, management and course in 55 patients. *American Journal of Diseases of Children, 132*, 605–608.

Panis, B., Forgot, P. P., Nieman, F. H., Van Kroonenburgh, M. J., & Rubio-Gozalbo, M. E. (2005). Body composition in children with galactosemia. *Journal of Inherited Metabolic Disease, 28*, 931–937.

Pietz, J., Kreis, R., Rupp, A., Mayatepek, E., Rating, D., Boesch, C., et al. (1999). Large neutral amino acids block phenylalanine transport into brain tissue in patients with phenylketonuria. *Journal of Clinical Investigation, 103*, 1169–1178.

Podskarbi, T., Kohlmetz, T., Gathof, B. S., Kleinlein, B., Bieger, W. P., Gresser, U., et al. (1996). Molecular characterization of Duarte-1 and Duarte-2 variants of galactose-1-phosphate uridyltransferase. *Journal of Inherited Metabolic Disease, 19*, 638–644.

Riazi, R., Rafii, M., Clarke, J. T. R., Wykes, L. J., Ball, R. O., & Pencharz, P. B. (2004). Total branched chain amino acids requirements in patients with maple syrup urine disease by use of indicator amino acid oxidation with L-$[1-^{13}C]$ phenylalanine. *American Journal of Physiology, Endocrinology and Metabolism, 287*, E142–E149.

Riviello, J. J., Rezvani, I., DiGeorge, A. M., & Foley, C. M. (1991). Cerebral edema causing death in children with maple syrup urine disease. *Journal of Pediatrics, 119*, 42–45.

Robinson, M., White, F. J., Cleary, M. A., Wraith, E., Lam, W. K., & Walter, J. H. (2000). Increased risk of vitamin B_{12} deficiency in patients with phenylketonuria on an unrestricted or relaxed diet. *Journal of Pediatrics, 136*, 545–547.

Roe, C. R., Millington, D. S., Maltby, D. A., Kahler, S. G., & Bohan, T. P. (1984). L-Carnitine therapy in isovaleric acidemia. *Journal of Clinical Investigation, 74*, 2290–2295.

Rouse, B., & Azen, C. (2004). Effect of high maternal blood phenylalanine on offspring congenital anomalies and developmental outcome at ages 4 and 6 years: The importance of strict dietary control preconception and throughout pregnancy. *Journal of Pediatrics, 144*, 235–239.

Scaglia, F., Marini, J., Rosenberger, J., Henry, J., Garlick, P., Lee, B., et al. (2003). Differential utilization of systemic and enteral ammonia for urea synthesis in control subjects and ornithine transcarbamylase deficiency carriers. *American Journal of Clinical Nutrition, 78*, 749–755.

Schwahn, B. C., Hafner, D., Hohfeld, T., Balkenhol, N., Laryea, M. D., & Wendel, U. (2003). Pharmacokinetics of oral betaine in healthy subjects and patients with homocystinuria. *British Journal of Clinical Pharmacology, 55*, 6–13.

Scriver, C. R., Kaufman, S., Eisensmith, R., & Woo, S. L. C. (2001). The hyperphenylalaninemias. In C. R. Scriver, A. L. Beaudet, W. S. Sly, & D. Valle (Eds.), *The Metabolic and Molecular Basis of Inherited Disease* (8th ed.). New York: McGraw-Hill.

Singh, R. H., Kruger, W. D., Wang, L., Pasquali, M., & Elsas, L. J. (2004). Cystathionine beta-synthase deficiency: Effects of betaine supplementation after methionine restriction in B_6-nonresponsive homocystinuria. *Genetic Medicine, 6*, 90–95.

Singh, R. H., Rhead, W. J., Smith, W., Lee, B., King, L. S., & Summar, M. (2005). Nutritional management of urea cycle disorders. *Critical Care Clinics, 21*, S27–S35.

Tada, H., Takanashi, J., Barkovich, A. J., Yamamoto, S., & Kohno, Y. (2004). Reversible white matter lesion in methionine adenosyltransferase I/III deficiency. *AJNR American Journal of Neuroradiology, 25*, 1843–1845.

Trefz, F. K., Scheible, D., Frauendienst-Egger, G., Korall, H., & Blau, N. (2005). Long-term treatment of patients with mild and classical phenylketonuria by tetrahydrobiopterin. *Molecular Genetics and Metabolism, 86*, 75S–80S.

Tyfield, L., Reichardt, J., Fridovich-Keil, J., Croke, D. T., Elsas, L. J., Strobl, W., et al. (1999). Classical galactosemia and mutations at the galactose-1-phosphate uridyl transferase (GALT) gene. *Human Mutation, 13*, 417–430.

Udenfriend, S. (1961). Phenylketonuria. *American Journal of Clinical Nutrition, 9*, 691–694.

Van den Berghe, H., Bruntman, M., Vannestes, R., & Hers, H. G. (1977). The mechanism of adenine triphosphate depletion in the liver after a load of fructose. A kinetic study of liver adenylate deaminase. *Biochemistry Journal, 134*, 637–645.

Waisbren, S. E., Schnell, R. R., & Levy, H. L. (1980). Diet termination in children with phenylketonuria: A review of psychologic assessments used to determine outcome. *Journal of Inherited Metabolic Disease, 3*, 149–153.

Walter, J. H., White, F. J., Hall, S. K., MacDondald, A., Rylance, G., Boneh, A., et al. (2002). How practical are recommendations for dietary control in phenylketonuria? *Lancet, 360*, 55–57.

Weese, S. J., Gosnell, K., West, P., & Gropper, S. S. (2003). Galactose content of baby food meats: Considerations for infants with galactosemia. *Journal of the American Dietetic Association, 103*, 373–375.

Weglage, J., Wiedermann, D., Denecke, J., Feldman, R., Koch, H. G., Ullrich, K., et al. (2001). Individual blood-brain barrier phenylalanine transport determines clinical outcome in phenylketonuria. *Annals of Neurology, 50*, 463–467.

Yaghmai, R., Kashani, A. H., Geraghty, M. T., Okoh, J., Pomper, M., Tangerman, A., et al. (2002). Progressive cerebral edema associated with high methionine levels and betaine therapy in a patient with cystathionine beta-synthase (CBS) deficiency. *American Journal of Medical Genetics, 108*, 57–63.

Yap, S., Boers, G. H., Wilcken, B., Wilcken, D. E., Brenton, D. P., Lee, P. J., et al. (2001). Vascular outcome in patients with homocystinuria due to cystathionine beta-synthase deficiency treated chronically: A multicenter observational study. *Arteriosclerosis, Thrombosis, and Vascular Biology, 21*, 2080–2085.

Yap, S., & Naughten, E. (1998). Homocystinuria due to cystathionine β-synthase deficiency in Ireland: 25 years' experience of a newborn screened and treated population with reference to clinical outcome and biochemical control. *Journal of Inherited Metabolic Disease, 21*, 738–747.

Yap, S., Rushe, H., Howard, P. M., & Naughten, E. R. (2001). The intellectual abilities of early-treated individuals with pyridoxine-nonresponsive homocystinuria due to cystathionine beta-synthase deficiency. *Journal of Inherited Metabolic Disease, 24*, 437–447.

Failure to Thrive

Corbett, S. S., & Drewett, R. F. (2004). To what extent is failure to thrive in infancy associated with poorer cognitive development? A review and meta-analysis. *Journal of Child Psychology and Psychiatry, 45*, 741–754.

Corrales, K. M., & Utter, S. L. (2004). Failure to thrive. In P. Q. Samour, K. K. Helm, & C. E. Lang (Eds.), *Handbook of Pediatric Nutrition* (2nd ed., pp. 395–412). Sudbury, MA: Jones and Bartlett Publishers.

Feldman, R., Keren, M., Gross-Rozval, O., & Tyano, S. (2004). Mother-touch patterns in infant feeding disorders: Relation to maternal, child, and environmental factors. *Journal of the American Academy of Child and Adolescent Psychiatry, 43*, 1089–1097.

Fomon, S. J., Haschke, F., Zeigler, E. E., & Nelson, S. E. (1982). Body composition of reference children from birth to age 10 years. *American Journal of Clinical Nutrition, 35*, 1169–1175.

Frank, D. A., & Zeisel, S. H. (1988). Failure to thrive. *Pediatric Clinics of North America, 35*, 1187–1207.

Homnick, D. N., Homnick, B. D., Reeves, A. J., Marks, J. H., Pimentel, R. S., & Bonnema, S. K. (2004). Cyproheptadine is an effective appetite stimulant in cystic fibrosis. *Pediatric Pulmonology, 38*, 129–134.

Kleinman, R. E. (Ed.). (2004). Failure to thrive (pediatric undernutrition). In *Pediatric Nutrition Handbook* (5th ed., pp. 443–458). Elk Grove, IL: American Academy of Pediatrics.

Mei, Z., Grummer-Strawn, L. M., Thompson, D., & Dietz, W. H. (2004). Shifts in percentiles of growth during early childhood: Analysis of longitudinal data from the California Child Health and Development Study. *Pediatrics, 113*, e717–e727.

Raynor, P., & Rudolf, M. C. (2000). Anthropometric indices of failure to thrive. *Archives of Disease in Childhood, 82*, 374–375.

Waterlow, C. (1972). Classification and definition of protein-calorie malnutrition. *British Medical Journal, 3*, 577–579.

University of Iowa. (2002). "Mealtime routine" suggestions. Adapted from Intensive Course in Pediatric Nutrition, University of Iowa, Iowa City, May 7–10, 2002.

Special Section: Neonatal Intensive Care Nutrition: Prematurity and Complications

Liesje Nieman, RD, CNSD, LDN

Reader Objectives

After studying this chapter and reflecting on the contents, you should be able to

1. Define prematurity and discuss the impact of prematurity on growth and nutrition.
2. Determine appropriate goals for growth for infants in the neonatal intensive care unit.
3. Identify enteral formulas that are inappropriate for infants born prematurely.
4. Explain the rationale for the use of postdischarge premature infant formulas.
5. Discuss the importance of evaluating developmental readiness, as opposed to just chronologic or corrected age, when introducing complementary foods.
6. Describe the impact of feeding disorders and reflux on nutrient intake.
7. Identify appropriate uses of parenteral nutrition in infants.
8. Discuss the limitations and risks of parenteral nutrition.
9. Explain under what circumstances a multivitamin supplement is appropriate when an infant is on enteral feedings.

Because of advancements in medical treatments and technology, survival of extremely premature infants (i.e., <26 weeks gestation) is improving (Chan, Ohlsson, Synnes, Chein, & Lee, 2001). This state of extreme **prematurity** brings about a host of unique nutrition-related issues. The importance of the nutritionist's role in the neonatal intensive care unit (NICU) has been brought to the forefront in recent years. Many find it quite rewarding to work with premature infants because of the clinician's ability to significantly impact outcomes, such as growth velocity, healing, and transition from parenteral to enteral nutrition support. Registered Dietitian involvement in the NICU has been associated with improved nutritional intake and infant growth, shortened hospital length of stay, and reduced related costs (Olsen, Richardson, Schmid, Ausman, & Dwyer, 2005).

Prematurity: Less than 37 weeks gestation at birth.

Nutrition Assessment

Premature infants are born at less than 37 weeks gestation. Infants are further classified by their birth weight as follows: low birth weight, less than 2,500 g; **very low birth weight** (VLBW), less than 1,500 g; **extremely low birth weight**, less than 1,000 g; and "micropremies," less than 750 to 800 g. To evaluate in utero growth, an infant's birth anthropometrics are plotted on the Lubchenco intrauterine growth chart. An infant is appropriate for gestational age if his or her weight plots between the 10th and 90th percentiles, **small for gestational age** (SGA) if below the 10th percentile, and large for gestational age if above the 90th percentile.

Very low birth weight (VLBW): Birth weight of less than 1,500 g.

Extremely low birth weight: Birth weight of less than 1,000 g.

Small for gestational age (SGA): Birth weight plots below the 10th percentile (see Appendix 1).

Symmetric growth restriction is defined as weight, length, and head circumference of an infant plotting below the 10th percentile; infants with this type of growth restriction are more prone to poor outcomes for later growth and development. An infant whose weight and length are SGA but whose head circumference is above the 10th percentile has asymmetric growth restriction (e.g., head spared). **Intrauterine growth restriction** is often used interchangeably with SGA, but these two terms have different denotations. An infant with intrauterine growth restriction has not achieved his or her full in utero growth potential, whereas an infant defined as SGA born to parents who are both less than the fifth percentile for height may have achieved his or her full genetic potential in utero and is therefore not defined as intrauterine growth restricted (Griffin, 2002). If an infant requires catch-up growth, generally the head circumference catches up first, followed by weight and then length. Catch-up growth in head circumference generally occurs in the first 3 to 8 months of life (Bernstein, Heimler, & Sasidharan, 1998).

Intrauterine growth restriction: When an infant has not achieved his or her full in utero growth potential.

There are several growth chart options for plotting premature infants. Using corrected age, infants may initially be plotted either on the Oregon growth record for infants (i.e., Babson Benda intrauterine and postnatal growth chart) or the Fenton growth chart. When plotting infants and children on growth charts, corrected age is generally used on average until 24 months, with a minimum of 18 months and maximum of 36 months.

Calculating Corrected or Adjusted Age

Calculating an infant's corrected age "adjusts" for the infant's prematurity. It may also be referred to as postconceptional or postmenstrual age. The calculation is as follows (Bernbaum, 2000):

(chronological age) − (weeks or months of prematurity) = corrected age

For example, an infant born at 28 weeks gestational age is 3 months (12 weeks) premature (based on a term pregnancy of 40 weeks). If the infant's actual age is 6 months, the corrected age is 3 months.

Example: (6 months) − (3 months) = 3 months

The Babson Benda chart represents cross-sectional data from a small group of newborns from 26 to 40 weeks gestation along with longitudinal data from over 4,000 term infants through the first year of life. Male and female data were combined (Babson & Benda, 1976). Its limits include the small sample size (which provides low confidence in the extremes of the data), the 26 weeks start, and the 500-g graph increments. Two standard deviations above the mean roughly corresponds with 97.5 percentile, two standard deviations below the mean corresponds with 2.5 percentile, 1 standard deviation above the mean corresponds with 84 percentile, and 1 standard deviation below the mean corresponds with 16 percentile (Groh-Wargo & Cox, 1997).

In creating the Fenton growth chart, the literature was searched from 1980 to 2002 for more recent data to complete the pre- and postterm sections of the chart. Data were selected from population studies with large sample sizes. Comparisons were made between the new chart and the Babson Benda graph. To validate the growth chart, the growth results from the National Institute of Child Health and Human Development Neonatal Research Network were superimposed on the new chart. The updated growth chart allows a comparison of an infant's growth as early as 22 weeks gestation, up to the term infant at 50 weeks postconceptional age (i.e., 10 weeks term). Comparison of the size of infants based on the National Institute of Child Health and Human Development data at a weight of 2 kg provides evidence that on average preterm infants are growth retarded with respect to weight and length, whereas their head size has caught up to birth percentiles. Other advantages of this chart include the 100-g graph increments and the percentile curves (3rd, 10th,

50th, 90th, and 97th) rather than standard deviation. As with all meta-analyses, the validity of this growth chart is limited by the heterogeneity of the data sources. Further validation is needed to illustrate the growth patterns of preterm infants to older ages (Fenton, 2003).

The Infant Health and Development Program charts (i.e., Casey charts) include separate charts for VLBW and low birth weight infants born prematurely and separate charts within each weight category for boys and girls. This growth chart starts at "−2 months of age." The benefit of using these charts over others is that growth is compared with other premature infants. However, these charts do not delineate "normal" or "abnormal" growth, and the data were collected before the availability of "enriched" formulas. Different from the NCHS growth charts, nutrition interventions should be initiated when measurements fall below the 50th percentile on the Infant Health and Development Program charts or when growth percentiles change rapidly (Groh-Wargo & Cox, 1997).

Growth Goals

Although most preterm infants demonstrate adequate growth before discharge, very few experience complete catch-up. At discharge, most premature infants are smaller than the fetus or newborn infant of comparable postconceptional age (Agosti, Vegni, Calciolari, Marini, & the Investigators of the "GAMMA" Study Group, 2003). During 38 to 48 weeks postconceptional age, prematurely born infants may show rates of weight gain similar to the rapid weight gain that normally occurs during 32 to 36 weeks gestation in utero (Groh-Wargo & Cox, 1997). This period of catch-up growth often correlates with optimal caloric intake and the absence of medical compromise. Until 1,800 g or 37 weeks gestation, expected growth velocity is 15 to 20 g/kg of current weight per day (Steward & Pridham, 2002; Ziegler, Thureen, & Carlson, 2002). Beyond 37 weeks gestation, growth velocity of premature infants is generally compared with the expected velocity of healthy reference standards. Catch-up growth may be 10% to 50% above expected. An infant should be referred for further nutrition evaluation if he or she is not gaining at least 20 g/day from term to 3 months corrected age, 15 g/day from 3 to 6 months corrected age, 10 g/day from 6 to 9 months corrected age, and 6 g/day from 9 to 12 months corrected age (Roche & Himes, 1982; Gairdner & Pearson, 1988; Giuo, Roche, & Moore, 1988). An infant should be referred to a dietitian if head circumference growth is less than 0.5 cm/wk from term to 3 months, less than 0.25 cm/wk from 3 to 6 months, and greater than 1.25 cm/wk at any time during infancy (Groh-Warg & Cox, 1997).

Estimating Nutrient Needs

Infants have a higher metabolic rate and energy requirement per unit of body weight than children and adults (Pierro, 2002). Energy requirements for infants are broken down as follows: 40 to 70 kcal/kg/day for maintenance metabolism, 50 to 70 kcal/kg/day for growth (tissue synthesis and energy stored), and up to 20 kcal/kg/day to cover losses via excrement (Pierro, 2002). Caloric needs for a newborn infant fed enterally are approximately 100 to 120 kcal/kg/day, whereas those who receive parenteral nutrition (PN) require fewer calories (i.e., 80 to 100 kcal/kg/day) because energy is not needed to cover losses in excrement nor is energy being used for the thermogenic effect of food.

The caloric needs of premature infants are even higher than the caloric needs of full-term newborn infants. Current research suggests that VLBW neonates require a daily minimum of 60 kcal/kg/day, including 2.5 g/kg/day of amino acids to prevent catabolism, and 80 to 90 kcal/kg/day, including 2.7 to 3.5 g/kg/day of amino acids to maintain growth rates similar to those observed in utero (Ibrahim, Jeroudi, Baier, Dhanireddy, & Krouskop, 2004). In contrast, other research demonstrated that preterm newborns are minimally anabolic with parenteral intakes of 2 g/kg/day of amino acids and 50 to 60 kcal/kg/day (Thureen & Hay, 2001). Enterally fed premature infants require approximately 110 to 130 kcal/kg/day and 90 to 110 kcal/kg/day via PN. Some medical circumstances may require even higher caloric intakes to support adequate growth (e.g., bronchopulmonary dysplasia, congenital heart disease).

Enteral Feeding and Prematurity

Breast milk produced by mothers who have given birth prematurely contains greater concentrations of the following as compared with term breast milk: immune proteins, total lipid, medium chain fatty acids, vitamins, some minerals (e.g., calcium and sodium), and trace elements (Rao & Georgieff, 2005). Breast milk is classified as preterm only for the 2 to 4 weeks after birth, regardless of how prematurely the infant was born. Studies have shown that **necrotizing enterocolitis (NEC)** occurs less frequently when human

Necrotizing enterocolitis (NEC): An inflammation or death of the intestinal tract.

milk is administered as compared with formula, which is especially pertinent to the preterm infant population (Lucas & Cole, 1990).

Some mothers are unwilling or unable to provide breast milk for their infant. Although pasteurized donor breast milk has not been studied as extensively as mothers' own milk, pasteurized donor human milk can provide many of the components and benefits of human milk while eliminating the risk of transmission of infectious agents. "Pasteurization does affect some of the nutritional and immunologic components of human milk, but many immunoglobulins, enzymes, hormones, and growth factors are unchanged or minimally decreased" (Wight, 2001). In addition, gastric emptying has been shown to be faster and feed tolerance better with human milk (Yu, 2005).

However, the exclusive feeding of unfortified breast milk in premature infants has been associated with poor growth velocity and nutritional deficits (Kashyap, Schulze, & Forsyth, 1990). It has been observed that formula-fed infants have a higher rate of growth than breast-fed infants. Premature human milk provides insufficient protein, sodium, calcium, and phosphate to meet the needs of the premature infant (Schanler, 2001). There are commercially available multicomponent human milk fortifiers that provide additional calories, protein, calcium, phosphate, and vitamins. A meta-analysis study (Kuschel & Harding, 2004) concluded the following:

- Infants receiving fortified human milk demonstrated greater weight gains, greater length gains, and greater head growth in the short term.
- There is no significantly increased risk of NEC in infants receiving fortified human milk.
- Mean serum alkaline phosphatase and bone mineral content values were not statistically different between control and treatment groups.
- No long-term advantage was shown in terms of either growth or neurodevelopmental outcomes.

Fortification of breast milk may be initiated when feeds are tolerated at 100 to 150 mL/kg/day, and a minimum intake of 150 mL/kg/day of preterm milk fortified to 24 calories/ounce (i.e., 120 kcal/kg/day) is required to achieve optimal nutrition.

When breast milk is not available, premature formulas are generally indicated for infants who weigh less than 1,850 to 2,000 g (Bernstein et al., 1998; AAP and American College of Obstetrics and Gynecology, 2002). Infants who require higher intakes of calcium and phosphorus (e.g., those with osteopenia) may continue to receive these formulas until they weigh 3,500 g (Carver, Wu, & Hall, 2001). The protein in premature infant formulas is whey predominant, which may result in greater cystine intake and retention as well as greater taurine stores. In addition, the use of whey-predominant formula may decrease the potential for development of lactobezoars in premature infants. Premature formulas contain greater amounts of protein than standard term infant formulas, and the fat content is a combination of vegetables oils, providing both long chain and medium chain triglycerides. The high medium chain triglyceride content may enhance calcium absorption; promote nitrogen retention, lipogenesis, and weight gain; and improve fat absorption. Mineral content (e.g., calcium, phosphorus, magnesium) of premature formulas is higher than term infant formulas to support optimal bone mineralization (Groh-Wargo, Thompson, & Cox, 2000).

It is the responsibility of the registered dietitian and the neonatologist to strictly monitor the use of these formulas and to transition to a postdischarge premature formula when medically appropriate. Intake of premature infant formula exceeding 500 mL/day will likely provide excessive amounts of vitamin A and vitamin D (Lucas, King, Bishop, & King, 1992; Nako, Fukushima, & Tomomasa, 1993). Examples of premature formulas include Enfamil Premature Lipil® (Mead Johnson Nutritionals) and Similac Special Care Advance® (Ross Products Division, Abbott Laboratories).

Premature infants should receive multivitamin supplementation if the daily volume intake of premature formulas is inadequate (i.e., <500 mL). Premature infants receiving postdischarge premature formulas (i.e., Enfacare Lipil®, Neosure Advance®) at intakes of less than 750 mL/day require multivitamin supplementation. There is no indication to provide multivitamin supplementation to full-term infants receiving term infant formulas (e.g., Enfamil Lipil®, Similac Advance®) to meet their caloric needs (i.e., 108 kcal/kg/day). Premature infants receiving full **enteral nutrition** via exclusive breast milk fortified with human milk fortifier do not require multivitamin supplementation, but supplementation with iron sulfate should be considered. Multivitamin supplementation is indicated for exclusively breast-fed premature infants to meet the recommended daily vitamin D intake of 400 IU.

Premature infants are prone to anemia because of their inadequate iron stores and iatrogenic blood losses. All premature infants should receive iron supplementation by 1 month of age at doses of 2 mg/kg/day for breast-fed infants and at doses of 1 mg/kg/day for those receiving preterm or postdischarge formulas. Iron may be administered to premature infants who are tolerating enteral feeds (i.e., >100 mL/kg/day) as early as 2 weeks of age. This early supplementation can reduce the incidence of iron deficiency and the need for blood transfusions, as compared with the late administration of iron starting at 2 months of age (Franz, Mihatsch, Sander, Kron, & Pohlandt, 2000).

Infants may not tolerate large volumes of breast milk or formula for a variety of reasons, such as disease of the pulmonary, cardiac, hepatic, renal, or GI systems. If adequate volumes cannot be provided by mouth, supplemental tube feedings are recommended. If fluid needs are met (i.e., >130 to 150 mL/kg/day for infants without medical conditions requiring fluid restriction) and additional caloric intake is needed, increasing the concentration of the breast milk or formula is recommended (Wheeler & Hall, 1996). Care should be taken to avoid administering a potentially excessive renal solute load (i.e., >30 to 35 mOsm/100 kcal). Often, formulas concentrated to 24 to 27 kcal/oz are tolerated, and infants with mature renal systems have been noted to tolerate formulas concentrated to 30 kcal/oz. If vitamin, mineral, and protein needs are met with the feeding volume and growth remains inadequate, modular products are often added. Modular products may be carbohydrate (e.g., Polycose®, Ross Products Division, Abbott Laboratories; Moducal®, Mead Johnson Nutritionals), fat (e.g., Microlipid®, Mead Johnson Nutritionals, vegetable oil), or protein (e.g., Beneprotein®, Novartis Medical Nutrition). When diverting from a standard formula dilution, it is essential to evaluate the final product's macronutrient distribution and to ensure that vitamin and mineral intake is appropriate. Recommended macronutrient distribution is as follows: 7% to 16% calories from protein, 30% to 55% calories from fat, and 30% to 60% calories from carbohydrate (Groh-Wargo et al., 2000).

Often referred to as postdischarge premature formulas or nutrient-enriched formulas, EnfaCare Lipil® (Mead Johnson Nutritionals) and Similac NeoSure Advance® (Ross Products Division, Abbott Laboratories) provide more calories, protein, vitamins, and minerals than standard term formulas to support rapid growth and prevent nutrient depletion without providing excessive nutrients (Groh-Wargo

Enteral nutrition: The delivery of nutrients into the digestive system.

et al., 2000). Carver et al. (2001) demonstrated that premature infants fed postdischarge formula had improved growth compared with those fed a term formula, with the most significant beneficial effects seen among infants with birth weights less than 1,250 g. Greater gains in weight and head circumference were seen in the infants fed postdischarge formula, especially within the first 1 to 2 months after discharge. This study and several others support the use of nutrient-enriched formulas for preterm infants after discharge (Groh-Wargo et al., 2000). For optimal growth and bone mineralization, providing postdischarge premature formulas to infants born prematurely is recommended until catch-up growth is completed or until 9 to 12 months corrected age, whichever occurs first (Lucas et al., 1992; Groh-Wargo et al., 2000; Henderson, Fahey, & McGuire, 2005).

For infants born appropriate for gestational age at 34 to 37 weeks gestation, clinical judgment should determine the appropriate duration for the use of postdischarge premature formulas, considering each patient case individually. Bhatia (2005) recommended transition from a postdischarge premature formula to a standard term formula at 4 to 6 months corrected age if all growth parameters are above the 25th percentile. A recent Cochrane Review concluded that "the limited available data do not provide strong evidence that feeding pre-term or low birth weight infants following hospital discharge with calorie and protein-enriched formula compared with standard term formula affects growth rates or development up to 18 months post-term" (Henderson et al., 2005). Further studies focusing on VLBW, extremely low birth weight, and micropremie infants are needed and may reveal a significant effect of postdischarge premature formulas on growth rates and development.

Ultimately, the primary care physician is responsible for ensuring that premature infants continue on a postdischarge formula for an appropriate duration. The current standard of practice is to use postdischarge premature formulas until the infant reaches 9 to 12 months corrected age. The cost for postdischarge premature formulas is approximately 10% to 30% more than standard formulas, depending on geographic location and place of purchase (e.g., grocery vs. drug store). Although these postdischarge formulas cost slightly more than term formulas, the benefits usually outweigh the costs. For patients who meet financial eligibility requirements, the Special Supplemental Nutrition Program for Women, Infants, and Children does cover these formulas.

Preterm infants with birth weights less than 1,800 g fed soy protein–based formulas had less weight gain, less linear growth, and lower serum albumin than those fed cow's milk–based formula. Preterm infants fed soy protein–based formulas also had lower phosphorus levels and higher alkaline phosphatase levels, thus increasing the risk for development of **osteopenia of prematurity** (Kulkarni, Hall, & Rhodes, 1980; Callenbach, Sheehan, Abramson, & Hall, 1981). Therefore the AAP concluded that soy protein–based formulas should not be fed to infants weighing less than 1,800 g at birth (Shenai, Jhaveri, & Reynolds, 1981; AAP, Committee on Nutrition, 1998).

Osteopenia of prematurity: Reduction in bone volume to below normal levels, often seen in infants born prematurely.

Feeding Evaluation

The introduction and maintenance of oral feeding in premature infants presents many unique challenges. One study recently surveyed NICU feeding practices, and results revealed inconsistent and often contradictory strategies in attempting to transition high-risk infants from gavage to oral feedings (Premji, McNeil, & Scotland, 2004). Effective sucking, intact gag reflex, and intact cough reflex are requirements for safe and successful oral feeding and generally correlate with an intact neurologic system and physiologic maturity. Preterm infants are particularly prone to feeding issues because of their difficulty coordinating the suck-swallow-breathe pattern, physiologic instability (i.e., respiratory or cardiac problems), behavioral state, and minimal energy reserve (Premji et al., 2004). Immature GI systems also contribute to feeding problems. A small percentage of premature infants never fully orally feed and require long-term enteral nutrition support (i.e., tube feedings) (Geggie, Dressler-Mund, Creighton, & Cormack-Wong, 1999).

Powdered Formula in the NICU

The following statement was released by the FDA in 2002 (available at http://www.cfsan.fda.gov/~dms/inf-ltr3.html):

The literature suggests that premature infants and those with underlying medical conditions may be at highest risk for developing *E. sakazakii* infection. Several outbreaks have occurred in neonatal intensive care units worldwide. . . . The Centers for Disease Control and Prevention (CDC) has communicated information to FDA about a fatal infection due to *E. sakazakii* meningitis in a neonatal intensive care unit in the United States. In CDC's subsequent investigation, a cluster of neonates with *E. sakazakii* infection or colonization were identified in association with a powdered infant formula containing these bacteria. As background information for health professionals, FDA wants to point out that powdered infant formulas are not commercially sterile products. Powdered milk-based infant formulas are heat-treated during processing, but unlike liquid formula products they are not subjected to high temperatures for sufficient time to make the final packaged product commercially sterile. FDA has noted that infant formulas nutritionally designed for consumption by premature or low birth weight infants are available only in commercially sterile liquid form. However, so-called 'transition' infant formulas that are generally used for premature or low birth weight infants after hospital discharge are available in both non-commercially sterile powder form and commercially sterile liquid form. Some other specialty infant formulas are only available in powder form. . . . In light of the epidemiological findings and the fact that powdered infant formulas are not commercially sterile products, FDA recommends that powdered infant formulas not be used in neonatal intensive care settings unless there is no alternative available.

Detailed guidelines for preparation of infant formula are available on the American Dietetic Association website (http://www.eatright.org/Public/Nutrition Information/92_formulaguide.cfm).

Enteral Nutrition

Early trophic feeding, also referred to as minimal feedings or GI priming, has been shown to decrease the time to attain full feeds, the time to regain to birth weight, the duration of PN, the number of days feedings are held for residuals or intolerance, and duration of hospital stay, without increasing the incidence of NEC (Landers, 2003; Tyson & Kennedy, 2005). In addition, benefits of trophic feeding into the intact intestine are maturation of neonatal intestinal digestive, absorptive, and motor and immune function; improved neonatal feeding tolerance and behavior; maintenance of intestinal function during starvation and catabolic states; and prevention of intestinal bacterial overgrowth and bacterial translo-

cation (Sondheimer, 2004). Trophic feedings also have been shown to improve nitrogen and mineral retention (Landers, 2003). Feedings are classified as trophic if they comprise less than 25% of the patient's nutritional needs or provide less than 20 mL/kg/day (Sondheimer, 2004). Delayed enteral feeding leads to gut mucosal atrophy, decreased enzyme activity, and impaired gut growth and immunity.

Premature infants often do not tolerate enteral feedings because of their small stomach capacity and immature GI tract (e.g., dysmotility, decreased digestive enzymes). Gastric emptying and intestinal transit times are significantly delayed when compared with the term infant (Weckwerth, 2004). "Organized" gut motility does not begin until 3 to 34 weeks gestation (Thureen & Hay, 2001). Supplemental PN is often required while enteral feedings advance to their goal volume.

Bolus Versus Continuous Feedings

In a study of infants with birth weights of 750 to 1,500, time to full feeds, time to regain birth weight, discharge, and nitrogen retention/balance studies were no different between the continuous and intermittent (e.g., gavage feeds every three hours) feeding groups (Silvestre, Morbach, Brans, & Shankaran, 1996). Another study assessing feeding tolerance in premature infants found the time to reach full feeds (160 mL/kg/day) was significantly higher in the continuous gastric infusion than in the intermittent gastric bolus. There was no significant difference noted in time to regain to body weight, however. Feeding intolerance was defined as gastric residuals greater than 21% of feed volume and/or emesis. Abdominal distention was also monitored. A plausible explanation is that there needs to be some stomach distention by a minimum volume of feeds to optimize gut peristalsis/gastric emptying (Dollberg, Kuint, Mazkereth, & Mimouni, 2000). Another study also reported less intolerance to intermittent feedings versus continuous infusions (Schanler, Shulman, Lau, O'Brian Smith, & Heitkemper, 1999). There are several advantages to intermittent feeds: easier to administer, facilitate monitoring of gastric residuals, provide optimal nutrient delivery, enhance surges of gut hormones, and allow easier transition to oral feeding schedule. Advantages of continuous feedings are minimal gastric distention, reduced adverse pulmonary effects (i.e., less pressure on the diaphragm), improved tolerance in infants with apnea and bradycardia, and increased nutrient absorption with GI disease.

Transpyloric Versus Gastric Feedings

Transpyloric feedings (e.g., nasoduodenal and oro-gastric jejunum) have been associated with increased mortality in preterm infants. Also, reports of GI disturbance were significantly higher in infants fed via transpyloric tubes. No evidence of significantly different rates of growth was found when comparing transpyloric with gastric feedings (McGuire & McEwan, 2004).

Introduction of Solid Foods

The introduction of solid foods should be based on a premature infant's developmental readiness, not chronologic age. Corrected age is a more true reflection of an infant's developmental stage than chronologic age, and many preterm infants are not developmentally ready for solid foods until at least 6 months corrected age. Feeding guidelines for the premature infant should also take into account the degree of immaturity at birth, because extremely premature infants are more likely to experience developmental delay. Anticipatory guidance for caregivers of neurologically impaired infants should stress the safe introduction of solids; introduction of solid foods before developmental readiness, based solely on corrected age, may result in "forced feedings" of solids and decreased intake of breast milk or formula, often reducing protein and mineral intake (Marino et al., 1995). Introducing solid foods or complex consistencies before developmental readiness may also increase the risk for aspiration. Reported inappropriate feeding practices include the early introduction of solids, early feeding of cow's milk, and feeding of low-fat cow's milk. These practices may have reflected infants who were perceived in terms of chronologic age rather than age corrected for prematurity (Dhillon & Ewer, 2004).

Feeding Disorders

Feeding problems are often encountered during follow-up of high-risk neonates (Groh-Wargo et al., 2000). A delay in feeding skills may be related to frequent or prolonged illness, oral defensiveness, decreased exposure to oral feeding, or parental misperception of infants' feeding cues. A common feeding aversion in infants with complex medical issues is "tactile defensiveness," in which infants have an adverse response to having objects placed in or near the oral cavity (Wheeler & Hall, 1996). Infants with neurologic or anatomic abnormalities may have poor suck–swallow coordination, excessive tongue thrust, problems with gag reflex, or gastroesophageal reflux (Groh-Wargo et al., 2000; Hawdon, Beauregard, Slattery, & Kennedy, 2000). Respiratory and cardiac diseases often increase the work of breathing, compromising an infant's ability to eat by decreasing feeding endurance (Bernstein et al., 1998). Marino et al. (1995) observed an increased incidence (63%) of gastroesophageal reflux in a group of preterm infants. Gastroesophageal reflux is commonly identified in infants born prematurely; however, there is a lack of randomized trials regarding the standardization of treatments for gastroesophageal reflux (Rommel, DeMeyer, Feenstra, & Veereman-Wauters, 2003). Treatment strategies range from using a "reflux sling" to medications to thickening feeds with cereal, depending on the belief of the neonatologist.

Neonates who have the most complex or severe conditions are most at risk for the development of "disorganized" or "dysfunctional feeding." In addition, medical interventions often delay the introduction and establishment of oral (sucking) feeding. It is possible that the interventions required and the disordered feeding patterns are both consequences of the degree of severity of illness or prematurity (Ritchie, 2002). Feeding disorders may be a consequence of improved neonatal survival. Rommel et al. (2003) demonstrated a significant correlation between prematurity/dysmaturity and feeding disorders. Children with feeding disorders had significantly lower birth weights for gestational age, which implies that feeding problems could be related to intrauterine growth restriction. Data showed that infants born before 34 weeks gestation had more GI and oral sensory problems (Rommel et al., 2003).

It may be difficult for premature infants to take adequate nutrients via oral feeds because effective feeding requires coordination of suck, swallow, and breathing. Feedings lasting more than 30 minutes may tire infants and result in a net energy loss. Supplemental tube feedings may be an effective adjunct therapy for these infants. Options for administering supplemental tube feedings include providing oral feedings followed by bolus tube feedings every 3 to 4 hours around the clock to meet a minimum daily volume requirement, or providing oral/bolus feedings during the day with supplemental continuous tube feedings via pump overnight. Several factors influence which method of supplemental tube feedings are chosen, including but not limited to parenteral preference, aspiration risk, compromised respiratory status, and dysmotility. Proposed criteria (Gray &

King, 1997) for referral to a feeding therapist include the following:

- Suck or swallow incoordination or weak suck
- Delayed or absent progress to spoon feedings or table foods within expected time
- Discomfort, increased fussiness, distress, severe irritability, and/or arching during feedings
- Disrupted breathing or apnea during feedings
- Lethargy, decreased arousal during feedings, or tires easily and has difficulty finishing a feeding
- Feeding lasting longer than 30 minutes for an infant or 45 minutes for a child
- Abnormal oral–motor anatomy or physiology: lips, tongue, jaw, or palate
- Choking, excessive gagging, or recurrent coughing during feedings, toward the end of feeding, or between feedings
- Recurrent vomiting during or after a feeding
- Unexplained food refusal or inability to take adequate nutrition to support growth
- Physical symptoms or conditions such as dysphagia, recurrent pneumonia, aspiration, hypertonicity, hypotonicity, and failure to thrive

Fluid and Electrolyte Management

It is essential to reevaluate an infant's fluid status daily, at least for the first week of life. In the first day of life a full-term infant requires as little as 60 mL/kg/day to meet fluids needs. As an infant matures, changes in renal solute load, stool water output, and infant growth increase fluid needs (Groh-Wargo et al., 2000). In preterm infants fluid needs are 80 mL/kg/day on day of life 1, increasing to 120–160 mL/kg/day as the infant matures (Groh-Wargo et al., 2000). Preterm infants have increased insensible water losses due to the immaturity of their skin and respiratory losses.

Close monitoring of electrolyte status is essential. Electrolytes are often not administered on the first day of life, with the exception of calcium (Groh-Wargo et al., 2000). Potassium is generally added once normal kidney status and good urine output are established, and sodium is often added once diuresis begins (Groh-Wargo et al., 2000). Daily adjustment to electrolyte intake is often necessary. Electrolyte requirements of preterm and full-term infants are generally similar.

Parenteral Nutrition

Parenteral nutrition (PN): The delivery of nutrients into the circulatory system.

Parenteral nutrition is the delivery of nutrients into the circulatory system. If one anticipates that an infant will not receive enteral feedings within the first 6 to 12 hours after birth, PN should be initiated once electrolyte and fluid stability is achieved. Infants in the NICU often require PN for at least the first days of life to maximize caloric intake until enteral feedings are adequate. Premature infants have very minimal caloric reserves given that most fetal nutrient stores are deposited during the last 3 months of pregnancy. For example, in a preterm infant weighing 1,000 g, fat contributes only 1% of total body weight as compared with a term infant (3,500 g), which is about 16% fat (Anderson, 1996). If adequate nutrition support cannot be achieved and fat and glycogen stores have been exhausted, infants begin to catabolize protein stores for energy.

PN support should be initiated immediately when medical conditions contraindicate enteral feedings. PN should be continued until the medical situation allows for safe initiation of enteral feedings, and then PN may be weaned as the enteral feedings are advanced to their goal. Timing of the discontinuation of PN varies, but many clinicians are comfortable doing so when enteral feedings are tolerated at 100 to 120 mL/kg/day.

Initiating Parenteral Nutrition

PN can be administered through a peripheral vein, which is called peripheral parenteral nutrition. Peripheral parenteral nutrition requires a relatively large volume to allow for adequate administration of nutrients. In the ill infant, nutrient requirements often cannot be met with peripheral parenteral nutrition because of fluid restriction. Limiting dextrose concentration to 10% to 12.5% with a final osmolality of 900 mOsm/kg is recommended to minimize risk of phlebitis and infiltration (AAP, Committee on Nutrition, 1983).

Total parenteral nutrition requires central vein access and allows for administration of a solution with a higher osmolality (i.e., >900 mOsm/kg). Venous access is not defined by the initial point of entry but by the position of the catheter tip. With central venous lines the catheter tip terminates in the superior vena cava or the right atrium of the heart. Examples of central venous lines that are found in infants include umbilical venous catheters, nontunneled lines, and tunneled lines. Umbilical venous catheters are generally placed after birth and are removed within 2 weeks because of increased risk of infection (Pereira, 1995). Nontunneled lines include femoral, jugular, subclavian, and peripherally/percutaneously inserted central catheters (PICCs). PICC lines are generally placed when a long-term intravenous access is needed and duration may vary from several days to months. PICC lines may be central or peripheral, depending on the placement of the catheter tip. If the PICC line terminates in the superior vena cava it is considered to be central, and termination in other vessels needs to be individually evaluated to determine the maximum dextrose concentration that can be safely infused. A Broviac line is the tunneled line typically used in pediatric patients, comparable with a Groshong or Hickman in adults. Broviac lines are often placed when an infant is expected to be discharged on home PN support. X-ray confirmation of central line placement is essential before administration of a solution with a high osmolality. Dextrose concentration is generally limited to a maximum of 25% to 30%.

Parenterally, carbohydrates are administered in the form of dextrose, which provides 3.4 calories per gram. For optimal brain function, initiating with 4 to 6 mg/kg/min a day is recommended (i.e., D7.5 10%). Typically, advancement of 1 to 2 mg/kg/min a day to a maximum of 11 to 14 mg/kg/min a day is tolerated; however, preterm neonates may have unpredictable glycemic control. Glucose intolerance (e.g., stress-induced hyperglycemia) persisting greater than 24 to 48 hours with a glucose infusion rate (i.e., mg dextrose/kg/min a day) of less than 4 to 6 may warrant the initiation of an insulin infusion to allow for provision of more dextrose.

Protein is administered as a crystalline amino acid solution, which provides four calories per gram. TrophAmine and Aminosyn PF are amino acid solutions most appropriate for use in infants because of the addition of taurine, N-acetyl-L-tyrosine, glutamic acid, and aspartic acid (Groh-Wargo et al., 2000). TrophAmine is formulated to promote growth in neonates and young infants and to achieve a plasma amino acid pattern similar to that of normal postprandial breast-fed infants (Heird, Dell, & Helms, 1987). Research has shown a potential decrease in PN-associated cholestasis with TrophAmine (Wright, Ernst, Gaylord, Dawson, & Burnette, 2003). Another benefit of TrophAmine is that when L-cysteine is added, there is an increased solubility of calcium and phosphorus to promote optimal bone mineralization (Schmidt, Baumgartner, & Fischlschweiger, 1986). TrophAmine is initiated with 2 to 3 g amino acid/kg/day for infants expected to have normal renal function, titrating by 1 g amino acid/kg/day as tolerated to a goal of 3 to 4 g amino acid/kg/day, the higher end of the range being most appropriate for the smallest infants (e.g., <1,000 g) (Porcelli & Sisk, 2002).

Parenteral fat is a lipid emulsion of either soybean oil or a combination of safflower and soybean oil. Intravenous lipids provide 10 calories per gram regardless of the product concentration and are available in 10% (1.1 calorie/mL) and 20% (2 calories/mL) concentrations. For infants, the 20% concentration is preferred over the 10% product because it allows adequate lipid intake in less volume and improved clearance of phospholipids and triglycerides (Groh-Wargo et al., 2000). Not only are lipids a concentrated source of calories, but they also provide essential fatty acids for cell membrane integrity and brain development. Lipids also help to prolong the integrity of peripheral lines because of their lower osmolality. It is crucial to provide a minimum of 0.5 to 1.0 g lipids/kg/day to prevent essential fatty acid deficiency, which can develop in premature infants during the first week of life and as early as the second day of life (Groh-Wargo et al., 2000). Essential fatty acid deficiency is defined as a triene-to-tetraene ratio of at least 0.4 (Kerner, 1996). Lipids are initiated with 1 to 2 g/kg/day, with titration as tolerated to a maximum of 3 to 3.5 g/kg/day. Premature infants have a maximum lipid oxidation rate of 0.125 g/kg/min, whereas term infants may tolerate up to 0.15 g/kg/min.

Most cases requiring PN support are due to either GI malformations or NEC. GI malformations include omphalocele, gastroschisis, intestinal atresia, volvulus, and Hirschsprung disease. An omphalocele is a congenital herniation of internal organs into the base of the umbilical cord, with a covering membranous sac. In contrast, gastroschisis is a defect in the abdominal wall resulting from rupture of the amniotic membrane, usually accompanied by protrusion of internal organs. Both conditions require surgical repair. Recovery from omphalocele is often quicker than gastroschisis because the bowel was protected by the membranous sac during pregnancy. In gastroschisis, the bowel is often quite dilated and inflamed because of exposure to amniotic fluids. Intestinal atresia is the absence of a normal opening (i.e., the intestinal lumen has a closure where it should be a continuous segment); this condition requires surgical repair as well. A volvulus is a twisting of the intestines, causing an obstruction. Hirschsprung disease (i.e., congenital megacolon) often presents as constipation and is characterized by the absence of ganglion cells in a distal intestinal segment. Various surgical treatments exist for treating Hirschsprung disease, such as a diverting colostomy or resection of the aganglionic bowel with a "pull through" of the normal bowel down to the distal rectum (Groh-Wargo et al., 2000).

NEC is an inflammation or death of the intestinal tract. Some cases of NEC are classified as "medical" because a period of bowel rest and administration of antibiotics is sufficient to promote a full recovery. Feedings are typically held for 7 to 14 days. Surgical NEC are those cases that require surgical intervention, such as peritoneal drain placement and/or intestinal resection.

The cause of NEC is unknown. Historically, rapid titration of feedings was implicated as the cause of NEC, but more recently this association has been questioned. Several retrospective studies suggested that rapid advancement of feedings was associated with increased NEC (Anderson & Kliegman, 1991; McKeown, Marsh, & Amarnath, 1992). Anderson and Kliegman (1991) concluded that "the feed increment rate from initiation of feeds to day of maximum feeds was 27.8 +/− 16 ml/kg/day for the NEC patients and 16.8 +/− 11 for the control patients." However, a recent prospective, randomized, controlled study concluded that among infants weighing between 1,000 and 2,000 g at birth, starting and advancing feedings at 30 mL/kg/day had no significant impact on incidence of development of NEC and resulted in fewer days to reach full volume feedings as compared with 20 mL/kg/day (Caple, Armentrout, & Huseby, 2004). That study confirmed earlier findings by Rayyis et al. (1999) that a 35 mL/kg/day feed advancement did not affect the incidence of NEC.

Because standards have not been set for evaluating gastric residuals in premature infants, there are many differences between NICUs in interpreting gastric residuals. A recent retrospective study concluded, however, that a gastric residual volume greater than 33% of a previous feed was associated with a higher risk for NEC (Cobb, Carlo, & Ambalavanan, 2004). A meta-analysis found that feeding with donor human milk was associated with a significantly reduced relative risk of NEC; infants who received donor human milk were three times less likely to develop NEC and four times less likely to have confirmed NEC than infants who received formula milk (McGuire & Anthony, 2003).

Short bowel syndrome (SBS):
A malabsorptive state due to a significant bowel resection or congenital defect.

GI malformations and NEC can lead to **short bowel syndrome** (SBS), also known as short gut syndrome, which may be composed of weight loss or inadequate weight gain, muscle wasting, diarrhea, rapid GI transit time,

malabsorption, dehydration, and hypokalemia. SBS is a malabsorptive state due to a significant bowel resection or congenital defect. SBS may present with a decreased ability to secrete GI regulatory peptides and trophic hormones as well as compromised GI immune function (Vanderhoof, 2004). Causes of SBS in the NICU often include NEC, gastroschisis, volvulus, or multiple intestinal atresias. Generally, a full-term infant has approximately 200 to 250 cm of small bowel (Vanderhoof, 2003). SBS may be defined as less than 75 to 100 cm of small bowel. After a bowel resection the remaining small bowel adapts in the following ways: mucosal hyperplasia, villus lengthening, increased crypt depth, and bowel dilatation (Andorsky et al., 2001). Provision of enteral nutrition is the main factor influencing bowel adaptation after a resection.

In some cases the postresection gut adaptation is sufficient to allow for a patient to wean off PN and sustain adequate growth on enteral nutrition. Given the complications of PN (e.g., line sepsis, cholestatic liver disease, poor bone mineralization) in the NICU, weaning from PN support should be a priority. Many SBS patients, however, require at least supplemental PN to sustain adequate growth and/or hydration. An infant with an intact ileocecal valve and at least 10 to 30 cm of small bowel may be able to wean from PN successfully. Without an ileocecal valve, at least 30 to 50 cm of small bowel are generally needed to wean from PN (Kurkchubasche, Rowe, & Smith, 1993; Quiros-Tejeira, Ament, & Reyen, 2004). Andorsky et al. (2001) observed that the mean residual bowel length in the group of patients able to be weaned from PN was 88.6 cm as compared with 71.7 cm in the group unable to be weaned from PN. Factors associated with a reduction in duration of PN include percentage of enteral feeding days when breast milk or an amino acid–based formula was given and percentage of caloric intake received by the enteral route 6 weeks after intestinal resection (Andorsky et al., 2001). Some studies associated the presence of an ileocecal valve with a decreased duration of PN, but at least four other studies did not support this theory (Andorsky et al., 2001). Early restoration of intestinal continuity (i.e., ostomy "takedown") appears to correlate with less severe PN-related cholestasis (Andorsky et al., 2001).

Patients with SBS are prone to morbidity and mortality from progressive liver failure and sepsis (Andorsky et al., 2001). PN cholestasis is defined as a conjugated bilirubin greater than 2 mg/dL. Typically, patients with cholestasis are jaundiced and may have pale clay-colored stools due to fat malabsorption. Neonates are especially prone to PN cholestasis because of their diminished bile acid pool size and key hepatobiliary transporters and their reduced enterohepatic circulation of bile acids (i.e., decreased bile flow) (Karpen, 2002). Karpen (2002) observed that patients with elevated conjugated bilirubin at approximately 4 months of age or older may have irreversible PN cholestasis. Recognizing end-stage liver disease as early as possible is essential, and referral for liver or liver plus small bowel transplantation should be made when medically appropriate (Karpen, 2002).

Goals of nutrition therapy for the infant with SBS should include promoting normal growth and development, maximizing intestinal adaptation, and minimizing complications. Initially, the focus of nutritional therapy is maintaining fluid and electrolyte balance, which is often accomplished through intravenous fluid (e.g., one-half normal saline with KCl) replacement of ostomy losses (Vanderhoof, 2004). Once fluid and electrolyte losses have resolved and GI function has returned (i.e., Salem sump is placed to gravity drainage without increased abdominal distention), trophic enteral feeds should be initiated. Andorsky et al. (2001) demonstrated that the use of breast milk showed the highest correlation with shorter PN courses. If breast milk is not available, hydrolyzed or amino acid–based formulas are generally used to facilitate absorption (Vanderhoof, 2004). Pasteurized donor breast milk should also be considered if the infant's mother is unable or unwilling to provide breast milk. Amino acid–based formulas may improve outcomes in SBS because there seems to be a higher incidence of allergy in children with SBS. Also, the infant amino acid–based formula used in several studies (e.g., Neocate, SHS, Inc.) contains a high percentage of fat from long chain fatty acid sources, which have been shown to stimulate mucosal adaptation better than medium chain triglycerides in animal models (Bines, Francis, & Hill, 1998; Andorsky et al., 2001). An amino acid–based formula recently approved for use in infants (e.g., Elecare®, Ross Laboratories) has also been administered to SBS patients with good tolerance. In comparing Elecare® with Neocate®, one observes a similar amino acid base; however, Elecare® contains significantly more medium chain triglycerides when compared with Neocate® (33% of total fat vs. 5%), facilitating optimal fat absorption during cholestasis.

Continuous enteral feedings are advantageous over bolus feedings due to enhanced absorption, which is facilitated by saturation of transporters in the gut 24 hours per day. Aggressive enteral nutrition reduces the need for PN as early as possible and helps to ameliorate the development and progression of PN cholestasis; moreover, aggressive enteral nutrition stimulates gut adaptation (Vanderhoof, 2004). Factors hindering advancement of enteral feeds include stool losses increasing more than 50% over baseline, ostomy output greater than 40 to 50 mL/kg/day, and ostomy output strongly positive for reducing substances (Vanderhoof, 2004).

Once weaned from PN support, SBS patients should routinely be screened for fat-soluble vitamins (A, D, E, and K), calcium, magnesium, and zinc deficiencies. Once a patient is tolerating full enteral feeds and PN has been discontinued, providing the following vitamin supplementation is recommended: TPGS-E (e.g., Liqui-E® or Nutr-E-Sol®) at 25 IU/kg/day plus 2 mL liquid multivitamin (e.g., Poly-vi-sol®) to provide adequate vitamins A and D and vitamin K (e.g., phytonadione) from 1 to 2.5 mg weekly up to 5 to 10 mg daily, according to need (Karpen, 2002; Francavilla, Miniello, Lionetti, & Armenio, 2003). Karpen (2002) stated that the "use of this combination vitamin treatment is superior to use of available water-soluble vitamin supplements" (e.g., A, D, E, and K). Dosing of vitamin supplements can be adjusted as needed based on the results of monthly measurements of vitamin A, 25-OH vitamin D, vitamin E, and coagulation profile.

Caring for infants with SBS is often a challenging undertaking. Daily or weekly changes are made to increase enteral nutrition support and to minimize the need for PN, with continual monitoring of growth and laboratory results as well as monitoring for symptoms of intolerance of enteral nutrition. NICU dietitians' close collaboration with the medical and surgical teams, as well as the gastroenterologist and hepatologist, is essential to facilitating a positive outcome for the SBS patient.

Other medical conditions that may warrant the use of PN support include intractable nonspecific diarrhea, extracorporeal membrane oxygenation, congenital diaphragmatic hernia, and vasopressor support (e.g., dopamine, dobutamine). Extracorporeal membrane oxygenation and vasopressor support are not absolute contraindications to enteral feedings; however, many neonatologists are hesitant to enterally feed infants with hemodynamic instability because of risk of bowel ischemia. Diaphragmatic hernia often requires PN until surgical repair of the hernia occurs and the stomach and/or intestines are returned to a lower place in the abdominal cavity and are functioning (e.g., "stooling").

Vitamins and Trace Elements in Parenteral Nutrition

Currently available pediatric parenteral multivitamins do not optimally meet the vitamin needs of preterm infants (Greene, Hambidge, Schanler, & Tsang, 1988). The available formulation provides higher amounts of thiamin, riboflavin, pyridoxine, and cyanocobalamin and lower amounts of fat-soluble vitamins (e.g., vitamin A) than recommended.

Available trace element products do not adequately meet the needs of preterm neonates either. Specifically, if sufficient zinc is administered, manganese is provided in excessive amounts. However, short-term use of a standard neonatal trace element product is considered to be safe. Many institutions with NICUs have begun developing their own trace element combinations from individual trace element products to better meet the needs of their smallest patients. In cases of specific medical conditions, such as renal (e.g., chromium, selenium) or hepatic (e.g., copper, manganese) disease, one may need to alter specific trace elements.

Zinc is important for the maintenance of cell growth and development. When PN is supplemental to enteral nutrition or of short duration, zinc is the only trace element that requires supplementation. Some conditions that require additional zinc intake include elevated urinary zinc excretion (e.g., high output renal failure) and increased GI excretion (e.g., high volume stool/ostomy losses, fistula/stoma losses).

Copper is an essential constituent of many enzymes. Current daily recommendations are adequate to prevent deficiency in preterm infants. Copper deficiency is more likely to occur with high dose zinc therapy because of their inverse relationship. Clinical manifestations of copper deficiency include hypochromic anemia that is unresponsive to iron therapy, neutropenia, and osteoporosis. Rapid growth in VLBW infants increases the risk of deficiency. Conditions requiring higher copper intake include increased biliary losses due to jejunostomy and losses via external biliary drainage. These conditions may require an additional 10 to 15 µg/kg/day. Historically, copper was withheld in PN for patients with cholestasis; however, cases of copper deficiency have recently been reported when copper was withheld in PN (Hurwitz, Garcia, Poole, & Kerner, 2004). It is recommended in patients with cholestasis to reduce supplementation by 50% (i.e., 10 µg/kg/day), monitor monthly serum copper levels and ceruloplasmin, and adjust supplementation accordingly.

Manganese is an important component of several enzymes. Manganese deficiency has not been documented in humans. However, manganese toxicity has been reported (Rao & Georgieff, 2005). Manganese supplementation in PN should be withheld in patients with cholestasis or other liver function impairment (Fok et al, 2001; Rao & Georgieff, 2005). Fok et al. (2001) provided evidence suggesting that high manganese intake contributes to the development of cholestasis. Manganese should therefore be used with caution in PN provided to infants because they are more susceptible to cholestasis (Fok et al., 2001). Monthly serum manganese levels should be monitored and supplementation adjusted as needed.

Selenium is a component of the enzyme glutathione peroxidase, which is involved in protecting cell membranes from peroxidase damage through detoxification of peroxides and free radicals (Rao & Georgieff, 2005). Supplementation with selenium is recommended in long-term PN (i.e., >1 month). Decreasing selenium intake when renal dysfunction is present is recommended.

Chromium potentiates the action of insulin and is required for growth in light of its role in glucose, protein, and lipid metabolism (Rao & Georgieff, 2005). Decreasing chromium intake with renal dysfunction is recommended.

Molybdenum supplementation is recommended in cases when exclusive PN exceeds 4 weeks. Deficiency of molybdenum has not been reported in premature infants; however, one adult case of deficiency has been documented (Rao & Georgieff, 2005).

Iodine is often omitted from PN given that iodine-containing disinfectants and detergents are used on the skin and absorbed. The Committee on Clinical Practice Issues of the American Society of Clinical Nutrition recommended parenteral intakes of iodine at 1.0 µg/kg/day for the preterm infant to avoid any risk of deficiency (Rao & Georgieff, 2005).

Iron supplementation should be considered only among long-term PN-dependent patients who are not receiving frequent blood transfusions. Iron supplementation of 100 µg/kg/day may be safely delayed until 3 months of age in term infants. Preterm infants *not* receiving blood products, with the exception of platelets, may benefit from iron supplementation of 100 to 200 µg/kg/day at 2 months of age (Rao & Georgieff, 2005). Monitoring iron status is imperative with iron supplementation because there is a risk of iron overload (Mirtallo et al., 2004).

Other Parenteral Nutrition Additives

Neonates and infants are unable to endogenously produce carnitine. Premature neonates also have limited tissue carnitine stores. Premature infants less than 34 weeks gestation receiving PN without carnitine can develop carnitine deficiency 6 to 10 days after birth (Schmidt-Sommerfield, Penn, & Wolf, 1982). Human milk is a good source of carnitine. PN does not contain carnitine unless it is added to the PN solution. A recent meta-analysis concluded that there was no evidence to support routine supplementation of parenterally fed neonates with carnitine (Cairns & Stalker, 2000). However, four of the six studies included in this review demonstrated positive effects on either growth or lipid tolerance. Clinicians may provide 10 to 20 mg carnitine/kg/day without risk of adverse effects (Putet, 2000; Crill, Christensen, Storm, & Helms, 2006).

Cysteine, a conditionally essential amino acid, is not a component of crystalline amino acid solutions because it is unstable and forms an insoluble precipitate (Groh-Wargo et al., 2000). In adults cysteine can be synthesized from methionine; however, preterm infants lack adequate hepatic cystathionase to facilitate this conversion. Commonly recommended dosing for L-cysteine hydrochloride is 40 mg/g amino acids (Mirtallo et al., 2004). One benefit of the addition of L-cysteine hydrochloride to PN is the decrease in the pH of the solution, which increases the solubility of supplemental calcium and phosphorus. It should be noted, however, that the addition of cysteine to PN warrants close monitoring of an infant's acid-base status because it may predispose infants to acidosis, and acetate may need to be added to the solution.

Addition of heparin to PN solutions "reduces the formation of a fibrin sheath around the catheter, may reduce phlebitis . . . and increases the duration of catheter patency" (Groh-Wargo et al., 2000). Heparin also stimulates the release of lipoprotein lipase, which may improve lipid clearance. Adding 0.25 to 1.0 units heparin per mL of PN solution is recommended. However, there is an increased risk of anticoagulation with the higher doses of heparin.

Parenteral Nutrition and Biochemical Monitoring

Before initiation of PN support, the following biochemical indices should be checked: basic metabolic panel, calcium, magnesium, phosphorus, liver function tests (i.e., alkaline phosphatase, alanine and aspartate aminotransferases, and gamma-glutamyltransferase), total bilirubin, conjugated or direct bilirubin, preal-bumin, albumin, and triglyceride. The basic metabolic panel, calcium, magnesium, phosphorus, and triglyceride levels should be checked daily for 3 days after the initiation of PN support, or until indices are stable. Weekly liver function tests, total bilirubin, conjugated or direct bilirubin, prealbumin, albumin, and triglyceride should be monitored. Other biochemical studies (e.g., iron status, vitamin levels, ionized calcium, serum zinc, copper, manganese) may be warranted on an individual basis. Patients on long-term PN, such as those with SBS, need monthly monitoring of vitamin and mineral status.

Parenteral Nutrition Complications

Short-term potential adverse effects of PN include infection, hyperglycemia, electrolyte abnormalities, disturbance of acid-base balance, hypertriglyceridemia, bacterial translocation, and compromised gut integrity. With long-term PN, adverse effects may include infection, PN cholestasis, metabolic complications, disturbance of acid-base balance, osteopenia, risk of vitamin/mineral deficiency or toxicity, and continued risk of bacterial translocation. Nosocomial infections appear to result either from improper care of the catheter and/or frequent use of the catheter for purposes other than delivery of nutrients (e.g., blood draws, medication administration).

Episodes of line infection can hasten the rising of the bilirubin level. Further, cholestasis may develop in 90% of infants after the first line infection (Beath et al., 1996; Sondheimer, Asturias, & Cadnapaphornchai, 1998). A multidisciplinary nutrition support service and early discharge on home PN has been shown to reduce the incidence of central venous catheter infection (Beath et al., 1996; Knafelz et al., 2003).

Often, the terms *osteopenia* and *rickets* are used interchangeably. However, osteopenia is defined as a "reduction in bone volume to below normal levels especially due to inadequate replacement of bone lost to normal lysis," whereas rickets is defined as "a deficiency disease that affects the young during the period of skeletal growth, is characterized especially by soft and deformed bones, and is caused by failure to assimilate and use calcium and phosphorus normally due to inadequate sunlight or vitamin D" (Medline Plus Medical Dictionary, 2003). Some experts proposed that the term *rickets* should be reserved for radiographic or physical findings. Fractures may occur in osteopenic premature infants, with or without radiologic features of rickets. The incidence of rickets or fractures in infants with a body weight less than 1,500 g ranges from 20% to 32%, increasing to 50% to 60% in infants with a body weight less than 1,000 g.

Fetal accretion rates of calcium and phosphorus reach their peak during the third trimester, with upward of about 80% of fetal skeletal mineralization taking place during this time period. It has been reported that the clinical onset of osteopenia of prematurity generally occurs in the 6th to 12th week postnatally. The diagnosis of rickets usually occurs between 2 to 4 months chronologic age (Greer, 1994; Groh-Wargo et al., 2000).

High 1,25-$[OH]_2$ vitamin D values are often associated with low serum phosphate levels, thus confirming phosphate insufficiency as a primary factor in the pathogenesis of osteopenia of prematurity. Vitamin D deficiency is quite rare in premature infants; exceptions to this include patients with liver disease, renal disease, and malabsorption.

Ideally, the goal of therapeutic interventions for osteopenia of prematurity is to achieve the intrauterine rate of bone mineralization. However, this would require enteral intakes of about 200 mg calcium/kg/day and about 90 mg phosphorus/kg/day, assuming 65% absorption of calcium (at best) and 80% absorption of phosphorus. In some instances the most realistic goal is to prevent severe osteopenia with fractures and rickets. In patients receiving PN support, maximal retention can be accomplished when providing between 1.3:1 and 1.7:1 Ca/P by weight, or 1.1 to 1.3:1 by molar ratio. Ca/P ratios less than 1:1 by weight (0.8:1 by molar ratio) and alternating daily infusions of calcium and phosphorus are not recommended (Prestridge, Schanler, Shulman, Burns, & Laine, 1993; Klein, 1998).

Emerging Issues

It has come to light that various products used during PN compounding have a high aluminum content, which can be especially dangerous for infants and children. Preterm infants are extremely vulnerable to aluminum toxicity because of immature renal function and the likelihood for long-term PN (Mirtallo et al., 2004). The FDA mandated that manufacturers of products used in compounding PN measure the aluminum content of their products and disclose it on the label by July 2004. The FDA identified 5 μg/kg/day as the maximum amount of aluminum that can be safely tolerated, and amounts exceeding this limit may be associated with central nervous system or bone toxicity (Miratallo et al., 2004). It is essential for pharmacists, dietitians, physicians, and nurses to collaborate to reduce the use of higher aluminum content products. However, it is difficult to achieve the recommended aluminum intake level set by the FDA when patients are receiving multiple medications and PN. A reasonable goal for clinicians is to minimize aluminum exposure.

Additional Neonatal Diagnoses and Nutritional Issues

Bronchopulmonary dysplasia is chronic lung disease that primarily affects premature infants with severe respiratory distress syndrome and is most commonly caused by intermittent positive pressure ventilation and oxygen therapy in the neonatal period. The lower the body weight and gestational age of the infant, the higher the incidence and severity of bronchopulmonary dysplasia. The etiology of growth impairment and compromised neurologic status in infants with bronchopulmonary dysplasia is multifactorial. Studies have shown reduced growth rates for weight, length, and head circumference during the first 2 years of life for patients with bronchopulmonary dysplasia (Davidson et al., 1990; Johnson, Cheney, & Monsen, 1998; Marks, 2006). Factors that contribute to this inadequate growth include elevated energy expenditure, fluid restrictions limiting nutrition intake, recurrent illnesses with periods of caloric and nutrient deficits, and chronic steroid use.

Osteopenia of Prematurity

Risk factors for osteopenia of prematurity:

- <30 weeks gestation
- <1,000 g body weight
- Delayed establishment of full enteral feeds and/or prolonged PN
- Enteral feeds with low mineral content or bioavailability (unfortified breast milk, standard term formula, soy formula)
- Chronic use of medications that increase mineral excretion
- Cholestatic jaundice

Etiology of osteopenia of prematurity:

- Increased mineral needs for growth and bone accretion
- Decreased calcium and phosphorus intake:
  - Parenteral nutrition
  - Fluid restriction
- Enteral feedings: unsupplemented formula or unfortified human milk
- Increased calcium and phosphorus losses:
  - Diuretics (furosemide and Aldactone) → hypercalcuria
  - Sodium bicarbonate → increases mineral excretion
- Corticosteroids → increase of bone resorption and a decrease of bone formation, increase of urinary calcium/creatinine, and decrease in serum phosphorus
- Decreased calcium and phosphorus reserves:
  - Prematurity
  - Placental insufficiency (severe preeclampsia)
- Other factors:
  - Aluminum contaminants (divalent cations) in PN components
  - Deposits in bone, displacing calcium and phosphorus
- Vitamin D deficiency:
  - Inadequate vitamin D intake (rare)
  - Liver/renal disease (affects vitamin D metabolism)

Summary

Advanced technologic and medical interventions enable clinicians to support infants born prematurely. It is a challenge to provide adequate nutrition to promote growth similar to fetal growth velocity and to support bone mineralization similar to fetal accretion rates. Neonatologists, registered dietitians, and neonatal clinical teams strive to provide optimal nutrition support to premature infants; however, clinicians sometimes are unable to provide optimal nutrition support because of barriers encountered throughout an infant's admission to the NICU. This special section defined prematurity, identified the potential adverse impact prematurity can have on oral feeding, described appropriate goals for growth, discussed feeding options, and explained appropriate uses of PN.

References

American Academy of Pediatrics (AAP) and American College of Obstetrics and Gynecology. (2002). *Guidelines for Perinatal Care* (5th ed.). Elk Grove Village, IL: American Academy of Pediatrics.

American Academy of Pediatrics (AAP) Committee on Nutrition. (1983). Commentary on parenteral nutrition. *Pediatrics, 71*, 547.

American Academy of Pediatrics (AAP) Committee on Nutrition. (1998). Soy protein-based formulas: Recommendations for use in infant feeding. *Pediatrics, 101*, 148–153.

Abad-Sinden, A., Verbrugge, K. C., and Buck, M. L. (2001). Assessment, prevention and management of metabolic bone disease in very low birthweight infants: the role of the neonatal nutritionist. *Nutrition in Clinical Practice*, 16, 13–19.

Agosti, M., Vegni, C., Calciolari, G., Marini, A., & the Investigators of the "GAMMA" Study Group. (2003). Post-discharge nutrition of the VLBW infant: Interim results of the multicentric GAMMA study. *Acta Paediatrica, 41*(Suppl.), 39–43.

Anderson, D. (1996). Nutrition in the care of the low birth weight infant. In: L. K. Mahan & S. Escott-Stump (Eds.), *Krause's Food, Nutrition, and Diet Therapy* (9th ed.). Philadelphia: W. B. Saunders.

Anderson, D., and Pittard, W. B. (1997). Parenteral nutrition for neonates. In R. Baker, S. Baker, and A. Davis (Eds.). *Pediatric Parenteral Nutrition*. New York: International Thomson Publishing.

Anderson, D. M., & Kliegman, R. M. (1991). The relationship of neonatal alimentation practices to the occurrence of endemic necrotizing enterocolitis. *American Journal of Perinatology, 8*, 62–67.

Andorsky, D. J., Lund, D. P., Lillehei, C. W., Jaksic, T., Dicanzio, J., Richardson, D. S., et al. (2001). Nutritional and other postoperative management of neonates with short bowel syndrome correlates with clinical outcomes. *Journal of Pediatrics, 139*, 27–33.

Babson, S. G., & Benda, G. I. (1976). Growth graphs for the clinical assessment of infants of varying gestational age. *Journal of Pediatrics, 89*, 814–820.

Beath, S. V., Davies, P., Papadopoulou, A., Khan, A. R., Buick, R. G., Corkery, J. J., et al. (1996). Parenteral nutrition-related cholestasis in postsurgical neonates: Multivariate analysis of risk factors. *Journal of Pediatric Surgery, 31*, 604–606.

Bernbaum, J. C. (2000). *Preterm Infants in Primary Care: A Guide to Office Management*. Columbus, OH: Ross Products Division, Abbott Laboratories.

Bernstein, S., Heimler, R., & Sasidharan, P. (1998). Approaching the management of the neonatal intensive care unit graduate through history and physical assessment. *Pediatric Clinics of North America, 45*, 79.

Bhatia, J. (2005). Post-discharge nutrition of preterm infants. *Journal of Perinatology, 25*, S15-S16.

Bines, J., Francis, D., & Hill, D. (1998). Reducing parenteral requirement in children with short bowel syndrome: Impact of an amino acid-based complete formula. *Journal of Pediatric Gastroenterology and Nutrition, 26*, 123–128.

Cairns, P. A., & Stalker, D. J. (2000). Carnitine supplementation of parenterally fed neonates. *Cochrane Database Syst Rev*, 4, CD000950.

Callenbach, J. C., Sheehan, M. B., Abramson, S. J., & Hall, R. T. (1981). Etiologic factors in rickets in VLBW infants. *Journal of Pediatrics, 98*, 800–805.

Caple, J., Armentrout, D., & Huseby, V. (2004). Randomized, controlled trial of slow versus rapid feeding volume advancement in preterm infants. *Pediatrics, 114*(6), 1597–1600.

Carver, J. D., Wu, P. K., & Hall, R. T. (2001). Growth of preterm infants fed nutrient-enriched or term formula after hospital discharge. *Pediatrics, 107*, 683–689.

Catache, M., and Leone, C. R. (2003). Role of plasma and urinary calcium and phosphorus measurements in early detection of phosphorus deficiency in very low birthweight infants. *Acta Paediatrica, 92*, 76–80.

Chan, K., Ohlsson, A., Synnes, A., Lee, D. S., & Chein, L. Y. (2001). Survival, morbidity, and resource use of infants of 25 weeks gestation or less. *American Journal of Obstetrics and Gynecology, 185*, 220–226.

Cobb, B. A., Carlo, W. A., & Ambalavanan, N. (2004). Gastric residuals and their relationship to necrotizing enterocolitis in very low birth weight infants. *Pediatrics, 113*, 50–53.

Crill, C. M., Christensen, M. L., Storm, M. C., & Helms, R. A. (2006). Relative bioavailability of carnitine supplementation in premature neonates. *JPEN: Journal of Parenteral and Enteral Nutrition, 30*, 421–425.

Davidson, S., Schrayer, A., Wielunsky, E., Krikler, R., Lilos, P., & Reisner, S. H. (1990). Energy intake, growth, and development in ventilated very-low-birth-weight infants with and without bronchopulmonary dysplasia. *American Journal of Diseases of Children, 144*, 553–559.

Dhillon, A. S., & Ewer, A. K. (2004). Diagnosis and management of gastro-oesophageal reflux in pre-term infants in neonatal intensive care units. *Acta Paediatrica, 93*, 88–93.

Dollberg, S., Kuint, J., Mazkereth, R., & Mimouni, F. B. (2000). Feeding tolerance in preterm infants: Randomized trial of bolus and continuous feeding. *Journal of the American College of Nutrition, 19*, 797–800.

Faerk, J., Peitersen, B., Petersen, S., & Michaelsen, K. F. (2002). Bone mineralisation in premature infants cannot be predicted from serum alkaline phosphatase or serum phosphate. *Archives of Disease in Childhood. Fetal and Neonatal Edition, 87*, F133–F136.

Fenton, T. R. (2003). A new growth chart for preterm babies: Babson and Benda's chart updated with recent data and a new format. *BMC Pediatrics, 16*, 13.

Fok, T. F., Chui, K. K. M., Cheung, R., Ng, P. C., Cheung, K. L., & Hjelm, M. (2001). Manganese intake and cholestatic jaundice in neonates receiving parenteral nutrition: A randomized controlled study. *Acta Paediatrica, 90*, 1009–1015.

Foman, S. J. (1993). *Nutrition of Normal Infants*. St. Louis, MO: Mosby.

Francavilla, R., Miniello, V. L., Lionetti, M. E., & Armenio, L. (2003). Hepatitis and cholestasis in infancy: Clinical and nutritional aspects. *Acta Paediatrica, 441* (Suppl.), 101–104.

Franz, A. R., Mihatsch, W. A., Sander, S., Kron, M., & Pohlandt, F. (2000). Prospective randomized trial of early versus late enteral iron supplementation in infants with a birth weight of less than 1301 grams. *Pediatrics, 106*, 700–706.

Gairdner, D., & Pearson, J. (1988). *Growth and Development Record: Preterm–2 Years, Length/Weight/Head Circumference*. Welwyn Garden City, Hertfordshire, England: Castlemead Press.

Geggie, J. H., Dressler-Mund, D. L., Creighton, D., & Cormack-Wong, E. R. (1999). An interdisciplinary feeding team approach for preterm, high-risk infants and children. *Canadian Journal of Dietetic Practice and Research, 60*, 72–77.

Giuo, S., Roche, A. F., & Moore, W. M. (1988). Reference data for head circumference and 1-month increments from 1 to 12 months of age. *Journal of Pediatrics, 113*, 490.

Gray, K., & King, W. (1997). Feeding assessment. In J. Cox (Ed.), *Nutrition Manual for At-Risk Infants and Toddlers*. Chicago: Precept Press.

Greene, H. L., Hambidge, K. M., Schanler, R., & Tsang, R. C. (1988). Guidelines for the use of vitamins, trace elements, calcium, magnesium, and phosphorus in infants and children receiving total parenteral nutrition: Report of the Subcommittee on Pediatric Parenteral Nutrition Requirements from the Committee on Clinical Practice Issues of the American Society for Clinical Nutrition. *American Journal of Clinical Nutrition, 48*, 1324–1342.

Greer, F. R. (1994). Osteopenia of prematurity. *Annual Reviews in Nutrition, 14*, 169–185.

Griffin, I. J. (2002). Postdischarge nutrition for high risk neonates. *Clinics in Perinatology, 9*, 327–344.

Groh-Wargo, S., & Cox, J. H. (1997). Prematurely born infants. In J. Cox (Ed.). *Nutrition Manual for At-Risk Infants and Toddlers.* Chicago: Precept Press.

Groh-Wargo, S., Thompson, M., & Cox, J. (2000). *Nutritional Care for High-Risk Newborns* (revised, 3rd ed.). Chicago: Precept Press.

Hatun, S., Ozkan, B., Orbak, Z., Doneray, H., Cizmecioglu, F., Toprak, D., et al. (2005). Vitamin D deficiency in early infancy. *Journal of Nutrition, 135*, 279–282.

Hawdon, J. M., Beauregard, N., Slattery, J., & Kennedy, G. (2000). Identification of neonates at risk of developing feeding problems in infancy. *Developmental Medicine and Child Neurology, 42*, 235–239.

Heird, W. C., Dell, R. B., & Helms, R. A. (1987). Amino acid mixture designed to maintain normal plasma amino acid patterns in infants and children requiring parenteral nutrition. *Pediatrics, 80*, 401–408.

Henderson, G., Fahey, T., & McGuire, W. (2005). Calorie and protein-enriched formula versus standard term formula for improving growth and development in pre-term or low birth weight infants following hospital discharge. *Cochrane Database Syst Rev, 18*, CD004696.

Hurwitz, M., Garcia, M. G., Poole, R. L., & Kerner, J. (2004). Copper deficiency during parenteral nutrition: A report of four pediatric cases. *Nutrition in Clinical Practice : Official Publication of the American Society for Parenteral and Enteral Nutrition, 19*, 305–308.

Ibrahim, H. M., Jeroudi, M. A., Baier, R. J., Dhanireddy, R., & Krouskop, R. W. (2004). Aggressive early total parenteral nutrition in the low-birth-weight infants. *Journal of Perinatology, 24*, 482–486.

Johnson, D. B., Cheney, C., & Monsen, E. R. (1998). Nutrition and feeding in infants with bronchopulmonary dysplasia after initial hospital discharge: Risk factors for growth failure. *Journal of the American Dietetic Association, 98*, 649–656.

Karpen, S. (2002). Update on the etiologies and management of neonatal cholestasis. *Clinics in Perinatology, 29*, 159–180.

Kashyap, S., Schulze, K. F., & Forsyth, M. (1990). Growth, nutrient retention, and metabolic response of low-birth-weight infants fed supplemented and unsupplemented preterm human milk. *American Journal of Clinical Nutrition, 52*, 254–262.

Kerner, J. A. (1996). Parenteral nutrition. In W. A. Walker, P. R. Durie, J. R. Hamilton, J. A. Walker-Smith, & J. B. Watkins (Eds.), *Pediatric Gastrointestinal Disease: Pathophysiology, Diagnosis, Management* (vol. 2). St. Louis, MO: Mosby.

Klein, G. L. (1998). Metabolic bone disease of total parenteral nutrition. *Nutrition, 14*, 149–152.

Knafelz, D., Gambarara, M., Diamanti, A., Papadatou, B., Ferretti, F., Tarissi De Iacobis, I., et al. (2003). Complications of home parenteral nutrition in a large pediatric series. *Transplantation Proceedings, 35,* 3050–3051.

Kulkarni, P. B., Hall, R. T., & Rhodes, P. G. (1980). Rickets in VLBW infants. *Journal of Pediatrics, 97,* 249–252.

Kurkchubasche, A. G., Rowe, M. I., & Smith, S. D. (1993). Adaptation in short-bowel syndrome: Reassessing old limits. *Journal of Pediatric Surgery, 28,* 1069–1071.

Kurl, S., Heinonen, K., and Lansimies, E. (2000). Effects of prematurity, intrauterine growth status, and early dexamethasone treatment on postnatal bone mineralisation. *Arch Dis Child Fetal Neonatal Ed,* 83, F109–F111.

Kuschel, C. A., & Harding, J. E. (2004). Multicomponent fortified human milk for promoting growth in preterm infants. *Cochrane Database Syst Rev,* (1), CD000343.

Ladhani, S., Srinivasan, L., Buchanan, C., and Allgrove, J. (2004). Presentation of vitamin D deficiency. *Arch Dis Child,* 89, 781–784.

Landers, S. (2003). Maximizing the benefits of human milk feeding for the preterm infant. *Pediatric Annals, 32,* 298–306.

Lucas, A., & Cole, T. J. (1990). Breast milk and neonatal necrotizing enterocolitis. *Lancet, 336,* 1519–1523.

Lucas, A., King, F., Bishop, N. B., & King, F. J. (1992). Randomized trial of nutrition for pre-term infants after discharge. *Archives of Disease in Childhood, 67,* 324.

Marino, A. J., Assing, E., Carbone, M. T., Hiatt, I. M., Hegyi, T., & Graff, M. (1995). The incidence of gastroesophageal reflux in pre-term infants. *Journal of Perinatology, 15,* 369–371.

Marks, K. A., Reichman, B., Lusky, A., Zmora, E., and Israel Neonatal Network. (1996). Fetal growth and postnatal growth failure in very-low-birthweight infants. *Acta Paediatrica, 95,* 236–242.

McGuire, W., & Anthony, M. Y. (2003). Donor human milk versus formula for preventing necrotising enterocolitis in preterm infants: Systematic review. *Archives of Disease in Childhood. Fetal and Neonatal Edition, 88,* F11–F14.

McGuire, W., & McEwan, P. (2004). Systematic review of transpyloric versus gastric tube feeding for preterm infants. *Archives of Disease in Childhood. Fetal and Neonatal Edition, 89,* F245–F248.

McKeown, R. E., Marsh, T. D., & Amarnath, U. (1992). Role of delayed feeding and of feeding increments in necrotizing enterocolitis. *Journal of Pediatrics, 121*(5 Pt 1), 764–770.

Medline Plus Medical Dictionary. (February 2003). Retrieved February 14, 2007, from http://www.nlm.nih.gov/medlineplus/mplusdictionary.html

Mirtallo, J., Canada, T., Johnson, D., Kumpf, V., Petersen, C., Sacks, G., et al. (2004). Safe practices for parenteral nutrition. *JPEN. Journal of Parenteral and Enteral Nutrition, 28,* S39–S70.

Nako, Y., Fukushima, N., & Tomomasa, T. (1993). Hypervitaminosis D after prolonged feeding with a premature formula. *Pediatrics, 92,* 862.

Olsen, I. E., Richardson, D. K., Schmid, C. H., Ausman, L. M., & Dwyer, J. T. (2005). Dietitian involvement in the neonatal intensive care unit: More is better. *Journal of the American Dietetic Association, 105,* 1224–1230.

Pereira, G. (1995). Nutritional care of the extremely premature infant. *Neonatal and Perinatal Nutrition, 22,* 61–75.

Pettifor, J. M. (2004). Nutritional rickets: deficiency of vitamin D, calcium, or both? *American Journal of Clinical Nutrition,* 80(6 Suppl.), 1725S–1729S.

Pierro, A. (2002). Metabolism and nutritional support in the surgical neonate. *Journal of Pediatric Surgery, 37,* 811–822.

Porcelli, P. J., Jr., & Sisk, P. M. (2002). Increased parenteral amino acid administration to extremely low-birth-weight infants during early postnatal life. *Journal of Pediatric Gastroenterology and Nutrition, 34,* 174–179.

Premji, S., McNeil, D. A., & Scotland, J. (2004). Regional neonatal oral feeding protocol: Changing the ethos of feeding preterm infants. *The Journal of Perinatal & Neonatal Nursing, 18,* 371–384.

Prestridge, L. L., Schanler, R. J., Shulman, R. J., Burns, P. A., & Laine, L. L. (1993). Effect of parenteral calcium and phosphorus therapy on mineral retention and bone mineral content in the very low birth weight infants. *Journal of Pediatrics, 122*(Pt 1), 761–768.

Putet, G. (2000). Lipid metabolism of the micropremie. *Clinics in Perinatology, 27,* 57–69.

Quiros-Tejeira, R. E., Ament, M. E., & Reyen, L. (2004). Long-term parenteral nutritional support and intestinal adaptation in children with short bowel syndrome: A 25-year experience. *Journal of Pediatrics, 145,* 157–163.

Rao, R., & Georgieff, M. (2005). Microminerals. In R. Tsang, A. Luca, R. Uauy, & S. Zlotkin (Eds.). *Nutritional Needs of the Preterm Infant: Scientific Basis and Practical Guidelines* (2nd ed.). Philadelphia: Lippincott Williams & Wilkins.

Rayyis, S. F., Ambalavanan, N., Wright, L., & Carlo, W. (1999). Randomized trial of "slow" versus "fast" feed advancements on the incidence of necrotizing enterocolitis in VLBW infants. *Journal of Pediatrics, 134,* 293–297.

Rigo, J., De Curtis, M., Pieltain, C., Picaud, J. C., Salle, B. L., and Senterre, J. (2000). Bone mineral metabolism in the micropremie. *Clin Perinatol,* 27, 147–170.

Ritchie, S. (2002). Primary care of the premature infant discharged from the neonatal intensive care unit. *MCN. The American Journal of Maternal Child Nursing, 27,* 76–85.

Ritz, E., Haxsen, V., and Zeier, M. (2003). Disorders of phosphate metabolism—pathomechanisms and management of hypophosphataemic disorders. *Best Pract Res Clin Endocrinol Metab,* 17, 547–558.

Roche, A., & Himes, J. H. (1982). Incremental growth charts. *American Journal of Clinical Nutrition, 35,* 629.

Rommel, N., DeMeyer, A., Feenstra, L., & Veereman-Wauters, G. (2003). The complexity of feeding problems in 700 infants and young children presenting to a tertiary care institution. *Journal of Pediatric Gastroenterology and Nutrition, 37*, 75–84.

Schanler, R. J. (2001). The use of human milk for premature infants. *Pediatric Clinics of North America, 48*, 207–219.

Schanler, R. J., Shulman, R. J., Lau, C., O'Brian Smith, E., & Heitkemper, M. M. (1999). Feeding strategies for premature infants: Randomized trial of gastrointestinal priming and tube-feeding method. *Pediatrics, 103*, 434–439.

Schmidt, G. L., Baumgartner, T. G., & Fischlschweiger, W. (1986). Cost containment using cysteine HCl acidification to increase calcium/phosphate solubility in hyperalimentation solutions. *JPEN. Journal of Parenteral and Enteral Nutrition, 10*, 203–207.

Schmidt-Sommerfield, E., Penn, D., & Wolf, H. (1982). Carnitine blood concentrations and fat utilization in parenterally alimented premature newborn infants. *Journal of Pediatrics, 100*, 260.

Shenai, J. P., Jhaveri, B. M., & Reynolds, J. W. (1981). Nutritional balance studies in VLBW infants: Role of soy formula. *Pediatrics, 67*, 631–637.

Silvestre, M. A., Morbach, C. A., Brans, Y. W., & Shankaran, S. (1996). A prospective randomized trial comparing continuous versus intermittent feeding methods in very low birth weight neonates. *Journal of Pediatrics, 128*, 748.

Sondheimer, J. M. (2004). A critical perspective on trophic feeding. *Journal of Pediatric Gastroenterology and Nutrition, 38*, 237–238.

Sondheimer, J. M., Asturias, E., & Cadnapaphornchai, M. (1998). Infection and cholestasis in neonates with intestinal resection and long term parenteral nutrition. *Journal of Pediatric Gastroenterology and Nutrition, 27*, 131–137.

Steward, D. K., & Pridham, K. F. (2002). Nutritional influences on the growth of extremely LBW infants. *Newborn and Infant Nursing Reviews, 2*, 159–165.

Thureen, P. J., & Hay, W. W. (2001). Early aggressive nutrition in preterm infants. *Seminars in Neonatology, 6*, 403–415.

Tyson, J. E., & Kennedy, K. A. (2005). Trophic feedings for parenterally fed infants. *Cochrane Database Syst Rev*, 20(3), CD000504.

Vanderhoof, J. (2004). New and emerging therapies for short bowel syndrome in children. *Journal of Pediatric Gastroenterology and Nutrition, 39*, S769–S771.

Vanderhoof, J. A. (2003). Enteral and parenteral nutrition in the care of patients with short-bowel syndrome. *Best Practice & Research Clinical Gastroenterology, 17*, 997–1015.

Weckwerth, J. A. (2004). Monitoring enteral nutrition support tolerance in infants and children. *JPEN. Journal of Parenteral and Enteral Nutrition, 19*, 496–503.

Weisberg, P., Scanlon, K. S., Li, R., and Cogswell, M. E. (2004). Nutritional rickets among children in the United States: review of cases reported between 1986 and 2003. *American Journal of Clinical Nutrition,* 80(6 Suppl.), 1697S–705S.

Wheeler, R. E., & Hall, R. T. (1996). Feeding of premature infant formula after hospital discharge of infants weighing less than 1,800 grams at birth. *Journal of Perinatology, 16*, 111.

Wight, N. E. (2001). Donor human milk for preterm infants. *Journal of Perinatology, 21*, 249–254.

Wright, K., Ernst, K. D., Gaylord, M. S., Dawson, J. P., & Burnette, T. M. (2003). Increased incidence of parenteral nutrition-associated cholestasis with Aminosyn PF compared to TrophAmine. *Journal of Perinatology, 23*, 444–450.

Yu, V. Y. (2005). Extrauterine growth restriction in preterm infants: Importance of optimizing nutrition in neonatal intensive care units. *Croatian Medical Journal, 46*, 737–743.

Ziegler, E. E., Thureen, P. J., & Carlson, S. J. (2002). Aggressive nutrition of the VLBW infant. *Clinics in Perinatology, 29*, 225–244.

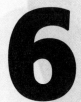

CHAPTER

6

Special Topics in Toddler and Preschool Nutrition: Vitamins and Minerals in Childhood and Children with Disabilities

Aaron Owens, MS, RD, and Harriet H. Cloud, MS, RD, FADA

CHAPTER OUTLINE

Neurologic Disorders
    Spina Bifida
    Cerebral Palsy
    Autism
    Attention Deficit Hyperactivity Disorder

Reader Objectives

After studying this chapter and reflecting on the contents, you should be able to

1. Recognize the purposes of vitamin and mineral functions in growth and development.
2. Review the definitions of developmental disabilities.
3. Identify the etiology and prevalence of various developmental disabilities.
4. Review the evidence-based practice for nutrition problems associated with selected syndromes and disabilities.
5. Compare legislative and community resources for children with developmental disabilities.

Vitamins and Minerals in Childhood

Aaron Owens, MS, RD

Vitamins and minerals are nutrients that are essential to life because of their involvement in cellular metabolism, maintenance, and growth throughout the life cycle. Vitamins and minerals are often called micronutrients because in comparison with the four major nutrients—carbohydrate, protein, fat, and water—they are needed in relatively small amounts. Changing life-styles and dietary patterns over the last two decades have conspired to increase a number of micronutrient imbalances in diets of children. Poor dietary patterns, such as skipping meals, a preference for low-nutrient-dense foods in place of nourishing ones, and frequent snacking, can contribute to suboptimal nutrition status during childhood (Kim, Kim, & Keen, 2005). The Commission on the Nutrition Challenges of the 21st Century (2000) stated that although protein–energy malnutrition remains a concern for many of the world's children, micronutrient malnutrition is recognized increasingly as a more widespread problem (Tanner & Finn-Stevenson, 2002).

Malnutrition permeates all aspects of health, growth, cognition, motor, and social development. Micronutrient deficiencies, such as iron deficiency anemia, have been shown to positively correlate with decreased school performance. Lack of adequate micronutrients, especially zinc, selenium, iron, and the antioxidant vitamins, can also lead to clinically significant immune deficiency and infections in children. More than 50% of deaths of children in developing countries are a result of infections related to malnutrition. Irreversible and lifelong sequelae may prevent children from reaching their fullest potential (Neuman, Gewa, & Bwibo, 2004). Therefore it is important that healthy dietary patterns are established during childhood.

Vitamins

Vitamins: Organic compounds that occur naturally in plants and animals and are not synthesized by the body in adequate amounts to meet physiologic needs.

Vitamins are organic compounds that occur naturally in plants and animals and are distinct from carbohydrates, fats, and proteins. Vitamins are also typically found naturally in foods in minute amounts and are not synthesized by the body in adequate amounts to meet physiologic needs. Vitamin needs are often dependent on energy intake or other nutrient levels. Therefore inadequate consumption of vitamins results in a specific deficiency syndrome. Vitamin functions are determined by their chemical and associated physical properties and serve essential roles in numerous metabolic processes. Few, however, show close chemical or functional similarities. By and large vitamins function as coenzymes, which are fundamental parts of enzymes.

Vitamins are usually classified into two groups, based on their solubility. Some are soluble in nonpolar solvents (i.e., vitamins A, D, E, and K), whereas others are soluble in polar solvents (i.e., vitamin C, thiamin, riboflavin, niacin, vitamin B_6, biotin, pantothenic acid, folate, and vitamin B_{12}). The **fat-soluble vitamins** tend to be absorbed and transported with dietary lipids, whereas the **water-soluble vitamins** are absorbed by passive and active processes. Vitamins remain in the body for varying amounts of time. Utilization of water-soluble vitamins begins the minute they are absorbed through the digestive system and remain in the body for 2 to 4 days. Water-soluble vitamins are not stored and are quickly excreted in the urine either intact or as water-soluble metabolites. Thus water-soluble vitamins must be replenished regularly, and toxicities are virtually unknown. Fat-soluble vitamins stay in the body for longer periods of time and are usually stored in lipid tissue of organs, especially the liver. In general, the fat-soluble vitamins are excreted with the feces via enterohepatic circulation. Toxicity is probable with some but only when taken in very large doses (Mahan & Escott-Stump, 2000).

Fat-soluble vitamins (e.g., A, D, E and K): Soluble in polar solvents, absorbed and transported with dietary lipids, and excreted in the feces.

Water-soluble vitamins (e.g., vitamin C, thiamin, riboflavin, niacin, vitamin B_6, biotin, pantothenic acid, folate, and vitamin B_{12}): Soluble in nonpolar solvents, absorbed by passive and active processes, and excreted in the urine.

Water-Soluble Vitamins

Vitamin B

Although each B vitamin has its own unique biological role and individual properties, as a group these nutrients are often thought of as a single entity because of their commonality. B vitamins work together in the body by maintaining healthy nerves, skin, hair, eyes, liver, and mouth and by preserving good muscle tone in the gastrointestinal tract. B vitamins are used as coenzymes in almost all parts of the body and also provide energy, because they are necessary for metabolism of carbohydrate, fat, and protein. Emotional stress, surgery, illness, pregnancy, and breast-feeding all increase B vitamin requirements. Deficiency in a single B vitamin is rare; rather, people tend to have multiple deficiencies, making subtle deficiency symptoms more difficult to diagnose yet more likely to be present. Because of competition for absorption in the intestines, high doses of a single B vitamin should be avoided. When considering supplementation, the ratio of B vitamins is most beneficial when 1:1. In general, no toxicity of B vitamins has been reported.

Vitamin B$_1$ (Thiamin)

Thiamin was the first B vitamin to be discovered in the 1920s, and it plays an essential role in metabolism of carbohydrates, a major source of energy in our cells. As daily intake of complex and simple carbohydrates increases, the need for thiamin increases as extra carbohydrates use more thiamin. The cells of the brain and central nervous system are the first to show signs of thiamin deficiency due to extreme sensitivity to carbohydrate metabolism. During periods of physical and emotional stress, including times of fever, muscular activity, overactive thyroid, pregnancy, and lactation, thiamin requirements increase. Thiamin is also involved in converting fatty acids into steroid hormones, such as cortisone and progesterone, necessary for proper growth and maintenance of healthy skin. Thiamine may play a role in resistance to disease (Libermann & Branning, 1997).

Beriberi: Classic thiamin deficiency disease that affects the gastrointestinal tract, cardiovascular system, and peripheral nervous system and is usually confined to alcoholics.

Classic thiamin deficiency disease is **beriberi,** a disease that affects the gastrointestinal tract, cardiovascular system, and peripheral nervous system and is usually confined to alcoholics. Advanced symptoms of deficiency are indigestion, constipation, headaches, insomnia, and heavy weak legs, which is then followed by cramping or numb feet. Thiamine deficiency can also produce ventricular dilatation and dysfunction resulting in a damaged, enlarged, or irregularly beating heart (Prabhu & Dalvi, 2000). Subclinical deficiency symptoms are fatigue, apathy, mental confusion, inability to concentrate, poor memory, insomnia, anorexia, weight loss, decreased strength, emotional instability, depression, and irrational fears. Such symptoms have been reported in children with B-cell leukemia lymphoma being treated with chemotherapy and total parenteral nutrition. In this group, profound lethargy developed because of severe lactic acidosis caused by an impairment of pyruvate dehydrogenase complex. This was due to a lack of its necessary cofactor, thiamine, in the total parenteral nutrition. Treatment with added thiamin resulted in an improved clinical and laboratory status (Svahn et al., 2003).

Significant food sources include organ meats, pork, dried beans, peas, soybeans, peanuts, whole grains, wheat germ, rice bran, egg yolk, poultry, and fish. Foods with anti-thiamin activity include blueberries, red chicory, black currants, brussel sprouts, red cabbage, and raw seafood. Ascorbic acid has been shown to protect against thiamin destruction in some of these foods.

Vitamin B$_2$ (Riboflavin)

Riboflavin plays an important role in the oxidation of amino acids, synthesis of fatty acids, and oxidation of glucose and thyroid hormone metabolism, processes that influence metabolism and energy production. An increased need for riboflavin is associated with tissue damage, including from burns, surgery, injuries, fever, and malignancies. The blood, too, requires riboflavin, a deficiency of which can lead to vitamin B$_2$ anemia. There is reasonably good evidence that poor riboflavin status interferes with iron handling and contributes to the etiology of anemia when iron intakes are low. Correcting a riboflavin deficiency in children improves the hematologic response of iron supplements. Riboflavin is also found in the pigment of the retina, enabling eyes to adapt to light with photophobia resulting in times of vitamin B$_2$ deficiency. Current interest is focused on the role that riboflavin plays in determining circulating concentrations of homocysteine, a risk factor for cardiovascular disease.

Biochemical signs of depletion arise within only a few days of dietary deprivation. Riboflavin deficiency among Western children seems to be largely confined to adolescents, primarily girls, despite the diversity of riboflavin-rich foods available. Classic deficiency symptoms are cheilosis (tiny lesions and cracks in the corners of the mouth); an inflamed purple tongue; tearing, burning, and itching of the eyes; flaking of the skin; and behavior changes. Riboflavin deficiency may exert some of its effects by reducing the metabolism of other B vitamins, notably folate and vitamin B$_6$. Some children may be marginally deficient as a result of taking antibiotics because antibiotics interfere with absorption and utilization of riboflavin. Phototherapy used to treat hyperbilirubinemia in neonates is also associated with transient deterioration in riboflavin status, although no functional deficits have been described. Riboflavin deficiency has also been implicated as a risk factor for cancer, although this has not been satisfactorily established.

Riboflavin is unique among the water-soluble vitamins in that milk and dairy products make the greatest contribution to its intake in Western diets. Meat and fish are also good sources of riboflavin, and certain fruits and vegetables, especially dark-green leafy vegetables, contain reasonably high concentrations. Breast milk concentrations of riboflavin are fairly sensitive to maternal riboflavin intake and can be moderately increased by riboflavin supplementation of the mother when natural intake is low. Even in well-nourished communities, concentrations of riboflavin in breast milk are considerably lower than in cow's milk. Infants receiving banked breast milk through nasogastric tubing may be at risk of developing transient riboflavin deficiency because of losses in the milk during collection, storage, and administration.

Intakes of riboflavin in excess of tissue requirements are excreted in the urine as riboflavin or other metabolites. Some urinary metabolites reflect bacterial activity in the gastrointestinal tract as well. Urinary excretion, however, is not a sensitive marker of very low riboflavin intakes (Powers, 2003).

Vitamin B₃ (Niacin)

There are two forms of niacin, nicotinic acid and niacinamide, which our bodies make from tryptophan. Nicotinic acid and niacinamide have identical vitamin activities but have very different pharmacologic activities. Niacin is a coenzyme in many important biochemical reactions involved in maintaining healthy skin, properly functioning gastrointestinal tract and central nervous system, and metabolism of lipids (Hendler & Rorvik, 2001). Because of niacin's role in the metabolism of fats, much of its use involves the treatment of elevated cholesterol. There is strong evidence that the onset of atherosclerosis occurs in childhood. Identifying and treating children and adolescents at risk for hypercholesterolemia should lead to a decrease in adult atherosclerotic disease. Studies show that niacin is effective in decreasing triglycerides in the blood. Long-term studies, however, are needed to determine if delivery of niacin truly provides long-term benefits for those children with hypercholesterolemia (Kronn, Sapru, & Satou, 2000).

Niacin deficiency can occur under certain conditions, which include malabsorption syndromes, cirrhosis, and the provision of total parenteral nutrition with inadequate niacin supplementation. The well-known disorder of niacin deficiency is **pellagra**. Pellagra is a nutritional wasting disease attributable to a combined deficiency of the essential amino acid

Pellagra: A nutritional wasting disease attributable to a combined deficiency of the essential amino acid tryptophan and niacin (nicotinic acid).

tryptophan and niacin (nicotinic acid). It is characterized clinically by four classic symptoms, often referred to as the four Ds: dermatitis, diarrhea, dementia, and death. Before the development of these symptoms, other nonspecific symptoms develop gradually and mostly affect dermatologic, neuropsychological, and gastrointestinal systems. Easily observable deficiency generally occurs only in severely malnourished people. A review of literature reveals several case reports describing pellagra in patients with anorexia nervosa, with the most common features being cutaneous manifestations such as erythema on sun exposed areas, glossitis, and stomatitis. Pellagra may be diagnosed if cutaneous symptoms resolve within 24 to 48 hours of oral niacin administration (Prousky, 2003). Although pellagra was commonly found in the United States through the 1930s, the disorder is rare today in industrialized countries. This is in large part due to the enrichment of refined flours with niacin (Hendler & Rorvik, 2001).

Niacin is found naturally in meat, poultry, fish, legumes, and yeast. Consumption of corn-rich diets has resulted in niacin deficiency in certain populations. The reason for this is that niacin contained in corn exists in bound forms, which exhibits little or no nutritional availability. Soaking corn in a lime solution, which releases the niacin, has prevented such a deficiency in parts of the world where corn-based diets are prevalent.

Flushing is the adverse reaction first observed after intake of a large dose of nicotinic acid because it causes vasodilatation of cutaneous blood vessels. Other adverse reactions of nicotinic acid include dizziness, shortness of breath, sweating, nausea, vomiting, insomnia, abdominal pain, and tachycardia. Excessive intake of niacin can also exacerbate gastric ulcers. With liver disorders, high-dose therapeutic supplementation needs to be monitored because of potential increased liver function tests (Hendler & Rorvik, 2001).

Vitamin B₆ (Pyridoxine)

Pyridoxine is one of the most essential and widely used vitamins in the body and participates as a coenzyme in more than 60 enzymatic reactions involved in the metabolism of amino acids and essential fatty acids. Vitamin B₆ is needed for proper growth and maintenance of almost all of our body structures and functions. One of the many systems dependent on vitamin B₆ is the nervous system. Pyridoxine is necessary for the production of serotonin and other neurotransmitters in the brain. Infants fed formulas low in vitamin B₆ have been reported to suffer from epileptic-like convulsions, weight loss, nervous irritability, and stomach disorders (Libermann & Branning, 1997). Pyridoxine-dependent epilepsy usually presents in the neonatal period or even in utero, is resistant to antiepileptic medications, and is treatable with lifelong administration of pyridoxine. The seizures are typically generalized as tonic-clonic, although myoclonic seizures or infantile spasms have been described (Yoshii, Takeoka, Kelly, & Krishnamoorthy, 2005).

Deficiency can cause anemia and depression of immune system responses. Symptoms of vitamin B_6 deficiency are dermatitis of the nose, eyes, and mouth; acne; cheilosis; stomatitis; and glossitis. Deficiency symptoms also include alteration of the nervous system, depression, confusion, dizziness, insomnia, irritability, nervousness, and convulsions.

All foods contain small amounts of vitamin B_6, but foods with the highest concentration are eggs, fish, spinach, carrots, peas, meat, chicken, brewer's yeast, walnuts, sunflower seeds, and wheat germ. The amount of vitamin B_6 in foods does not necessarily represent the amount that is bioavailable or active in the tissues after ingestion. Studies have shown that bioavailability is quite limited (Libermann & Branning, 1997).

Vitamin B_6 is relatively nontoxic, but some problems with the nervous system have been reported when consumed in huge doses of 2,000 to 6,000 mg/day, with reversal of side effects when dosage is discontinued. Inconclusive studies have suggested that social isolation, verbal delays, and self-stimulating behaviors of autistic children have been shown to improve when given high doses of vitamin B_6 along with magnesium (Libermann & Branning, 1997; Samour & King, 2005). The use of megavitamin intervention began in the 1950s with the treatment of schizophrenic patients. A number of studies attempted to assess the effects of vitamin B_6 magnesium (Yoshii et al., 2005). It is thought that total vitamin B_6 is abnormally high in children with autism due to impaired conversion of pyridoxine to pyridoxal-5-phosphate. This may explain the published benefits of high-dose vitamin B_6 supplementation (Adams, George, & Audhya, 2006). Because of the small number of studies, the methodologic quality of studies, and small sample sizes, no recommendation can be advanced regarding the use of high doses of vitamin B_6 as a treatment for autism.

Vitamin B_{12} (Cobalamin)

Recent data indicate that cobalamin status undergoes marked changes during childhood, particularly during the first year. During the first year of life vitamin B_{12} uptake may be limited because of low vitamin B_{12} content in breast milk and immature intrinsic factor system, but the estimated vitamin B_{12} stores in the neonatal liver are assumed to be sufficient for normal growth. Serum cobalamin has been shown to be lower during the first 6 months of life, with total homocysteine and methylmalonic acid particularly high, suggesting impaired cobalamin function. Children have the ability to produce vitamin B_{12} in the intestines, but it is not definite how much can be absorbed by the body. Older children with an omnivorous diet are thought to ensure daily dietary requirement for vitamin B_{12}.

Cobalamin is a coenzyme in a methyl transfer reaction that converts homocysteine to methionine, which is later converted to L-methylmalonyl-coenzyme A to succinyl-coenzyme A. This explains why increased total homocysteine and methylmalonic acid in the blood are measures of impaired cobalamin status, which may occur even in the presence of normal serum cobalamin concentrations. The reported occurrence of low serum cobalamin and increased methylmalonic acid in a significant portion of healthy infants, as reported by newborn screening tests, may be more prevalent than once recognized. The increased metabolite concentrations in infants may be a harmless phenomenon related to developmental, physiologic, or nutritional factors or may reflect the common occurrences of impaired cobalamin function in infants. Because impaired cobalamin function may have long-term effects related to psychomotor development, intervention studies with cobalamin supplementation in pregnancy and infancy may be warranted (Monsen, Refsum, Markestad, & Ueland, 2003).

Some causes of deficiency are various forms of intestinal malabsorption, inborn errors of cobalamin metabolism, exposure to nitrous oxide, infants born to vitamin B_{12}–deficient mothers, and children adhering to strict vegetarian diets (Korenke, Hunneman, Eber, & Hanefeld, 2004; Kim et al., 2005). Vitamin B_{12} is absorbed from the terminal ileum, which is the commonly affected segment of gut in Crohn disease. Its absorption may be compromised in these children secondary to inflammatory lesions, ileal bacterial overgrowth, and surgical resection. Prolonged depletion of vitamin B_{12} is one of the major causes of megaloblastic anemia and ultimately leads to neuropathy (Ahmed & Jenkins, 2004). An example of such a disorder characterized by megaloblastic anemia due to malabsorption of cobalamin is Imerslund-Grasbeck disease (Eitenschenck, Armari-Alla, Plantaz, Pagnier, & Ducros, 2005). Cobalamin deficiency is prevalent in vegetarian teens and has been associated with increased risk of osteoporosis. In adolescents, signs of impaired cobalamin status, as judged by elevated concentrations of methylmalonic acid, have been associated with low bone mineral density. This is especially true in adolescents fed a macrobiotic diet during the first years of life, where cobalamin deficiency is more prominent (Dhonukshe-Rutten, van Dusseldorp, Schneede, de Groot, & van Staveren, 2005). Childhood pernicious anemia is exceedingly rare; etiology is varied and may result despite adequate dietary intake.

Deficiency in infancy presents as failure to thrive, developmental delay, progressive neurologic disorders, or hematologic changes. Symptoms may be evident as early as 3 to 4 months of age but are often nonspecific and difficult to diagnose. Because the age at onset and the duration of neurologic symptoms may contribute to the development of long-term symptoms, early diagnosis and treatment is important for vitamin B_{12}–deficient children (Monsen et al., 2003; Korenke et al., 2004).

The amount of vitamin B_{12} in food sources is small, with good sources including beef, herring, mackerel, egg yolk, milk, cheese, clams, sardines, salmon, crab meat, and oysters. Vegetarian teens should be counseled on the need to identify and regularly consume dietary sources of vitamin B_{12}, especially breast-feeding teen girls. Infants of vegan mothers should also receive vitamin B_{12} supplements starting at birth while breast-feeding if the mother's diet is not supplemented.

Folic Acid (Folate)

One of the most important roles of folate is that it works closely with vitamin B_{12} in metabolism of amino acids, synthesis of proteins, and production of genetic material such as RNA and DNA. Abnormal metabolism of homocysteine and methylmalonic acid, which is directly related to folate metabolism, has been associated with neurologic disorders, such as autism (Miller, 2003; Muntjewerff et al., 2003). The observed imbalance of folate metabolism in autistic children is complex and not easily explained by one single pathway or isolated genetic or nutritional deficiency (James et al., 2004).

The greatest attention received by folic acid is secondary to its ability to prevent **neural tube defects**.

Neural tube defects (NTDs): Defects in the structure of the embryo that give rise to the brain, spinal cord, and other parts of the central nervous system as a result of inadequate folic acid intake during pregnancy.

The neural tube is the structure of the embryo that gives rise to the brain, spinal cord, and other parts of the central nervous system. Neural tube defects occur in 1 to 2 per 1,000 births and are the most significant fetal anomalies leading to long-term morbidity. Evidence from a number of studies demonstrated that periconceptional use of vitamin supplements containing folic acid reduces the risk of neural tube defects by at least 60% (Lumley, Watson, Watson, & Bower, 2000; Persad, Van den Hof, Dube, & Zimmer, 2002). Although the mechanism of action of this nutrient in influencing the risk of neural tube defects is poorly understood, the evidence of the benefit of folic acid has led many health organizations to recommend periconceptional supplementation at a level of 400 µg/day. Because of the concern that public education campaigns alone cannot achieve optimal periconceptional intake of folic acid, food fortification has been proposed as a strategy to encourage all women of childbearing age. The fortification of grain products with folic acid has been controversial because of the potential to mask vitamin B_{12} deficiency. A study in Newfoundland implemented the food fortification strategy with a marked decrease (78%) in the rate of neural tube defects. No evidence of adverse effect of folic acid fortification on the detection of vitamin B_{12} deficiency was identified (Liu et al., 2004).

Because of folic acid's vital role in healthy cell division, replication, and tissue growth, deficiency of this nutrient is associated with dysplasia, an abnormal growth of tissues that is considered precancerous. Acute lymphoblastic leukemia is the most common childhood cancer in developed countries. Little is known about its causes, although its early age at diagnosis has focused interest on maternal and perinatal factors. The second most common pediatric tumor is neuroblastoma, an embryonic tumor, which is also the most prevalent extracranial solid tumor in children. Results of previous studies suggested a protective effect of maternal folate supplementation during pregnancy against acute lymphoblastic leukemia and neuroblastoma tumors. Other studies of genes and environment interaction in acute lymphoblastic leukemia and other cancers provided contradictory results, perhaps because of varying definitions of folate exposure (French et al., 2003; Milne et al., 2006). Further investigation into the interaction of folate intake and the role of metabolism in the formation and prevention of embryonically determined cancers is needed.

Like vitamin B_{12}, folic acid is needed for formation of red blood cells. Without adequate amounts of folic acid, specific types of anemia result, characterized by oversized red blood cells. Symptoms of deficiency are irritability, weakness, sleep difficulty, and pallor. When testing for anemia it is imperative to use diagnostic tests to distinguish vitamin B_{12} anemia from folic acid anemia. If folic acid is supplemented when a child is deficient in vitamin B_{12}, severe vitamin B_{12} deficiency will develop, because the body needs vitamin B_{12} to use folic acid. The reverse, severe folic acid deficiency, occurs if vitamin B_{12} is given to a child deficient in folic acid (Libermann & Branning, 1997).

Cerebral folate deficiency is defined by low active folate metabolites in the presence of normal folate metabolism. Cerebral folate deficiency could result from either disturbed folate transport or increased folate turnover in the central nervous system. Typical features begin to manifest from age 4 months, starting with irritability, sleep disturbances, psychomotor retardation, cerebellar ataxia, spastic paraplegic, and epilepsy. Children often show signs of decelerated head growth from ages 4 to 6 months. Visual disturbances begin around age 3 years with progressive hearing loss starting at age 6 years. Cerebral folate deficiency has been treated with carefully titrated doses of folinic acid to prevent over- or underdosage of folinic acid. Various conditions such as Rett syndrome, Aicardi-Goutieres syndrome, and Kearns-Sayre syndrome may also be related to cerebral folate deficiency (Ramaekers & Blau, 2004).

Food sources include beef, lamb, pork, chicken liver, deep-green leafy vegetables, asparagus, broccoli, whole wheat, and brewer's yeast. Twenty-five percent to 50% of folic acid in food is bioavailable.

Vitamin C (Ascorbic Acid)

The usefulness of vitamin C in the diet stems from its role as an antioxidant, preventing free radical damage and other antioxidant vitamins from being oxidized and thus keeping them potent. It is also essential for growth and repair of tissues in all parts of the body, such as formation of collagen, bone, and cartilage. The skin may also be protected from free radical damage associated with ultraviolet light with adequate intake of vitamin C. Synthesis of hormones in the adrenal glands requires vitamin C, with vast amounts of this micronutrient depleted during times of stress such as surgery, illness, and infection. Studies have shown that ascorbic acid may help prevent increased blood pressure, atherosclerosis, and decreased serum cholesterol. Vitamin C also plays a role in the bioavailability of other micronutrients, such as converting folic acid to its active form and increasing the body's ability to absorb iron from nonheme sources.

Both cross-sectional and follow-up studies have shown an association between decreased intake of vitamin C–containing fruits during the winter and an increased risk of wheezing symptoms in children. Asthma has been associated with oxidant and antioxidant imbalance. Patients with asthma have been shown to have decreased plasma concentrations of vitamin C and increased oxidative stress. Protective effects of citrus fruit consumption do not seem to follow a dose-related response, with positive effects shown with as little as fruit once a week. Results, however, of various experimental studies regarding the effect of vitamin C supplementation on lung function and bronchial responsiveness are conflicting (Forastiere et al., 2000).

> **Vitamin C Research**
> Research into the effects of the antioxidant properties of vitamin C and the risk of childhood leukemia, the leading cause of cancer morbidity under age 15 years, has shown promising results. A two-phase study in California including over 500 children found that regular consumption (>4 to 6 days per week) of oranges, bananas, or orange juice during the first 2 years of life was associated with reduced risk of leukemia in children diagnosed younger than age 15 years. Oxidative damage to DNA may be prevented due to the antioxidant properties of vitamin C, thus precluding an initiating event in carcinogenesis (Kwan, Block, Selcin, Month, & Buffler, 2004).

Vitamin C deficiency in the United States is rare, with the classic disease being **scurvy**. Symptoms are often subtle and difficult to diagnose, with early signs being listlessness, weakness, irritability, vague muscle and joint pain, and weight loss. Late symptoms of deficiency include bleeding gums, gingivitis, loosening of teeth, and fatigue. Unlike most other animals, humans are incapable of producing vitamin C in their bodies and depend on the daily food supply. The level at which tissue saturation occurs is approximately 1,500 mg/day. Concentrated food sources include broccoli, Brussels sprouts, black currants, collards, guava, horseradish, kale, turnip greens, parsley, and sweet peppers. Interestingly enough, citrus fruits are not the most concentrated sources of vitamin C. The bioflavonoids in the skin are responsible for increased vitamin C absorption from citrus fruits. Few people realize that an orange loses 30% of its vitamin C concentration after being squeezed, with nonfortified commercial juice almost having no natural vitamin C left. No proven toxicity has been identified. However, there is a potential

> **Scurvy:** Classic vitamin C deficiency in which symptoms are often subtle and difficult to diagnose, with early signs being listlessness, weakness, irritability, vague muscle and joint pain, and weight loss.

for formation of kidney stones, intestinal gas, and loose stools when extremely large doses are consumed (Libermann & Branning, 1997).

Fat-Soluble Vitamins

Vitamin A

Vitamin A has essential roles in the proper function of the eye, growth and maintenance of epithelial tissue, protection from cardiovascular disease and cancer, immune system function, and reproduction. Vitamin A is especially useful in the prevention of both infectious and noninfectious diseases of the respiratory system.

Each function of vitamin A can be satisfied by ingesting the compounds that form vitamin A, which are retinoids (preformed vitamin A) and carotenoids (precursor to vitamin A that the body converts into active vitamin A). Over 400 carotenoids exist, such as beta-carotene, lutein, canthaxanthin, zeaxanthin, lycopene, alpha-carotene, and cryptoxanthin. Although not all have vitamin A activity, many have powerful antioxidant properties. All forms of active vitamin A, both fat and water soluble, are stored in the liver where they can be mobilized for distribution to peripheral tissues. Because active vitamin A and beta-carotene have slightly different functions in the body, a combination should be consumed. Palmitate, a synthetic form of vitamin A, is water miscible and appropriate for children experiencing fat malabsorption. Chain-shortened and oxidized forms of vitamin A are excreted in the urine with intact forms excreted in the bile and lost with the feces (Mahan & Escott-Stump, 2000).

An estimated 250 million children globally are at risk for vitamin A deficiency. Traditionally recognized symptoms of deficiency are night blindness, skin disorders, suboptimal growth, and reproduction failure. In 1991 nearly 14 million preschool children, most from South Asia, had clinical eye disease (xerophthalmia) due to vitamin A deficiency. Xerophthalmia involves atrophy of the periocular glands, hyperkeratosis of the conjunctiva, and finally involvement of the cornea, leading to softening of keratomalacia and blindness. Although the condition is rare in the United States, where it is usually associated with malabsorption, it is more common in developing countries where it is a major source of blindness among children. Two-thirds of new patients die within months of going blind, due to enhanced susceptibility to infections. Even subclinical vitamin A deficiency increases child morbidity and mortality (Mahan & Escott-Stump, 2000).

Measles is also a major cause of childhood morbidity and mortality, with vitamin A deficiency recognized as a risk factor for severe measles infections. The World Health Organization recommends administration of an oral dose of vitamin A (200,000 IU for children or 100,000 IU for infants) each day for 2 days to children with measles when they live in areas where vitamin A deficiency may be present. When comparing several studies, there was no evidence that vitamin A in a single dose was associated with a reduced risk of mortality among children with measles (Huiming et al., 2005).

Vitamin A deficiency produces characteristic changes in skin texture. These involve follicular hyperkeratosis in which blockage of the hair follicles with plugs of keratin causes "goose flesh" or "toad skin." The skin becomes dry, scaly, and rough. At first the forearms and thighs are involved, but in advanced stages the whole body is affected. Subsequently, deficiency leads to failures in systemic functions characterized by anemia and impaired immunocompetence. A deficiency also leads to the keratinization of the mucous membranes that line the respiratory tract, alimentary canal, urinary tract, skin, and epithelium of the eye. These changes hinder the roles that these membranes play in protecting the body against infections. Clinically, these conditions are manifest as poor growth, blindness, periosteal overgrowth of the cranium, or increased

Vitamin A Research

Chronic infection and illness can decrease the body's level of vitamin A, thereby weakening the mucous membranes and making them more susceptible to viral infection. Randomized controlled trials have shown inconsistent responses of childhood pneumonia with the use of vitamin A as an adjunct to the standard treatment of pneumonia (Huiming, Chaomin, & Meng, 2005; Rodriguez et al., 2005). There is growing evidence that vitamin A and beta-carotene provide some protection against various forms of cancer.

Beta-carotene may also offer hope to children infected with HIV where the infection has a devastating impact on children in developing countries. Poor nutrition and HIV-related adverse health outcomes contribute to a vicious cycle that may be slowed down by using nutritional interventions, including supplemental vitamin A. Periodic supplementation with vitamin A starting at age 6 months has been shown to be beneficial in reducing both mortality and morbidity among HIV-infected children (Fawzi, Msamanga, Spiegelman, & Hunter, 2005).

Vitamin A has been proposed as a nutrient for which infants at risk for chronic pulmonary insufficiency may have special requirements. There is suggestive evidence that high doses when given intramuscularly may reduce the incidence of death from chronic lung disease. Exogenous steroid therapy, which is often used to improve pulmonary compliance in ventilated premature infants, may compromise vitamin A status and induce restricted somatic and bone mineral growth (Atkinson, 2001). Further studies are needed to verify the role that vitamin A may play in preventing severe chronic lung disease in premature infants.

susceptibility to infections. Primary deficiencies result from inadequate intakes of preformed vitamin A and provitamin A carotenoids. Secondary deficiencies can result from malabsorption due to insufficient dietary fat, biliary or pancreatic insufficiency, liver disease, protein–energy malnutrition, or zinc deficiency.

Acute vitamin A deficiency is treated with large oral doses of vitamin A. When it is part of concomitant protein–energy malnutrition, correction of this condition is needed to realize benefits of vitamin A treatment. The signs and symptoms of vitamin A deficiency respond to vitamin A supplementation in the same order as they appear: Night blindness resolves quickly, whereas the skin abnormalities may take several weeks to resolve. Treatment with single doses of 200,000 IU of vitamin A has reduced child mortality by 35% to 70%. This approach is very costly, which has stimulated interest in increasing vitamin A content of local food systems as a more sustainable approach to preventing the deficiency (Mahan & Escott-Stump, 2000).

Active vitamin A is only found in food sources with preformed vitamin A present in foods of animal origin, either in storage areas such as the liver or associated with the fat of milk and eggs. Very high concentrations occur in fish liver oil from cod, halibut, salmon, and shark. Provitamin A carotenoids are found in dark leafy, green, and yellow-orange vegetables and fruit; deeper colors are associated with higher carotenoid levels. In much of the world carotenoids supply most of the dietary vitamin A.

Persistent large doses of vitamin A, which overcome the capacity of the liver to store the vitamin, can produce intoxication. Hypervitaminosis A can be induced by single doses of retinal greater than 330,000 IU in children, potentially resulting in liver disease. Vitamin A toxicity is characterized by changes in the skin and mucous membranes. Early signs of toxicity include fatigue, nausea, vomiting, muscular incoordination, and dryness of the lips. Dryness of the nasal mucosa and eyes, erythema, scaling and peeling of the skin, hair loss, and nail fragility follow. Chronic hypervitaminosis can result from chronic intakes, usually from misuse of supplements, greater than at least 10 times the Recommended Dietary Allowance of 14,000 IU for an infant (Mahan & Escott-Stump, 2000). Reversal of symptoms occurs when supplementation is discontinued. On the other hand, beta-carotene, a naturally occurring pigment, can be given for long periods of time virtually without risk of toxicity. Carotenemia, a harmless condition, is a sign that the body converted as much beta-carotene to active vitamin A as it can, leaving the excess as an orange-yellow pigment in the skin (Libermann & Branning, 1997).

Vitamin D

Vitamin D is not truly a vitamin and can be described as a steroid hormone because it does not need to be supplied from a source outside the body. Now recognized as the "sunshine vitamin," it is a hormone produced in the body by the photoconversion of 7-dehydrocholesterol in the skin. With adequate exposure to solar ultraviolet B radiation (290 to 320 nm), no dietary supplement is needed (Mughal, 2002). There are two forms of vitamin D: vitamin D_2 (ergocalciferol) and vitamin D_3 (cholecalciferol), which is the preferred form because of its natural occurrence in the body. Both vitamin D_2 and D_3 become active hormone vitamin D after passing through the liver and kidneys. The bioactive form of vitamin D is produced not only in the kidneys but also in the placenta during pregnancy. In the active form it is considered to be a hormone because of its roles in calcium and phosphorous homeostasis, cell differentiation, and bone formation and maintenance. As compared with the knowledge of vitamin D in calcium homeostasis and skeletal growth, very little is known about its role in the central nervous system. Vitamin D may also have anticancer properties and play a role in treatment of immunologic disorders, mood behavior, and improvement in muscle strength (Libermann & Branning, 1997; Chaudhuri, 2005).

Life-style, skin pigmentation, clothing, degree of air pollution, and geographic latitude affect the degree of exposure to the sun and therefore the amount of vitamin D internally produced by the body. It is also speculated that iron deficiency may affect vitamin D handling in the skin, gut, or its intermediary metabolism (Wharton & Bishop, 2003). It is difficult to determine amount of sun exposure needed; however, modest exposure to sunlight is sufficient for most children to produce their own vitamin D. Light sun exposure to the hands and face for 20 to 30 minutes two to three times per week has been shown to release approximately 50,000 IU into circulation within 24 hours of exposure (Hollis & Wagner, 2004). Most vitamin D in older children and adolescents is supplied by sunlight exposure. Ethnic populations living in geographic areas with high levels of solar exposure throughout the year have darkly pigmented skin, a feature associated with reduced rate of cutaneous vitamin D. It is also questionable whether any vitamin D is synthesized during the winter months and whether the body's stores of this vitamin are able to meet the daily requirements during this period because the half-life of 25-hydroxyvitamin D is only 19 days (Mughal, 2002; Chaudhuri, 2005). As a population, dermatologists discourage unprotected exposure to sun due to the increased risk of skin cancer and premature aging.

Nutritional rickets: Vitamin D deficiency that was thought to have vanished but is reappearing.

The incidence of vitamin D deficiency, also known as **nutritional rickets,** was thought to have vanished, but it is reappearing. Concerns about vitamin D resurfaced because of the promotion of exclusive breast-feeding for long periods without vitamin D supplementation, particularly for infants whose mother are vitamin D deficient; reduced opportunities for production of the vitamin within the skin because of cultural practices and fear of skin cancer; and the high prevalence of rickets in groups in more temperate regions (Gartner, Greer, & Section on Breastfeeding and Committee on Nutrition, 2003; Pawley & Bishop, 2004). Rickets has been reported in children with chronic problems of lipid malabsorption and in those receiving long-term anticonvulsant therapies. Rickets can also be secondary to disorders of the gut, pancreas, liver, kidney, or metabolism; however, it is most likely due to nutrient deprivation of not only vitamin D but also of calcium and phosphorus (Wharton & Bishop, 2003).

Clinical features of rickets vary in severity and age at onset, with symptoms present for months before diagnosis. Juvenile deficiency affects ossification at the growth plates, resulting in deformity and impaired linear growth of long bones (Pawley & Bishop, 2004). A state of deficiency occurs months before structural abnormalities of the weight-bearing bones and is associated with bone pain, muscular tenderness, and hypocalcemic tetany. Soft, pliable, rachitic bones cannot withstand ordinary stresses, resulting in the appearance of bowlegs, knock-knees, pigeon breast, and frontal bossing of the skull. Improvement in clinical symptoms, such as aches and pains, occurs within 2 weeks of supplementation. Full correction of bowlegs and knock-knees can take up to 2 years. Adolescents are usually left with residual skeletal deformities that require surgical correction (Mughal, 2002).

Regular sources of dietary vitamin D are recommended for those otherwise at risk for deficiency. The National Academy of Sciences recommends the regular intake of a multiple vitamin with 200 IU vitamin D per day for all infants who are breast-fed unless weaned to 500 mL/day of formula, for all non–breast-feeding infants with less than 500 mL/day formula or milk, and for children not regularly exposed to sunlight and not ingesting 500 mL fortified milk. It is generally accepted that nutritional rickets can be prevented by dietary supplementation of 400 IU/day. In the past human milk was thought to be an adequate source of vitamin D for neonates and growing infants (Hollis & Wagner, 2004). However, it has been determined that human milk typically contains 25 IU/L or less of vitamin D. Thus the recommended intake cannot be met with expressed breast milk as a sole source (Gartner et al., 2003). More data are needed to support adequacy of present recommendations and possibly even higher recommendations for vitamin D daily intake.

Vitamin D deficiency has also been associated with **osteopenia** in adults with cystic fibrosis and is potentially related to childhood deficiency. Studies have shown, however, that most children with cystic fibrosis had normal 25-hydroxyvitamin D levels. Interpretation is difficult due

Osteopenia: Bone mineral density that is lower than normal peak bone mineral density but not low enough to be classified as osteoporosis; often present in preterm infants, resulting in fractures.

Vitamin D Research

It has been previously hypothesized that vitamin D deficiency in early life may be a risk factor for various neurologic and psychiatric diseases, including multiple sclerosis (MS), which is a demyelinating disease of the central nervous system that runs a chronic course and disables young people. The suggestion that vitamin D may have a protective effect on MS is not new. In areas of high latitudes where MS is common, ultraviolet radiation is too low to produce sufficient vitamin D in the fair-skinned population throughout the year. Vitamin D supplementation may significantly reduce the incidence of MS. The protective roles of sunlight exposure in early life and cutaneous vitamin D synthesis on the lifetime risk of developing MS is probably not without genetic predisposition because the population prevalence of MS does not parallel the prevalence of rickets. Although subclinical vitamin D deficiency is more common in dark-skinned races, MS is more common in fair-skinned races of European decent. Low vitamin D, however, appears to be an important modifiable external risk factor for MS (Chaudhuri, 2005).

to a lack of knowledge of optimal levels of 25-hydroxyvitamin D required for healthy bone accretion. Lower levels in adolescents may be a precursor to low levels in adulthood and do not seem to be simply related to poor compliance with supplementation. This may, however, reflect normal physiology (Chavasse, Francis, Balfour-Lynn, Rosenthal, & Bush, 2004). Excessive intake of vitamin D can produce intoxication characterized by hypercalcemia and hyperphosphatemia and, ultimately, calcinosis of the kidney, lungs, heart, and even the tympanic membrane of the ear, which can result in deafness. Infants given excessive amounts of vitamin D may have gastrointestinal upsets, bone fragility, poor appetite, and retarded growth. Nutritional hypervitaminosis results from pharmacologic doses of vitamin D consumed over a long period of time and is defined by large increase in circulating 25-hydroxyvitamin D concentration. The tolerable upper level has been established at 1,000 IU day for infants and 2,000 IU day for children. Amount consumed to cause toxicity is thought to be 20,000 IU/day. Hypervitaminosis of vitamin D is a serious, albeit, very rare condition with mild cases being treatable (Hollis & Wagner, 2004). Evidence exists that synthetic active forms of vitamin D, available by prescription, may be better in individuals with malabsorption because smaller doses can be used and thus decrease the risk of toxicity. Currently available solitary vitamin D preparations (containing up to 800 IU) are too concentrated for use in children when the recommendation is filled by standard multiple vitamin preparation (1 mL = 400 IU) (Gartner et al., 2003).

Calcium and magnesium, as well as other vitamins and minerals, should be taken with vitamin D, because these nutrients all work together in the body to form and maintain bone mass. Vitamin D_3 occurs naturally in animal products, the richest sources being fish liver oils and eggs. However, approximately 98% of all fluid milk sold in the United States is fortified with vitamin D_2 (usually at the level of 400 IU per quart), as is most dried whole milk and evaporated milk, as well as some margarines, butter, soy milk, certain cereals, and infant formulas. A typical American diet does not supply the recommended 200 to 400 IU/day, requiring supplementation or fortification (Mughal, 2002; Samour & King, 2005). In many European countries, supplemented foodstuffs with vitamin D are limited; therefore solar exposure is responsible for providing most of the body's vitamin D.

Vitamin E

Vitamin E is now recognized as having a fundamental role in the normal metabolism of all cells as a powerful antioxidant and anticarcinogen. Benefits may be due to its ability to protect vitamin A and C from oxidation, thus keeping them potent. In addition, vitamin E helps to increase the body's level of superoxide dismutase, an enzyme that is a powerful free radical scavenger. The antioxidant function of vitamin E can be affected by the nutritional status of a child with respect to one or more other nutrients that, collectively, protect against the potentially damaging effects of oxidative degradation. Therefore deficiency can affect several different organ systems. The absorption of vitamin E is highly variable, with efficiencies in the range of 20% to 70% (Mahan & Escott-Stump, 2000). Vitamin E actually consists of eight substances, with alpha, beta, delta, and gamma tocopherols being the most active forms. The naturally occurring form is D-alpha-tocopherol, which appears to be the most absorbable.

Vitamin E Research

A variety of studies has provided inconclusive, but promising, results identifying additional roles vitamin E may play in childhood. The results of a study in China (*n* = 120) suggest that chronic childhood constipation causes oxidative stress, in which levels of vitamin C and E were both decreased (Wang, Wang, Zhou, & Zhou, 2004). Because of its antioxidant capability, vitamin E also helps protect the body from mercury, lead, carbon tetrachloride, benzene, ozone, and nitrous oxide exposure that bring about harm through their ability to act as free radicals. The use of vitamin E during cancer treatment to enhance the ability of radiation treatment to shrink cancer cells has been considered. Vitamin E may also play a role in wound healing and reduction of scar formation (Libermann & Branning, 1997).

Deficiencies of vitamin E in childhood present in a variety of ways. Children with progressive neuromuscular diseases are reported to have vitamin E deficiency, which may take 5 to 10 years to develop. Deficiency is manifested clinically as abnormal reflexes, impaired ability to walk, changes in balance and coordination, muscle weakness, and visual disturbances, which are improved after vitamin E supplementation. Additional deficiency symptoms include anemia caused by premature aging and death of red blood cells. These symptoms generally only appear when severe fat malabsorption results due to disorders of the pancreas, celiac disease, and cystic fibrosis. The limited transplacental movement of vitamin E results in newborn infants having low tissue concentrations of vitamin E. Premature infants may therefore be at increased risk of vitamin E deficiency because they typically have limited lipid absorptive capacity for some time (Mahan & Escott-Stump, 2000). Premature infants may also suffer from disorders of the retina, which can lead to blindness, as a result of vitamin E deficiency.

Vitamin E is synthesized only by plants and therefore is found primarily in plant products, the richest sources being oils such as cottonseed, corn, soybean, safflower, and wheat germ having the highest concentration. Smaller amounts may be found in whole grains, green leafy vegetables, nuts, and legumes. Animal tissues tend to contain low amounts of vitamin E, the richest source being fatty tissues and tissues of animals fed large amounts of the vitamin.

Vitamin E is one of the least toxic of the vitamins. Humans appear to be able to tolerate relatively high intakes, at least 100 times the nutritional requirement. At very high doses, however, vitamin E can antagonize the utilization of other fat-soluble vitamins (Mahan & Escott-Stump, 2000). Many supplements contain only alpha-tocopherols. However, it is recommended that a mixture of tocopherols be provided because this is how they exist in foods. For children experiencing fat malabsorption, vitamin E succinate is an alternative, synthetic, oil-free powder that is water miscible and well tolerated. With very high doses of more than 1,200 IU/day some adverse effects result, such as nausea, flatulence, diarrhea, heart palpitations, and fainting, which are reversible upon decrease in dose. To avoid adverse side effects, the recommendation is to begin with the provision low dose and increase gradually (Libermann & Branning, 1997).

Vitamin K

Vitamin K is a general term used to describe a group of similar compounds. Vitamin K_1 is found in food, vitamin K_2 is made by intestinal bacteria, and vitamin K_3 is a synthetic form only available by prescription. For this reason vitamin K is not strictly considered a vitamin, with its most important function being the role it plays in production of coagulation factors in the body. Vitamin K is required to make prothrombin, which is converted to thrombin, which converts fibrinogen to fibrin and creates a blood clot. Newborn infants, particularly those who are premature or exclusively breast-fed, are susceptible to hypoprothrombinemia during the first few days of life as a result of poor placental transfer of vitamin K and failure to establish a vitamin K–producing intestinal microflora. This is associated with hemorrhagic disease of the newborn, which is treated prophylactically by administering vitamin K intramuscularly on delivery, which has been a standard of care since 1961 (Committee on Fetus and Newborn, 2003; Samour & King, 2005).

Vitamin K is also essential for development of normal bone density during childhood and is thought to be important in preventing the development of osteoporosis in later life. There has been relatively little research emphasis on the effect of vitamin K on bone health during childhood. Better vitamin K status is associated with lower levels of markers of bone resorption and bone formation, suggesting a lower rate of bone turnover. There is a need for randomized supplementation trials to better understand the role of vitamin K on bone acquisition in growing children (Cashman, 2005). A marked reduction in bone mineral density has also been observed in children on long-term use of warfarin, a vitamin K antagonist. The etiology for reduced bone density is likely to be multifactorial; however, screening children on long-term warfarin for reduced bone density should be considered (Barnes et al., 2005).

Because vitamin K is easily obtained from the diet and synthesized in the body, deficiencies are rare and usually occur only with lipid malabsorption, destruction of intestinal flora as with chronic antibiotic therapy, and liver disease in which supplementation is recommended. The predominant sign of vitamin K deficiency is hemorrhage, which in severe cases can cause a fatal anemia. The underlying condition is hypoprothrombinemia, which manifests as prolonged clotting time (Mahan & Escott-Stump, 2000).

Vitamin K is found in large amounts in green leafy vegetables, especially broccoli, cabbage, turnip greens, and dark lettuces. Breast milk tends to be low in vitamin K content, providing insufficient amounts of the vitamin for infants less than 6 months of age. An important source of vitamin K is a result of microbiologic synthesis in the gut, which is affected by long-term antibiotic treatment by altering the gut flora (Samour & King, 2005). The synthetic form, vitamin K_3, is known to potentially result in toxicity when consumed in large doses. Major symptoms of overdose include hemolytic anemia, in which red blood cells die more quickly than the body can replace them.

Multiple Vitamin Supplementation

Multiple vitamin supplementation is a common practice in the United States, with approximately 54% of preschool children taking a supplement, typically a multiple vitamin and mineral preparation with iron. Use of supplementation generally decreases in older children and adolescents. Children taking supplements do not necessarily represent those who need them the most. Higher rates of use are found in families of higher socioeconomic status and education levels. Supplements may be taken inappropriately when the marginal or deficient nutrient is not supplied. For example, a child may be taking a children's vitamin but may actually need extra calcium, not always provided in a supplement. Except for fluoride supplementation in nonfluoridated areas, the American Academy of Pediatrics (AAP) does not recommend routine supplementation for normal healthy children. The American Medical Association and the

American Dietetic Association recommend that nutrients for a healthy child come from food, not supplements. Dietary evaluation determines the need for supplementation. The AAP identifies six groups of children or adolescents at nutrition risk who might benefit from supplementation: (1) those with anorexia, poor appetites, and fad dieting; (2) those with chronic disease states such as cystic fibrosis or irritable bowel syndrome; (3) those from deprived families involving abuse or neglect; (4) those who use diet to manage obesity; (5) those who have an inadequate consumption of dairy products; and (6) those who have limited sun exposure or no consumption of vitamin D fortified milk. Children with food allergies, those who omit entire food groups, and those with limited food acceptances may also be likely candidates for supplementation. Megadose levels of nutrients should be discouraged and parents counseled regarding dangers of toxicity, especially with fat-soluble vitamins. The Dietary Reference Intakes include the tolerable upper limit levels, which can be used to detect excess levels of vitamins and minerals from supplemental sources. Because many children's vitamins look and taste like candy, parents should be educated to keep them out of reach of children. Megavitamin therapy has been promoted, despite the lack of controlled studies, for many disorders, such as attention deficit hyperactivity disorder (ADHD), autism, and various behavioral problems.

> **● Learning Point** Except for fluoride supplementation in nonfluoridated areas, the AAP does not recommend routine supplementation for normal healthy children. The American Medical Association and the American Dietetic Association recommend that nutrients for a healthy child come from food, not supplements. Dietary evaluation determines the need for supplementation.

| Minerals

Minerals: Inorganic elements not produced by plants and animals and primarily stored in bone and muscle tissues.

Macrominerals: Needed in large amounts (calcium, magnesium, and phosphorus).

Trace minerals: Needed in much smaller amounts (iron, zinc, copper, selenium, iodine, manganese, molybdenum, chromium, and cobalt).

Minerals are inorganic elements not produced by plants and animals and are primarily stored in bone and muscle tissues. Like vitamins, many minerals function as coenzymes enabling chemical reactions to occur throughout the body. Minerals belong to two groups: **macrominerals,** which are needed in large amounts (calcium, magnesium, and phosphorus), and microminerals or **trace minerals,** which are needed in much smaller

amounts (zinc, iron, and potassium). Currently, nine trace minerals are considered to have a nutrient requirement: iron, zinc, copper, selenium, iodine, manganese, molybdenum, chromium, and cobalt. Notable differences between trace elements are the availability of biomarkers such as tissue concentration, mineral homeostasis and metabolism, body stores, functional indices, and response to increased intake.

Calcium

Calcium is an essential mineral with a wide range of biological roles. Apart from being a major constituent of bones and teeth, calcium is crucial for muscle contraction and relaxation, transmission of nerve impulses, the beating of the heart, blood coagulation, glandular secretion, and the maintenance of immune function. Calcium is also used to activate enzymes involved in fat and protein digestion and production of energy. Calcium also aids in the absorption of many nutrients, especially vitamin B_{12}. Studies have also shown potential anticarcinogenic, antihypertensive, and hypocholesterolemia activity (Hendler & Rorvik, 2001).

Bodies contain approximately 2½ pounds of calcium, 99% of which is stored in the bones and teeth with the remaining 1% (13 ounces) distributed throughout the body in the bloodstream and fluids surrounding our cells. Calcium is primarily found in bone and teeth in the form of the calcium phosphate compound hydroxyapatite (Hendler & Rorvik, 2001). The skeleton functions as a bank from which the body can draw the calcium it needs for various purposes. Therefore identifying skeletal growth is a dynamic process. Approximately 100 mg of calcium per day is retained as bone during the preschool years. This triples and quadruples for adolescents during peak growth. Normally, sufficient calcium absorption from diet, blood, and bone calcium levels remain in balance and fluctuate only slightly. From the body's point of view, however, it is more important to maintain enough calcium in the blood to keep the heart beating regularly than it is to keep the bones strong. Because the body gives top priority to the maintenance of normal calcium levels in the blood, blood tests are an ineffective means of determining calcium levels in either the bone or diet. The concentration of calcium in the blood may be perfectly normal, whereas bone mineral density is suboptimal. If a child's diet is deficient in calcium, the body will always choose to maintain plasma calcium concentration by drawing it out of the bone, often resulting in osteopenia (Libermann & Branning, 1997; Samour & King, 2005).

Optimal dietary calcium and possibly vitamin D intake throughout childhood and adolescence may enhance bone mineral accrual and is central to osteoporosis prevention. During adolescence, children often receive less calcium because of rapid growth, dieting, and substitution of carbonated beverages for milk. From early childhood to late adolescence it has been reported that milk intake decreases by 25%. Mean calcium intake from ages 5 to 9 is positively related to bone mineral density at 9 years of age and is weakly related to bone mineral content after control for pubertal development and height at age 9. Adolescence is a critical period for optimal calcium retention to achieve peak bone mass, especially for females at risk for osteoporosis in later years. During this period of rapid bone mineral acquisition, adolescent girls' calcium intakes are reported to be 30% to 40% below the 1,300 mg/day recommendation (Fisher, Mitchell, Smiciklas-Wright, Mannino, & Birch, 2004; Samour & King, 2005), placing these adolescents at risk for calcium deficiency. Studies have also shown that gender, life-style factors, and socioeconomic status are significant predictors of calcium and vitamin D intake (Salamoun et al., 2005). Children who are vegetarians and do not consume fortified foods may also be at risk for not consuming the recommended calcium requirement. These findings have important implications regarding the institution of public health strategies to promote skeletal health during a critical time for bone mass accrual.

Bone health is now recognized to contribute to overall lifetime management of children and adolescents with disabling conditions, including physical and intellectual disability and with many chronic disease processes. Increased skeletal fragility in the disabled child is well recognized. Strategies to address bone health, including public and medical education concerning consumption of calcium, appropriate selection of vitamin D preparations, and possible use of newer drugs, such as bisphosphonates, are changing the outlook for this large group (Zacharin, 2004).

Nutrition and oral health are also closely related. Micronutrients such as calcium, vitamin D for mineralization, and fluoride for enamel formation are critical to developing and maintaining oral structures. Because of individual variability, children receiving less than the recommended allowance of calcium may not necessarily be at risk.

Clinical signs of calcium depletion from bone gradually develop and are not usually apparent until the symptoms of osteopenia begin to appear. Even x-rays are incapable of picking up bone loss until 30% to 40% of bone has disappeared. Calcium-deficient diets, over long periods of time, result in bones that become porous, brittle, and weak. Children may easily suffer fractures from normal activity such as sneezing, bending over, or receiving a hug. The spinal vertebrae have also been reported to compress or fracture. Inconclusive studies have linked diets high in protein and fat with loss of calcium from the bone. Medications, such as antibiotics, anticonvulsants, and laxatives, can also affect absorption and utilization of calcium (Libermann & Branning, 1997).

Needs are determined by growth velocity, rate of absorption, and phosphorus and vitamin D status. The absorption efficiency of calcium varies throughout the life cycle. It is highest during infancy when it is about 60% with a decrease to approximately 28% in prepubescent children. During early puberty, at the time of the growth spurt, it increases to about 34% and then again drops to 25% 2 years later where it remains for several years. The efficiency of absorption from a calcium supplement is greatest when taken in doses of 500 mg or lower (Hendler & Rorvik, 2001). Genetics and life-style also affect bone mineral density and possible calcium requirements. When assessing calcium status, vitamin D intake should be considered because of its major role in calcium metabolism. Concomitant use of vitamin D and calcium may increase absorption of calcium. The ratio of calcium to phosphorus has also been advised by researchers to be at least 1:1 to improve calcium absorption (Hambridge, 2003). Concomitant use of iron and calcium may inhibit the absorption of iron. Similarly, concomitant use of fluoride, magnesium, phosphorus, or zinc and calcium may decrease the absorption of these minerals (Hendler & Rorvik, 2001).

Food sources include dairy, canned salmon or sardines including the bones, green leafy vegetables, clams, oysters, shrimp, broccoli, soybeans, and soy products. Although unfortified plant foods have less calcium than milk, increased absorption rate makes them good sources of this nutrient overall. Vitamin D fortified milk is a primary source of this nutrient. It has been estimated that humans actually absorb as little as 20% to 40% of the calcium in our food. This may be a result of the presence of oxalic acid, a substance that has been shown to bind with calcium, preventing its absorption in the colon. Limited known toxic effects have been reported, such as the rare development of kidney stones as a result of extremely large doses (Libermann & Branning, 1997).

Iron

Iron is an essential trace mineral that is involved in the entire process of respiration due to its role in the synthesis of hemoglobin, which carries oxygen in the blood. In addition to its fundamental roles in energy production, iron is involved in DNA synthesis and may also play roles in normal brain development and in immune function. Iron is also involved in the synthesis of collagen, serotonin, dopamine, and norepinephrine.

Iron is the most notable example of a mineral that is stored by the body, as ferritin, when intake of bioavailable iron is generous and released as required when intake is less adequate. Serum ferritin is highly correlated with total body iron stores, making it the most sensitive index of iron status among healthy children. Requirements are determined by rate of growth, iron stores, increased blood volume, and rate of absorption from food sources. Menstrual loss and rapid growth increases the need in adolescent girls. Reliable biomarkers of the total quantity of dietary iron are unavailable because of the wide variation in bioavailability and especially due to the large difference in absorption of heme iron versus inorganic iron. In contrast, a range of biomarkers is available that in combination allows for reliable assessment of iron status, therefore identifying the adequacy of iron intake, especially in noninfected nonstressed individuals. Biomarkers can distinguish three generally accepted levels of iron deficiency and are also useful in the evaluation of iron overload. The three levels of iron deficiency are depleted iron stores, early functional iron deficiency, and iron deficiency anemia (Pollitt, 2001; Hambridge, 2003).

Iron deficiency: The most common nutritional disorder in the world, with approximately 25% of the world's population being deficient.

Iron deficiency is the most common nutritional disorder in the world, with approximately 25% of the world's population being deficient. Iron deficiency anemia is most common in children between ages 1 and 3 years, with a prevalence of approximately 9%. Over the last two decades there has been an overall decrease in prevalence of iron deficiency anemia. Factors that have influenced this are prolonged used of iron-fortified infant formulas, increased breast-feeding, iron intake in the form of food sources, and Special Supplemental Nutrition Program for Women, Infants, and Children food program. The AAP recommends universal or selective screening for infants between 9 and 12 months of age and with a second screening 6 months later. Universal screening up to age 2 years for communities with significant levels of iron deficiency or infants whose diets put them at risk is also recommended. Selective screening may be based on risk factors such as prematurity, low birth weight, and dietary intake. Routine screening is not recommended for children over 2 years of age except when risk factors such as poor diet, poverty, and special needs are present (Samour & King, 2005).

The relationship between iron deficiency and cognition has been debated for many years. Much of the research has been focused on the idea that even in the early stages of iron deficiency, iron dependent neurotransmitters can be altered, which in turn can impair learning ability and behaviors. It is plausible that some cerebral changes occur soon after the reserve of iron is depleted and there is a decreased activity in nutrient-dependent enzymes. This could be followed by constraint in motor development and physical activity secondary to a drop in the oxygen supply to muscle fibers. Iron deficiency during infancy may have long-term consequences, as demonstrated by impaired cognitive development and impaired learning ability. Anemic children have been reported to be at risk of delayed acquisition of developmentally appropriate emotional regulation (Pollitt, 2001). It is not certain, however, whether iron status is the major factor contributing to poor school performance of children with general lack of nutrition, such as that which often occurs in rural areas. For these children, cumulative overall nutrient intake may affect school performance more significantly than their iron intake. Despite the improving trends, iron deficiency is especially common among children from low-income families, with many of these children having the more severe form of the disorder, iron deficiency anemia (Kim et al., 2005).

Rapid growth during the first year of life requires an adequate supply of iron for synthesis of blood, muscle, and other tissues. Preterm infants have an increased requirement for dietary iron needed to facilitate appropriate growth. Most health authorities recommend exclusively breast-feeding for 4 to 6 months, a practice thought to prevent development of iron deficiency anemia in term healthy infants. Iron in human milk, however, is low, but it is thought that the high bioavailability partly compensates for decreased concentration. Iron absorption is regulated by recent dietary iron intake, independent of the size of iron stores and the rate of erythropoiesis. Observational studies suggest that dietary regulation of iron absorption is immature in an infant less than 6 months of age and is subject to developmental changes between 6 and 9 months of age. Changes in the regulation of iron absorption between 6 and 9 months of age enhance the infant's ability to adapt to a low-iron diet and provide a mechanism by which some, but not all, infants avoid iron deficiency despite low iron intake in late infancy. This adaptation may not be sufficient to prevent iron deficiency in exclusively breast-fed infants, especially those who were born prematurely. To prevent this, iron supplements are often recommended for breast-fed infants after 4 to 6 months if not consuming adequate amounts of iron-rich complementary foods. Iron supplementation is also often recommended for older breast-feeding infants who are not consuming iron-rich infant cereals. Little, however, is known about factors affecting iron absorption from human milk or supplements (Domellof, Lonnerdal, Abrams, & Hernell, 2002).

Different stages of iron deficiency involve different systemic changes, which in turn affect different psychobiological domains. During early iron deficiency the supply of iron to the bone marrow is marginal, not causing measurable decline in hemoglobin. Iron deficiency anemia is associated with variation in red blood cell width. Hemoglobin and hematocrit are the main biological screening tests because of the simplicity of measurements. Low values only occur during later stages of deficiency and result in impairment of normal physiology (Hambridge, 2003). Acute blood loss, acute and chronic infection, micronutrient deficiency (vitamin B_{12} or folate), and defects in red blood cell production (sickle cell or thalassemia) may also cause low values. An advantageous side effect of correcting low iron levels with iron supplements has been shown to be improved appetite (Pawley & Bishop, 2004).

Iron absorption from food depends on iron status of the individual (those with low iron stores have increased absorption rate) and increased absorption rate from heme iron versus non-heme sources. It is uncertain if excessive dietary iron levels result in abnormally high ferritin levels. A typical American mixed diet contains approximately 6 mg iron per 1,000 calories. Adolescents dieting to lose weight will likely have minimal iron intake, especially if animal protein is limited. The best dietary sources of iron are green vegetables, legumes, and meat. Much of the iron ingested in the American diet in the form of bread and cereals is not well absorbed. Although iron is clearly essential for a wide range of vital biological processes, it is also a potentially toxic substance. Iron overload disorders, which can lead to cirrhosis, coronary heart disease, and congestive heart failure, are also a public health concern (Hendler & Rorvik, 2001).

Magnesium

Magnesium is an essential mineral involved with over 300 metabolic reactions. It is necessary for every major biological process, including the production of cellular energy and the synthesis of nucleic acids and proteins. It is also important for the electrical stability of cells, the maintenance of membrane integrity, muscle contraction, nerve conduction, and regulation of vascular tone. About 50% to 60% of the body's magnesium content is in the bone, whereas a mere 1% is found extracellularly. Magnesium is the second most abundant intracellular cation, with potassium being the most abundant. There is much about the pharmacokinetics of magnesium that is not known.

Magnesium deficiency is associated with the pathogenesis of numerous serious disorders, notably ischemic heart disease, congestive heart failure, sudden cardiac death, diabetes, and hypertension. Treatment with supplemental magnesium is often helpful in these conditions. It may help prevent or reduce the incidence of cerebral palsy (CP) and mental retardation in preterm infants. Symptoms and signs of magnesium deficiency include anorexia, nausea and vomiting, diarrhea, generalized muscle spasticity, confusion, seizures, and cardiac arrhythmias. Magnesium deficiency may be found in diabetes mellitus, malabsorption syndromes, and hyperthyroidism. Long-term use of diuretics may also result in magnesium deficiency. Magnesium deficiency itself is an important cause of hypokalemia (Hendler & Rorvik, 2001).

Magnesium is associated with a low risk of adverse effects that are

> **Magnesium and Respiratory Illness: A Connection?**
>
> Randomized controlled trials assessing the use of magnesium sulfate in asthmatic children with moderate exacerbation have produced contradictory results. Higher intakes of magnesium are associated with lower incidence of airway reactivity and respiratory symptoms. There is evidence that magnesium functions, in part, by antagonizing calcium in membrane channels of smooth muscle cells, thus decreasing uptake of calcium and leading to smooth muscle relaxation. In addition, magnesium may inhibit release of histamine and other inflammatory mediators. More research is needed to further determine the relative value of supplemental magnesium in the prevention and treatment of asthma and related conditions. There is poor correlation between serum and tissue magnesium levels. Therefore children who have serum levels falling within a normal range may be total body magnesium deficient. Because magnesium deficiency is difficult to diagnose, one question that has proved difficult to answer is whether all asthmatic patients may potentially benefit from magnesium's physiologic effects.

most often related to the rate of administration and the dose given. The most common adverse reaction from the use of magnesium supplements is diarrhea. Other gastrointestinal symptoms that may occur with the use of magnesium supplements are nausea and abdominal cramping. Magnesium, excreted by the kidney, is contraindicated in patients with renal failure. Those with renal failure may develop hypermagnesemia with use of magnesium supplements. Magnesium seems to have a wide therapeutic window in which doses expected to produce clinical benefits should not result in significant adverse effects. There is currently very little information to guide physicians regarding the frequency with which magnesium boluses may be administered (Scarfone, 1999).

Foods rich in magnesium include unpolished grains, nuts, and green leafy vegetables, which are particularly good sources because of their chlorophyll content. Refined and processed foods are generally poor sources of magnesium. The efficiency of absorption of magnesium is inversely proportional to the amount of magnesium ingested.

Potassium

Potassium is an essential micromineral that is important in the transmission of nerve impulses; contraction of the cardiac, smooth, and skeletal muscles; production of energy; and synthesis of nucleic acids. Its antihypertensive properties were first identified in 1928. Evidence suggests that high intakes of potassium also protect against strokes and cardiovascular disease (Hendler & Rorvik, 2001).

The major cause of potassium depletion is excessive losses through the alimentary tract and kidneys. Depletion typically occurs as a result of chronic diuretic use, from severe diarrhea, or in children receiving long-term total parenteral nutrition inadequately supplemented with potassium. The effects of potassium depletion on the rapidly growing infant have not been well studied. Chronic hypokalemia has been associated with renal hypertrophy, interstitial disease, and hypertension in adults. Additional symptoms of depletion include metabolic alkalosis, anorexia, fatigue, and cardiac arrhythmias (Hendler & Rorvik, 2001). Animal studies, including in young rats, have shown significant growth retardation and increased renin-angiotensin system activity. Potassium depleted kidneys also showed early fibrosis. Systolic blood pressure was also elevated in potassium depleted rats, which persisted even after the serum potassium was normalized (Ray, Suga, Liu, Huang, & Johnson, 2001).

Foods that are rich in potassium include fresh fruits and vegetables. Therefore children following vegetarian diets tend to higher intakes of potassium. The efficiency of absorption of supplementary potassium is significant at approximately 90% via the gastrointestinal tract. Dietary potassium is absorbed at a similar rate. The most common adverse effects of potassium supplementation include nausea, vomiting, abdominal discomfort, and diarrhea. Oral potassium supplements rarely result in hypokalemia when normal renal function is present.

Phosphorus

Phosphorus is an essential macromineral that plays a pivotal role in the structure and function of the body. Phosphorus is essential for the process of bone mineralization and makes up the structure of the bone. Phosphorus in the form of phospholipids makes up the structure of cellular membranes. Phosphorus also makes up the structure of nucleic acids and nucleotides, including adenosine triphosphate. During the last trimester of pregnancy, the human fetus accrues about 80% of the calcium, phosphorus, and magnesium present at term. Therefore infants born prematurely require higher intakes of these minerals per kilogram of body weight than do term infants. Providing adequate amounts of these nutrients, particularly phosphorus, to very low birth weight infants during the first few weeks of life is not always possible. As a result, osteopenia is frequent in these infants, with fractures developing in some. Preterm human milk is low in phosphorus and has been associated with impaired bone mineralization and rickets. The addition of human milk fortifiers has improved bone mineralization (Kleinman, American Academy of Pediatrics Committee on Nutrition, & Kleinmad, 2003).

Phosphorus deficiency states are usually a result of malabsorption syndromes and diseases causing renal tubular losses of phosphorus. In addition, those with malnutrition and critically ill patients, such as those being treated for diabetic ketoacidosis, are at risk for phosphorus deficiency and phosphorus imbalance. The so-called refeeding syndrome can cause hypophosphatemia, which may be life threatening. Phosphorus deficiency can result in anorexia, impaired growth, osteomalacia, skeletal demineralization, proximal muscle atrophy, cardiac arrhythmias, respiratory insufficiency, susceptibility to infectious rickets, nervous system disorders, and even death.

Phosphorus supplements, in the form of phosphate salts, are not widely used in the United States to treat phosphorus deficiency. The one exception is calcium phosphate, which is mainly used as a delivery form of calcium. The most common adverse reaction to use of sodium or potassium phosphate is diarrhea. The salts are less likely to cause diarrhea when they are used by phosphorus-deficient individuals than when used by those with normal phosphorus status. Those with renal failure may develop hyperphosphatemia, which can result in ectopic calcification (Hendler & Rorvik, 2001).

Phosphorus, mainly in the form of phosphates, is widely distributed in the food supply, and phosphorus intake from the normal diet is usually sufficient to meet the body's needs. Milk and milk products are particularly good sources of phosphorus.

Copper

Copper essentiality was first demonstrated in the late 1920s when malnourished children with anemia were nonresponsive to iron supplementation. Anemia, neutropenia, and osteopenia are found with frank copper deficiency. Twenty years later the essentiality of Cu for fetal development was reestablished when it was shown that deficits of this nutrient during pregnancy can result in gross structural malformations in the fetus and persistent neurologic and immunologic abnormalities. Copper is required for normal infant development, red and white blood cell maturation, iron transport, bone strength, cholesterol metabolism, myocardial contractility, brain development, and immune function. Premature and small for gestational age infants who are born with low Cu stores can exhibit signs of Cu deficiency, including neutropenia, normocytic hypochromic anemia, osteopenia, pathologic bone fractures, depigmentation of the skin and hair, and distended blood vessels. During the past decade there has been increasing interest in the concept that marginal deficits of this element can contribute to the development and progression of a number of disease states, including cardiovascular disease and diabetes.

Menkes disease: X-linked genetic disorder that is responsible for Cu deficiency. Symptoms are characterized by hypothermia; neuronal degeneration; mental retardation; abnormalities in hair, skin, and connective tissue; bone fractures; and widespread vascular abnormalities, with death typically occurring by age 4.

Several human disorders with genetic mutations in Cu transporters have further defined the role of Cu in human health. Infants with the X-linked genetic disorder, **Menkes disease**, have a gene mutation that is responsible for Cu deficiency. Symptoms are characterized by hypothermia; neuronal degeneration; mental retardation; abnormalities in hair, skin, and con-

nective tissue; bone fractures; and widespread vascular abnormalities, with death typically occurring by age 4 years. Some of the above symptoms may be likely secondary to excessive iron accumulation and subsequent oxidative stress (Uriu-Adams & Keen, 2005).

Plasma copper and ceruloplasmin levels are the most frequently used biomarkers of copper status and are depressed in Cu deficiency states. Levels plateau when copper intake reaches an adequate level, and these biomarkers do not reflect the magnitude of copper intake beyond this point (Hambridge, 2003). Low intakes of Cu in the diet can result in marginal Cu deficiency in young children. Although the mean dietary intake of Cu in most countries is close to the Recommended Dietary Allowance, a substantial percentage of individuals have intakes less than the recommendation, fueling the concern that marginal Cu deficiency may be a common public health concern. Moreover, high dietary intakes of iron or zinc can adversely affect Cu status. For example, infants consuming infant formula with high iron absorb less Cu that those consuming formulas with low iron level. Manifestations of mild copper deficiency may include abnormal glucose intolerance, hypercholesterolemia, myocardial disease, arterial disease, cardiac arrhythmias, loss of pigmentation, and neurologic symptoms.

Although copper is clearly essential for a wide range of biochemical processes, which are necessary for the maintenance of good health, it is also a potentially toxic substance. There are a number of case reports of acute Cu toxicity in the literature. Typically, these case reports represent instances when the acute toxicity is due to ingestion of beverages (including water) that have been contaminated with Cu. Acute Cu toxicity can result in a number of pathologies and, in severe cases, death. **Wilson disease** is an inherited disorder of copper metabolism characterized by a failure of the liver to excrete copper, leading to its accumulation in the liver, brain, cornea, and kidney, with resulting chronic degenerative changes. Cu toxicity, typically due to genetic disorders, can also be a significant health concern (Uriu-Adams & Keen, 2005).

Wilson disease: An inherited disorder of copper metabolism characterized by a failure of the liver to excrete copper, leading to its accumulation in the liver, brain, cornea, and kidney, with resulting chronic degenerative changes.

The richest food sources of copper include nuts, seeds, legumes, liver, kidneys, and shellfish. Absorption efficiency appears to depend on the level of dietary copper intake with a range of approximately 15% to 97%. As dietary copper increases, the fractional absorption of copper decreases. Excessive intake of non-heme iron, zinc, and vitamin C may decrease copper status (Hendler & Rorvik, 2001).

Zinc

Zinc is an essential nutrient that because of its fundamental role in many aspects of cellular metabolism is critical for normal immune function and physical growth. Zinc is critically involved in several biological mechanisms related to growth, including protein synthesis, gene expression, and hormonal regulation. Zinc is a trace mineral that is involved with RNA and DNA synthesis and is critical to cellular growth, differentiation, and metabolism. The body also appears to have the ability, though much more modest, to store zinc. As the global public health importance of zinc deficiency has attracted increasing attention during the past decade, so have the limitations of current biomarkers. Plasma zinc is currently the most widely used and accepted biomarker despite poor sensitivity and imperfect specificity. Investigators often use indirect measures of zinc status because only a small percentage of the body's zinc is in plasma. Most of the body's zinc is located in muscle, bone, and liver, where it turns over slowly (Black, 2003; Hambridge, 2003).

Animal studies have shown that zinc deficiency probably begins to affect the growth process before birth (Merialdi et al., 2004). Zinc deficiency may be particularly relevant to early development because it is an essential trace element that plays fundamental roles in cell division and maturation and in the growth and function of many organ systems, including the neurologic system. Zinc deficiency may also influence child development by altering a child's ability to elicit or use nurturing interactions from caregivers. Low birth weight infants have been noted to have low zinc concentrations in cord blood, and zinc deficiency in childhood is associated with reduced immunocompetence and increased infectious disease morbidity (Sazawal et al., 2001). With a small liver and thus very limited hepatic stores of zinc and increased requirements for catch-up growth, they are at risk for zinc deficiency. Healthy infants are usually able to get an adequate amount of zinc from breast-feeding during the first 6 months of life, as long as the mother's milk supply is adequate and breast milk is not displaced by complementary foods. However, infants who are small for gestational age and premature infants may benefit from zinc supplementation in addition to the zinc they receive from breast-feeding. During the second 6 months of life when complementary foods are introduced, the risk for zinc deficiency increases because most traditional complementary foods are low in bioavailable zinc (Black, 2003).

Zinc Research

Investigations of zinc supplementation on infants' development have yielded inconsistent findings. There are suggestions that perhaps zinc supplementation may promote activity and perhaps motor development in the most vulnerable infants. Although motor development is thought to promote cognitive development by enabling children to be more independent and to explore their surroundings, the only evidence linking zinc supplementation to cognitive development is counterintuitive (Black et al., 2004). Long-term follow-up studies among zinc-supplemented infants are needed to examine whether early supplementation leads to developmental or behavioral changes that have an impact on school performance.

Zinc deficiency is regarded as a major public health problem with multiple health consequences. Zinc deficiency appears to be widespread in low-income countries because of low dietary intake of zinc-rich animal source foods and a high consumption of cereal grains and legumes, which contain inhibitors of zinc. The prevalence of zinc deficiency throughout childhood is estimated to be high, primarily related to the low consumption of foods high in bioavailable zinc. Children in poor countries are also frequently affected by diarrhea, which causes excess fecal losses of zinc (Penny et al., 2004). In such settings zinc supplementation trials among nutritionally deficient infants have demonstrated beneficial effects on mortality and on health indicators, including growth, diarrhea, and pneumonia morbidity (Brown, Peerson, Rivera, & Allen, 2002). Improved zinc status has been associated with improved appetites in young stunted children. Randomized trials are necessary to examine the specificity of zinc deficiency on children's behavior and development (Sanstead, Frederickson, & Penland, 2000; Bhatnagar & Taneja, 2001). Most of the research linking zinc to child development has not addressed the possibility of interactions with other micronutrient deficiencies.

The small rapidly exchangeable pool of zinc is dependent on a steady source of zinc from the diet. The optimal source of zinc is from animal sources, such as beef, lamb, and oysters, which are also important sources of iron and vitamin B_{12}. This suggests that children who are zinc deficient are also likely to be deficient in iron and vitamin B_{12}. All three micronutrients have been associated with deficits in cognitive functioning. On the other hand, it is possible that simultaneous administration of multiple other micronutrients could interfere with zinc absorption or utilization. For example, adverse reactions between iron and zinc have been described (Penny et al., 2004).

Selenium

Selenium is a trace mineral involved in the regulation of thyroid hormone metabolism, healthy immune function, antioxidant activity, and prevention of coronary artery disease. Recognition of selenium's importance in the diet has long been impeded by its fear of toxicity and potential carcinogenic effects.

The quality of biomarkers of dietary intake of selenium and selenium status is quite favorable relative to that of most trace minerals. These biomarkers are in increasing demand principally because of the antioxidant role of this micromineral. Plasma selenium responds rapidly to selenium supplementation and is regarded as a biomarker of short-term selenium status, although in reasonably stable circumstances it also provides a biomarker of long-term intake. Whole blood selenium is of potential value as a biomarker of relatively long-term intake and status. Hair selenium has also been used to assess selenium status. Selenium homeostasis is regulated by excretion via the kidneys with increased intakes resulting in increased urinary metabolites (Hendler & Rorvik, 2001).

A limited number of studies identified children with severe neurodevelopmental delays and elevated liver function tests after developing intractable seizures during the first year of life. At the time of seizures, evidence of systemic selenium deficiency was documented. Findings support the hypothesis that the presence of selenium depletion in the brain among patients with epilepsy constitutes an important trigger of intractable seizures and neuronal damage (Ramaekers, Calomme, Berghe, & Makropoulos, 1994).

The amount of selenium found in foods is based on the concentration of selenium in the soil in which they were grown. Because of the uneven distribution of selenium in the soil throughout the world, disorders of deficiency and excesses have been reported. China, for example, is known to have the lowest and highest concentrations of soil selenium in the world. Reported adverse reactions to toxic levels of selenium are skin rash, brittle hair and nails, garlic-like breath, irritability, nausea, and vomiting (Kleinman et al., 2003).

Iodine

Iodine is required for the production of thyroid hormones, which are necessary for normal brain development and cognition. Iodine deficiency is the main cause of potentially preventable mental deficit in childhood and causes goiter and hypothyroidism in people of all ages. Environmental iodine deficiency causes a wide spectrum of devastating mental and physical disorders, collectively described as iodine deficiency disorders, which are a major public health problem all over the world (Chandria, Tripathy, Ghosh, Debnath, & Mukhopadhyay, 2005). Although endemic goiter is the most visible consequence of iodine deficiency, the most significant and profound consequences are on the developing brain. Congenital hypothyroidism and endemic iodine deficiency are a common cause of mental retardation (Simsek, Karabay, Safak, & Kocabay, 2003). Impaired intellectual development of people living in iodine-deficient regions is of particular concern, especially when all the adverse effects can be prevented by long-term sustainable iodine prophylaxis. Information processing, fine motor skills, and visual problem solving are improved by iodine repletion in moderately iodine-deficient school children (Zimmermann et al., 2006). Adverse effects of supplementation are generally minor and transient, including adolescent acne, rashes, arrhythmias, numbness, weakness in the hands, hypothyroidism, hyperthyroidism, parotitis (iodide mumps), and small bowel lesions. Children with cystic fibrosis appear to have an exaggerated susceptibility to the goitrogenic effect of high doses of iodide. High-quality controlled studies investigating long-term outcome measures are needed to address the best form of iodine supplementation in different population groups and settings (Angermayr & Clar, 2004).

The mean serum thyroid-stimulating hormone is increased in iodine deficiency, although absolute values may remain within the normal range. Thyroid function tests provide useful functional biomarkers of longer term iodine intake and iodide status. Urinary iodine is the standard biochemical indicator used worldwide that shows current state of iodine nutrition. It is also used as a valuable indicator for the assessment of iodine deficiency disorders because 90% of the body's iodine is excreted through the urine (Hambridge, 2003; Chandria et al., 2005). Urine iodine excretion reflects intake within the past few days.

Percutaneous absorption of topically applied substances and the potential for systemic toxicity are important considerations in the child. Most cases of percutaneous drug toxicity have been reported in newborns, although cases in infants and young children have also been noted. Iodine-containing compounds such as povidone-iodine have long been used for topical antisepsis, and it has been suggested they may carry a significant risk to infants. Percutaneous toxicity is of greatest concern in the premature infant, in whom immaturity of the epidermal permeability barrier results in disproportionately increased absorption. Immature drug metabolism capabilities may further contribute to the increased risk in this population. Elevations in both plasma and urinary iodine have been documented in premature infants exposed to these agents. The potential for transient hypothyroxinemia and hypothyroidism has been a concern of many clinicians. This concern stems from the known risks of abnormal thyroid function in the infant, including growth and motor retardation, cognitive delay, and intraventricular hemorrhage. The surface area of the treated skin seems to correlate directly with the risk (Mancini, 2000). In addition to iodized salts, rich sources of iodine include fish and sea vegetables. Iodine is also available in animal products such as eggs, milk, meat, and poultry.

Chromium

Chromium is believed to be an essential trace mineral in human nutrition. Evidence suggests that it plays an important role in normal carbohydrate metabolism. The mechanism of chromium's possible glucose regulatory activity is not well understood. It has also been suggested that chromium may decrease hepatic extraction of insulin and improve glucose tolerance. It has been found that patients receiving long-term total parenteral nutrition without chromium develop glucose intolerance, weight loss, and peripheral neuropathy. These symptoms reverse when given intravenous chromium chloride (Hendler & Rorvik, 2001). Suggestive but poorly substantiated evidence that chromium deficiency may be widespread, especially in individuals with some degree of glucose intolerance, points to a need for reliable biomarkers of dietary chromium and chromium status. It has been concluded that plasma chromium is unlikely to offer a useful indicator in part because normal values are so near the limit of detection. There are conflicting data on the relationship of urine chromium excretion to dietary intake. Only one study, in which controlled quantities of dietary chromium were given, provided some evidence for deterioration in glucose tolerance with a severely chromium-restricted diet (Hambridge, 2003).

The efficiency of absorption of chromium from inorganic or organic compounds is minimal at approximately 2%. Chromium is distributed to various tissues in the body but appears to have a preference for bone, spleen, liver, and kidney. Most of the ingested chromium is excreted in the feces. Chromium that has been absorbed is excreted mainly in the urine. There is much that remains unknown regarding the pharmacokinetics of chromium. Dietary intake is approximately 25 µg/day, with the recommended adequate daily dietary intake being 10 to 120 µg for children under the age of 7 (Hendler & Rorvik, 2001).

Good food sources of chromium include whole grains, cereals, mushrooms, brown sugar, and brewer's yeast. Fruits and vegetables are generally poor sources of chromium, as are most refined foods.

Children with Disabilities

Harriet H. Cloud, MS, RD, FADA

Increasing numbers of children with developmental disabilities enter the health care system each year. It is reported by the Centers for Disease Control and Prevention (CDC, 2003) that 17% of all children less than 18 years of age have some type of developmental disability. This is the result of improved care for many disorders that were once fatal and the developmental of new management techniques. Many of the changes apparent today began in the 1960s as a result of legislation that brought children with developmental disabilities into the educational and health care systems. Nutrition is an important component of the care of these children in treating their chronic diseases but also in the prevention of poor growth, obesity, gastrointestinal disorders, feeding problems, and metabolic problems. In 2004, The American Dietetic Association published a position paper stating the need for nutrition services being available for all age groups with developmental disabilities.

Definitions

The Developmental Disabilities and Assistance and Bill of Rights Act defines a developmental disability as a severe chronic disability of a person that is attributable to a mental or physical impairment or combination of mental and physical impairments. Characteristically, a developmental disability

- Manifests before age 22
- Is likely to continue indefinitely
- Results in substantial functional limitations in three or more of the following areas of major life activity: self-care, receptive and expressive language, learning, mobility, self-direction,

capacity for independent living, and economic self-sufficiency

- Reflects the individual's need for a combination and sequence of special interdisciplinary or generic services, supports, or other assistance that is of lifelong or of extended duration

When applied to the younger population, ages 0 to 5 years, it means the probability of resulting in developmental disabilities if services are not provided (Developmental Disabilities Act, 2000).

Mental retardation is defined as a substantial limitation in present functioning. It is characterized by significantly subaverage intellectual function, existing concurrently with related limitations in two or more areas: communication self-care, home living, social skills, and community use; self-direction; health and safety; functional academics; leisure; and work. *Children with special health care needs* is used to describe children who have or are at increased risk for a chronic physical, developmental, behavioral, or emotional condition and who require health and related services of a type or amount beyond that required by children generally.

Etiology and Incidence

Chromosomal aberration: A change in the makeup of a chromosome, often leading to a developmental disability.

Down syndrome: An aberration of the 21st chromosome causing mental retardation, low muscle tone, and other physical abnormalities.

Congenital anomaly: Malformation present at birth that can affect various organs or structure of the body, such as a cleft lip or palate.

Syndromes: A term used to identify a developmental disability with a cluster of distinctive features, such as Down syndrome.

The etiologies of developmental disabilities are multifactorial. They can include **chromosomal aberrations** such as **Down syndrome** (trisomy 21), neurologic insults in the prenatal period, **congenital anomalies**, prematurity, infectious diseases, untreated inborn errors of metabolism, trauma, neural tube defects (such as spina bifida), and other **syndromes** of lesser incidence. The incidence of the various conditions included under the umbrella of developmental disabilities varies. It is estimated for example that Down syndrome has an incidence of 1 in 600-800 live births, whereas spina bifida has an incidence of 1 in 1,000. The CDC (2003) reported that 17% of children under 18 years of age have some type of developmental disability. Other surveys reported that 3 to 4 million Americans have a developmental disability and another 3 million have a milder form of cognitive disabilities or mental retardation (American Dietetic Association, 2004).

Nutrition Considerations

The nutritional needs of the child with developmental disabilities are the same as those for a nonaffected child from the standpoint of energy needs, nutrients, and fluids. The needs may vary depending on a particular syndrome involving growth in height, energy needs being lower or greater, and metabolic factors. As a result there are nutritional risk factors such as growth deficiency, obesity, gastrointestinal disorders, feeding problems, and drug–nutrient interaction problems.

As a result of varying nutritional needs, nutrition considerations include an assessment of growth and energy needs, feeding issues (such as oral–motor problems), developmental delays of feeding skills, and behavioral problems. Other areas of nutrition consideration include drug–nutrient interaction, constipation, dental caries, urinary tract infections, allergies, and food or nutrition misinformation related to various types of developmental disabilities. These issues are addressed separately under each condition.

Nutrition Assessment

Assessment of the child with developmental disabilities includes anthropometric measures, biochemical measures when indicated by a particular syndrome, dietary intake, and inclusion of an evaluation of feeding development. Anthropometric measures can be extensive or are limited in most clinical settings to height, weight, head circumference, arm circumference, and triceps skinfold measures. Although a number of growth charts exist for specific conditions and syndromes, the CDC recommends using the current CDC charts (see Appendix 1). Information for accurately measuring the child with disabilities and the limitations of the specific use of the growth curves can be found on the CDC website (www.cdc.gov).

Obtaining special equipment for determining height and weight is often necessary for accurate assessment. Weight measuring devices may include chair scales, bucket scales, or wheelchair scales. Obtaining height for the nonambulatory individual requires either a recumbent board or alternative measures such as arm span, knee height, or sitting height.

Biochemical Assessment

Laboratory assessment of the child with developmental disabilities is generally the same as the nonaffected child, with the exception of the individual who is receiving medication. Children with seizures or epilepsy receiving anticonvulsant medications are at risk for low blood levels of folic acid, carnitine, ascorbic acid, calcium, vitamin D, alkaline phosphatase, phosphorus, and pyridoxine. Assessment of thyroid status is recommended for the child with Down syndrome and a glucose tolerance test for Prader-Willi syndrome (PWS).

Dietary Information and Feeding Assessment

Dietary information may be difficult to obtain regarding the child with developmental disabilities, just as it is for the nonaffected child related to the various environments where children are fed. Diet histories obtained from the parent can be helpful in revealing diet progression and texture issues that may exist. Often written diaries are required.

Many children with developmental disabilities display feeding problems that decrease their ability to eat an adequate diet. The problems may include oral motor difficulties, positioning problems, sensory issues, tactile resistance postintubation, and conflict in parent–child relationship (Tobin et al., 2005). Evaluation of the feeding process is an important component of nutrition assessment for the child with a developmental disability, because it may result in poor weight gain, decreased immunity, poor growth, anemia, and mineral and vitamin deficiencies. The problems should be assessed with an understanding of the normal development of feeding and the physical makeup of the mouth and pharynx (Cloud, Ekvall, & Hicks, 2005). Collaboration with other disciplines such as occupational therapy, physical therapy, and speech pathology is often indicated.

Once the nutrition assessment has been completed, problems should be identified and priorities set for addressing them. This information should be shared with the parents and other disciplines working with the child before the intervention process begins. For the child in an early intervention program (ages 0 to 3 years), the nutrition intervention plan should become part of the **individualized family plan**. If the child is of school age, the nutrition component should be a part of the **individualized education plan**.

Individualized family plan: Used for children in early intervention programs.

Individualized education plan: Mandated for children in special education.

Although intervention will vary depending on the particular condition, there are general rules that should govern all intervention. These include programs that are comprehensive, family centered, culturally appropriate, and community based. A second consideration is the need for follow-up, either by the dietitian or another health care professional, and it is important to clarify information provided or to answer questions. A third consideration involves the cost of the nutrition therapy required and possibly finding resources for special nutrition products if indicated.

Chromosomal Aberrations

Down Syndrome

Down syndrome (also called trisomy 21) is a chromosomal aberration involving chromosome 21 that results in the presence of an extra chromosome in each cell of the body. There is an incidence of 1 in 600–800 live births, and there are three processes by which this anomaly can occur: nondysfunction, translocation, and mosaicism. In nondysfunction the chromosome (21) fails to separate before conception and the abnormal gamete joins with a normal gamete at conception to form a fertilized egg with three of chromosome 21. Distinguishing features include short stature, congenital heart disease, mental retardation, **hypotonia**, hyperflexibility of the joints, upward slant of the eye, Brushfield spots (speckling of the iris of the eye), epicanthal folds, small oral cavity, and short broad hands with the single palmar crease and a wide gap between the first and second toes. The National Down Syndrome Congress developed a chart of health concerns that should be addressed by those providing care to children with Down syndrome, and many have nutritional concerns (available at http://downsyn.com/guidelines/health99.txt).

Hypotonia: Low tone of the muscles frequently found in Down syndrome, Prader-Willi syndrome, and other conditions such as prematurity.

Growth in children with Down syndrome differs markedly from nonaffected children. Typically, growth is at the third percentile for height when compared with the general population. Birth weights can be in a normal range of greater than 2,500 g; however, longitudinal follow-up indicates a sloping off of height after the child is 15 months of age. As a result of the differences in height from the general population, special growth curves have been developed. Cronk et al. (1988) developed Down syndrome curves in the 1970s using a population of children with Down syndrome followed over time. Children with heart defects, one of the common findings in Down syndrome, were included. Studies completed in Sweden (Myerlid, Gustafsson, Ollars, & Anneren, 2002) led to the development of growth specific curves as an aid to diagnosing celiac disease and hypothyroidism. The growth charts were developed from longitudinal and cross-sectional data from 4,532 examinations of 354 males and females from 1970 to 1977. The mean birth length in both sexes was 48 cm, and a final height of 161.5 cm for boys and 147.5 cm for girls ages 15 and 16 was found. Average height at age 16 years developed by Crocker et al. (1988) for girls with Down syndrome was 145 cm and for boys, 155 cm. The Swedish study found that European boys with Down syndrome are taller than corresponding American boys, although European girls with Down syndrome have similar height to corresponding American girls. Specific growth curves have now been developed in the United Kingdom, Saudi Arabia, and Japan.

Various factors have been listed as contributing factors for less growth in height, including congenital heart disease, hypotonia, hypothyroidism, and hip dysplasia. Growth hormone (GH) therapy has become a clinical option for the child with Down syndrome, but research studies are in the beginning stages. Annernen et al. (2000) compared the use of GH therapy between PWS and Down syndrome and found the mean height of the Down syndrome child changing from –1.7 to –0.8 standard deviations. The mean height of the control group fell from –1.7 to 2.2 standard deviations. One of the conclusions of this study was that GH is not recommended for children with Down syndrome who have not been diagnosed with GH deficiency. Although height increased in the study, there was no change in head circumference, gross motor development, or mental development. There was some improvement in fine motor development.

Energy Needs

Children with Down syndrome have a high prevalence of obesity related to their metabolic rate, lowered gross motor activity, low muscle tone, and poor dietary practices. Recent studies on the energy needs of the Down syndrome child are limited. Luke and colleagues (1994) investigated the relationship between energy expenditure and obesity in a study exploring body composition, resting metabolic rate, and total energy expenditure for 13 prepubescent children with Down syndrome and in 10 control subjects matched for age, weight, and percentage of fat. Indirect calorimetry and doubly labeled water were used. Measurement of resting metabolic rate was complicated by excessive movement by both the

Down syndrome subjects and the control subjects. The investigators calculated a corrected resting metabolic rate and found the value significantly lower in the Down syndrome children than in the control group when expressed as a percentage of the World Health Organization basal metabolic rate: 79.5% ± 10.4% and 96.8% ± 7.8%, respectively. No significant differences were detected in daily energy expenditure or non–resting metabolic rate expenditure between the subject groups.

In contrast to the work of Luke et al. (1994), a more recent study of adults with Down syndrome (Fernhall et al., 2005) comparing the basal metabolic rate of 22 individuals with Down syndrome to 20 nondisabled control subjects of similar age (25.7 and 27.4, respectively) showed no differences in basal metabolic rate. One older study was completed to investigate energy intake related to body composition in the Down syndrome population (Luke, Sutton, Schoeller, & Roizen, 1996). They measured nutrient intake and body composition in prepubescent children and 10 nondisabled children. The subjects with Down syndrome were significantly shorter than the control subjects, body composition did not differ between the groups, and reported energy intake was low in subjects with Down syndrome, at less than 80% of the Recommended Dietary Allowance. The investigators concluded that the tendency for obesity in the Down syndrome child should be treated with a balanced diet with no energy restriction and increased physical activity.

> **Down Syndrome Research**
>
> Whitt-Glover, O'Neill, and Stettler (2006) investigated physical activity in Down syndrome children and their siblings between 3 and 10 years of age. Results of this study, which used accelerometers for 7 days, were that the Down syndrome children accumulated less vigorous intensity activity than their siblings ($p = 0.04$) and for shorter periods of time ($p < 0.01$). Child feeding practices were also evaluated (O'Neill, Shults, Stallings, & Stettler, 2005) to find their relationship to weight status among children with Down syndrome and their unaffected siblings. The study included 36 children with Down syndrome and 36 children without Down syndrome between 3 and 10 years of age. A child feeding questionnaire was completed assessing six aspects of control in feeding. Anthropometric measures were completed with height and weight and calculation of a body mass index (BMI) score and the BMI z-score. Mean BMI z-scores were higher for the children with Down syndrome than for their siblings. Parents' perceptions of feeding included greater use of restriction, greater feelings of responsibility for feeding and concern about child weight status, and lower pressure for the child with Down syndrome to eat than for their siblings. It was concluded that differences in child feeding practices may play a role in the development of obesity in Down syndrome.

Nutrient Needs

Numerous studies have shown biochemical and metabolic abnormalities in individuals with Down syndrome; however, many have involved small samples and were difficult to interpret (Capone, Muller, & Ekvall, 2005). Although serum concentrations of albumin have been found to be low, the guidelines from the Down Syndrome Medical Congress do not list serum albumin assessment as routine. Increased glucose levels have been reported, with one study reporting an increased incidence of diabetes mellitus (Van Goor, Massa, & Hirasing, 1997).

A number of studies looked at zinc, copper, and selenium status, with some reporting reduced zinc and selenium levels and conflicting plasma levels of copper (Anni et al., 2000). These studies, along with multiple studies involving vitamin A, carotene, and vitamin D, concluded that these deficiencies do not exist. Studies involving vitamin E reported decreased concentrations in Down syndrome (Shah & Johnson, 1989). It is suggested that trisomy 21 predisposes to increased oxidative stress and the increased use of antioxidants protect against the stress, thus the low levels of vitamin E, an antioxidant. This theory of oxidative stress has led parents of individuals with Down syndrome to purchase many vitamin supplements with the expected outcome of improved cognitive ability and growth. At this point there is no conclusive evidence that supplementation is effective.

Dietary Intake

During infancy the food intake of the infant with Down syndrome may differ from the normal infant. Although human breast milk is recommended, many infants with Down syndrome are formula-fed. Pisacane et al. (2003) found that of 560 children with Down syndrome, 57% were formula fed versus 24% of nonaffected infants. The main reasons reported by the mothers were infants' illness and admission to the neonatal unit, frustration or depression, perceived milk insufficiency, and difficulty in suckling by the infant. It has been this author's experience that the problems with sucking and latching onto the breast have been the deciding factors in the use of formula rather than breast-feeding, although use of the pump is an option.

Progression to solid food has been found to be delayed in children with Down syndrome, mostly due to delays in feeding and motor development (Hopman et al., 1998). Introduction of solid food may not be offered at 4 to 6 months if the infant has poor head control or is not yet sitting up. Low tone and sucking problems also delay weaning from the breast or bottle to the cup. Early intervention programs include feeding and feeding progression instruction and practice.

Feeding Skills

Feeding skills are delayed in the infant and child with Down syndrome. Some parents found difficulty in initiating oral motor skills such as suckling and sucking. The infant with Down syndrome often has difficulty in coordinating sucking, swallowing, and breathing, the foundation for early feeding. When the infant has a congenital heart defect, which occurs in 40% to 60% of the Down syndrome infants, sucking is weakened and fatigue interferes with the feeding process. Gastrointestinal anomalies are found in 8% to 12% of infants with Down syndrome, and these infants often require nasogastric or gastrostomy feedings.

Other physical factors that make feeding difficult in the first years of life include a midfacial hypoplasia, a small oral cavity, a small mandible, delayed or abnormal dentition, malocclusion, nasal congestion, small hands, and short fingers. Weaning and self-feeding are usually late when compared with the nonaffected infant and frequently do not emerge until 15 to 18 months of age. The Down syndrome infant strives for independence and autonomy about 6 months later than the child without Down syndrome.

Nutrition Problems and Intervention

Weight Status

The most effective intervention for the overweight child with Down syndrome is to design a well-balanced diet

---

Special Olympics Serves Diversity

Special Olympics is a program for children and adults with special needs that now reaches 2,256,733 participants across the world. Areas involved include Africa, Asia Pacific, East Asia, Europe/Eurasia, Latin America, Middle East, and North America.

More than 67% of the participants are under age 22. Sports training and athletic competitions constitute the core of the organization's activities and include athletics, basketball, football, bowling, and aquatics.

The global Special Olympics movement began in July 1968 when the first international games were held in Chicago. The concept for Special Olympics began in 1962 through the efforts of Eunice Kennedy Shriver when she started a day camp for people with intellectual disabilities at her home. Through the efforts of the Kennedy Foundation and her leadership, Special Olympics began and grew. Many associations such as the American Dental Association and the American Dietetic Association are involved in the various competitions providing evaluations and nutrition education.

---

without energy restriction, with vitamin and mineral supplementation, and with increased physical activity (Luke et al., 1996). Dietary management includes assessing the feeding developmental level of the child, working with a physical therapist related to gross motor skills to determine possible activity levels, and making environmental changes. Environmental changes should include following a regular eating schedule of three meals at regular times with the child sitting either in a high chair or at the table and planned low-fat and low-sugar snacks, matching the child's feeding development. Soft drinks should be drastically limited, and milk should be low fat (after age 2). Physical activity should be encouraged. Counseling with the parent helps determine a realistic plan that focuses on serving sizes and food preparation and decreases the number of times meals are purchased in fast food restaurants. If the child or

adolescent is school age, a special meal at school can be obtained by using the school food service prescription (see Sidebar: Community Resources).

Feeding Skills

Often, parents erroneously expect different feeding development for the child with Down syndrome. Behavioral problems related to feeding usually develop based on what happens between the parent and child at mealtime. An example of this is the unnecessary delay of weaning to a cup or avoidance of progression of food textures because of inadequate effort or education needed to enable this in the Down syndrome child. During intervention programs the feeding team can guide the parent in positioning the child and working toward attainable feeding skills related to the developmental level of the child. Close attention should be paid to feeding and the development of self-feeding skills.

Constipation

This is a frequent problem for the child with Down syndrome because of overall low tone, followed by lack of fiber and fluid in the diet. Treatment should involve increasing fiber and fluid, with water consumption emphasized. Fiber content of the diet for children after age 3 is 5 to 6 g per year of age per day. For adults the recommendation is 25 to 30 g dietary fiber/day (see Case Study 1, below).

Prader-Willi Syndrome

Prader-Willi syndrome was first described in 1956 by Drs. Prader, Willi, and Lambert. It is a genetic condition caused by the absence of chromosomal material from chromosome 15. PWS occurs with a frequency of 1 in 10,000 to 25,000 live births. Characteristics of the syndrome include developmental delays, poor muscle tone, short stature, small hands and feet, incomplete sexual development, and unique facial features. Insatiable appetite leading to obesity is the classic feature of PWS; however, in infancy the problem of hypotonia interferes with feeding and leads to failure to thrive (McCune & Driscoll, 2005).

The genetic basis of PWS is complex. Individuals with PWS have a portion of genetic material deleted from chromosome 15 received from the father. Seventy percent of the cases of PWS are caused from the paternal deletion, occurring in a specific

> **Prader-Willi syndrome (PWS):** A genetic condition caused by an absence of material from the 15th chromosome. Characteristics include developmental delays, low motor tone, and an insatiable appetite.

region on the q arm of the chromosome. PWS can also develop if a child receives both chromosome 15s from the mother. This is seen in approximately 25% of the cases of PWS and is called maternal uniparental disomy. Early detection of PWS is now possible due to the use of DNA methylation analysis, which can correctly diagnose 99% of the cases (McCune & Driscoll, 2005). This is an important development in the early identification and subsequent treatment of these children to prevent obesity and growth retardation. It is selected for use at birth for the infant born with the features and characteristics described above (McCune & Driscoll, 2005).

GH Research

GH therapy was approved by the U.S. Food and Drug Administration in 2000. In a 5-year study in Japan (Obata, Sakazume, Yoshino, Murakami, & Sakuta, 2003), 37 children with PWS from ages 3 to 21 years were evaluated for height velocity, final height, BMI, and Röhrer index. After 1 year of treatment, the mean height velocity improved significantly from 4.32 to 8.69 cm/yr ($p < 0.0001$). After 5 years the mean standard deviation score increased from –0.99 to + 0.88 ($p = 0.003$). A U.S. study (Carrel et al., 2004) investigated body composition and motor development in 29 infants and toddlers with PWS aged 4 to 37 months who were randomized for GH treatment for 12 months. The GH treated subjects, compared with control subjects, demonstrated decreased percent body fat ($p < 0.001$), increased lean body mass ($p < 0.001$), and increased height velocity z-scores ($p < 0.001$). Children who started GH treatment before 18 months of age showed higher mobility skill acquisition compared with control subjects in the same age range ($p < 0.05$). These data have encouraged the use of GH in children with PWS.

Metabolic Abnormalities

Short stature in the individual with PWS has been attributed to GH deficiency. In addition to decreased GH release, children have low serum insulin-like growth factor-I, low insulin-like growth factor binding protein-1, and low insulin compared with normal obese children.

In addition to GH deficiency, individuals with PWS have a deficiency in the hypothalamic-pituitary-gonadal axis causing delayed and incomplete sexual development. Finally, there is a decreased insulin response to a glucose load in children with PWS compared with age-matched obese children without PWS (Schuster, Osei, & Zipf, 1996).

Appetite and Obesity

Appetite control and obesity are common problems with individuals with PWS. After the initial period of failure to thrive, children begin to gain excessively between the ages of 1 and 4, and appetite is excessive. This uncontrollable appetite, a classic feature of PWS, when combined with overeating, a low basal metabolic rate, and decreased activity, leads to the characteristic obesity. The cause of the uncontrollable appetite involves the hypothalamus and the parvocellular oxytocin neurons, which are decreased in the brains of those afflicted with PWS (Swaab, Purba, & Hofman, 1995). Other hormones and peptides related to appetite control in animals were not found to be increased in the hypothalamus of individuals with PWS (Goldstone et al., 2002). Developmental delays (affecting 50% of the population), learning disabilities, and mental retardation (affecting 10%) are associated with PWS.

Body composition is an important consideration in the evaluation of individuals with PWS. They have abnormal body composition, decreased lean body mass, and increased body fat, even in infancy. In a study of 16 infants (Bext et al., 2003) the percent of body fat was significantly increased ($p < 0.001$) and the percent of fat-free mass significantly decreased in both male and female subjects ($p \leq 0.001$, $p = 0.04$) with decreased energy expenditure. The conclusion was that the lower energy expenditure is caused by the decreased fat-free mass. Body fat is generally deposited in the thighs, buttocks, and abdominal area. The lowered energy expenditure is also found in young children, adolescents, and adults with PWS. One study found adolescents with PWS having a total energy expenditure 53% of that of nonaffected obese adolescents (McCune & Driscoll, 2005). The low muscle tone contributes greatly to the lack of interest in physical activity.

Nutrition Assessment

Anthropometrics

As stated earlier, height measurements tend to be lower in infants and young children with PWS, with the rate of height gain tapering off between the ages of 1 and 4. The usual measurements of length or height, weight, and head circumference should be taken and plotted on the CDC growth curves (see Appendix 1). Other measures of interest include arm circumference and triceps skinfold measures. BMI may be distorted for the individual with PWS due to short stature; however, plotting the BMI over time is useful in determining unusual changes. It is important that anthropometric measures are done frequently and reported to the parents or caregiver.

Biochemical Measures

Biochemical studies are generally the same for the PWS individual with the exception of either fasting blood glucose tests or glucose tolerance tests. These are added because of the risk for diabetes mellitus, possibly related to the obesity that usually accompanies PWS.

Dietary Intake

Dietary information varies for individuals with PWS depending on their age. In infancy the dietary information should be obtained with a careful dietary history and analyzed for energy and nutrient intake. Infants are commonly difficult to feed because of their hypotonia, poor suck, delayed motor skills, and failure to thrive. Breast-feeding has been limited due to their sucking difficulties. Generally, their feeding development is slower than in normal infants, and transitioning to food at 4 to 6 months of age may be difficult. Many of these infants have gastroesophageal reflux that requires medication or thickening of their formula. During the toddler years, weight gain may increase rapidly as intake increases. Appetite may increase around 1 year of age and continue. This requires careful assessment of portion sizes, frequency of feeding, and types of foods served. Although some parents may report that the child with PWS does not eat more than other children in the family, they need to be informed that energy needs are lower due to the reduced lean muscle mass and slow development of motor skills and activity. As the children get older their interest in food increases, and starting around 5 through 12 they may be hungry all the time and display difficult behaviors such as tantrums, stubbornness, and food stealing. Many parents have found it necessary to lock cabinets, refrigerators, and the kitchen door to control food intake (Dimitropoulos et al., 2001). Information gathered during the dietary interview should include environmental control techniques.

Whitman and colleagues (2002) investigated the impact of GH therapy on behavior problems that have been attributed to the appetite and compulsive desire for food. Previous studies were reported to improve alertness, activity level, endurance, irritability, tendency to worry, and extroversion, resulting in better personal relationships. This study included 54 children with PWS from ages 4 to 16 years. Children with previous GH therapy were excluded as were children with scoliosis greater than 20 degrees. Behavior was monitored at 6-month intervals using the Offord Survey Diagnostic Instrument, which is a 165-item behavioral checklist, and was modified to include 10 items specifically designed for PWS. No differences were found between treatment and control groups for attentional symptoms, anxiety, violence, or psychotic symptoms. A significant positive effect (reduction of depressive symptoms) was noted for the treatment group. The study conclusions were that GH therapy contributes to behavioral improvement, an important outcome related to programs designed to prevent or treat obesity in this population.

Determination of energy needs for the infant with PWS is the same as for a normal infant. However, as the child enters the toddler years he or she needs fewer calories to maintain weight gain along the growth curve. This also applies in adulthood, when fewer calories are needed to maintain weight. Energy needs have been calculated according to centimeters of height from 2 years on. The macronutrient intake of the diet should be 25% protein, 50% carbohydrate, and 25% fat.

Feeding Skills

The infant with PWS often presents with weak oral skills and poor sucking skills in the first year of life. As the child matures feeding skills are not a problem, but they may be delayed. Chewing and swallowing problems are not widely found, although they may be associated with low muscle tone. Behavioral feeding issues are associated with an insatiable appetite and not being provided with food. As stated earlier, this can bring about tantrums.

Intervention Strategies

Intervention for PWS involves several age stages: infancy, toddler and preschool age, school age, and adult. In infancy, providing adequate nutrition as established by the AAP related to breast-feeding or formula feeding is recommended. Because feeding may be difficult related to sucking, concentrating the formula or breast milk may be necessary to promote adequate weight gain. Feeding intervention assists in improving the sucking problems caused by hypotonia. As the infant matures a concentrated formula is not necessary, and foods can be added when head control and trunk stability are achieved, usually around 4 to 6 months.

Most toddler and preschool age children begin to gain excessive weight between 1 and 4 years of age. Beginning a structured dietary protocol for the child and the family is important so that the toddler learns that meals are provided at specified times and a pattern of grazing does not develop. Parents should be taught to provide small servings of meats, vegetables, grains, and fruits and limited intakes of sweets. The importance of early intervention for these children in the preschool years is very important in working with feeding issues and intake control as they grow older. Weight, height, and nutrient intake should be monitored monthly and energy needs adjusted if weight gain becomes excessive. Concurrently, physical activity must be encouraged as a part of early intervention programs and physical therapy services made available if necessary.

For the school age child, collaboration with the school food service program becomes important. Energy needs should be calculated per centimeter of height and are generally 50% to 75% of the energy needs of unaffected children. This may require using the prescription for special meals through the school food service program. At home, environmental controls may be required with locked cupboards and refrigerators, because the child and adolescent have limited satiety and search for food away from mealtime. Some parents say that GH therapy for their child helps, but it does not seem to change the child's lack of satiety. Appetite suppressing medications have been used but are largely unsuccessful.

Medical nutrition therapy of children and adults with PWS requires follow-up through many health care providers and schools. Fortunately, parents of the individual with PWS now have access to a number of support groups and organizations dedicated to education, research, and establishing treatment programs.

Neurologic Disorders

Spina Bifida

Spina bifida: A neurologic tube defect caused by a lesion in the spinal cord that occurs during the formation of the spinal cord.

Spina bifida is a neurologic tube defect that presents in a number of ways: meningocele, myelomeningocele, and spina bifida occulta. Myelomeningocele is the most common derangement in the formation of the spinal cord and generally occurs between 26 and 30 days gestation with the date of occurrence affecting the location of the lesion. The lesion may occur in the thoracic, lumbar, or sacral area and influences the amount of paralysis. The higher the lesion, the greater the paralysis. Manifestations range from weakness in the lower extremities to complete paralysis and loss of sensation. Other manifestations include incontinence and hydrocephalus. The incidence of spina bifida is 1 per 1,000 births, whereas the incidence of myelomeningocele is 5 per 10,000 in the United States. It is found more frequently in whites than in African-Americans or Asian-Americans and more frequently in girls than in boys, with a ratio of 1.25:1.00 (Ekvall & Cerniglia, 2005). The spinal lesion may be open and can be surgically repaired shortly after birth, usually within 24 hours to prevent infection. Although the spinal opening can be surgically repaired, the nerve damage is permanent, resulting in the varying degrees of paralysis of the lower limbs. In addition to physical and mobility issues, most individuals have some form of learning disability.

Prevention of spina bifida is now possible (Stevenson, Allen, & Pai, 2000). In 1983 Smithells and coworkers published results of a multilevel study involving the preconceptional supplementation of mothers with folic acid plus multivitamins. This reduced the risk of a second pregnancy with spina bifida as an outcome. As a result of numerous studies showing folic acid supplementation before conception to be effective, the national recommendation is 400 μg/day for all women of childbearing age. These studies resulted in the addition of folic acid to many flours and other cereal and grain products in the food supply (U.S. Department of Health and Human Services, U.S. Food and Drug Administration, 1996). These public health measures have resulted in increased folic acid blood levels in U.S. women of childbearing age and a decrease of 20% in the national rate of spina bifida (Williams et al., 2005).

Health Concerns

The spinal lesion affects many systems of the body and can result in weakness in the lower extremities, paralysis and nonambulation, poor skin condition due to pressure sores, loss of sensation and bladder incontinence, hydrocephalus, urinary tract infections, constipation, and obesity. Seizures occur in approximately 20% of children with myelomeningocele and require medication. Chronic medication is also required for prevention and treatment of urinary tract infections and for bladder control. The resulting nutrition problems include obesity, feeding problems, constipation, and drug–nutrient interaction problems. Children with spina bifida can become allergic to latex brought about by multiple surgeries. It is recommended that children with spina bifida avoid certain foods, such as bananas, kiwi, and avocados. Mild reactions can occur from apples, carrots, celery, tomatoes, papaya, and melons (Cloud et al., 2005).

Nutrition Assessment

Anthropometrics

Infants and children with neural tube defects are usually shorter because of reduced length and atrophy of the lower extremities, although other problems such as hydrocephalus, scoliosis, renal disease, and malnutrition may contribute to it. The level of the lesions can also affect the length and height of the individual.

Obtaining accurate length and height measures can be difficult, especially as the child grows older. An alternate measure for determining height, the arm span to height ratio, is used and modified depending on leg muscle mass. Arm span can be used directly as a height measure (arm span $\times$ 1.0) if there is no leg muscle mass loss, as in a sacral lesion. Arm span $\times$ 0.95 can be used to determine height if there is partial leg muscle loss, and arm span $\times$ 0.90 is used for a height measurement when there is complete leg muscle loss, such as with a thoracic spinal lesion (Ekvall & Cerniglia, 2005).

Weight measures can be obtained for the child unable to stand by using chair scales, bucket scales, and wheelchair scales. In a clinical situation weight should be obtained in a consistent manner, with the person in light clothing or undressed to obtain an accurate weight. Triceps skinfold measurements can also be used along with subscapular and abdominal and thorax measurements to determine the amount of body fat.

Head circumference should be measured in infants and toddlers up to age 3. A high percentage of children with spina bifida have head shunts due to their hydrocephalus. Unusual changes in the size of the head may indicate a problem with the shunt.

Biochemical Measures

Most protocols in the treatment of spina bifida include iron status tests, measurements of vitamin C and zinc levels, and other tests related to the nutritional consequences of medications needed for seizures and urinary tract infection control.

Dietary Intake

Many children with spina bifida eat a limited variety of foods and are frequently described as "picky eaters" by the parents. When doing a dietary history it is important to ask about the variety of foods, particularly of high fiber foods. The school age child may be prone to skipping breakfast because early morning preparations for school require more time than for the nonaffected child.

Energy needs are lower for the child with spina bifida, and calorie requirements must be carefully determined to prevent the obesity to which many are prone. Ekvall and Cerniglia (2005) found that for children 8 years or older with myelomeningocele, the caloric need is 7 kcal/cm of height for weight loss and 9 to 11 kcal/cm of height to maintain weight. It is important to evaluate how the mother or caregiver perceives food for the child, because it represents sympathy and love for many parents.

Fluid intake is very important to evaluate because so many children have urinary tract infections and may be drinking inadequate amounts of water and excessive amounts of soft drinks, tea, and so on. Physical activity must also be evaluated and may be found to be very limited, particularly when the child is nonambulatory. Ambulatory individuals with a shunt may be restricted from contact sports but can be involved in walking and running.

Feeding skills need to be evaluated, along with oral motor function in particular. Many children with spina bifida are born with the **Arnold-Chiari malformation of the brain** that affects the brainstem and swallowing. Swallowing may be difficult and contributes to the child avoiding certain foods later in life. Because of this there may be delays in weaning from the breast or bottle to the cup, but there should be no delays in gaining self-feeding skills.

Arnold-Chiari malformation of the brain: A structural disorder affecting the cerebellum, frequently found in spina bifida; can affect swallowing and gagging.

Clinical Evaluation

This evaluation should include examination of the skin due to pressure sores, along with asking the amount and type of fluids consumed. Cranberry juice has been recommended along with vitamin C to provide a urine pH of 5.5 to 6; however, cranberry juice has been discounted by some literature reviews. Constipation may be caused by the neurogenic bowel and a diet low in fiber and fluids. The evaluation should include a review of food intake, fiber content, and fluids.

Intervention Strategies

From a nutritional standpoint, many children with spina bifida have obesity as the number one problem because of the impact of other physical problems. It usually occurs when ambulation is a problem and there is a lack of awareness of energy needs coupled with a lack of exercise. Other problems include inadequate fluids and fiber and refusal to accept a wide variety of foods. Feeding is frequently a problem and can be both behavioral and oral motor. Early intervention and counseling about introducing foods around age 6 months, limiting the intake of high sucrose infant jar foods, and training the child in accepting a wide variety of flavors and textures is important.

Obesity prevention should include addressing the problems with limited physical activity and lack of fluids and fiber and should begin with a calculation of the appropriate amount of calories and fluid. If the child is overweight, the food service manager should be provided with a prescription for a low calorie breakfast and lunch, and weight management should be listed as a part of the individualized education plan. Enrollment in a group weight management program has been used successfully with modification of the accompanying physical exercise. The ideal program uses a team approach with involvement of the physician, dietitian, nurse, occupational therapist, physical therapist, educator, and psychologist.

In many clinics serving the child or adult with spina bifida, clients are seen on semiannual or annual basis. This frequent follow-up is necessary and should include monitoring of growth, particularly weight; food and fluid intake; and medication use. School programs and early intervention programs are excellent follow-up sites; however, often the school lacks appropriate scales for weighing a non-ambulatory student. In this situation parents should be encouraged to bring the child to the clinic for weight checks or, if distance is a problem, to find a long term care facility that permits using their scales. Follow-up by phone contact or e-mail can be done for evaluating dietary intake and fluid management.

Cerebral Palsy

Cerebral palsy: A disorder of motor control or coordination resulting from injury to the brain during its early development.

Cerebral palsy is a disorder of motor control or coordination resulting from injury to the brain during its early development. Among the causative agents of CP are prematurity, blood type incompatibility, placental insufficiency, maternal infection that includes German measles or other viral diseases, neonatal jaundice, anoxia at birth, and other bacterial infections of the mother, fetus, or infant that affect the central nervous system. The problem in CP lies in the brain's inability to control the muscles, even though the muscles themselves and the nerves connecting them to the spinal cord are normal. The extent and location of the brain injury determine the type and distribution of CP. The incidence of CP varies with different studies, but the most commonly used rate is 1.5 to 2 per 1,000 live births. The increasing prevalence of premature births has contributed to an increase in this figure (Winter, Autry, Boyle, & Yeargin-Allsop, 2002).

Various types of CP are classified according to the neurologic signs involving muscle tone, abnormal motor patters, and postures. The diagnosis of CP is generally made between 9 and 12 months of age and as late as 2 years with some types. The various types of CP include spastic, dyskinetic, mixed, and ataxia of CP (Ekvall & Cerniglia, 2005).

Health Concerns

Poor nutritional status and growth failure, often related to feeding problems, are common in children with CP. Meeting energy needs is particularly difficult in those children and adults with more severe forms of CP, such as **spastic quadriplegia** and athetoid CP. Assessment of the bone mineral density of children and adolescents with moderate to severe CP showed lower scores associated with gross motor function and feeding difficulty (Henderson, Kairalla, Barrington, Abbas, & Stevenson, 2005). One hundred seven participants (aged 2 years, 1 month to 21 years, 1 month) with moderate to severe spastic CP were assessed for anthropometric measures of growth and nutrition and dual energy x-ray absorptiometry measures of bone mineral density. Seventeen participants were ambulatory, and 90 had little or no ambulation. The weight z-score proved to be the best predictor of bone mineral density, an important indicator of a nutritional risk factor. Other factors related to the bone mineral density score included a history of fractures, anticonvulsant medication, and feeding difficulties.

Spastic quadriplegia: Spastic paralysis of the arms and legs.

Constipation is another health problem and may be caused by inactivity, lack of fiber and fluids, and feeding problems. Dental problems occur and are often related to malocclusion, dental irregularities, and fractured teeth. Lengthy and prolonged bottle feedings of milk and juice promote the decay of the primary upper front teeth and molars. Hearing problems and especially visual impairments, mental retardation, respiratory problems, and seizures impact nutritional status. Seizures are controlled with anticonvulsants, and a number of drug nutrient interaction problems occur.

Nutrition Assessment

Anthropometrics

This is an important area of assessment because of the growth failure of the more severely involved child or adult with CP. Children with CP are often shorter, and depending on the level of severity, some children with CP may need to be measured for length using **recumbent length** boards or standing boards even as they grow older. However, some of

Recumbent length: Measuring the length of an individual lying down.

the measuring devices are inappropriate for the child with contractures and inability to be stretched out full length. Arm span can be used when the individual's arms are stretchable, as well as upper arm length and lower leg length. Hogan (1999) and Stevenson (2005) recommended lower leg length or knee height as a possible measure for determining height for both children and adults with lower leg CP. Krick et al. (1996) developed growth charts for children with CP using weight and length data on 360 children; however, the CDC training module on use of the growth curves for children from birth to 20 years of age recommends using the CDC curves, designed for nonaffected children, and plotting sequentially for indications of malnutrition rather than using the disease specific curves.

Stevenson et al. (2006) completed a six-site, multicentered, region-based, cross-sectional study of children with moderate or severe CP. There were 273 children enrolled (71% white) and the anthropometric measures included weight, knee height, upper arm length, upper arm muscle area, triceps skinfold, and subscapular skinfold. Growth curves were developed and z-scores published for each of the six measures. Pilot studies will be conducted on the validity of the growth curves before they are distributed. Current results indicated that from the growth data collected, the most positive measures were found in children with the fewest days of health care use and fewest days of social participation missed.

Weight measures should be collected over time. Scales may require modifications with positioning devices for the individual with CP who has developed scoliosis, contractures, and spasticity. Working with a physical therapist to find a positioning device that can be placed in a chair scale or using a bucket scale often works well. Mid-upper arm circumference and triceps skinfold measures are reported by Samson-Fang and Stevenson (2000) as the recommended way to screen for fat stores in children with CP. Head circumference should be measured regularly from birth to 36 months and plotted on the CDC growth curves.

Biochemical Measures

Although there are no specific laboratory values indicated for the child with CP, a complete blood count, including hemoglobin and hematocrit, should be done when food intake is limited and malnutrition is a possibility. Because bone fractures are a significant problem for many children and adults with spastic quadriplegia, bone mineral density may need to be evaluated. Medications for seizures may be given, and many have nutrition interaction problems. Evaluation of vitamin D, calcium, carnitine, and vitamin K levels may be indicated (King, Levin, Schmidt, Oestreich, & Heubi, 2003).

Dietary Intake

Feeding may be an important problem that limits the intake of food and fluid, and caregivers may not provide sufficient food to meet nutritional needs. The energy needs of the individual with CP vary according to the type of CP. Studies show that the resting metabolic rate and total energy expenditure are lower in those with spastic quadriplegic CP than in normal control subjects (Bandini, Schneller, Fukagana, Wykes, & Dietz, 1991; Stallings, Zemel, Davies, Cronk, & Charney, 1996). Bandini et al. (1995) recommended that measures of energy intake should be adjusted for changes in body weight to determine energy requirements for the individual with severe CP. Stallings et al. (1996) found total energy expenditure in the child with spastic quadriplegic CP in a ratio to resting energy expenditure significantly lower in the spastic quadriplegic CP children compared with a control group. Dietary intake was markedly over-reported by caregivers. Stallings et al. concluded that growth failure and an abnormal pattern of resting energy expenditure were related to inadequate energy intake.

Feeding Problems

A high percentage of children with CP have feeding problems that are largely due to oral motor, positioning, and behavioral factors. As infants they have difficulty swallowing and coordinating swallowing and chewing, so the normal progression to solid foods is difficult. All this may lead to inadequate intake and growth limitations. Early detection of the feeding problem was demonstrated by Motion et al. (2002), who investigated the prevalence of feeding difficulties at 4 weeks and 6 months of age in 33 children with CP. Feeding difficulties at 4 weeks of age were associated with a pattern of functional impairment at age 4 years and at 8 years and being clinically underweight and having speech and swallowing difficulties at 8 years of age. Sullivan et al. (2002) studied 100 children (mean age, 9 years) with disabilities related to the impact of feeding problems on nutritional status and growth. Ninety children had a diagnosis of CP. Results confirmed the significant impact of neurologic impairment and oral motor problems on energy intake, leading to poor growth and nutritional status.

Increasing numbers of children with CP with severe feeding problems are tube fed. This usually follows swallowing studies such as the modified barium swallow where there is video fluoroscopy indicating aspiration. Sullivan et al. (2005) reported a longitudinal, prospective, multicenter, cohort study designed to measure the outcomes of gastrostomy tube feeding in children with CP. The study included 57 children with CP (28 girls and 29 boys, median age 4 years 4 month, range 5 months to 17 year 3 months). The children were assessed before gastrostomy placement and at 6 months and 12 months. At baseline, half of the children were more than 3 standard deviations below the average weight for age and gender, when compared with standards for normally developing children. Weight increased over the study period from a median weight z-score of −3 to −2.2 at 6 months and −1.6 at 12 months.

CRITICAL Thinking

Use of Feeding Teams

For those infants and children in early intervention programs, the team of dietitian, speech therapist, occupational therapist, and physical therapist should evaluate the feeding problems and work together in planning therapy. Providing an appropriate formula requires the dietitian to evaluate the caloric and nutritional value of the product selected, determine the amount needed, and work with the parent in obtaining insurance funding. Working out an intervention plan is most successful when it involves the parent as part of the team, addresses cultural issues, and recognizes the importance of the feeding problem (Spiker, 2004).

Children with CP have complex problems that require follow-up with the family and in the community and take time to correct. There are agencies within the state that provide tube feeding formulas, special wheelchairs, and equipment to assist with feeding problems.

Autism

Autism is one of five disorders under the category of pervasive developmental disorder (PDD). PDD was first used in the 1980s to describe a class of disorders: autistic disorders, Rett disorder, childhood disintegrative disorder, Asperger disorder, and PDD not otherwise specified (American Psychiatric Association, 1994). In general, children with PDD have a neurologic disorder usually evident by age 3 characterized by difficulty in talking, playing with other children, and relating to others, including family.

Autism spectrum disorders (ASDs) affect 3.4 per 1,000 (Yeargin-

Autism spectrum disorders (ASDs): A number of disorders that involve poor social interaction, impaired communication skills, a tendency to be repetitive, and sometimes mental retardation; found more in males than in females.

Allsopp et al., 2003) and are diagnosed by the presence of qualitatively impaired reciprocal social interaction, impaired communication skills, and restricted, repetitive, stereotypical interests and behaviors. Many children with autism also have mental retardation. Autistic disorder is four times more common in boys than in girls. Asperger syndrome is most often used to describe children with the problems of ASDs but who have normal to high cognitive level (Autism Society of America, 1995).

ASDs may occur with other developmental or physical disabilities. They have been associated with tuberous sclerosis, maternal rubella, and mental retardation. Macrocephaly has been a common finding in large surveys of individuals with autism and also among their relatives. Overall growth is usually normal and medical problems nonexistent. It is possible that with the limited variety of foods usually eaten by these children, that vitamin and mineral intake could be inadequate.

Efforts to find the cause of ASDs have led to many studies to look at a possibly toxic environment, toxic food, a nutritionally deficient diet, immune system problems, oxidative stress, and emotional stress as important factors. Other studies have studied neurotransmitters such as elevated serotonin levels and disturbances in gamma-aminobutyric acid receptors, glutamate transmitters, and cholinergic activity.

Research studies are needed to find a major link between heredity and neuropathology and autism. Some treatment and research programs are using genomic panels to identify specific intervention protocols. The genomic panel identifies single nucleotide polymorphisms that are identified from blood samples or cell cultures. This work has revealed that the child with autism may need additional essential fatty acids; nutrients with antioxidant qualities such as vitamins A, C, and E and selenium; mineral supplementation with zinc, calcium, and magnesium; a mercury-free diet; or an allergy elimination diet.

Interest in a neurochemical cause of ASDs was started in 1979 when Jaak Panksepp proposed that ASDs simulated brain opioid dysfunction. Earlier studies discovered a unique urinary peptide pattern in adults with ASDs and hypothesized that brain opioids came from an exogenous source. Gluten and casein were the suspected sources, and in the 1980s researchers found these urinary peptides in the urine and cerebrospinal fluid of autistic individuals (Reichelt & Knivsberg, 2003). The condition of the intestine has played a role in this theory, with constipation and diarrhea common in the individual with ASDs. Intestinal inflammation has been reported in children with ASDs and has reportedly improved with dietary restriction of gluten and casein (Knivsberg et al., 2003).

Nutrition Assessment

Anthropometrics

Height and weight are determined for the child and adult with ASDs using the equipment and growth charts for nonaffected individuals. Head circumference should be taken and has been found to be larger than for the individual without ASDs.

Biochemical Measures

These tests vary depending on the clinic where the child is followed. There is no standard pattern of tests that should be given, other than the regular blood work for health monitoring. However, amino acid screening shortly after birth is indicated along with thyroid testing. For some children allergy testing may be indicated.

Dietary Intake

Evaluations are sometimes difficult to complete for the child with a very limited intake. An effective measure may be to have parents and caregivers keep a food diary for several days to determine the macronutrient intake in addition to the vitamin and mineral intake. Obtaining information related to when food is presented and the amounts eaten is important along with fluid consumption. Often, excessive fluids are provided to compensate for limited food consumption.

Evaluations should include an observation of the child during mealtime. Some children will be slow in arriving at developmental milestones for self-feeding and will require feeding. Others will finger feed or insist on self-feeding. The texture of the food presented should be recorded because sensory integration is difficult for children with ASDs, and they may be very resistant to texture progression or variety. This is reflected in their fixation on one food, for example, crackers, dry cereal, or chips. Fugassi et al. (2003) found that 70% of 87 children with autism had food jags and were picky eaters. The feeding evaluation should also include a description of the feeding environment, whether there is a high chair or age-appropriate toddler chair, the timing of meals, and the location for meals.

Intervention Strategies

No one therapy or method works for all individuals with ASDs. Conventional treatments include behavior management and medications, whereas others consist of structured educational approach, speech therapy, and occupational therapy. Popular nutrition interventions include mineral and vitamin therapy, elimination diets such as the gluten-free casein-free diet, allergy identification, adding essential fatty acids, megavitamins (Lucas, 2002), and specific diets. Very little has been published to demonstrate the value of the diets, although there are anecdotal reports of success. The exclusion diets are now used in some treatment centers and are publicized on various websites. It is important for the nutrition professional to understand these various forms of therapy to counsel the parent effectively. In addition, with the increasing prevalence of ASDs, research of potential medical nutrition therapy should be promoted based on evidence-based practice.

One of the problems with the gluten-free casein-free diet is cost, because special foods needed to provide sufficient food choices are expensive and sometimes difficult to find. When medical nutrition therapy is used, taking a team approach and working with the occupational therapist, speech therapist, and other members of the team is important for success. Parents also should be members of the team and counseled that changes take time.

> **● Learning Point** Follow-up is an important component of all therapy. From a nutritional standpoint, routine measures of height and weight should be scheduled, and there should be regular evaluation of eating and feeding behavior related to increasing ability to self-feed and to accept new and different foods. Children with autism and PDD are at increased nutritional risk because of the limited variety of foods eaten, mealtime behavior problems, elimination diets, food allergy/sensitivity/intolerance, and chronic gastrointestinal disorders.

Attention Deficit Hyperactivity Disorder

Attention deficit hyperactivity disorder is a neurobehavioral problem seen in children with increasing frequency. It has been associated with learning disorders and inappropriate degrees of impulsiveness, hyperactivity, and attention deficit. Diagnostic criteria developed by the American Psychiatric Association have designated three types: (1) combined type of hyperactivity and attention deficit, (2) predominately inattentive type, and (3) predominately hyperactive-impulse type. ADHD affects the child at home, in school, and in social situations.

> **Attention deficit hyperactivity disorder (ADHD):** Neurobehavioral problem associated with learning disorders, hyperactivity, attention deficit, and inappropriate degrees of impulsiveness.

Nutrition Assessment

Many factors should be considered along with the usual anthropometric measures, particularly when the individual is on medication.

Anthropometric Measures

Measurements of height and weight should be taken and recorded on a regular basis, because the medications used in treatment may cause anorexia if given at inappropriate times, resulting in inadequate energy intake and potential slowing of growth.

Biochemical Measures

These measurements should include a complete blood count and blood and tissue levels of vitamin and minerals if megavitamin therapy is used.

Dietary Intake

A detailed dietary history should be taken to include infant feeding history, food likes and dislikes, behavior at mealtimes, snacking behavior, food allergies or food intolerances, and special diets. If the individual is on medications, the time of administration in relation to mealtime is important. Information should be obtained regarding any specific diet for the child or individual and how closely it is being followed.

Feeding evaluations should include observing the individual at mealtime. Generally, the problems around feeding are behavioral and do not include oral motor or positioning peculiarities. Evaluating the environment around mealtime is important because distractions can be problematic.

Intervention Strategies

Current treatment may include psychotropic medications and following consistent behavioral management techniques. The timing and type of medication must be adjusted so that there is minimal influence on the child's dietary intake.

For the child or adult who is up and down throughout the meal, behavior modification may be indicated, and it should be a part of the overall behavioral management program. Distractions should be eliminated.

The most effective treatment for the individual with ADHD is a diet based on wholesome foods as outlined in the Dietary Guidelines or My Pyramid. The food should be served at regular times, with small servings followed by refills. This is an important concept because of the tendency of the child or individual to eat very small amounts and leave the table, planning to return or graze throughout the day. Some programs recommend removing the food and returning it only once after explaining why this is being done. The intervention requires that the child or individual sit at the table in the high chair away from television or other distractions. These suggestions are most applicable to children in preschool settings and in the school cafeteria or classroom.

It has been suggested that a lack of essential fatty acids is a possible cause of hyperactivity in children. It is more likely the result of varying biochemical influences. These children have a deficiency of essential fatty acids either because they cannot metabolize linoleic acid normally, cannot absorb essential fatty

Special Diets

Specific diets have been used for many years, but they are not based on scientific research. For example, parents have been advised to use the Feingold diet (Feingold, 1974), which states that foods containing synthetic food colors and naturally occurring salicylates be removed from the diet because of their neurologic effect. Other recommendations have included the elimination of sugar, the elimination of caffeine, or the addition of large doses of vitamins (megavitamin therapy). A series of well-designed studies to evaluate the effectiveness of these recommendations has generally had negative results, and successful outcomes are largely anecdotal (Lucas, 2002).

Controversial Nutrition Therapies

An important factor in providing medical nutrition therapy for children with developmental disabilities is realizing that counseling may have been inadequate in helping the parent accept the limitations of the disorder. These limitations may include growth, feeding, and cognitive ability. As a result many parents look for unusual medical or nutritional therapies. A major source of information is often the Internet and parent support groups. Recent media coverage has promoted the use of antioxidant vitamins (A, C, and E) and minerals (zinc, copper, manganese, and selenium) along with the amino acids, glucosamine, tyrosine, and tryptophan. The expected outcome is improved growth; increased cognition, alertness, and attention span; and changed facial features.

There is little scientific information to back these therapies. Research studies have addressed the vitamin needs of children with Down syndrome, spina bifida, fragile X syndrome, and ASDs and findings do not indicate that the vitamin and mineral needs of these child with developmental disabilities are higher than normal (Ani, Grantham-McGregor, & Muller, 2000; Salman, 2002). Numerous historical studies (Bennett, McClelland, Kriegsmann, Andrus, & Sells, 1983) have searched for nutritional deficiencies as causative factors in Down syndrome. Traditionally, the studies have included looking at numerous vitamins, minerals, fatty acids, digestive enzymes, lipotropic nutrients, and numerous drugs with no definitive results.

The key concept in the proposed nutritional interventions for Down syndrome is metabolic correction of genetic overexpression. It is postulated that presence of the third chromosome 21 causes overproduction of superoxide dismutase and cystathionine beta-synthase, which disrupts active methylation pathways. Vitamin supplements of antioxidants counteract this and are considered key to the treatment. However, these are just theories, and at this point nutritional supplements are considered an expensive questionable approach.

Parents of children with ADHD report that omitting sugar from the children's diets decreases hyperactivity, but there is no scientific evidence to support this (MTA Cooperative Group, 1999). However, it probably is a good idea to eliminate or at least reduce the sugar intake in any child's diet to promote better nutritional intake. Blue green algae have been promoted for children with Down syndrome and other developmental disabilities, and monitoring is part of the initiation of these treatments. High dose supplementation of vitamin B_6 and magnesium has been proposed for autism to diminish tantrums and self-stimulation activities and to improve attention and speech (Martineau, Barthelemy, Cheliakine, & Lelord, 1988). Another proposed treatment is dimethyl glycine. Limited research is available to substantiate anything other than anecdotal reports of success (Cornish, 2002).

acids effectively from the intestine, or their essential fatty acid requirements are higher than normal. Older studies showed lower levels of docosahexaenoic acid and arachidonic acid in children with hyperactivity, which have been replicated in more recent studies (Burgess, Stevens, Zhang, & Peck, 2000).

Summary

Generally, healthy infants and toddlers can achieve recommended levels of vitamins and minerals from food alone. Dietetic professionals should encourage caregivers to use foods rather than supplements as the primary source of nutrients in a child's diet. Vitamin and mineral supplements can help infants and toddlers with special nutrient needs or marginal intakes achieve adequate intakes, but care must be taken to ensure supplements do not lead to excessive levels. This is especially important for nutrients that are widely used as food fortifiers, including vitamin A, zinc, and folate.

Despite the success of child survival programs, approximately 12 million children under 5 years old in developing countries still die of preventable causes, half of them of diarrheal diseases and respiratory infections. It is becoming clear that a large portion of the risk of infectious disease morbidity and mortality attributed to malnutrition may result primarily from deficiencies of a few critical micronutrients. Actions needed to control micronutrient deficiencies include prevention strategies, extensive nutrition, and health education through innovative materials to support program-specific problems and strengthening of various state government programs. Interventions to reduce infant and preschool morbidity are a public health priority globally.

The nutritional needs of individuals with developmental disabilities are unique because of differences in body composition, growth, metabolic functions, physical activity, medications, and behavioral issues. Nutrition is an important component of preventing developmental disabilities from occurring; however, more research is needed to identify the role of nutrition as part of the etiology of developmental disorders along with effective intervention strategies.

Issues to Debate

1. Growth charts exist for a number of syndromes such as Down syndrome, CP, PWS, and many others. It has been the position of the CDC that the CDC curves were more appropriate for everyone to use instead of the special growth charts. How would you debate this issue?
2. Many children with developmental disabilities have feeding problems that affect their intake of an adequate diet. Under the regulations for school food service and IDEA the feeding problem would be a part of the child's individualized education plan. Debate the issue of where the intervention should take place: in the school lunch room or in the classroom?
3. Discuss the issue of the most appropriate site for physical activity or physical education for the child with developmental disabilities. Often, this is not adequately addressed in the school system and as a result the child may receive no physical education.

Case Study 1: Developmental Disabilities

MP is a 23 months old boy with Down syndrome who was seen in an early intervention program. He was referred to a dietitian for feeding problems. His history indicated that he was born at 30 weeks gestation with a birth weight of 3 lb 9 oz and birth length of 15¼". Feeding problems at birth consisted of a very weak suck, severe gastroesophageal reflux, and poor weight gain. A gastrostomy tube was placed at 10 days of age and the baby formula iron was given. He was referred to the early intervention program at 4 months of age and services were provided by nutrition, speech therapy, physical therapy, occupational therapy, and special education.

The clinical concerns are as follows:

1. Gastric esophageal reflux was a continuous problem although treated with medication. At 7 months of age fundoplication surgery was completed.
2. Respiratory problems were treated with medications as well.
3. Constipation occurred and was treated with lactulose. Many of his problems were related to extreme hypotonia even for Down syndrome. The hypotonia also contributed to delays in gross motor development.
4. MP's growth was typical for children with Down syndrome and although a major family concern he more than tripled his birth weight (16 lb). He also grew 10 inches in length during the first year. Tube feeding intake was adequate for 100 kcal/kg of body weight, but at 7 months of age (corrected to 4.5 months for prematurity) no food had been introduced for oral intake, which was permissible because head control was good. At that time cereal, strained fruit, and oral formula intake was started along with the tube feeding. Consumption of baby food was never greater than one jar per day. At 16 months, 1 kcal/cc became the tube feeding at the rate of 21 oz/day with discontinuation of the pump at night and some by bottle. Table food was introduced, but acceptance was poor.

5. Feeding problems identified were weak suck and swallow, gagging on food before the fundoplication surgery, tube feeding with progression to oral feeding difficult due to refusal to drink formula and other fluids, and poor appetite due to tube feeding.

What interventions can the medical team make to improve this situation for MP?

Case Study 2: Developmental Disabilities

LR is an infant with PWS, diagnosed shortly after birth and first evaluated by a dietitian at age 2 months. He had a birth weight of 7 lb 5 oz and birth length of 20". Typical of infants with PWS, LR was very hypotonic and had a weak suck and micrognathia. These problems interfered with his ability to breast-feed so his mother pumped her milk and supplemented with formula.

LR's intake at 2 months of age consisted of 9 oz of breast milk and 9 oz of baby formula for a total intake of 360 calories and 9 g of protein. His weight was 8 lb 1.7 oz at the 3rd percentile with his length of 22.5" at the 10th percentile. His intake was approximately 100 kcal/kg. Both parents were extremely concerned with the prevention of obesity and not providing too many calories.

Feeding was observed during the first visit, and the weak suck was very apparent along with leakage from the sides of the mouth. Positioning was inappropriate for promoting good sucking and better head and trunk control.

What recommendations could be made by the medical team?

Websites for Developmental Disabilities

Centers for Disease Control and Prevention www.cdc.gov/ncbdd

National Down Syndrome Society www.ndss.org

Autism Society of America www.autism-society.org

United Cerebral Palsy www.ucp.org

Spina Bifida Association of America www.sbaa.org

Cleft Palate Foundation www.cleftline.org

National Dissemination Center for Children with Disabilities www.nichcy.org

Asperger Syndrome Coalition of the United States www.irsc.org (Interstate Resource for Special Children)

The ARC (advocates for rights and full participation of all children and adults with intellectual and developmental disabilities) www.thearc.org

References

Vitamins and Minerals in Childhood

Adams, J. B., George, F., & Audhya, T. (2006). Abnormally high plasma levels of vitamin B_6 in children with autism not taking supplements compared to controls not taking supplements. *Journal of Alternative and Complementary Medicine, 12*, 59–63.

Ahmed, M., & Jenkins, H. R. (2004). Vitamin B-12 in Crohn's disease patients with small bowel surgery. *Archives of Disease in Childhood, 89*, 293.

Angermayr, L., & Clar, C. (2004). Iodine supplementation for preventing iodine deficiency disorders in children. *Cochrane Database Syst Rev,* (2), CD003819.

Atkinson, S. A. (2001). Special nutritional needs of infants for prevention of and recovery from bronchopulmonary dysplasia. *Journal of Nutrition, 131*, 942S–946S.

Berseth, C. L., Van Aerde, J. E., Gross, S., Stolz, S., Harris, C. L., and Hansen, J. W. (2004). Growth, efficacy and safety of feeding an iron-fortified human milk fortifier. *Pediatrics, 114*, 699–706.

Black, M. M. (2003). Evidence linking zinc deficiency with children's cognitive and motor functioning. *Journal of Nutrition, 133*, 1473S–176S.

Black, M. M., Sazawal, S., Black, R. E., Khosla, S., Kumar, J., & Menon, V. (2004). Cognitive and motor development among small-for-gestational-age infants: Impact of zinc supplementation, birth weight, and caregiving practices. *Pediatrics, 113*, 1297–1305.

Briefel, R., Hanson, C., Fox, M. K., Novak, T., and Ziegler, P. (2006). Feeding Infants and Toddlers Study: do vitamins and mineral supplements contribute to nutrient adequacy or excess among US infants and toddlers? *Journal of the American Dietetic Association, 106*(1 Suppl. 1), S52–S65.

Brown, K. H., Peerson, J. M., Rivera, J., & Allen, L. H. (2002). Effect of supplemental zinc on the growth and serum zinc concentrations of prepubertal children: A meta-analysis of randomized controlled trials. *American Journal of Clinical Nutrition, 75*, 1062–1071.

Cashman, K. D. (2005). Vitamin K status may be an important determinant of childhood bone health. *Nutrition Reviews, 63*, 284–289.

Chakravarty, I., and Sinha, R. K. (2002). Prevalence of micronutrient deficiency based on results obtained from the national pilot program on control of micronutrient malnutrition. *Nutrition Reviews, 60*(5 Pt. 2), S53–S58.

Chandria, A. K., Tripathy, S., Ghosh, D., Debnath, A., & Mukhopadhyay, S. (2005). Iodine nutritional status and prevalence of goiter in Sundarban delta of South 24-Parganas, West Bengal. *The Indian Journal of Medical Research, 122*, 419–424.

Chaudhuri, A. (2005). Why we should offer routine vitamin D supplementation in pregnancy and childhood to prevent multiple sclerosis. *Medical Hypotheses, 64,* 608–618.

Chavasse, R. J., Francis, J., Balfour-Lynn, I., Rosenthal, M., & Bush, A. (2004). Serum vitamin D levels in children with cystic fibrosis. *Pediatric Pulmonology, 38,* 119–122.

Commission on the Nutrition Challenges of the 21st Century. (2000). Ending malnutrition by 2020: An agenda for change in the millennium. *Food and Nutrition Bulletin, 21,* 1–88.

Committee on Fetus and Newborn. (2003). Controversies concerning vitamin K and newborn. *Pediatrics, 112,* 191–192.

Cunningham-Rundles, S., McNeeley, D. F., and Moon, A. (2005). Mechanisms of nutrient modulation of the immune response. *J Allergy Clin Immunol, 115,* 1119–1128.

Dhonukshe-Rutten, R. A., van Dusseldorp, M., Schneede, J., de Groot, L. C., & van Staveren, W. A. (2005). Low bone mineral density and bone mineral content are associated with low cobalamin status in adolescents. *European Journal of Nutrition, 44,* 341–347.

Domellof, M., Lonnerdal, B., Abrams, S. A., & Hernell, O. (2002). Iron absorption in breast-fed infants: Effects of age, iron status, iron supplementation and complementary foods. *American Journal of Clinical Nutrition, 76,* 198–204.

Eitenschenck, L., Armari-Alla, C., Plantaz, D., Pagnier, A., & Ducros, V. (2005). Belated decompensation of an Imerslund-Grasbeck disease. *Archives of Pediatrics, 12,* 1729–1731.

Fawzi, W., Msamanga, G., Spiegelman, D., & Hunter, D. J. (2005). Studies of vitamins and minerals and HIV transmission and disease progression. *Journal of Nutrition, 135,* 938–944.

Fisher, J. O., Mitchell, D. C., Smiciklas-Wright, H., Mannino, M. L., & Birch, L. L. (2004). Meeting calcium recommendations during middle childhood reflects mother-daughter beverage choices and predicts bone mineral status. *American Journal of Clinical Nutrition, 79,* 698–706.

Forastiere, F., Pistelli, R., Sestini, P., Fortes, C., Renzoni, E., Rusconi, F., et al. (2000). Consumption of fresh fruit rich in vitamin C and wheezing symptoms in children. *Thorax, 55,* 283–288.

French, A. E., Grant, R., Weitzman, S., Ray, J. G., Vermeulen, M. J., Sung, L., et al. (2003). Folic acid food fortification is associated with a decline in neuroblastoma. *Clinical Pharmacology and Therapeutics, 74,* 288–294.

Gartner, L. M., Greer, F. R., & Section on Breastfeeding and Committee on Nutrition. (2003). Prevention of rickets and vitamin D deficiency: New guidelines for vitamin D intake. *Pediatrics, 111,* 908–910.

Greer, F. R. (2004). Issues in establishing vitamin D requirements for infants and children. *American Journal of Clinical Nutrition, 80*(6 Suppl.), 1759S–1762S.

Hambridge, M. (2000). Human zinc deficiency. *Journal of Nutrition, 130*(Suppl. 5), 1344S–1349S.

Hambidge, M. (2003). Biomarkers of trace mineral intake and status. *Journal of Nutrition, 133,* 948S–955S.

Hendler, S. S., & Rorvik, D. (2001). *PDR for Nutritional Supplements.* Montvale, NJ: Medical Economics Company.

Hollis, B. W., & Wagner, C. L. (2004). Assessment of dietary vitamin D requirements during pregnancy and lactation. *American Journal of Clinical Nutrition, 79,* 717–726.

Huiming, Y., Chaomin, W., & Meng, M. (2005). Vitamin A treating measles in children. *Cochrane Database Syst Rev, 19*(4), CD001479.

James, S. J., Cutler, P., Melnyk, S., Jernigan, S., Janak, L., Gaylor, D. W., et al. (2004). Metabolic biomarkers of increased oxidative stress and impaired methylation capacity in children with autism. *American Journal of Clinical Nutrition, 80,* 1611–1617.

Juval, R., Osmamy, M., Black, R. E., Dhingra, U., Sarkar, A., Dhingra, P., et al. (2004). Efficacy of micronutrient fortification of milk on morbidity in pre-school children and growth—a double blind randomized controlled trial. *Asia Pac J Clin Nutr, 13*(Suppl.), S44.

Kapil, U., and Bhavna, A. (2002). Adverse effects of poor micronutrient status during childhood and adolescence. *Nutrition Reviews, 60*(5 Pt. 2), S84–S90.

Kim, S., Kim, J., & Keen, C. (2005). Comparison of dietary patterns and nutrient intakes of elementary school children living in remote rural and urban areas in Korea: Their potential impact on school performance. *Nutrition Research, 25,* 349–363.

Kleinman, R. E., American Academy of Pediatrics (AAP) Committee on Nutrition, & Kleinmad, R. (2003). *Pediatric Nutrition Handbook* (5th ed.). Elk Grove Village, IL: American Academy of Pediatrics.

Korenke, G. C., Hunneman, D. H., Eber, S., & Hanefeld, F. (2004). Severe encephalopathy with epilepsy in an infant caused by subclinical maternal pernicious anemia: Case report and review of literature. *European Journal of Pediatrics, 163,* 96–201.

Kronn, D. F., Sapru, A., & Satou, G. M. (2000). Management of hypercholesterolemia in childhood and adolescence. *Heart Disorders, 2,* 348–353.

Kwan, M. L., Block, G., Selcin, S., Month, S., & Buffler, P. A. (2004). Food consumption by children and the risk of childhood acute leukemia. *American Journal of Epidemiology, 160,* 1098–1107.

Li, M., Eastman, C. J., Waite, K. V., Ma, G., Zacharin, M. R., Topliss, D. J., et al. (2006). Are Australian children iodine deficient? Results of the Australian National Iodine Nutrition Study. *MJA, 184,* 165–169.

Libermann, S., & Branning, N. (1997). *The Real Vitamins and Minerals Book* (2nd ed.). Garden City Park, New York: Avery Publishing Group.

Liu, S., West, R., Randell, E., Longerich, L., O'Connor, K. S., Scott, H., et al. (2004). A comprehensive evaluation of food fortification with folic acid for the primary prevention of neural tube defects. *BMC Pregnancy and Childbirth, 4,* 20.

Lumley, J., Watson, L., Watson, M., & Bower, C. (2000). Periconceptional supplementation with folate and/or multivitamins for preventing neural tube defects. *Cochrane Database Syst Rev*, (2), CD001056.

Mancini, A. J. (2000). Skin. *Pediatrics, 113*, 1114–1119.

Mahan, L. K., & Escott-Stump, S. (2000). *Krause's Food, Nutrition and Diet Therapy* (10th ed.). Philadelphia: W. B. Saunders.

Marcellini, M., Di Ciommo, V., Callea, F., Devito, R., Comparcola, D., Sartorelli, M. R., et al. (2005). Treatment of Wilson's disease with zinc from the time of diagnosis in pediatric patients: a single-hospital 10-year follow-up study. *J Lab Clin Med, 145*, 139–143.

Merialdi, M., Caulfied, L. E., Zavaleta, N., Figueroa, A., Costigan, K. A., Dominici, F., et al. (2004). Randomized controlled trial of prenatal zinc supplementation and fetal bone growth. *American Journal of Clinical Nutrition, 79*, 826–830.

Miller, A. L. (2003). The methionine-homocysteine cycle and its effects on cognitive diseases. *Alternative Medicine Reviews, 8*, 7–19.

Milne, E., de Klerk, N. H., van Bockxmeer, F., Kees, U. R., Thompson, J. R., Baker, D., et al. (2006). Is there a folate-regulated gene-environment interaction in the etiology of childhood acute lymphoblastic leukemia? *International Journal of Cancer, 119*, 229–232.

Monsen, A. L., Refsum, H., Markestad, T., & Ueland, P. M. (2003). Cobalamin status and its biochemical markers MMA and homocysteine in different age groups from 4 days to 19 years. *Clinical Chemistry, 49*, 2067–2075.

Morgan, J. (2005). Nutrition for toddlers: the foundation for good health—toddler's nutritional needs: what are they and are they being met? *J Fam Health Care, 15*, 56–59.

Mughal, Z. (2002). Rickets in childhood. *Seminars in Musculoskeletal Radiology, 6*, 183–190.

Muntjewerff, J. W., Van der Put, N., Eskes, T., Ellenbroek, B., Steegers, E., Blom, H., et al. (2003). Homocysteine metabolism and B-vitamins in schizophrenic patients: Low plasma folate as a possible independent risk factor for schizophrenia. *Psychiatry Research, 121*, 1–9.

Murphy, S. P., Gewa, C., Liang, L., Grillenberger, M., Bwibo, N. O., and Neumann, C. G. (2003). School snacks containing animal source foods improve dietary quality for children in rural Kenya. *Journal of Nutrition, 133*, 3950S–3956S.

Neumann, C. G., Gewa, C., & Bwibo, N. O. (2004). Child nutrition in developing countries. *Pediatric Annals, 33*, 658–674.

Pawley, N., & Bishop, N. J. (2004). Prenatal and infant predictors of bone health: The influence of vitamin D. *American Journal of Clinical Nutrition, 80*(6 Suppl.), 1748S–1751S.

Penland, J. G. (2000). Behavioral data and methodology issues in studies of zinc nutrition in humans. *Journal of Nutrition, 130*, 147S–153S.

Penny, M. E., Marin, R. M., Duran, A., Peerson, J. M., Lanata, C. F., Lonnerdal, B., et al. (2004). Randomized controlled

trial of the effect of daily supplementation with zinc or multiple micronutrients on the morbidity, growth and micronutrient status of young Peruvian children. *American Journal of Clinical Nutrition, 79*, 457–465.

Persad, V. L., Van den Hof, M. C., Dube, J. M., & Zimmer, P. (2002). Incidence of open neural tube defects in Nova Scotia after folic acid fortification. *CMAJ: Canadian Medical Association Journal, 167*, 241–245.

Pollitt, E. (2001). The developmental and probabilistic nature and functional consequences of iron-deficiency anemia in children. *Journal of Nutrition, 131*, 669S–675S.

Powers, H. J. (2003). Riboflavin (vitamin B-2) and health. *American Journal of Clinical Nutrition, 77*, 1352–1360.

Prabhu, S. S., & Dalvi, B. V. (2000). Treatable cardiomyopathies. *Indian Journal of Pediatrics, 67*(3 Suppl.), S7–S10.

Prousky, J. E. (2003). Pellegra may be a rare secondary complication of anorexia nervosa: A systematic review of the literature. *Alternative Medicine Reviews, 8*, 180–185.

Ramaekers, V. T., & Blau, N. (2004). Cerebral folate deficiency. *Developmental Medicine and Child Neurology, 46*, 843–851.

Ramaekers, V. T., Calomme, M., Berghe, V., & Makropoulos, W. (1994). Selenium deficiency triggering intractable seizures. *Neuropediatrics, 25*, 217–223.

Ray, P. E., Suga, S., Liu, X. H., Huang, X., & Johnson, R. J. (2001). Chronic potassium depletion induces renal injury, salt sensitivity, and hypertension in young rats. *Kidney International, 59*, 1850–1858.

Rodriguez, A., Hamer, D. H., Rivera, J., Acosta, M., Salgado, G., Gordillo, M., et al. (2005). Effects of moderate doses of vitamin A as an adjunct to the treatment of pneumonia in underweight and normal-weight children: A randomized, double-blind, placebo-controlled trial. *American Journal of Clinical Nutrition, 82*, 1090–1096.

Salamoun, M. M., Kizirian, A. S., Tannous, R. I., Nabulsi, M. M., Choucair, M. K., Deeb, M. E., et al. (2005). Low calcium and vitamin D intake in healthy children and adolescents and their correlates. *European Journal of Clinical Nutrition, 59*, 177–184.

Samour, P. Q., & King, K. (2005). *Handbook of Pediatric Nutrition* (3rd ed.). Sudbury, MA: Jones and Barlett Publishers.

Sanstead, H. H., Frederickson, C. J., & Penland, J. G. (2000). Zinc nutriture as related to brain. *Journal of Nutrition, 130*, 140S–146S.

Sazawal, S., Black, R. E., Menon, V. P., Dinghra, P., Caulfield, L. E., Dhingra, U., et al. (2001). Zinc supplementation in infants born small for gestational age reduces mortality; a prospective, randomized, controlled trial. *Pediatrics, 108*, 1280–1286.

Scarfone, R. J. (1999). Use of magnesium sulfate in the treatment of children with acute asthma. *Clinical Pediatric Emergency Medicine, 1*, 6–12.

Simsek, E., Karabay, M., Safak, A., & Kocabay, K. (2003). Congenital hypothyroidism and iodine status in Turkey: A comparison between the data obtained from an epidemiological study in school-aged children and neonatal screening for congenital hypothyroidism in Turkey. *Pediatric Endocrinology Reviews: PER, 1*(Suppl. 2), 155–161.

Svahn, J., Schiaffino, M. C., Caruso, U., Calvillo, M., Minniti, G., & Dufour, C. (2003). Severe lactic acidosis due to thiamine deficiency in a patient with B-cell leukemia lymphoma on total parenteral nutrition during high-dose methotrexate therapy. *Journal of Pediatric Hematology/Oncology: Official Journal of the American Society of Pediatric Hematology/Oncology, 25*, 965–968.

Tanner, E. M., & Finn-Stevenson, M. (2002). Nutrition and brain development: Social policy implications. *American Journal of Orthopsychiatry, 72*, 182–193.

Uriu-Adams, J. Y., & Keen, C. L. (2005). Copper, oxidative stress, and human health. *Molecular Aspects of Medicine, 26*, 268–298.

Wang, J. Y., Wang, Y. L., Zhou, S. L., & Zhou, J. F. (2004). May chronic childhood constipation cause oxidative stress and potential free radical damage to children? *Biomedical and Environmental Sciences: BES, 17*, 266–272.

Wharton, B., & Bishop, N. (2003). Rickets. *Lancet, 362*, 1389–1400.

Yoshii, A., Takeoka, M., Kelly, P. J., & Krishnamoorthy, K. S. (2005). Focal status epilepticus as atypical presentation of pyridoxine-dependent epilepsy. *Journal of Child Neurology, 20*, 696–698.

Zacharin, M. (2004). Current advances in bone health of disabled children. *Current Opinion in Pediatrics, 16*, 545–551.

Zimmermann, M. B., Connolly, K., Bozo, M., Bridson, J., Rohner, F., & Grimci, L. (2006). Iodine supplementation improves cognition in iodine-deficient schoolchildren in Albania: A randomized, controlled, double-blind study. *American Journal of Clinical Nutrition, 83*, 108–114.

Zinc Investigators' Collaborative Group. (2000). Therapeutic effects of oral zinc in acute and persistent diarrhea in children in developing countries: pooled analysis of randomized controlled trials. *American Journal of Clinical Nutrition, 72*, 1516–1522.

Children with Disabilities

American Dietetic Association. (2004). Position of the American Dietetic Association: Providing nutrition services for infants, children, and adults with developmental disabilities and special health care need. *Journal of the American Dietetic Association, 104*, 97–107.

American Psychiatric Association. (1994). *Diagnostic and Statistical Manual of Mental Disorders* (4th ed.). Washington, DC: Author.

Ani, C., Grantham-McGregor, S., & Muller, D. (2000). Nutritional supplementation of Down syndrome: Theoretical considerations and current status. *Developmental Medicine and Child Neurology, 42*, 207.

Anneren, G., Tuveno, T., and Gustafsson, J. (2000). Growth hormone therapy in young children with Down syndrome and a clinical comparison of Down and Prader-Willi syndrome. *Growth Horm IGF Res, 10*(Suppl. B), S87–S91.

Autism Society of America. (1995). *Asperger's Syndrome Information Package*. Bethesda, MD: Author.

Bandini, L. G., Puelzll-Quinn, H., Morelli, J. A., & Fukagawa, N. K. (1995). Estimation of energy requirements in persons with severe central nervous system impairment. *Journal of Pediatrics, 126*, 828.

Bandini, L. G., Schneller, D. A., Fukagana, N. K., Wykes, L., & Dietz, W. H. (1991). Body composition and energy expenditure in adolescents with cerebral palsy or myelodysplasia. *Pediatric Research, 29*, 70–77.

Bekx, M. R., Carrel, A. L., Shriver, T. C., and Allen, J. B. (2003). Decreased energy expenditure is caused by abnormal body composition in infants with Prader-Willi syndrome. *Journal of Pediatrics, 143*, 372–376.

Bennett, F. C., McClelland, S., Kriegsmann, E., Andrus, L., & Sells, C. (1983). Vitamin and mineral supplementation in Down syndrome. *Pediatrics, 72*, 707–713.

Bidder, R. T., Gray, P., Newcombe, R. G., Evans, B. K., and Hughes, M. (1989). The effects of multivitamins and minerals on children with Down syndrome. *Dev Med Child Neurol, 31*, 532–537.

Burgess, J. R., Stevens, L., Zhang, W., & Peck, L. (2000). Long chain poly unsaturated fatty acids in children with attention-deficit hyperactivity disorder. *American Journal of Clinical Nutrition, 71*(Suppl.), 327–330.

Capone, G., Muller, D., & Ekvall, S. W. (2005). Down syndrome. In S. Ekvall & V. Ekvall (Eds.), *Pediatric Nutrition in Chronic Disease and Developmental Disorders*. New York: Oxford University Press.

Carrel, A. L., Moerchen, V., Myers, S. E., Bekx, M. T., Whitman, B. Y., & Allen, D. B. (2004). Growth hormone improves mobility and body composition in infants and toddlers with Prader-Willi syndrome. *Journal of Pediatrics, 145*, 744–749.

Centers for Disease Control and Prevention (CDC). (2003). Developmental disabilities. Retrieved August 21, 2006, from http://www.cdc.gov/ncbdbb/dd/default.htm

Cloud, H. H. (2001). Recent trends in care of children with special needs: Nutrition services for children with developmental disabilities and special health care needs. *Topics in Clinical Nutrition, 16*, 28–40.

Cloud, H. H., Ekvall, S. W., & Hicks, L. (2005). Feeding problems of the child with special health care needs. In S. V. Ekvall & V. K. Ekvall (Eds.), *Pediatric Nutrition in Chronic Disease and Developmental Disorders* (2nd ed.). New York: Oxford University Press.

Cornish, E. (2002). Gluten and casein free diets in autism: A study of the effects on food choice and nutrition. *Journal of Human Nutrition and Dietetics: The Official Journal of the British Dietetic Association, 15*, 261–269.

Cronk, C., Crocker, A. C., Pueschel, S. M., Shea, A. M., Zackai, E., Pickens, G., et al. (1988). Growth charts for children with Down syndrome: 1 month to 18 years of age. *Pediatrics, 81*, 102–110.

Demitropoulas, A., Feurer, I. D., Butler, M. G., and Thompson (2001). Emergence of compulsive behavior and tantrums in children with Prader-Willi syndrome. *American Journal of Mental Retardation, 106*, 208–201.

Developmental Disabilities Assistance and Bill of Rights Act, 20002, Public Law 106-402.

Ekvall, S. W., & Cerniglia, F. (2005). Myelomeningocele. In S. V. Ekvall & V. K. Ekvall (Eds.), *Pediatric Nutrition in Chronic Disease and Developmental Disorders* (2nd ed.). New York: Oxford University Press.

Fernhall, B., Figueroa, A., Collier, S., Goulopoulou, S., Giannopoulou, I., & Baynard, T. (2005). Resting metabolic rate is not reduced in obese adults with Down syndrome. *Mental Retardation, 43*, 391–400.

Fugassi, P., Stevens, F., & Ekvall, S. (2003). The characteristics of autism and nutrition in children. *American Journal of the College of Nutrition, 22*, 481.

Glenn, C. C., Driscoll, D. J., Yang, T. P., and Nicholls, R. D. (1997). Genomic imprinting: potential function and mechanism revealed by the Prader-Willi and Angelman syndromes. *Mol Human Reprod, 3*, 321.

Golds, A. P., Unmehopa, U. A., Bloom, S. R., and Swaab, D. F. (2002). Hypothalmic NPY and agouti-related protein are increased in human illness but not in Prader-Willi syndrome and other obese subjects. *J Clin Endocrinol Metab, 87*, 927.

Green, N. S. (2002). Folic acid supplementation and prevention of birth defects. *Journal of Nutrition,* 132(Suppl.), 2356S–2360S.

Henderson, R. C., Kairalla, J. A., Barrington, J. W., Abbas, A., & Stevenson, R. D. (2005). Longitudinal changes in bone density in children and adolescents with moderate to severe cerebral palsy. *Journal of Pediatrics, 146*, 769–775.

Hogan, S. E. (1999). Knee height as a predictor of recumbent length for individuals with mobility-impaired cerebral palsy. *Journal of the American College of Nutrition, 18*, 201–205.

Hopman, E., Csizmadia, C. G., Bastiani, W. F., Engels, Q. M., de Graaf, E. A., Cessie, S., et al. (1998). Eating habits of young children with Down syndrome in the Netherlands: Adequate nutrient intakes but delayed introduction of solid food. *Journal of the American Dietetic Association, 98*, 790–794.

King, W., Levin, R., Schmidt, R., Oestreich, A., & Heubi, J. E. (2003). Prevalence of reduced bone mass in children with spastic quadriplegia. *Developmental Medicine and Child Neurology, 45*, 12.

Krick, J., Murphy-Miller, P., Zeger, S., & Wright, E. (1996). Pattern of growth in children with cerebral palsy. *Journal of the American Dietetic Association, 97*, 680.

Lucas, B. (2004). Nutrition in childhood. In K. Mahan and S. E. Stump (Eds.). *Krause's Food Nutrition and Diet Therapy* (11th ed.). Philadelphia: Elsevier.

Lucas, B., and Feucht, S. (1998). *The Benefits of Nutrition Services for a Case Series of Children with Special Health Care Needs.* Seattle: Washington State University of Human Development and Disability.

Luckasson, R., Borthwick-Duffy, S., Buntinx, W. H. E., Coulter, D., Craig, E. M., Reeve, A., et al. (2002). *Mental Retardation: Definition, Classification, and Systems of Supports* (10th ed.). Washington, DC: American Association on Mental Retardation.

Luke, A., Sutton, M., Schoeller, D. A., & Roizen, N. J. (1996). Nutrient intake and obesity in prepubescent children with Down syndrome. *Journal of the American Dietetic Association, 96*, 1262–1267.

Luke, D. A., Roizen, N. J., Sutton, M., & Schoeller, D. A. (1994). Energy expenditure in children with Down syndrome: Correcting metabolic rate of movement. *Journal of Pediatrics, 125*(5 Pt. 1) 829–838.

Martineau, J., Barthelemy, C., Cheliakine, C., & Lelord, G. (1988). Brief report: An open middle-term study of combined vitamin B_6–magnesium in a subgroup of autistic children selected on their sensitivity to this treatment. *Journal of Autism and Developmental Disorders, 18*, 435–446.

McCrary, J. M. (2006). Improving access to school based nutrition services for children with special health care needs. *Journal of the American Dietetic Association, 106*, 133–136.

McCune, H., & Driscoll, D. (2005). Prader-Willi syndrome. In S. W. Ekvall & V. K. Ekvall (Eds.), *Pediatric Nutrition in Chronic Disease and Developmental Disorders* (2nd ed.). New York: Oxford University Press.

Myerlid, A., Gusfasson, J., Ollars, B., & Anneren, G. (2002). Growth charts for Down syndrome from birth to 18 years of age. *Archives of Disease in Childhood, 86*, 97–103.

Obata, K., Sakazume, S., Yoshino, A., Murakami, N., & Sakuta, R. (2003). Effects of 5 years growth hormone treatment in patients with Prader-Willi syndrome. *Journal of Pediatric Endocrinology & Metabolism: JPEM, 16*, 155–162.

O'Neill, K. L., Shults, J., Stallings, V., & Stettler, N. (2005). Child feeding practices in children with Down syndrome and their siblings. *Journal of Pediatrics, 146*, 234–238.

Piscane, A., Toscano, E., Pirri, I., Continisio, P., Zoli, B., Andria, G., et al. (2003). Down syndrome and breastfeeding. *Acta Paediatrica, 92*, 1479–1481.

Reichelt, K., & Knivsberg, A. M. (2003). Why use the gluten-free and casein free diet? What results have shown so far. Presented at the Autism Research Institute Conference. Retrieved October 29, 2007, from www.autismwebsite.com/ARI/dan/reichelt.htm

Salman, M. (2002). Systematic review of the effect of therapeutic dietary supplements and drugs on cognitive function in subjects with Down syndrome. *European Journal of Paediatric Neurology: EJPN: Official Journal of the European Paediatric Neurology Society, 6*, 213.

Samson-Fang, L. J., & Stevenson, R. D. (2000). Identification of malnutrition in children with cerebral palsy: Poor performance of weight for height percentiles. *Developmental Medicine and Child Neurology, 43*, 162–168.

Schoeller, D. A., Levitsky, L. L., Bandini, L. G., Dietz, W. W., and Walczak, A. (1988). Energy expenditure and body composition in Prader-Willi syndrome. *Metabolism, 37,* 115.

Schuster, D. P., Osei, K., & Zipf, W. B. (1996). Characterizations of alterations in glucose and insulin metabolism in Prader-Willi subject. *Metabolism, 45,* 1514.

Shah, S., & Johnson, R. (1989). Antioxidant vitamin A and E status in children with Down syndrome subjects. *Nutrition Research, 9,* 709.

Smithells, R. N., Seller, M. J., Harris, R., Fielding, D. W., Schorah, C. J., Nevin, N. C., et al. (1983). Further experience of vitamin supplementation for prevention of neural tube defect recurrences. *Lancet, 1,* 1027.

Spiker, D., Hebbeler, K., Wagner, M., Cameto, R., and McKenna, P. (2000). A framework for describing variations in state early intervention systems. *Topics in Early Childhood Special Education, 20,* 195–218.

Stallings, V. A., Zemel, B. S., Davies, J. C., Cronk, C. E., & Charney, E. B. (1996). Energy expenditure of children and adolescents with severe disabilities: A cerebral palsy model. *American Journal of Clinical Nutrition, 64,* 627–634.

Stevenson, R. D. (2005). Use of segmental measures to estimate stature in children with cerebral palsy. *Archives of Pediatrics & Adolescent Medicine, 149,* 658–662.

Stevenson, R. D., Allen, W. P., & Pai, G. S. (2000). Decline in prevalence of neural tube defects in a high risk region of the United States. *Pediatrics, 106,* 677–683.

Stevenson, R. D., Conaway, M., Chumlea, W. C., Rosenbaum, P., Fung, E. B., Henderson, R. C., et al. (2006). Growth and health in children with moderate to severe cerebral palsy. *Pediatrics, 118,* 1010–1018.

Sullivan, P. B., Juszczak, E., Bachlet, A. M., Lambert, B., Vernon-Roberts, A., Grant, H. Q., et al. (2005). Gastrostomy tube feeding in children with cerebral palsy: A prospective longitudinal study. *Developmental Medicine and Child Neurology, 47,* 77–85.

Sullivan, P. B., Juszczak, E., Lambet, B. R., Rose, M., Ford-Adams, M. E., & Johnson, A. (2002). Impact of feeding problems on nutritional intake and growth: Oxford Feeding Study II. *Developmental Medicine and Child Neurology, 44,* 461–467.

Swaab, D. F., Purba, J. S., & Hofman, M. A. (1995). Alterations in the hypothalamic paraventricular nucleus and its oxytocin neurons (putative satiety cells) in Prader-Willi syndrome—a study of five cases. *The Journal of Clinical Endocrinology and Metabolism, 80,* 573.

Tobin, S. P., Cheng, V., Schumacher, C., Barsky, D., Greis, S. M., Siemon, J., et al. (2005). The role of an interdisciplinary feeding team in the assessment and treatment of feeding problems. Building blocks for life. Pediatric Nutrition Practice Group, American Dietetic Association. 28, 3.

U.S. Department of Health and Human Services, U.S. Food and Drug Administration. (1996). Food standards amendment of the standards of identity for enriched grain products to require addition of folic acid. *Federal Register, 61,* 8781–8807.

Van Goor, J., Massa, G., & Hirasing, R.(1997). Increased incidence and prevalence of diabetes mellitus in Down syndrome. *Archives of Disease in Childhood, 77,* 186.

Whitman, B. Y., Myers, S., Carrel, A., & Allen, D. (2002). The behavioral impact of growth hormone treatment for children and adolescents with Prader-Will syndrome: A 2 year controlled study. *Pediatrics, 109,* E35.

Whitt-Glover, M. C., O'Neill, K. L., & Stettler, N. (2006). Physical activity patterns in children with and without Down syndrome. *Pediatric Rehabilitation, 9,* 158–164.

Winter, S., Autry, A., Boyle, C., & Yeargin-Allsop, M. (2002). Trends in the prevalence of cerebral palsy in a population based study. *Pediatrics, 110,* 1220.

Yeargin-Alsopp, M., Rice, C., Karapurkar, T., Doernberg, N., Boyle, C., and Murphy, C. (2003). Prevalence of autism in a US metropolitan area. *Journal of the American Medical Association, 289,* 49–55.

CHAPTER 7

Special Topics in School-Aged Nutrition: Pediatric Vegetarianism, Childhood Overweight, and Food Allergies

Reed Mangels, PhD, RD, Inger Stallmann-Jorgensen, MS, RD, LD, Edna Harris-Davis, MS, MPH, RD, LD, and Shideh Mofidi, MS, RD, CSP

With a Special Section: Celiac Disease
Anne R. Lee, MS Ed, RD

CHAPTER OUTLINE

Reader Objectives

After studying this chapter and reflecting on the contents, you should be able to

1. Describe the similarities and differences between lacto-ovo-vegetarian, lacto-vegetarian, vegan, macrobiotic, fruitarian, and raw foods diets.
2. List potential health and nutritional benefits of vegetarian diets for the pediatric population.
3. Describe possible motivations for following a vegetarian diet.
4. Contrast growth of lacto-ovo-vegetarian, vegan, and nonvegetarian children and adolescents.
5. Identify key nutrients for vegetarian infants, children, and adolescents and suggest acceptable food sources for each nutrient.
6. Identify major nutritional issues for pediatric vegetarians and describe appropriate approaches for working with these issues.
7. Describe specific considerations for counseling vegetarians of various ages and their families.
8. List the growing problems related to overweight in children.
9. Describe the paradigm shift that occurred over the years to cause increased rates of overweight children.
10. Articulate some steps that families may take to help prevent overweight in children.
11. List overweight prevention strategies that could be incorporated into existing federal programs.
12. Realize the difference between food allergy and food intolerances.

13. Comprehend the principles of diagnosis and management of food allergies.
14. Understand the use and limitations of diagnostic tests for food allergy.
15. Recognize various manifestations of food allergic disorders.
16. Understand basic principles of nutritional management of children with food allergies.
17. Discern the impact of and appreciate the role of diet in the treatment of food allergies
18. Recognize the proper use of elimination diets and oral food challenges in the diagnostic and/or therapeutic management of food allergies.

Pediatric Vegetarianism

Reed Mangels, PhD, RD

Today, about a million school-aged children in the United States consistently follow a vegetarian diet (Vegetarian Resource Group, 2001) and say that they never eat meat, fish, or poultry. Many more children and adolescents eat a mostly vegetarian diet that may include limited amounts of animal products (Perry, McGuire, Neumark-Sztainer, & Story, 2002). Attitudes toward vegetarian diets for children have changed markedly. In the 1970s vegetarian diets were labeled a form of child abuse (Roberts, West, Ogilvie, & Dillon, 1979). Compare this with the 2003 statement by the American Dietetic Association and Dietitians of Canada that states, "Appropriately planned vegan, lacto-vegetarian, and lacto-ovo-vegetarian diets satisfy nutrient needs of infants, children, and adolescents and promote normal growth" (Mangels, Messina, & Melina, 2003).

Types of Vegetarian Diets

When working with vegetarians it is important to understand what a vegetarian diet is and to realize there are several different kinds of vegetarians. In the broadest sense a **vegetarian** is a person who does not eat meat, fish, or poultry (Mangels et al., 2003). **Lacto-ovo-vegetarians** include dairy products and eggs in their diets. **Lacto-vegetarians** include dairy products but not eggs. **Vegans** avoid eating any animal products.

Other types of vegetarian (or near-vegetarian) diets that may be encountered include **macrobiotic**, raw foods, and **fruitarian** diets (Messina, Mangels, & Messina, 2004). Macrobiotic diets are based largely on grains along with vegetables, especially **sea vegetables**; beans; fruits; nuts; soy products; and possibly fish. A number of studies have reported serious nutrient deficiencies with long-term consequences in children following macrobiotic diets (Dagnelie et al., 1989b, 1990; Louwman et al., 2000; Dhonukshe-Rutten, van Dusseldorp, Schneede, de Groot, & van Staveren, 2005). Depending on food and supplement choices, with careful planning, macrobiotic diets can be used by children (Mangels & Messina, 2001; Messina et al., 2004). Practitioners of a raw foods diet only consume foods in their raw state. Foods used include fruits, vegetables, nuts, seeds, sprouted grains, and sprouted beans; raw dairy products may be used. Fruitarian diets are based on fruits, nuts, and seeds and often include vegetables that are botanically fruits like avocado and tomatoes. Use of extremely restrictive diets such as raw foods and fruitarian diets has not been studied in infants and children. These diets can be very low in protein, energy, some vitamins, and minerals and cannot be recommended for infants and children (Messina et al., 2004). Some self-described vegetarians eat fish, chicken, or even meat (Barr & Chapman, 2002; Perry et al., 2002). This can have a significant impact on food choices and nutrient intake, so individual assessment of the diets of vegetarian clients is essential.

How Many Vegetarians Are There?

Approximately 2% of children and adolescents in the United States consistently follow a vegetarian diet, whereas about 0.5% consistently follow a vegan diet according to a Roper Poll conducted in 2000

Vegetarian: A person who does not eat meat, fish, or fowl or products containing those foods.

Lacto-ovo-vegetarian: A vegetarian who eats dairy products and eggs.

Lacto-vegetarian: A vegetarian who eats dairy products but not eggs.

Vegan: A vegetarian who avoids all animal products, including dairy products and eggs.

Macrobiotic: A person following a vegetarian or near-vegetarian diet based largely on grains, legumes, and vegetables; may include limited amounts of fish.

Fruitarian: A person following a diet based on fruits, nuts, and seeds that often includes vegetables that are botanically fruits like avocado and tomatoes.

Sea vegetables: Wild ocean plants, including nori, kelp, hiijiki, and dulse, that are often purchased in dried form.

(Vegetarian Resource Group, 2001). Similar results were obtained in a poll conducted in 1995 (Vegetarian Resource Group, 2001).

Reasons for Vegetarianism

Children and adolescents have a variety of motivations for following a vegetarian diet. Some are members of vegetarian families. Others cite an assortment of reasons, including health, animal welfare, and environmental concerns (Worsley & Skrzypiec, 1998; Larsson, Ronnlund, Johansson, & Dahlgren, 2003).

Health Benefits of Vegetarian Diets

There are numerous health benefits for adults following a vegetarian diet, including a lower body mass index (BMI), reduced risk of cardiovascular disease, lower blood pressure and lower rates of hypertension, reduced risk of type 2 diabetes, and a lower risk for prostate and colorectal cancer (Messina et al., 2004). Less is known about benefits for vegetarian children. Vegetarian children do tend to be leaner than nonvegetarian children (Hebbelinck & Clarys, 2001), and at least one study reported lower serum cholesterol concentrations in vegetarian children (Krajcovicova-Kudlackova, Simonic, Bederova, Grancicova, & Megalova, 1997a). Positive food patterns of vegetarian children and adolescents include greater consumption of fruits, vegetables, nuts, and legumes and lower consumption of sweets, fast food, and salty snack foods (Neumark-Sztainer, Story, Resnick, & Blum, 1997; Donovan & Gibson, 1996; Perry et al., 2002; Larsson & Jo-

hansson, 2005). In addition, diets of vegetarian children and adolescents tend to be lower in cholesterol, saturated fat, and total fat and higher in fiber than diets of nonvegetarians (Thane & Bates, 2000; Larsson & Johansson, 2002; Perry et al., 2002).

Growth and Energy Needs of Vegetarian Children

A limited number of studies have examined growth of vegetarian children in developed countries. Many of these studies were conducted more than 20 years ago when the availability of many foods frequently used by vegetarian families, such as fortified soy milk and veggie burgers, was much less than today. Generally, studies of lacto-ovo-vegetarian school-aged children and adolescents show that their height is similar and their weight is similar to or slightly lower than nonvegetarians (Sabaté, Linsted, Harris, & Johnston, 1990; Sabaté, Linsted, Harris, & Sanchez, 1991; Nathan, Hackett, & Kirby, 1997; Hebbelinck & Clarys, 1999). Some studies have suggested that vegetarian girls enter puberty later than nonvegetarians and therefore are shorter than similarly aged nonvegetarian girls (Kissinger & Sanchez, 1987; Sabaté, Llorca, & Sanchez, 1992), whereas other studies have not found this (Hebbelinck & Clarys, 1999). Vegan children tend to be leaner than nonvegetarian children but are typically within normal ranges of standards for height and weight (Sanders, 1988; Sanders & Manning, 1992). Markedly lower heights and weights have been reported in children following macrobiotic diets (Dagnelie, van Staveren, van Klaveren, & Burema, 1988; Dagnelie et al., 1989a), with lower heights persisting even after some relaxation of dietary practices (van Dusseldorp et al., 1996).

Lacto-ovo-vegetarian and vegan diets can support appropriate growth and development of children. If a child's growth rate is below what is expected, an increased energy intake may be necessary. This can be accomplished by providing concentrated energy sources, including soy products and other legumes, nuts and nut butters, and oils. In addition, some children may benefit from a somewhat lower fiber intake (Mangels et al., 2003).

Nutritional Considerations

Key nutrients for vegetarian children and adolescents include protein, iron, zinc, calcium, vitamin D, vitamin B_{12}, and omega-3 fatty acids. In the nonvegetarian diet these nutrients are frequently largely obtained from animal products, so questions have

---

Vegetarianism and Cultural Diversity

**Seventh-Day Adventists
Did you know?**

- Seventh-day adventists (SDAs) are a conservative religious group with more than 13 million members worldwide.
- SDAs are strongly encouraged to abstain from meat. About 27% are lacto-ovo-vegetarians, 3% are vegans, and 20% eat meat less than once a week.
- They tend to have healthy life-styles, eating more fruits and vegetables and exercising more frequently than their neighbors.
- Less than 2% use any form of tobacco; less than 10% use alcohol and those who do generally only drink small amounts.
- SDAs have been studied extensively and have provided a wealth of information about the health advantages of a healthy life-style. Significant findings include
  - Lower rates of coronary disease than non-SDAs with even lower rates in vegetarian SDAs.
  - Lower incidence of lung, colon, stomach, bladder, and other cancers than nonSDAs.
  - SDAs live longer than non-SDAs; vegetarian SDAs live longer than nonvegetarian SDAs.
  - Vegetarian SDAs weigh less than nonvegetarian SDAs.
  - Vegetarian SDAs are less likely to develop diabetes, hypertension, and arthritis than nonvegetarian SDAs.

Compiled from Fraser, G. E. (2003). *Diet, Life Expectancy, and Chronic Disease: Studies of Seventh-Day Adventists and Other Vegetarians.* New York: Oxford University Press.

been raised about their adequacy in vegetarian or vegan diets. Other nutrients, including folate, vitamin C, and vitamin A (as beta-carotene), are generally not considered problematic for vegetarians due to many vegetarians' higher consumption of fruits and vegetables.

Protein

Protein is rarely below recommendations in vegetarian children's diets that contain adequate energy and a variety of plant foods (Dagnelie, van Staveren, Verschuren, & Hautvast, 1989c; Thane & Bates, 2000; Leung et al., 2001). The Institute of Medicine (IOM, Food and Nutrition Board, 2002) concluded that the protein requirement for vegetarians who consume a variety of plant proteins is not different from that of nonvegetarians. Plant proteins contain varying amounts of essential amino acids. For example, compared with the Amino Acid Scoring Pattern developed by the Food and Nutrition Board and IOM, wheat is low in lysine (IOM, 2002). Chickpeas and other legumes are relatively low in the sulfur amino acids (methionine and cysteine). By eating a variety of protein sources over the course of a day, differences in amino acid content are satisfied (Young & Pellett, 1994; Mangels et al., 2003).

Iron and Zinc

Iron intakes of vegetarian children and adolescents vary. Some studies reported iron intakes by vegetarian children that are similar to or higher than those of nonvegetarian children (Houghton et al., 1997; Thane & Bates, 2000; Larsson & Johansson, 2002; Perry et al., 2002), whereas others identified lower iron intakes in vegetarians (Donovan & Gibson, 1995, 1996). Lower hemoglobin and ferritin levels have been reported in vegetarian children (Donovan & Gibson, 1995, 1996; Nathan, Hackett, & Kirby, 1996; Thane & Bates, 2000; Thane et al., 2003), suggesting that iron is not as well absorbed from a vegetarian diet.

Non-heme iron is the only form of iron found in vegetarian diets. Inhibitors and enhancers affect the absorption of non-heme iron. **Phytate,** found in whole grains, legumes, and to a lesser extent vegetables (Hallberg & Hulthen, 2000), is the main inhibitor of iron absorption in vegetarian diets. Although no information is available with regard to the phytate content of pediatric vegetarian diets, adult vegan diets may contain two to three times as much phytate as non-

Non-heme iron: The form of iron found in plants and the portion of iron from animal foods that is not part of hemoglobin or myoglobin.

Phytate: A phosphorus-containing compound found in whole grains and dried beans that binds with minerals, particularly iron and zinc, and interferes with their absorption.

vegetarian diets; lacto-ovo-vegetarian diets have a phytate content intermediate between vegan and nonvegetarian diets (Ellis et al., 1987; Hunt, Matthys, & Johnson, 1998).

Because of the lower **bioavailability** of iron from vegetarian diets, a separate iron Recommended Dietary Allowance (RDA) has been established for vegetarians that assumes an iron bioavailability of 10% compared with 18% for nonvegetarian diets (IOM, Food and Nutrition Board, 2001). Adjustments do not need to be made to the RDA for infants from birth to 12 months (IOM, Food and Nutrition Board, 2001), because recommendations for infants from birth to 6 months are based on the iron content of breast milk. The RDA for infants ages 7 to 12 months is based on a bioavailability of 10% rather than the higher bioavailability that is used for other age groups (IOM, Food and Nutrition Board, 2001). Iron recommendations for older vegetarian children can be found in Table 7.1.

Bioavailability: A measure of how available to the body a nutrient is after it is ingested.

Iron absorption from a vegetarian diet can be enhanced even in the presence of phytate by consuming a vitamin C source at the same time as the iron source (Hallberg & Hulthen, 2000; Sandstrom, 2001). Leavening of bread reduces its phytate content and enhances iron absorption (Hunt, 2002). Iron sources for vegetarian children include iron-fortified breakfast cereals, soy foods, dried beans, and whole grains. Table 7.2 provides more information about vegetarian iron sources, whereas Table 7.3 shows a sample menu that would meet a vegetarian adolescent girl's high iron requirements. Laboratory assessment of iron status is appropriate if a child's diet is low in iron and iron supplements are not regularly used.

Limited information suggests that the zinc content of diets of vegetarian children is similar to that of nonvegetarian children (Sanders, 1995; Thane & Bates, 2000). However, because phytate also inhibits

TABLE 7.1	Iron RDA for Vegetarian Children and Adolescents*
Age, Gender	**Iron RDA (mg)**
1–3 yr, M/F	12.6
4–8 yr, M/F	18
9–13 yr, M/F	14.4
14–18 yr, M	19.8
14–18 yr, F	27

*Values calculated based on 1.8 times RDA for nonvegetarians. From IOM (2001).

TABLE 7.2	Food Sources of Iron* for Vegetarians		
Food, Standard Amount		**Iron (mg)**	**Calories**
Fortified ready-to-eat cereals (various), ~1 oz		1.8–21.1	54–127
Fortified instant cooked cereals (various), 1 packet		4.9–8.1	Varies
Soybeans, mature, cooked, ½ cup		4.4	149
Pumpkin and squash seed kernels, roasted, 1 oz		4.2	148
White beans, canned, ½ cup		3.9	153
Blackstrap molasses, 1 T		3.5	47
Lentils, cooked, ½ cup		3.3	115
Spinach, cooked from fresh, ½ cup		3.2	21
Kidney beans, cooked, ½ cup		2.6	112
Chickpeas, cooked, ½ cup		2.4	134
Prune juice, ¾ cup		2.3	136
Cowpeas, cooked, ½ cup		2.2	100
Tomato puree, ½ cup		2.2	48
Lima beans, cooked, ½ cup		2.2	108
Soybeans, green, cooked, ½ cup		2.2	127
Navy beans, cooked, ½ cup		2.1	127
Refried beans, ½ cup		2.1	118
Tomato paste, ¼ cup		2.0	54

*Food sources of iron ranked by milligrams of iron per standard amount; also calories in the standard amount.

Adapted from DHHS and USDA. (2005). *Dietary Guidelines for Americans*. Washington, DC: DHHS and USDA. Nutrient values from Agricultural Research Service (ARS) Nutrient Database for Standard Reference, Release 17. Foods are from ARS single nutrient reports, sorted in descending order by nutrient content in terms of common household measures. Food items and weights in the single nutrient reports are adapted from those in 2002 revision of USDA Home and Garden Bulletin No. 72, Nutritive Value of Foods. Mixed dishes and multiple preparations of the same food item have been omitted from this table.

zinc absorption, vegetarian children are likely to have higher requirements for zinc than nonvegetarian children. The IOM has not specified a zinc RDA for vegetarians but suggests that the dietary requirement for zinc may be as much as 50% greater for vegetarians, especially for those relying mainly on grains and legumes (IOM, Food and Nutrition Board, 2001). Techniques that can enhance zinc absorption include using yeast-leavened breads, using fermented soy products like tempeh and miso, and soaking dried beans and discarding the soaking water before cooking the beans (Gibson, Yeudall, Drost, Mtitmunit, & Cullinan, 1998). Zinc supplements should be considered for children on vegan diets, especially those based on high-phytate cereals and legumes (Allen, 1998).

Calcium and Vitamin D

Children following lacto-ovo-vegetarian diets tend to have adequate intakes of calcium and vitamin D because of their use of dairy products (Thane & Bates, 2000; Perry et al., 2002). Limited data suggest that calcium intakes of vegan children are lower than recommendations (Messina et al., 2004). Rickets, due to a deficiency of vitamin D, has been seen in some children following macrobiotic diets (Dagnelie et al., 1990) and in infants and toddlers fed unfortified soy or rice milk (Carvalho, Kenney, Carrington, & Hall, 2001; Imataka, Mikami, Yamanouchi, Kano, & Eguchi, 2004). Adequate calcium and vitamin D are important for all children to promote bone growth and to reduce risk of fracture (Black, Williams, Jones, & Goulding, 2002; Kalkwarf, Khoury, & Lanphear, 2003). There is no evidence that vegan children need less calcium than nonvegetarians, and increased calcium intakes (342 vs. 1,056 mg/day) have been shown to improve bone mineral status of children on near-vegan diets (Dibba, Prentice, & Ceesay, 2000). The adequate intake for calcium is 500 mg/day for 1- to 3-year-olds, 800 mg/day for 4- to 8-year-olds, and 1,300 mg/day for 9- to 18-year-olds (IOM, Food and Nutrition Board, 1997).

There are a number of reliable sources of calcium for children and adolescents who limit or avoid dairy products. These include soy milks and juices that have been fortified with calcium (Heaney, Dowell, Rafferty, & Bierman, 2000; Heaney, Rafferty, & Bierman, 2005). Low-oxalate vegetables, like kale, broccoli, and collard greens, contain generous amounts of well-absorbed calcium (Weaver & Plawecki, 1994), and although these foods may not be the major source of calcium in children's diets, they can significantly increase calcium intake. Tofu processed with calcium sulfate, almonds, almond butter, and dried figs are another source of calcium (Mangels et al., 2003). Vegan products that have been developed to resemble dairy products, such as

TABLE 7.3	Example of an Iron-Rich Menu

	Iron (mg)
1 cup oatmeal 1.6	
¼ cup raisins	1.4
8 oz fortified soy milk	0.7
6 oz orange juice	0.3
2 slices whole-wheat toast	1.7
Bean burrito:	
1 flour tortilla	1.0
½ cup kidney beans	2.6
2 T salsa	0.0
1 cup watermelon chunks	0.4
Stir-fry:	
¾ cup tofu	10.0
1 cup cooked broccoli	1.0
1 cup brown rice	1.0
½ cup cooked carrots	0.3
¾ cup strawberries	0.6
1 cup fortified soy milk	0.7
Trail mix:	
¼ cup pumpkin seeds	8.5
2 T sunflower seeds	0.6
¼ cup dried apricots	0.9
Total	33.3

From U.S. Department of Agriculture, Agricultural Research Service. (2005). USDA Nutrient Database for Standard Reference, Release 18, and manufacturers' information.

soy yogurt and soy cheese, do not always contain the same amount of calcium as their dairy counterparts. Label reading is essential to determine the nutrient content of these products. Table 7.4 provides more information about nondairy sources of calcium for vegetarians.

Fortified soy milks and juices also frequently contain vitamin D. Some breakfast cereals are fortified with vitamin D as well. Although cutaneous synthesis can be an important vitamin D source, factors like age, limited sunlight exposure, skin tone, season, and sunscreen use can lead to concerns about adequate vitamin D production (Holick, 2004). Vitamin D supplements can also be used to ensure adequate vitamin D intakes.

Vitamin B$_{12}$

Vitamin B$_{12}$ is only found in significant amounts in foods derived from animals or in fortified foods. Lacto-ovo-vegetarians who consume an adequate amount of cow's milk, yogurt, or eggs regularly can meet recommendations for vitamin B$_{12}$. Vegans must obtain their vitamin B$_{12}$ from fortified foods (some brands of soy milk, breakfast cereals, meat analogs, and nutritional yeast) or from vitamin B$_{12}$ supplements. Table 7.5 provides information about recommendations, food sources, and serving sizes of vitamin B$_{12}$–rich foods. Foods such as sea vegetables, fermented soy products, and Spirulina are sometimes promoted as sources of vitamin B$_{12}$; these cannot be counted on as reliable sources because they have been shown to contain analogues of vitamin B$_{12}$ that can interfere with the absorption of active vitamin B$_{12}$ (van den Berg, Dagnelie, & van Staveren, 1988; Dagnelie, van Staveren, & van den Berg, 1991; Watanabe et al., 1999).

Adequate vitamin B$_{12}$ is especially important during pregnancy and lactation because the maternal diet during these times is the major influence on the infant's vitamin B$_{12}$ status (IOM, Food and Nutrition Board, 1998). Breast-fed infants whose mothers do not consume dairy products, vitamin B$_{12}$–fortified foods, or vitamin B$_{12}$ supplements regularly need vitamin B$_{12}$ supplements at the adequate intake level from birth (IOM, Food and Nutrition Board, 1998).

Although the RDA for vitamin B$_{12}$ is extremely low, failure to achieve an adequate intake can lead to serious consequences. Marginal vitamin B$_{12}$ status in adolescents has been associated with impaired cognitive function (Louwman et al., 2000) and gait disturbances (Licht, Berry, Brooks, & Younkin, 2001), whereas vitamin B$_{12}$ deficiency in infants and children has led to failure to thrive, developmental delay, and seizures (Centers for Disease Control and Prevention [CDC], 2003).

Vegetarians eating few or no animal foods and not using vitamin B$_{12}$–fortified foods or vitamin B$_{12}$ supplements should have their **cobalamin** status assessed (CDC, 2003). Serum or urine methylmalonic acid is one test for cobalamin deficiency; holotranscobalamin II, total homocysteine, and serum B$_{12}$ also can be used (Hermann & Geisel, 2002).

Cobalamin: Vitamin B$_{12}$.

Omega-3 Fatty Acids

Vegetarian diets are generally low in **alpha-linolenic acid,** an omega-3 fatty acid, whose essential role appears to be as a precursor for the synthesis of the long chain omega-3 fatty acids, **eicosapentaenoic acid (EPA)** and **docosahexaenoic acid (DHA).** DHA is found in high

Alpha-linolenic acid: An essential 18-carbon omega-3 fatty acid.

Eicosapentaenoic acid (EPA): A 20-carbon omega-3 fatty acid found in fish oil.

Docosahexaenoic acid (DHA): A 22-carbon omega-3 fatty acid found in fish oil.

TABLE
7.4

Nondairy Food Sources of Calcium* for Vegetarians

Food, Standard Amount	Calcium (mg)	Calories
Fortified ready-to-eat cereals (various), 1 oz	236–1,043	88–106
Soy beverage, calcium fortified, 1 cup	368	98
Tofu, firm, prepared with nigari,† ½ cup	253	88
Collards, cooked from frozen, ½ cup	178	31
Molasses, blackstrap, 1 T	172	47
Spinach, cooked from frozen, ½ cup	146	30
Soybeans, green, cooked, ½ cup	130	127
Turnip greens, cooked from frozen, ½ cup	124	24
Oatmeal, plain and flavored, instant, fortified, 1 packet prepared	99–110	97–157
Cowpeas, cooked, ½ cup	106	80
White beans, canned, ½ cup	96	153
Kale, cooked from frozen, ½ cup	90	20
Okra, cooked from frozen, ½ cup	88	26
Soybeans, mature, cooked, ½ cup	88	149
Beet greens, cooked from fresh, ½ cup	82	19
Pak-choi, Chinese cabbage, cooked from fresh, ½ cup	79	10
Dandelion greens, cooked from fresh, ½ cup	74	17

*Nondairy food sources of calcium ranked by milligrams of calcium per standard amount; also calories in the standard amount. The bioavailability may vary. Both calcium content and bioavailability should be considered when selecting dietary sources of calcium. Some plant foods have calcium that is well absorbed, but the large quantity of plant foods that would be needed to provide as much calcium as in a glass of milk may be unachievable for many. Spinach, Swiss chard, beet greens, and rhubarb are high oxalate vegetables, and the calcium in these foods is largely unavailable. Many other calcium fortified foods are available, but the percentage of calcium that can be absorbed is unavailable for many of them.

†Calcium sulfate and magnesium chloride.

Adapted from DHHS and USDA. (2005). *Dietary Guidelines for Americans*. Washington, DC: DHHS and USDA.

Nutrient values from Agricultural Research Service (ARS) Nutrient Database for Standard Reference, Release 17. Foods are from ARS single nutrient reports, sorted in descending order by nutrient content in terms of common household measures. Food items and weights in the single nutrient reports are adapted from those in 2002 revision of USDA Home and Garden Bulletin No. 72, Nutritive Value of Foods. Mixed dishes and multiple preparations of the same food item have been omitted from this table.

TABLE
7.5

Recommendations, Food Sources, and Serving Sizes of Vitamin B_{12}–Rich Foods

Age Group	Vitamin B_{12} RDA (?g/day)	Servings of Vitamin B_{12}–Rich Foods
0–6 mo	0.4 (AI)	Vitamin B_{12} should be obtained from breast milk, infant formula, or supplements
7–12 mo	0.5 (AI)	Vitamin B_{12} should be obtained from breast milk, infant formula, or supplements
1–3 yr	0.9	1
4–8 yr	1.2	1.5
9–13 yr	1.8	2
14–18 yr	2.4	3

AI, adequate intake. From IOM (2001).

concentrations in the membrane lipids of the brain and the retina (IOM, 2002) and appears to play a role in visual and cognitive performance (Birch, Garfield, Hoffman, Uauy, & Birch, 2000; SanGiovanni, Parra-Cabrera, Colditz, Berkey, & Dwyer, 2000), although results of supplementation studies are mixed (McCann & Ames, 2005). Unless vegetarians eat eggs or generous amounts of sea vegetables, their diets will also lack direct sources of

EPA and DHA. Requirements for alpha-linolenic acid may be higher for many vegetarians than for nonvegetarians because vegetarians must rely on conversion of alpha-linolenic acid to EPA and DHA rather than obtaining these **n-3 fatty acids** from their diet (Davis & Kris-Etherton, 2003). The conversion of alpha-linolenic acid to EPA and subsequently to DHA is very limited (Davis & Kris-Etherton, 2003; Francois, Connor, Bolewicz, & Connor, 2003).

n-3 fatty acid: A polyunsaturated fatty acid in which the first double bond is three carbons from the methyl end of the carbon chain. Important sources in the U.S. diet include certain fish tissues, canola and soybean oils, and seeds and nuts such as flax seeds and walnuts.

Vegetarians' lower dietary intakes of EPA and DHA are reflected in blood and breast milk concentrations. Adult lacto-ovo-vegetarians and vegans have lower blood concentrations of EPA and DHA than nonvegetarians (Krajcovicova-Kudlackova, Simoncic, Babinska, & Bederova, 1995; Geppert, Kraft, Demmelmair, & Koletzko, 2005; Rosell et al., 2005), and adolescent vegans have lower concentrations than lacto-ovo-vegetarians or nonvegetarians (Krajcovicova-Kudlackova, Simoncic, Bederova, & Klvanova, 1997b). Breast milk concentrations of alpha-linolenic acid, EPA, and DHA reflect the amounts present in the mother's diet and are lower in breast milk of vegetarian and vegan women (Sanders & Reddy, 1992; Uauy et al., 1996). Breast-fed infants of vegetarian and vegan women have lower plasma and red blood cell DHA concentrations than breast-fed infants of nonvegetarian women (Sanders & Reddy, 1992).

DHA supplements derived from microalgae are one option for vegetarians (Conquer & Holub, 1996; Davis & Kris-Etherton, 2003; Geppert et al., 2005). Because some EPA can be synthesized from alpha-linolenic acid, good sources of alpha-linolenic acid such as flaxseed and flaxseed oil, canola oil, soybean oil, walnuts, and soy products should be promoted (Mangels et al., 2003). The conversion of alpha-linolenic acid to EPA can be enhanced by limiting use of oils high in linoleic acid and trans-fats (Davis & Kris-Etherton, 2003).

Nutritional Counseling of Vegetarian Infants, Children, and Adolescents and Their Families

The Position of the American Dietetic Association and Dietitians of Canada: Vegetarian Diets states, "Dietetics professionals have an important role in supporting clients who express an interest in adopting vegetarian diets or who already eat a vegetarian diet" (Mangels et al., 2003, p. 759). Families

---

Critical Thinking About a Vegetarian Diet for a Child

- What tools and techniques would you use to assess a 3-year-old vegan's nutritional status?
- What are some "red flags" for an eating disorder in a vegetarian adolescent? What would you do if you suspected that a client had an eating disorder?
- Why is it important to ask a vegetarian client to tell you specifically about foods eaten and avoided rather than relying on their characterization of their diet as "vegetarian"?
- When would you recommend supplements for a vegetarian child? Which supplements and what amounts? Would your recommendations differ for a lacto-ovo-vegetarian and a vegan child?

---

with vegetarian infants, children, and adolescents seek nutrition counseling for a variety of reasons. Perhaps a child or adolescent has decided to become vegetarian but the rest of the family wants to continue eating meat. Perhaps a health care provider has referred the family because of concerns about dietary adequacy. Perhaps a family that is already following a vegetarian diet is seeking advice on dietary modifications to improve their diet or to cope with a condition such as renal disease or diabetes. In any case, dietetics professionals need to be able to provide information about food sources of key nutrients for infants, children, and adolescents; to adapt guidelines for individuals with allergies, chronic diseases, or other factors necessitating dietary modifications; to assist with meal planning, food purchases, and food preparation decisions; and to give current information about vegetarian nutrition for the pediatric age group (Mangels et al., 2003). Table 7.6 lists some tips for effective counseling of vegetarian clients. Although key nutrients are important at every age, there are some considerations that vary by age group.

Infants and Toddlers

In early infancy, vegetarian infants do not differ from nonvegetarian infants in terms of feeding practices. Exclusive breast-feeding for 6 months and breast-feeding with complementary foods until at least 12 months of age are the ideal feeding patterns for infants (Dobson & Murtaugh, 2001).

● Learning Point If there is any question about adequate vitamin B₁₂ in a lactating woman's diet, a vitamin B₁₂ supplement is recommended for her infant.

Commercial infant formula is recommended for infants who are not breast-fed or who are weaned

TABLE
7.6   Tips for Effective Counseling of Vegetarian Clients

- Develop vegetarian-specific counseling materials. These might include handouts on good sources of iron for vegetarians and good sources of calcium and vitamin D for vegans.
- Respect the client's food preferences. Suggesting that a vegetarian include fish or fish oil or that a vegan use some dairy products can alienate clients and compromise the practitioner's credibility.
- Be aware of current research. Many vegetarians have a strong interest in nutrition and may ask detailed questions regarding studies they have heard or read about.
- Create lists of resources for additional information: family-friendly cookbooks, credible websites, and vegetarian organizations.
- If you believe you are not familiar enough with vegetarian nutrition to counsel a vegetarian client, it is your responsibility as a professional to assist this client in finding another registered dietitian with expertise in vegetarian nutrition or to inform the client about reliable vegetarian nutrition resources.

Compiled from Mangels et al. (2003, p. 760).

A Word on Vegetarianism and Adolescents

Vegetarian diets are somewhat more common among adolescents with eating disorders (Neumark-Sztainer et al., 1997; Perry, McGuire, Newmark-Sztainer, & Story, 2001). Possibly, adolescents who have issues with food and body weight choose vegetarian or partial vegetarian diets as a socially acceptable way to restrict their food intake (Janelle & Barr, 1995; Barr, 1999; Martins, Pliner, & O'Connor, 1999). The use of a vegetarian diet does not appear to increase the risk of developing an eating disorder (Janelle & Barr, 1995; Barr, 1999). Dietetics professionals should be aware of vegetarian clients who exhibit symptoms of an eating disorder.

Adolescents (and some children) may choose to follow a vegetarian diet even though their family is not vegetarian. Depending on the age and ability of the child or adolescent, parental participation may be needed in the areas of menu planning, food purchases, and food preparation (Messina et al., 2004). Dietetics professionals can help families to identify vegetarian meals that the whole family enjoys, to plan meals that can be served with vegetarian options, and to find foods that the child or adolescent can prepare independently.

before 1 year of age. Lacto-ovo-vegetarian families who use infant formula can use a cow milk–based formula, whereas for vegan families who use infant formula, soy formulas are the only option. Commercial soy beverages do not provide adequate nutrition for infants and should not be used, except for small amounts in cooking, during the first year (Messina et al., 2004). Other formulas such as those based on rice, nut, or seed milks; nondairy creamer; cereal gruels; or mixtures of fruit or vegetables juices should not be used to replace breast milk or commercial infant formula (Mangels & Messina, 2001). After the first year, either fortified full-fat soy milk or whole cow's milk can be used as the primary

beverage for a child who is growing normally and eating a variety of foods (Mangels & Messina, 2001).

Solid foods can be introduced to vegetarian infants in the same order that they would be introduced to nonvegetarian infants (Scott, 2003). At around 7 to 8 months when higher protein foods would typically be introduced, vegetarian infants can start to eat cooked and pureed legumes, well-mashed tofu, or soy yogurt. Infants in lacto-ovo-vegetarian families can also have pureed cottage cheese, yogurt mixed with mashed fruit, or egg yolks. Foods that will eventually play a significant role in the diets of vegetarian children (e.g., legumes, tofu, and leafy green vegetables) should be introduced in infancy so that the child becomes familiar with the flavor of these foods.

As toddlers are weaned from breast milk or infant formula, energy intake may decrease. Foods that are both nutrient and energy dense, like soy products, bean spreads, and avocado, are often recommended to maintain energy intake during weaning.

Meal Planning Guidelines

A variety of meal planning guidelines has been developed for vegetarian children and adolescents (Truesdell & Acosta, 1985; Messina & Mangels, 2001; Stepaniak & Melina, 2003; Messina, Melina, & Mangels, 2003; Messina et al., 2004). The ideal plan should achieve the following goals (Messina et al., 2003):

- Meet the needs of different types of vegetarian diets
- Help vegetarians meet the most recent nutrient recommendations
- Focus on specific nutrients identified as being of special importance to vegetarians
- Include a wide variety of foods
- Meet the needs of different age groups

Childhood Overweight

Inger Stallmann-Jorgensen, MS, RD, LD, and
Edna Harris-Davis, MS, MPH, RD, LD

Obesity and obesity-related diseases are some of the biggest health challenges of the 21st century. The rapidly increasing rate of excessive weight in children is especially alarming. Thus now is the time for health care professionals to accept the urgent challenge of addressing overweight and obesity through prevention-based approaches. To maximize effectiveness, overweight and obesity prevention efforts must target children and their families and focus on policy and environmental interventions.

The topic of overweight children is a large and complex issue; it is not possible to address every aspect of the problem and its prevention and treatment in this chapter. Rather, the aim of this chapter is to provide an overview of overweight children and to guide the entry-level practitioner in addressing this challenging health issue.

Assessment of Overweight Children

In the pediatric population the BMI is used as a screening tool and is not a diagnosis for overweight children. The CDC revised and published the growth charts for children ages 2 to 20 years: BMI-for-Age, Weight-for-Age, and Stature-for-Age. The BMI-for-Age nutrition status indicators for *At Risk for Overweight* and *Overweight* children are ≥85th percentile to <95th percentile and ≥95th percentile, respectively (CDC, n.d.-b) (see Appendix 1). There is evidence that many overweight children will become obese adults (Serdula et al., 1993; Freedman, Khan, Dietz, Srinivasan, & Berenson, 2001). However, the BMI-for-Age assessment should be applied carefully so as to not label children as obese in error. It is important to determine whether a child indeed has extra fat mass and not extra muscle mass, particularly across genders and ethnicity (Ellis, Abrams, & Wong, 1999; Taylor, Jones, Williams, & Goulding, 2002). In addition, labeling as "obese" carries a stigma for many people. Therefore, as CDC has defined, the terms "overweight" and "at-risk for overweight" should be used when addressing the pediatric population and to establish some consistency when making comparisons between various groups of children, particularly in research literature.

Overweight Rates in the United States

For adults, there has been a rapid increase in our nation's prevalence rate of overweight status over the past two decades. The United States is not alone in facing this serious health problem. Obesity has been declared one of the top 10 health risk conditions in the world and the top 5 in the developed world by the World Health Organization. Recent data from the 2003–2004 National Health and Nutrition Examination Survey (NHANES) found 66.3% of the U.S. adult population to be overweight or obese as defined by a BMI of greater than 25 kg/m^2 (Ogden et al., 2006). This represents an increase of 1.8% from the rates in 1999–2000 and more than 10% since the NHANES III (1988–1994). Obesity rates among children are lower than adult rates but have increased rapidly to levels not seen before. Between NHANES I (1971–1974) and NHANES II (1976–1980) the prevalence of excessive weight among children was unchanged overall, but between NHANES II and NHANES III (1988–1994), the prevalence rose within all age and gender groups (Ogden, Flegal, Carroll, & Johnson, 2002).

The rising trend of overweight children has since continued through NHANES 1999–2000, 2001–2002, and 2003–2004. Compared with 1988–1994 data, overweight rates in NHANES 2003–2004 increased by 6.9% for 12- to 19-year-olds, 7.5% for 6- to 11-year-olds, and 6.7% for 2- to 5-year-olds. Most recent rates now stand at 17.4% for 12- to 19-year-olds, 18.8% for 6- to 11-year-olds, and 13.9% for 2- to 5-year-olds for all racial/ethnic and gender groups combined. When children and adolescents (2 to 19 years of age) who are at risk for excessive weight are included, the overall prevalence rate is 33.6%. However, the increases in overweight rates have not occurred to the same extent among all age and race groups. Most affected by the rising trend in rates of at-risk for overweight and overweight combined are Mexican-American boys ages 6 to 11 (47.9%) and 2 to 5 (38.5%), followed by non-Hispanic African-American girls ages 6 to 11 (45.6%), 12 to 19 (42.1%), and 2 to 5 (27%). Thus, for some of these groups, almost half of the children and youth are either at risk for or are overweight (Ogden et al., 2006). The trend for increasing overweight prevalence among children is illustrated in Figure 7.1.

Health Effects of the Overweight

The recent trends of overweight children are especially disturbing because of the predicted health consequences

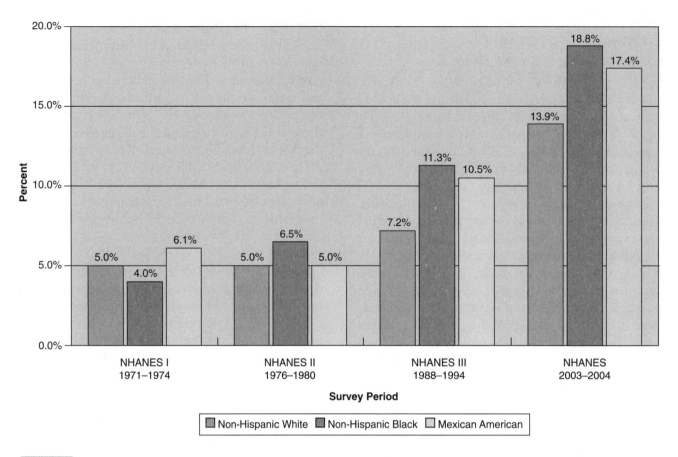

Figure 7.1 Prevalence of Overweight Among U.S. Children and Adolescents (Aged 2–19 Years) National Health and Nutrition Examination Surveys. *Source:* National Health and Nutrition Examinations Survey. Available at nutrition.gov.

of being overweight. Freedman et al. (2001) studied the longitudinal relationship between children's BMI and their adult levels of lipids, insulin, and blood pressure. The mean time interval between first and follow-up measurements was 17 years. Over this time period 77% of overweight children remained so as adults. The persistence of excessive weight, once it occurs, is of great concern because being overweight is more strongly linked to chronic disease than is living in poverty, smoking, or drinking. The impact of obesity on overall health has been likened to aging by 20 years (Hill, Wyatt, Reed, & Peters, 2003). "[C]hildhood obesity precedes insulin resistance/hyper-insulinemia and strongly predicts the risk of developing a constellation of metabolic, hemodynamic, thrombotic, and inflammatory disorders of syndrome X" (Berenson, 2002).

Although there is well-justified concern for overweight in children tracking into adulthood and in-

creasing the risk of adult health problems, one must not ignore the acute, both physical and psychological, health issues that affect the overweight child. Many body functions are affected by being overweight, including the nervous, pulmonary, cardiovascular, skeletal, gastrointestinal, endocrine, and reproductive systems. In addition, overweight children suffer from mental health problems, such as depression, anxiety, lowered self-esteem, and sometimes eating disorders (Erickson, Robinson, Haydel, & Killen, 2000; Raman, 2002; Hassink, 2003). Pediatricians are diagnosing the most obese children and adolescents with hypertension, dyslipidemia, and non–insulin-dependent diabetes (NIDDM).

> **Health Disparities in Cultural Diversity**
> Ethnic, cultural, gender, genetic, socioeconomic, and regional differences exist that influence which children are at greater risk for being overweight. Especially boys of Hispanic-American origin, African-Americans, and those residing in the South experience higher rates of being overweight (Strauss & Pollack, 2001; Nelson, Chiasson, & Ford, 2004). The ethnic differences in the degree to which certain population groups are affected by overweight prevalence may exacerbate long-term health outcomes and economic disparities that already exist in the United States (Strauss & Pollack, 2001).

> **● Learning Point** Even if the overweight status does not track into adulthood, there may be long-lasting medical and psychosocial effects in overweight children (Hill & Trowbridge, 1998).

Environmental Influences on Overweight Children

Societal Factors Influencing Overweight Children

Some overweight people have experienced discrimination because of the negative attitudes and judgmental behaviors of others who may see them as lazy and lacking will power. Such attitudes have contributed to a social stigma and caused psychological pain for those suffering from the condition. Viewing overweight children, within a construct of "personal responsibility," has allowed past treatment interventions to focus on the child and perhaps the family unit. Experience shows that this treatment model often fails because many overweight children have

> ### 2005 Dietary Guidelines for Physical Exercise
> The 2005 Dietary Guidelines Advisory Committee recommends that children engage in at least 60 minutes of physical activity on most (preferably all) days of the week. Physical activity may include short bouts (i.e., 10 minutes each) of moderately intense activity. In this way exercise can be accumulated through three to six bouts over the course of the day. The accumulated total of physical activity is what is important for health.

grown up to be overweight adults. Today, it is widely recognized that the micro-environment (home and family setting) and the macro-environment, in which it is imbedded, either promote healthy weight or overweight. Thus altering both the micro- and macro-environments is vital to prevention and treatment of overweight in children. The dynamics between individuals and their near, intermediate, and distal environments influence their food choices and physical activity levels, both of which play important roles in the development of overweight (Booth et al., 2001).

Overweight Status and Energy Balance

The environmental factors underlying the recent increase in obesity rates in the United States are multiple; however, diet and physical activity play a crucial role. Basic to this concept is the fact that to maintain a stable weight, energy intake and output must be balanced. Thus when physical activity level is low, weight status can be maintained with a diet appropriately lower in calories. However, if an adjustment is not made to keep energy intake and expenditure in balance, through either increased physical activity or decreased energy intake or a combined approach, excessive weight gain is the result. The alarming rise in overweight among U.S. children begs the question: What changes have occurred in our life-styles that could have contributed to this problem?

Dietary Trends Affecting Overweight Status in Children

Historical Perspective

Today's life-styles are very different from the life-styles of our hunter–gatherer ancestors. Genetically, humans evolved during the Paleolithic period 2.6 million to 10,000 years ago and were biologically adapted to survive under the prevailing conditions of that time. Today's Western-style diet is in sharp contrast to the diet of the hunter–gatherers. Yet our human genome has changed little since that period to help us adapt to our present-day life-styles. Now, most of us "dwell in mechanized urban settings, leading sedentary lives and eating a highly processed, synthetic diet" (O'Keefe & Cordain, 2004). The differences in today's diets from that of the hunter–gatherers are that they consumed foods higher in fiber content and lower in energy density and with a different diet composition of the long chain fatty acids. The long chain fatty acids of the n-6 and n-3 families were consumed in a ratio about 1:1. Today's Western-type diet can provide less of the omega-3 fatty acids with an n-6 to n-3 ratio of 1:15–17 (Simopoulos, 2002). The diet of the hunter–gatherer was rich in plant foods, supplemented by fish and lean meats and nuts. Indications are that these early ancestors did not experience obesity. Changes in agricultural practices, as well as food processing and manufacturing, have resulted in a vastly different food supply that has evolved over a relatively short time, historically. The development of agricultural societies led to diets based on grains. With this change from a plant-based to a grain-based diet, vitamin and mineral deficiencies began to appear as evidenced by studying bones and teeth. Our natural preference for foods that are calorie dense is rooted in the conditions of our ancestors where obtaining food for survival through hunting, fishing, and gathering food required high levels of physical activity and a correspondingly high expenditure of energy.

In contrast, obtaining food today means a car ride to the grocery store and little connection between energy intake and expenditure (O'Keefe & Cordain, 2004). The typical American diet today is lower in fiber and plant foods, higher in meat and high in highly refined carbohydrates (i.e., of high glycemic load) and possibly contains a much higher ratio of the n-6 relative to the n-3 long chain fatty acids. Sources of n-3 fatty acids that are diminished in our typical diet include fish, shellfish, wild game, and plant foods. Potassium intakes are much lower today, whereas sodium intakes are much higher than in the diets of our distant ancestors. In short, most people consume a diet they were not genetically designed to eat. Calcium is an important mineral to human health, yet calcium intakes are not adequate for adolescent girls, older women, and older men. Although calcium intake has increased a little for women aged 20 to 74 since NHANES III, recommendations for milk and dairy intake are not met by 70% of the population over 2 years of age according to the NHANES 1999–2000 data (Briefel & Johnson, 2004). Researchers contend that these dietary changes, combined with sedentary life-styles, play a significant role in the etiology of chronic diseases affecting developed countries: heart disease, diabetes, cancer, and obesity (Simopoulos, 1999; Conner, 2000).

Changes in the Food Environment

One of the most noticeable changes affecting our food environment during the past two decades is the rapid growth in the number of restaurants and, especially, of fast food establishments, currently numbering about 250,000 outlets nationally. Fast food restaurants are found throughout our communities, even inside public schools and hospitals. The effective marketing and advertising of these restaurants to adults and children have fueled the growth of this industry. Unfortunately, fast food restaurant fare is usually high in calories, fat, salt, and sugars and low in fiber content (Bowman, Gortmaker, Ebbeling, Pereira, & Ludwig, 2004). This is especially true for menu items offered as special value promotions. Often, the more healthful selections on fast food menus are more expensive and are not subject to the low price offers that might otherwise encourage customers to buy them.

Fast food items are convenient and relatively low cost. These factors appeal to working and single parents, and the percentage of children eating fast food meals will likely increase (Bowman et al., 2004). The amount of food dollars spent outside the home has increased significantly to now comprise about 46% of total household food budgets. Fast food meals consume about 34% of the family food dollar. Meals eaten outside the home tend to be of large portion sizes and higher energy content and include fewer fruits and vegetables than meals eaten in the home. As a result, the increase in out-of-home-meal consumption may have a negative impact on diet quality and on the obesity and health risk of children and their families (Nicklas, Baranowski, Cullen, & Berenson, 2001; American Dietetic Association, 2002).

Product innovations launched during the past two decades have included many products designed to lower the fat content of popular foods to address consumers' concerns about dietary fat and unwanted weight gain. In spite of an explosive growth in low-fat food products in many food categories, these food supply changes have seemingly not had the desired effect on our obesity rates. Many food manufacturers offset the lower fat content of the reformulated foods by increasing sugar and carbohydrate contents to maintain product acceptance by consumers. In the end, the caloric content of the lower-fat product is often similar to the original version. There is also concern that so-called low-fat foods may encourage the consumer to actually eat more calories overall because the low-fat food provides a "license to eat more" (Kurtzweil, 1996).

Energy intakes in children's diets have remained fairly stable since 1971–1974 (NHANES I), except for increases for children ages 1 to 2 years and for adolescent girls ages 12 to 19 years. The macronutrient composition of children's diets has changed, reflecting changes in the food supply. Fat intake as a percentage of energy intake fell from 38% to 33% since 1973, whereas carbohydrate and protein intakes increased. Still, about 75% of children did not meet the fat intake recommendations in 1994 (Munoz, Krebs-Smith, Ballard-Barbash, & Cleveland, 1997; Nicklas et al., 2001).

Children's diets have changed in respect to the types of carbohydrate they consume. In a 1998 roundtable and national briefing on child nutrition, the Director of the National Institute of Child Health and Human Development was quoted as saying that children's diets are characterized by "too much energy . . . too much sugar, and too little fiber" (fruits and vegetables) and could be described as an inverted My Pyramid (McBean & Miller, 1999). Easily digestible highly refined carbohydrates from foods and beverage sources have increased in consumption recently. Much scientific interest has been focused on the possible role of high **glycemic index** foods in the childhood and adult obesity epidemic. An effect of the glycemic index of breakfast foods on subsequent unrestricted food intake at lunch has been studied. Lunch intake after a breakfast of foods high in glycemic index (i.e., a meal of high glycemic load) was greater than after a breakfast of low **glycemic load** (Warren, Henry, & Simonite, 2003). In a review of the high

Glycemic index: The effect of carbohydrate in a food on blood glucose, as a percentage of the effect of an equal amount of glucose.

Glycemic load: Calculated by multiplying the glycemic index by the amount of carbohydrate provided by a food and dividing the total by 100. Dietary glycemic load is the sum of the glycemic loads for all foods consumed in the diet.

glycemic index foods, hunger, and obesity connection Roberts (2000) concluded that compared with similar low glycemic index carbohydrates, high glycemic index carbohydrates promote a more rapid return of the hunger sensation and increase subsequent caloric intake. Foods of high glycemic index may, therefore, contribute to maintenance of excess weight in the obese and to weight gain in susceptible individuals. Many children start their day with high sugar content breakfast cereals of high glycemic index. Over the longer term, a diet of high glycemic load could lead to higher energy intake and contribute to excess weight gain (Augustin, Franceschi, Jenkins, Kendall, & La Vecchia, 2002).

High sugar beverage intake is linked with fast food consumption because soft drinks are usually marketed and bundled with meal packages in fast food restaurants. Twice as many children and adolescents drank carbonated soft drinks if they had consumed fast foods on one of two survey days than if they did not (Paeratakul, Ferdinand, Champagne, Ryan, & Bray, 2003). So-called super-sized meal offers upgrade beverage serving size along with food portions. "Super-sizing" of meal packages may have contributed to increased intakes of sweetened beverages by children. Between 1977–1979 and 1994 the proportion of children who consumed soft drinks on a given day increased by 74% for boys and 65% for girls. High consumption of soft drinks among children and adolescents has been shown to be associated with higher energy intake (Harnack, Stang, & Story, 1999). An association between school children's sugar-sweetened drink consumption and their BMI has been demonstrated, although more research is ongoing. For example, a study conducted prospectively over 19 months showed that for each additional serving of sugar-sweetened beverage consumed, both BMI and propensity to become obese increased. This was after controlling for anthropometric, demographic, dietary, and life-style variables (Ludwig, Peterson, & Gortmaker, 2001).

The typical 12 fluid ounce can of soda is rapidly being replaced by the 20 fluid ounce bottle at convenience stores and in vending machines, encouraging increased consumption of these drinks. Many brands offer a 32 fluid ounce version that is packaged in a bottle shape that is easy to tote around, thereby encouraging frequent and increased consumption. Average portion sizes of soft drinks have increased by 12% to 18% for persons ages 2 and older (Briefel & Johnson, 2004). Soft drink consumption (per capita) has increased about 500%

over the past 50 years, with adolescents consuming between 36 and 58 g of sugar daily from this source (Ludwig et al., 2001).

Food portions have increased as well. Most consumers recognize portion inflation among baked goods, such as bagels and muffins. Also, hamburger sandwiches are both larger and offered with two and three servings of meat with cheese.

Regulation of Energy Intake

Although very young children possess innate abilities to regulate energy intake based on their needs, children tend to lose some of this ability as they age and become more responsive to environmental influences and increasingly take their behavioral cues from their surroundings. Children vary in their ability to self-regulate energy intakes (Johnson, 2000), but children who have experienced so-called restrictive feeding practices appear to be less able to respond appropriately to internal signs of hunger and satiety and may be more susceptible to overeating (Birch & Fischer, 1998). Also, as children learn from their environment, food portion sizes influence their intake. Thus, children may overeat when presented with excessive food and beverage portions, risking excessive weight gain over time.

Family Eating Environment

Genetic differences are estimated to account for about 30% to 50% of the variance of BMI within a population, but these estimates do not describe the complex interactions taking place between genetics and the environment (Allison & Faith, 2000). For example, parents contribute both genetics and environment to the equation. Their own eating behaviors help shape the child's eating environment and to an extent may be influenced by the parents' own genetic makeup. In turn, the child's or adolescent's eating environment helps to shape the development of the child's own eating behaviors. These learned (eating) behaviors in turn influence whether any genetic predispositions toward obesity are expressed in the child (Birch & Fischer, 1998).

Parents who are struggling with personal weight issues may hamper their children's ability to self-regulate energy intake. Because many adults suffer from overweight or obesity (National Center for Health Statistics, 1999), some parents are understandably concerned about their children's risk of also becoming overweight or obese. Aiming to avoid overweight in their children, parents may impose greater restrictions on their children's intake. If these same parents exhibit uninhibited eating styles themselves, they serve as poor role models. These behaviors in combination can cause the transfer of eating styles that pose an increased risk for the development of an overweight child. As a result well-intentioned parents may actually produce the very outcome they sought to avoid (Johnson, 2000). A common strategy used to control children's intake is to restrict their access to high calorie foods or to use favorite foods as a reward to shape behavior. At first, these behaviors may seem reasonable enough; however, restricting certain foods has been shown to increase the child's desire to consume these foods. When available, these desirable foods will likely be consumed in greater amounts. Again, such family dynamics around food may set up patterns of poor self-control of energy intake in the child (Fischer & Birch, 1999).

An optimal environment for children to develop self-control of energy intake is when parents provide nutritious food and allow children to determine if and how much to eat. These principles of division of responsibility are discussed extensively elsewhere (Satter, 1987, 1999, 2000; Johnson & Birch, 1994).

Household Food Insecurity

Although seemingly paradoxical, low-income compared with higher income households appear to experience increased rates of overweight individuals. Proposed mechanisms for this effect include higher intakes of cheaper more calorie-dense foods that may lead to excessive energy intakes (Alaimo, Olson, & Frongillo, 2001; Drewnowski & Specter, 2004). Persons from low-income, food-insecure households may overeat during periods of relative abundance and gain weight as a result. Food insecurity in low-income households appears to play a role in the increased overweight rates among older white girls (8 to 16 years of age) compared with children from low-income households that do not experience food insecurity (Alaimo et al., 2001). However, family participation in programs, such as the National School Breakfast and Lunch Programs and in the Food Stamp Program, may be protective for these girls. Girls who participated in all three programs were at a 68% reduced odds of becoming overweight when compared with nonparticipants from families experiencing food insecurity (Jones, Jahns, Laraia, & Haughton, 2003). On the other hand, a more recent study found a 42.8% increase for young girls and a 28.8% decrease for young boys in the predicted probability of obesity with participation in Food Stamp Program for the previous 5 years. This study did not control for food insecurity within households, which may help to explain the differing results (Gibson, 2004). Additional retrospective longitudinal studies that included assessment of food security and hunger status of each household member might help explain why some children are affected more than others. This is important because not all members of a household may experience food insecurity to the same extent. A better understanding of these dynamics can focus attention on those within a household who may be at a greater risk of being overweight.

Breast-Feeding

New mothers returning to work may decide against breast-feeding or may nurse their infants for only a very limited time because of the real and/or perceived obstacles to breast-feeding their infants while working outside the home. This is unfortunate because breast milk is the ideal food for infants. Evidence is emerging that breast-feeding may offer some protection against obesity (Armstrong & Reilly, 2002). Proposed mechanisms for this effect include more normal growth patterns (lower early weight gain), possibly associated with lower basal insulin levels in the breast-fed versus the formula-fed infant, and the inherent control of food intake maintained by the breast-fed infant (Dietz, 2001).

Breast-feeding on demand is thought to teach infants to regulate their intakes appropriately, based on internal cues for hunger and satiety and in response to their individual growth needs. Formula-fed infants may have fewer opportunities to develop this important skill. Reasons for this may be that parents or caregivers may want to follow a set feeding schedule or may encourage the infant to consume a certain amount of formula. Both of these feeding behaviors override the infant's internal cues and may result in overfeeding and lessen the infant's ability to self-regulate energy intake (Birch & Fischer, 1998).

Physical Inactivity Affecting Overweight Status in Children

Physical inactivity among children is one of the major health concerns regarding overweight children. Children learn physical inactivity from their adult role models and environment through limited access to recreational activities in their community, lack of safe neighborhoods, and, perhaps, unlimited access to television viewing and other media outlets, including computers. In addition, many newly developed communities are poorly planned when "built-in" access to physical activity is left out of the design. Often, children are bused to school because walking to school is not an option due to safety issues and distance. In many towns and cities, sidewalks were once common, but now some urban and suburban developments have shaped many residential areas into "unwalkable" communities. Although further research is needed for a better understanding of the influence of the human-built environment on physical activity, it appears clear that urban sprawl has caused some relationship between land use, transportation, and health, particularly children's health (Frumkin, 2002).

School Physical Education

At school, children are challenged to find opportunities to be physically active on a daily basis. Often, school academic curriculums and programs take priority over physical education and recess time. Physical education curriculums and recess have slowly diminished over the last few years (Burgenson, Wechsler, Brener, Young, & Spain, 2001).

Data from the Youth Risk Behavior Surveillance System show that 55.7% of students nationwide were enrolled in physical education classes 1 or more days in an average week, whereas only 28.4% of students nationwide attended physical education classes 5 days in an average week. Of the 55.7% of students enrolled in physical education classes nationwide, 80.3% of students actually exercised or played sports more than 20 minutes. Improvements in physical education are also needed to decrease inappropriate teaching practices, such as prohibiting physical activity as a form of punishment or physical activity games that may cause embarrassment or aggressive behavior (i.e., dodge ball) (Burgenson et al., 2001). Although some physical education improvements are needed, a nationwide effort to establish laws or policies to increase student enrollment and participation in daily physical education is desirable, especially in the older student population. The goal is for children to establish healthy life-style habits that may carry over into adulthood.

Because most children spend much of their waking hours in school, it is a threat to children's health and fitness when the school schedule and curriculum does not include daily opportunities for physical activity. Advocacy for increasing student participation in daily recess and physical activity should be a top priority of schools and health and community leaders to help prevent overweight children.

Television Viewing

Television viewing and other media outlets to an extent have displaced a more natural environment of family interactions for growing children, such as learning and playing. Children, who spend more time in sedentary activities, tend to weigh more and to be at greater risk of being overweight. Several studies conclude that children who watch 4 or more hours of television are more likely to be overweight than those who watch less television (Gortmaker et al., 1996; Andersen, Crespo, Bartlett, Cheskin, Pratt, 1998; Dowda, Ainsworth, Addy, Saunders, & Riner, 2001). In addition, African-American (30%) and Hispanic-American (22%) children are both more likely than white (12%) children to spend more than 5 hours a day watching television. Similarly, African-American (69%) and Hispanic-American (60%) children are more likely than white (48%) children to have a television in their bedroom (Kaiser Family Foundation, n.d.).

One cross-sectional study failed to find a relationship between television viewing and overweight status in adolescent girls (Robinson et al., 1993). Another study questioned the leisure activities in the United States, indicating that U.S. children overall are less active than children in other countries and cultures (Crawford et al., 2004). The trend toward increasingly sedentary life-styles is obvious to many older adults, as they compare the children's activity level in this current generation with that of children two or three generations earlier. Learning, playing, and physical activity were an integral part of family life, and television viewing was a special occasion. However, today, television viewing is a prominent part of family life, and it is a sedentary behavior.

Excessive television viewing not only leaves less time for positive family interactions and activities, but the actual programs and advertisements may be questionable for young viewers. Granted, there are many educational and worthwhile programs to watch on television. Unfortunately, not all programs and advertisements have children's health as a priority. One major challenge is the multimillion dollar advertising industry that promotes products between and during television programming (Borzekowski & Robinson, 2001). Appealing and enticing advertising segments are targeted at children to increase their desire to choose unhealthy foods. Food products advertised directly to young children during children's television programming have contributed to an impressive growth in sales of high-sugar breakfast cereals and snack foods. The young consumers predictably request these products (or may even purchase these themselves) during trips to the grocery store, because they recognize their favorite cartoon characters on the colorful packages strategically placed at their eye level when riding in the grocery cart. Excessive television viewing by children creates a cycle of physical inactivity and high calorie consumption due to the influence of television food advertising; this combination of factors adds up to a perfect formula for fueling the rising trend of overweight status in children.

An important part of treating overweight children is to decrease sedentary behavior and increase physical activity (Steinbeck, 2001). These are important factors in the intervention process; however, children are still challenged with real barriers to being physically active existing in their physical environment. Limited access to safe physical activity in the community, unlimited television viewing, fewer opportunities for physical activity in the schools, and adults who may not view physical activity as a priority are important barriers to physical activity. Thus U.S. children live in an **obesigenic** society with various barriers that make healthy living choices, such as daily physical activity, difficult to achieve.

Obesigenic: An environment that encourages obesity by features, including unlimited quantities of a variety of foods high in caloric density together with minimal need of energy expenditure.

Opportunities to Intervene and Prevent Childhood Obesity

Health care practitioners are challenged to think of new and creative ways to address the problem of childhood obesity within existing venues and frameworks. To be most successful and cost effective, the emphasis must be on population-based approaches and prevention, as traditional and clinic-based services alone clearly have failed to adequately address the obesity epidemic. Thus the health care practitioner should examine existing nutrition, social, and other programs and seize opportunities to intervene to prevent overweight in children. Some suggestions for opportunities are listed below.

Nutrition Programs

Special Supplemental Program for Women, Infants, and Children

Developing policies and conducting outreach activities to recruit pregnant women into prenatal care during the first trimester promotes early intervention and nutrition care for the expectant woman. This may improve nutrition delivery to her unborn child and help to avoid under- or over-nutrition, thereby lowering the risk of future obesity in the child (Dietz, 2004). Some clinics conduct grocery store tours to teach shopping skills to Special Supplemental Program for Women, Infants, and Children, also known as WIC, program participants to help them establish healthy eating patterns.

It is important to assess monitoring systems and develop policies or protocols to identify participant children older than 2 years of age who exhibit rapid weight gain and to target efforts to ensure they receive culturally appropriate interventions and guidance intervention to lower their risk of becoming overweight. Training clinic health care practitioners in anticipatory guidance and counseling will enable the team to provide infant and child feeding and physical activity advice consistent with evidence-based obesity prevention strategies and to serve as positive role models. The clinic environment should convey clear and consistent messages to encourage healthy eating and physical activity for both program participants and staff; this would include policies and environmental interventions that promote, support, and protect breast-feeding.

Social Programs

Preschool and Day Care

Policies to support healthy eating and physical activity should include strategies such as these: (1) serving healthy menu items within a positive eating environment for children, (2) opportunities for and encouragement of children (and adults caregivers) to be physically active daily, and (3) training of childcare providers and the food service team in obesity prevention strategies through nutritious food choices and daily physical activity appropriate for the children's age and development. Grants can provide resources to fund environmental intervention (i.e., playground, equipment for physical activity, and policy interventions for staff and parents to attend training in overweight prevention for children). Involving families and staff in fun events that encourage adoption of healthy living practices, such as less sedentary behavior and more physical activity, can help to reinforce the message.

School Systems

Advocating for daily recess and active physical education for all children through school boards, parent and teacher organizations, school administrators, and elected officials can help to bring needed changes to our children's daily environment. Such improvements should include policies that limit competitive foods and beverages and serve fruits and vegetables daily on the breakfast and lunch menus, nutrition standards for food and beverages sold from vending machines and school stores, and a unified message for healthy eating and physical activity throughout the school (no candy fundraisers, no food and or candy rewards for good behavior in the classroom, healthy snacks at parties, school events, and a campus that is friendly to physical activity, such as walkways, bicycle racks, and safe outdoor play equipment). Promotion of school breakfast and lunch program participation can help to ensure appropriate nutrition for students within the school, whereas nutrition education curricula from pre-kindergarten through 12th grade (50 hours a year minimum has been suggested) can influence student eating behaviors outside the school as well (American Dietetic Association, Society for Nutrition Education, and the American School Food Service Association, 2003). Systems to assess children's health and behaviors (i.e., height and weight, BMI, blood pressure, fruit and vegetable consumption, television viewing, transportation modes to school, and actual physical activity during recess and physical education classes) are important to monitor progress and regress in these health promotion efforts and target areas for change.

After School Care

The after school setting offers opportunities for promotion of healthy eating and adequate physical activity that are very similar to those in childcare and school settings: staff training to support obesity prevention efforts, consistent messages regarding a healthy life-style, limited availability of competitive foods of low nutritional quality, and an environment friendly to physical activity for all children and youth. Again, grants can help provide funds to make environmental improvements as needed.

Other Possible Venues

Children of low-income households who participate in federal and state-supported summer food service programs may secure a nutritious alternative to the fast food and snacks of low nutritional quality that often comprise a significant part of their diet between school years. Advocating for a healthy environment in various setting for children, such as Boys and Girls Clubs, YMCA/YWCA, and summer camps, can help children establish and maintain healthy life-styles year around. Directors and staff in these settings who are trained in overweight prevention strategies can strengthen their influence on the health behaviors of

the children and youth in their care when they model healthy behaviors themselves.

Programs and Resources That Support Evidence-Based Practices in Preventing Childhood Obesity

The CDC Nutrition, Physical Activity and Obesity Prevention Program established three evidence-based goals to prevent and control obesity (CDC, 2003):

1. To increase physical activity
2. To reduce television viewing
3. To improve nutrition through increased breast-feeding and increased fruit and vegetable consumption

Although research is limited on successful practices in various settings, programs and resources that may be used by a health care practitioner when addressing overweight children follow.

Physical Activity

KidsWalk-to-School

KidsWalk-to-School is a community-based program developed by the CDC Nutrition and Physical Activity Program. It "encourages children to walk to and from school in groups accompanied by adults" (CDC, n.d.-a). This program mobilizes community members, such as school staff, the Parent Teacher Association, police departments, businesses, civic associations, and other groups to work together to increase safe routes to and from school for children to walk or ride their bicycles. The program raises community awareness of the importance of daily physical activity for children and the barriers to activity they encounter. In this way the program helps to change an "unwalkable" community into a "walkable" community, bringing about an environmental intervention. This program supports the *Healthy People 2010* objectives related to children's trips to school by walking or bicycling (U.S. Department of Health and Human Services, 2000).

Television Viewing

TV Turnoff Network

The TV Turnoff Network encourages children and adults to turn off the television and replace that time with enjoyable family activities that promote healthy living. It sponsors two programs: TV Turnoff Week and More Reading, Less TV. TV Turnoff Week is held during the last week of April of every year. TV

Turnoff Week encourages physical activity, such as gardening, skating, dancing, walking, bicycling, or playing a sport along with other nonphysical activities. More Reading, Less TV encourages reading as a replacement to television viewing among children and adults. Because of the link between excessive television viewing and increased BMI in children, decreasing television viewing may encourage children to be more physically active (TV Turnoff Network, n.d.). This program supports the *Healthy People 2010* objectives related to increasing the number of adolescents watching 2 hours or less of television on school days (U.S. Department of Health and Human Services, 2000).

Nutrition

Breast-Feeding

Breast-feeding may serve as an early intervention to prevent childhood obesity, and breast-feeding promotion can occur in various settings. For instance, the health care practitioner may develop a breast-feeding coalition that focuses on developing breast-feeding policies in work sites, hospitals, and community sites. In addition, coalition members may monitor and evaluate the interventions implemented. Or, a health care practitioner may collaborate with partners or participate in coalitions to increase breast-feeding awareness and promotion through World Breastfeeding Week, health fairs, or other community events. In addition, a health care practitioner may train nutritionists, nurses, doctors, and other medical professionals on breast-feeding management and supportive ways to increase breast-feeding initiation and duration rates.

In a clinical setting a health care practitioner may provide one-on-one breast-feeding education, counseling, and support of pregnant and lactating women to increase the breast-feeding initiation and duration rates. This initiative supports the *Healthy People 2010* objectives related to increasing the proportion of women who breast-feed their babies (U.S. Department of Health and Human Services, 2000).

Promoting Healthy Eating Practices

Beyond breast-feeding, healthy eating habits among toddlers and children are vitally important, because these lay the foundation for lifelong eating patterns. There are good sources of information on healthy eating practices among toddlers. An example is Children's Healthcare of Atlanta (Buechner, 2001), which has developed a Stress-Free Feeding© curriculum that advocates healthy eating habits and environments for both the parent and child. This initiative supports

the *Healthy People 2010* objective (developmental) related to increasing the proportion of children and adolescents who consume meals and snacks that are of good overall dietary quality (U.S. Department of Health and Human Services, 2000).

5-A-Day

The Produce for Better Health Foundation is a consumer education foundation that chairs the national 5-A-Day for Better Health Program. The 5-A-Day for Better Health Program is the nation's largest public–private nutrition education initiative. The national 5-A-Day Month is observed in September, and this initiative encourages people to consume five to nine servings of colorful fruits and vegetables daily. Researchers have studied the relationship between fruit and vegetable intake and weight maintenance and loss, especially in the pediatric population. For example, one study found that families who increased fruit and vegetable intake tended to consume fewer calories and were better able to mange their weight than those families who focused on decreasing fat and sugar intake in their diet. In addition, 5-A-Day campaigns are timely and useful because they have adaptable toolkits and other promotional items that fit various settings. In particular, There Is a Rainbow on My Plate is a good resource. It is designed to educate children on the importance of healthy eating by consuming a variety of colorful fruits and vegetables. This initiative supports the *Healthy People 2010* objective related to persons 2 years and older who consume two servings of fruit and three servings of vegetables daily (U.S. Department of Health and Human Services, 2000).

The programs and resources discussed above are only a few avenues to explore and recommend to partners and perhaps focus groups. To accomplish the ultimate goal of healthy children in healthy communities, the health care practitioner should be resourceful when suggesting programs, initiatives, and campaigns related to overweight children. The practitioner should have a "toolbox" ready when entering various settings: coalition, community, school, worksite, health care facility, or other organizations. This toolbox of information and resources will vary depending on the target population. Nevertheless, health care practitioners must be creative and timely in sharing their vision and potential solutions to address childhood obesity. The authors encourage health care practitioners and students to research other resources and participate in Internet "listservs" for best practices and new findings in preventing and controlling overweight status among children.

Food Allergies

Shideh Mofidi, MS, RD, CSP

Food allergy: An immune-mediated abnormal response to food (specifically food proteins) triggered by the body's immune system with involvement of multiple systems in the body, including the skin, respiratory, cardiovascular, and/or the gastrointestinal tract.

Over the past 20 years the prevalence of **food allergy** has almost doubled, resulting in increased awareness among the general public and the scientific community. This has led to significant advances not only in the diagnostic evaluation of food allergy but also in the development of therapeutic modalities for the treatment of food allergy. Although 20% to 25% of the general public believe they have food allergies, studies have shown that 3% to 4% of adults and 6% to 8% of children have food allergies. Any food can provoke a reaction, although relatively few foods are responsible for most food-induced allergic reactions. Currently, management of food allergies is educating the food allergic individual to avoid the identified food allergen completely and to initiate therapy in case of an accidental ingestion.

Definitions

Adverse food reaction is a broad term defined as any abnormal reaction resulting from the ingestion of a food that might be the result of **food intolerance** (nonallergic food hypersensitivities) or food hypersensitivity (food allergy) (Sampson, 2004a) Sicherer & Teuber, 2004). Food intolerances do not involve the immune system and are usually limited to the gastrointestinal system. In contrast, food allergy is an immune-mediated abnormal response to food with involvement of multiple systems in the body.

Food intolerance: Any abnormal reaction to food that does not involve the immune system and is usually limited to the gastrointestinal system, such as lactose intolerance.

To correctly diagnose food allergies, it is critical to be aware of and be able to differentiate the symptoms of food allergy from other adverse reactions to foods. Adverse food reactions can be divided into those that are toxic and those that are nontoxic. Toxic reactions do not rely on individual sensitivity and can occur in virtually anyone who ingests sufficient quantities of a tainted food. Examples of toxic reactions include bacterial food poisoning resulting in diarrhea and vomiting, pharmacologic effects such as jitteriness from caffeine or headaches from tyramine-containing foods, or scombroid fish poisoning whereupon ingestion of sufficient quan-

tities of the fish, the histidine in the spoiled fish is metabolized to histamine, resulting in itching, flushing, and angioedema. In contrast, nontoxic adverse reactions to foods depend on individual sensitivity and can be further divided to non–immune mediated (food intolerance) and immune mediated (food allergy). Food intolerance includes conditions such as lactose intolerance, in which sufficient lactase enzyme is not present and nausea, abdominal cramps, bloating, gas, and diarrhea result when lactose, the major sugar found in milk, is ingested. Other conditions categorized as food intolerance are metabolic disorders such as galactosemia, in which deficiency of an enzyme that converts galactose to glucose results in a myriad of significant complications; pancreatic insufficiency such as in cystic fibrosis; and neuronally mediated illness such as in gustatory rhinitis-rhinorrhea from spicy or hot foods or auriculotemporal syndrome where there is facial flushing after ingestion of tart foods (Sampson, 2004b; Sicherer & Sampson, 2006).

Food allergy is different from food intolerance in that the reactions are specifically related to food proteins, not to fat or carbohydrate. The offending allergens are typically small glycoproteins that are heat resistant and acid stable (Sampson, 2004b). Food hypersensitivity can be further classified based on the role of IgE antibody as **IgE mediated, non–IgE mediated** (cell mediated), and mixed IgE and cell mediated (**Table 7.7**). Typically, the IgE-mediated food allergies are characterized by an acute onset of symptoms that typically involve the skin, respiratory and cardiovascular systems, and/or the gastrointestinal tract (**Table 7.8**) (Sampson, 2004b).

IgE- and non–IgE-mediated food allergies: IgE-mediated allergies are characterized by an acute onset of symptoms that typically involve the skin, respiratory, cardiovascular, and/or the gastrointestinal tract. Non–IgE-mediated or cell-mediated allergies are slower in onset and primarily are gastrointestinal reactions.

When a food protein is ingested, the IgE recognizes it on the surface of these cells; mediators such as histamine are released, and symptoms occur. These symptoms usually occur within minutes and up to 2 hours after the ingestion of the food. The severity of the reaction depends on many factors, including the disease pathophysiology, host factors, the quantity of allergen ingested, and other ancillary factors such as exercise and intake of other foods and/or alcohol (Sicherer & Teuber, 2004; Sicherer & Sampson 2006). The non–IgE-mediated food allergies are generally slower in onset and primarily produce gastrointestinal reactions but can affect the same organ systems that the IgE form affects.

TABLE 7.7	Spectrum of Food Allergy Disorders

IgE mediated
  Oral allergy syndrome
  Anaphylaxis
  Urticaria
Mixed IgE and non–IgE (cell) mediated
  Allergic eosinophilic esophagitis
  Allergic eosinophilic gastroenteritis
  Atopic dermatitis
  Asthma
Non–IgE mediated
  Protein-induced enterocolitis
  Protein-induced enteropathy
  Eosinophilic proctocolitis
  Contact dermatitis
  Dermatitis herpetiformis

A single food is composed of many proteins, and these proteins have several areas to which the immune system can respond. These areas, called epitopes, can behave differently in response to a food protein de-

TABLE 7.8	Symptoms of an Allergic Reaction

Cutaneous (skin symptoms)
- Itchy rash
- Urticaria (hives)
- Erythema (redness)
- Angioedema (swelling of the face, lips and tongue)
- Atopic dermatitis (eczema)

Gastrointestinal
- Itching of the lips, tongue, or mouth
- Nausea and vomiting
- Abdominal cramping and pain
- Diarrhea

Respiratory
- Watery and/or itchy eyes
- Rhinitis (nasal congestion)
- Sneezing
- Dry cough
- Itching or tightness in the throat
- Tightness in the chest or shortness of breath
- Wheezing

Cardiovascular
- Hypotension (low blood pressure)
- Syncope
- Shock
- Arrhythmia

pending on the way the protein is folded. Further investigations of these epitopes are underway in an attempt to determine the difference in outcome and outgrowing of food allergies (Beyer et al., 2003, 2005).

Prevalence

Food allergy affects about 6% to 8% of infants and young children and approximately 3% to 4% of adults (Sampson, 2003; Sicherer, Munoz-Furlong, & Sampson, 2004; Sicherer & Sampson, 2006). Prevalence of IgE-mediated food allergy in children with moderate to severe atopic dermatitis is higher and has been reported at about 35% (Eigenmann, Sicherer, Borowski, Cohen, & Sampson, 1998). Adverse reactions to food additives (nonprotein colors and preservatives) are rare, at about less than 1% (Sicherer & Teuber, 2004).

The prevalence of an allergy to a specific food depends on societal eating patterns such as increased incidence of fish allergy in Scandinavian countries. In the United States, 2.5% of infants have milk allergy and 1.1% of the general population has peanut or tree nut allergy (Sampson, 2003; Sicherer et al., 2004). The specific food and food proteins in question and the mechanism of reactivity determine the clinical course and natural history of food allergy.

The most common food allergens in the pediatric population are milk, egg, wheat, soy, peanuts, tree nuts, fish, and shellfish, whereas peanuts, tree nuts, fish, and shellfish predominate in adults (Sampson, 2003; Sicherer & Teuber, 2004; Sicherer & Sampson, 2006). A 5-year follow-up study of peanut and tree nut allergy using a random-digit dial telephone survey found a doubling of prevalence of peanut allergy in American children aged 5 years and younger from 0.4% in 1997 to 0.8% in 2002 (Sicherer, Munoz-Furlong, & Sampson, 2003). About 85% of childhood food allergies to cow's milk, egg, wheat, and soy are outgrown by 5 years of age; however, allergy to peanut, tree nuts, and seafood are not commonly outgrown (Sicherer & Teuber, 2004).

Allergy Incidence and Immediate Treatment

Although 20% to 25% of the general public believes they have food allergies, studies have shown that 3.5% to 4% of adults and 6% to 8% of children have food allergies. Virtually any food protein can cause a reaction; however, only a small number of foods account for most adverse food reactions. The foods that most commonly cause allergic reactions in children are egg, milk, soy, wheat, peanuts, tree nuts, and fish. Adults most often react to peanuts, tree nuts, fish, and shellfish. The drug of choice for the treatment of severe or potentially severe food allergic reactions is epinephrine.

Other Reactions to Food Proteins

There are several other types of reactions to food proteins that may or may not be IgE mediated. In this section, anaphylaxis, oral allergy syndrome, celiac disease, and allergic eosinophilic esophagitis/gastroenteritis are briefly described as a representative of these other allergic disorders.

Food-Induced Anaphylaxis

Anaphylaxis: Sudden, severe, potentially fatal systemic allergic reaction that can involve various areas of the body, such as the skin, respiratory tract, gastrointestinal tract, and the cardiovascular system.

Anaphylaxis is a rapid multisystem IgE-mediated food allergic reaction that potentially can be fatal. Fatal food-induced anaphylaxis in the United Stated has a frequency of about 200 per year and accounts for approximately 30,000 emergency room visits every year (Sampson, 2004b; Sampson et al., 2006). Any food protein can in essence cause anaphylaxis; however, the foods responsible for 80% to 90% of life-threatening anaphylactic reactions are peanuts, tree nuts (almond, brazil nuts, cashew, hazelnut, pecan, walnuts), and seafood (Sampson, 2004b; Sampson et al., 2006). Individuals are at higher risk for fatal anaphylaxis when they delay treatment with epinephrine, have asthma, have experienced prior severe reactions, or deny ongoing symptoms (Sicherer & Teuber, 2004). In up to 20% of food-induced anaphylactic episodes, symptoms recur within 2 to 4 hours (Sampson et al., 2006).

Food-associated exercise-induced anaphylaxis is a disorder in which eating a particular food (such as celery) before exercising results in anaphylaxis. Less common is when anaphylaxis occurs after the ingestion of any food. Individuals with this disorder are able to eat any food, even the offending food, and exercise as long as each one is done separately and not in combination (Sampson, 2004b).

Oral Allergy Syndrome

Oral allergy syndrome is an IgE-mediated condition that is characterized by pruritus (itching) and edema of the oral mucosa occurring after the ingestion of certain fresh fruits and vegetables (Ortolani, Ispano, Pastorello, Bigi, & Ansaloni, 1988; Ortolani, Ispano, Pastorello, Ansaloni, & Magri, 1989). The symptoms typically do not progress beyond the mouth. Individuals with sensitivity to pollens are susceptible because proteins found in pollens and in the fruits and vegetables are similar. For example, individuals with birch pollen allergy may experience symptoms after the ingestion of apple, peach, plum, nectarine, cherry, almond, hazelnut, carrots, and celery, whereas individuals with ragweed allergy may experience symptoms with banana, melons, and tomato (Ortolani et al., 1988, 1993). These proteins are heat labile; hence, cooked versions of these foods are typically tolerated. The cooking process denatures the responsible cross-reacting proteins in the foods and there is no reaction. Differentiation of symptoms of oral allergy syndrome from early symptoms of a systemic reaction to food (anaphylaxis) is critical.

Celiac Disease or Gluten-Sensitive Enteropathy

Celiac disease is a non–IgE-mediated immunologic reaction to foods caused by hypersensitivity to gluten presenting with flatulence, steatorrhea, and weight loss. Diarrhea, anemia, or metabolic bone disease can also be presenting symptoms of celiac disease. Hypersensitivity to gluten causes the disease, and the characteristic diagnostic feature is flattening of the villi in a biopsy of the jejunal mucosa upon gluten challenge. Improvement of symptoms upon initiation of a gluten-free diet has been noted in 2 to 3 weeks, although histologic improvements may take up 2 to 3 months (Jones, Robins, & Howdle, 2006).

Allergic Eosinophilic Esophagitis/Gastroenteritis

These are a group of disorders of the gut characterized by eosinophilic inflammation and infiltration of the esophagus, stomach, and/or the small intestine. Symptoms in allergic eosinophilic esophagitis/gastroenteritis do overlap with other gastrointestinal disorders and may include dysphagia, vomiting, diarrhea, obstruction, and malabsorption (Kelly et al., 1995; Kelly, 2000; Orenstein et al., 2000; Sampson & Anderson, 2000; Rothenberg, Mishra, Collins, & Putnam, 2001; Sampson, Sicherer, & Birnbaum, 2001; Liacouras, 2003, 2006; Rothenberg, 2004). However, they are unresponsive to antireflux medications and most often have normal pH probe studies (Justinich, 2000; Liacouras, 2006). A subset of these patients does not exhibit specific IgE antibody to foods (Spergel, Andrews, Brown-Whitehorn, Beausoleil, & Liacouras, 2005). Histopathologic confirmation of significant eosinophilic infiltration of the esophagus, stomach, or small intestine via an endoscopy and biopsy is needed, although it does not identify the responsible allergen (Sampson et al., 2001; Liacouras et al., 2005). Currently, treatment with a strict avoidance diet eliminating all incriminating foods has been suggested, although the number of foods involved may prohibit the long-term use of such a diet. Use of an elemental formula has been shown to be efficacious in some patients (Kelly et al., 1995; Justinich et al., 1996; Markowitz, Spergel, Ruchelli, & Liacorous, 2003; Liacouras, 2006).

Diagnostic Evaluation

Once food allergy is identified as a likely cause of symptoms, confirmation of the diagnosis and identification of the implicated food(s) can proceed. Diagnosis of food allergy requires obtaining a careful history (including a thorough medical and reaction history), physical examination, a food and symptom diary, allergy testing (prick skin and food specific IgE antibody testing), and food challenges to confirm the identified or suspected offending allergens (Bock, 2000; Sicherer, 2002; Sampson, 2004b; Sicherer & Teuber, 2004). In cases of acute reactions, as in urticaria or anaphylaxis, the history is very important and may clearly identify the causal food. In chronic disorders, such as asthma or atopic dermatitis, identification of a particular food may be more difficult. In cases of gastrointestinal reactions, similar problems exist because most often delayed reactions after ingestion of causal foods is noted, making the identification of the food somewhat difficult.

History and Physical Examination

Diagnosis is a team effort, and involvement of the child, the child's family, the dietitian, and the physician are all instrumental in correctly identifying the allergenic foods. The physician should be able to conclude from the history and physical examination whether an allergy or food intolerance is part of the differential diagnosis. The history should provide a description of symptoms, the length of time between ingestion and the development of symptoms, whether ingesting the suspected food produces similar symptoms on different occasions, quantity of food required to produce symptoms, whether other factors such as exercise or alcohol ingestion are necessary to induce symptoms, and the length of time since the last reaction occurred (Sampson, 1999, 2004b; Bock, 2000). The physical examination focuses on the exclusion of nonallergic causes of food-induced symptoms in addition to evaluating disease severity. Also, in performing the physical examination, the overall nutritional status of the child should be assessed, particularly if the child has undergone a prolonged overly restrictive diet.

Diet and Symptom Diaries

Diet diaries are an important component of the diagnostic process. Besides providing the ability to determine adequacy of the diet, they serve as another form of recall of foods eaten and timing of symptoms provoked. Details such as time of the meal or snack, brand name if commercially prepared and/or specific ingredients if homemade, amount consumed and also symptoms noted are recorded in the diary. If the parent can provide the actual labels from the foods consumed during the time the diary was kept, it would further enhance the evaluation. Reviewing the diet diaries can be a starting point for the dietitian and the physician to identify a particular food that is common to different products and is repeatedly causing similar symptoms. It can also help reveal hidden sources of the food allergen or unknown sources of contamination and provide a listing of foods that can help facilitate directive counseling. Utilizing alternative foods similar to what is recorded in the diet diary can enhance compliance to the restricted diet significantly.

Laboratory Studies

Food-specific IgE antibody testing can help provide more information regarding either identifying or excluding IgE-mediated food allergies. Prick–puncture skin tests (PST) and radioallergosorbent (RAST) tests are useful standardized screening tools that establish presence of food allergen-specific IgE. (Sampson & Ho, 1997; Bock, 2000; Sicherer & Teuber, 2004; Sicherer & Sampson, 2006). It is important to stress that these tests do not indicate symptomatic clinical reactivity. These test results must be interpreted in combination with information from the child's history, physical examination, and diet/symptom diaries.

In PSTs, commercial food antigen extracts (foods being tested) and positive (histamine) and negative (saline) controls are applied by the prick or puncture method using a bifurcated needle or multipurpose plastic device. In a sensitized individual, food allergen binds to specific IgE antibody present on the surface of the mast cells in the skin and causes degranulation of mast cells. Histamine released from mast cells leads to a flare or erythema and wheal response within 10 to 15 minutes. Wheals equal to or greater than 3 mm compared with the negative control are considered positive with the rest, less than 3 mm, as negative. In infants and young children a wheal greater than 8 to 10 mm is associated with a greater than 95% likelihood of clinical reactivity to cow's milk, egg, and peanuts (Sporik, Hill, & Hosking, 2000).

There is a high false-positive rate associated with skin tests (about 50%), although negative predictive accuracy is greater than 95% (Sampson, 2004b). Hence, a negative PST to a particular food excludes an IgE-mediated reaction and a positive PST in isolation cannot be proof of clinical reactivity. However, a positive PST in an individual with a history of systemic anaphylactic reactions after ingestion of the isolated food may be considered diagnostic (Sampson, 2004b; Sicherer & Teuber, 2004). Commercial fruit and vegetable extracts may lack the proteins responsible for IgE-mediated sensitivity because they are susceptible to protein degradation (Ortolani et al., 1989; Sampson, 2004b). Fresh food extracts can be especially useful in detecting sensitivity to fruits and vegetables. The prick–prick method, which involves pricking the fresh food and then pricking the skin of the child, is most beneficial in situations where raw fruits and/or vegetables are symptomatic but cooked versions are tolerated without any problems.

The child undergoing skin testing (PST) should be off antihistamines; otherwise, it may result in a false-negative test to the particular food tested. Histamine wheals less than 3 to 5 mm in diameter may indicate the presence of an interfering antihistamine.

Food-specific IgE antibody blood testing (CAP RAST system) also measures the presence of food-specific IgE antibodies, although they are not as sensitive as PSTs. A negative test (food-specific IgE antibody < 0.35 kIU/L) has a greater than 95% predictive value; however, a positive blood test has low specificity (Sampson, 2004b; Sicherer & Teuber, 2004). The advantage of blood tests in the evaluation of a food allergic child is that levels are not affected by antihistamine use. Although these tests also have the same inherent problems as do PSTs, a negative blood test virtually excludes an IgE-mediated sensitivity but a positive result in isolation cannot be proof of clinical reactivity.

Studies have looked at the positive predictive value of the CAP RAST system in children undergoing oral food challenges (Sampson & Ho, 1997; Sampson, 2001). Clinical decision points indicating greater than 95% likelihood of reaction have been established for the most common food allergens, including milk (15 kU/L), egg (7 kU/L), peanut (14 kU/L), tree nuts (~ 15 kU/L), and fish (20 kU/L). These numbers indicate that a child older than 2 years with a milk IgE antibody of at least 15 kU/L is highly likely (> 95%) to react if milk was ingested accidentally or during a milk challenge. This would, in addition, infer that a milk challenge should be deferred unless there is convincing history that the child tolerates a significant quantity of milk without a reaction. Milk-specific IgE of 5 kU/L for a child aged 12 months or less and egg-specific IgE of 2 kU/L for a child aged 24 months or less has been shown to have a 95% positive predictive value (Sampson, 2001).

At this point in time current diagnostic laboratory methods such as PST and food-specific IgE cannot distinguish between individuals who will outgrow their food allergies. Ongoing research using the microarray technology is focusing on epitope recognition patterns that can be used to identify markers of persistent food allergy. This information can be significant when therapy for food allergy other than dietary avoidance becomes available (Beyer et al., 2003, 2005).

Other forms of skin testing, such as intradermal or patch testing, can be used in the diagnostic process; however, there are inherent problems with these tests. Intradermal allergy skin tests are contraindicated because they have high false-positive rates and have been associated with systemic reactions (Sampson, 2004b; Sicherer & Teuber, 2004). The atopy patch test has been recently proposed as a useful screening tool in children with atopic dermatitis in diagnosing late-phase clinical reactions (Niggemann, Reibel, & Wahn, 2000; Roehr et al., 2001). More studies are needed to study other subject groups, such as adults, and also to study the atopy patch test more closely in relation to optimum concentration of the food used in the patch test and in correlation with double-blind placebo-controlled food challenges before using this as another widespread screening tool for diagnosing food allergies.

A number of unproven tests should not be used, and they include provocation neutralization, cytotoxic test, applied kinesiology, hair analysis, and IgG₄ testing, among others (Terr & Salvaggio, 1996; Ortolani et al., 1999; Sicherer & Teuber, 2004; Beyer & Teuber, 2005).

A negative prick skin test or food-specific IgE in the blood essentially excludes IgE-mediated reactivity. A positive prick skin test or food-specific IgE in the blood indicates the presence of IgE antibody and does not represent symptomatic clinical reactivity. However, a positive PST or food-specific IgE in the blood in an individual with a history of systemic anaphylactic reactions after ingestion of the isolated food may be considered diagnostic. Any food, whether it has a negative or positive skin and/or blood result, that has been identified through the history to have provoked a serious reaction should only be reintroduced under physician supervision with emergency medication immediately available.

Elimination Diets and Oral Food Challenges

The next step in the diagnostic evaluation is confirming that the foods identified through testing are in fact problem foods. Elimination diets and oral food challenges both have a significant role in this process. Selection of single-ingredient foods without any contamination with other allergens is critical in this verification process.

A negative prick skin test or a negative food-specific IgE blood test (<0.35 kU/L) essentially excludes IgE-mediated reactivity, and reintroduction of the particular food is not likely to elicit a reaction, at least acutely. However, if that same food with negative skin and/or blood test results has been identified through the history to have provoked a serious reaction, it should only be reintroduced under physician supervision with emergency medication immediately available (Mofidi & Bock, 2005).

If test results are positive, an elimination diet can be considered to determine if the symptoms are caused by the foods that tested positive on either skin or blood test. If the elimination diet fails to show resolution of the underlying disorder, the foods can be reintroduced to the diet unless, again, a convincing history warrants a supervised food challenge. The possibility that the wrong foods were eliminated or the presence of some level of contamination has to also be accounted for if there is no resolution of symptoms.

If the elimination diet results in resolution of symptoms, an oral food challenge should be considered so that foods can be added back to the diet one by one. Oral food challenges would not be appropriate for severe reactions of isolated food ingestion with a positive food-specific IgE antibody. These patients are at high risk for severe and potentially life-threatening reactions. Any food, whether it is one of the major allergens or not, that has been reported to provoke a serious reaction should only be reintroduced under physician supervision with emergency medications immediately available (Sicherer, 1999; Mofidi & Bock, 2005).

If any foods were eliminated from the child's diet based on positive skin and/or blood results even though there is a history of tolerance of those specific foods before the allergy testing, possible reintroduction of those foods to the child's diet should be discussed with the physician. If reintroduction of the foods is suggested, each food should be introduced one at a time over 5 to 7 days so that any adverse reaction can be identified and further investigated. Some of the foods may also need to be introduced under physician supervision with emergency medication available.

There is no simple supporting laboratory test for non–IgE-mediated disease, and in many cases histopathologic confirmation via an endoscopy is required (Kelly, 2000; Noel et al., 2004a; Potter et al.,

2004; Liacouras, 2006). However, a positive biopsy for eosinophils does not specifically identify the responsible allergen in the diet. Elimination diets and oral food challenges are therefore needed to support this diagnosis as well. If an elimination diet results in resolution of symptoms, an oral food challenge is performed to identify the particular foods involved. Symptoms from ingestion of particular foods in enteropathy syndromes or eosinophilic esophagitis/gastroenteritis may require several days of ingestion to elicit symptoms. In these cases, foods are added one at a time with at least 1 to 2 weeks between each food introduction. The length of time between each food introduction depends on the specific food and the reported history in relation to that food (Mofidi & Bock, 2005). In food protein–induced enterocolitis syndrome, which is a symptom complex of profuse vomiting and diarrhea, symptoms completely resolve when the responsible food protein is removed from the diet. Most often cow's milk or soy are responsible for the symptoms observed in food protein–induced enterocolitis syndrome, although other food proteins such as egg, wheat, rice, oat, chicken, and fish have also been noted to induce enterocolitis symptoms (Sicherer, 2000; Nowak-Wegrzyn, Sampson, Wood, & Sicherer, 2003).

Elimination Diets

Elimination diets: A diet in which suspected foods are eliminated in an attempt to identify and/or confirm offending allergenic foods.

Elimination diets are central to the diagnosis and treatment of food allergies and when used in the diagnostic process should be for a specified trial period. The symptoms attributed to the food should resolve and then reappear when the food is reintroduced. The duration of the diet can be from 1 week (for acute symptoms such as hives) to 8 weeks (for chronic symptoms such as vomiting and diarrhea), depending on the underlying suspected disorder. Success of the elimination diet depends on the correct identification of the allergen(s) and complete exclusion of the allergen(s) from the diet. In some gastrointestinal food allergies, an elemental diet using amino acid-based formulas may be required before significant resolution of gut pathology can be noted via endoscopy and biopsy.

When elimination diets are used in the management and essentially as the treatment of food allergies, education becomes the focal point for not only the health care providers but also for the child and the child's family. The physician and the dietitian teach the food allergic individual and his or her family the principles of daily management of food allergies. The individual or his or her family will take on the role of the educator to teach other family members, teachers, and staff at day cares, schools, and camps and others involved in the day-to-day life of the food allergic individual (Munoz-Furlong, 2003). All involved in the care of the allergic individual need to be educated on the basic principles of food allergy because an accident or a simple mistake can lead to a reaction ranging from mild discomfort to life-threatening anaphylaxis.

The principles of management are quite simple in theory but can be quite complicated upon implementation. The identified allergenic food(s) must be removed from the diet while adequate nutrition is provided to promote appropriate growth and development despite the limitations of some of the major contributors to the diet. This is most critical in the management of food allergies in infants and children. The nutritional quality of the diet depends on the number of major foods restricted, the availability of appropriate food substitutes, and the palatability of the diet (Mofidi, 2003). It is certainly not necessary to limit an entire food family; the focus of the treatment plan is to minimize the list of restricted foods.

There are three types of elimination diets:

1. Elimination of one or several foods suspected of provoking symptoms
2. Elimination of all but a defined group of "allowed" foods, also called the "eat only" diet
3. Use of an amino acid-based formula, or the elemental diet

The type of elimination diet used depends on the clinical situation being evaluated, the age of the child, the reported history, and the results of tests for food-specific IgE antibody (skin and blood). The first type of an elimination diet is useful when an isolated food ingestion provokes a sudden acute reaction and there is a positive IgE to the food. By avoiding the specific food in all forms, symptoms should resolve (Mofidi, 2003).

When more than one particular food allergen is suspected, then a limited "eat only" diet is prescribed. The foods allowed are those that cannot be related to an isolated reaction or were negative on skin and/or blood testing. Individualization is critical in this type of an elimination diet, not only for selection of the allowed foods but also for compliance. If the symptoms attributed to the foods still persist, a thorough review of the diet is necessary to ensure that no other food allergens have been inadvertently added to the diet. If a source of contamination or mistake cannot be found, reassessment of the allowed foods may be necessary to determine if the causal food is still in the diet (Mofidi, 2003).

In the elemental diet, all nutrient needs are essentially obtained from the amino acid-based formula. Occasionally, one or two foods are allowed to provide textures to the individual on the elimination diet.

Allergic eosinophilic esophagitis: A disease involving patchy infiltration of one or more layers of the esophagus with eosinophils.

Allergic eosinophilic gastroenteritis: A disease involving patchy infiltration of one or more layers of the stomach and/or small intestine with eosinophils.

Elemental diets are generally required for gastrointestinal food allergies such as **allergic eosinophilic esophagitis** and **allergic eosinophilic gastroenteritis**. Studies have looked at the use of systemic and inhaled corticosteroids in allergic eosinophilic esophagitis and have both clinical and histologic improvements (Liacouras, Wenner, Brown, & Ruchelli, 1998). However, the symptoms often recur upon the discontinuation of the medications (Noel et al., 2004b; Liacouras et al., 2005). The elemental diet has become a fundamental part of the treatment of these gastrointestinal food allergies (Kelly et al., 1995; Kelly, 2000; Markowitz et al., 2003; Spergel et al., 2005; Liacouras, 2006). It allows healing of the gut during the elimination process and further allows the identification and hence restriction of the offending food allergen during the slow introduction of foods. Upon accurate identification and restriction of the suspect foods, these individuals are symptom free and do not require medications. Even though all foods have been implicated in allergic eosinophilic esophagitis, the most common foods have been milk, eggs, nuts, beef, wheat, fish, shellfish, corn, and soy (Spergel et al., 2005; Liacouras, 2006).

Label Reading

Dietary elimination of any of the major allergens, such as egg, milk, soy, wheat, or peanut, is not a simple procedure. Particular allergens may be hidden in unsuspected foods, such as milk or egg proteins in bread products, milk or soy protein in canned tuna, peanut flour in cakes, sauces, or chili, and peanut butter as the glue that holds egg rolls together (Steinman, 1996). Education regarding, for example, elimination of egg protein from the diet includes not only avoidance of egg-based foods (mayonnaise, ice cream, and quiche), but also learning to identify words used on food labels that may indicate the presence of egg protein as a "hidden ingredient" in the food (Mofidi, 2003). When looking at a food label the parent

should be able to recognize terms that can be easily identified to be an egg byproduct (egg white), terms that are not so obvious (ovomucoid), or terms that may or may not be egg based (lecithin, natural flavor). There are "How to read a label" cards available from the Food Allergy and Anaphylaxis Network (FAAN, a nonprofit organization located in Fairfax, VA) to assist patients, their families, dietitians, and physicians in this very difficult task of eliminating particular food allergens (Table 7.9). FAAN provides accurate and current information on food allergies with resources ranging from handouts and cookbooks to videos and bimonthly newsletters. In addition, FAAN sponsors conferences to educate professionals and individuals about managing food allergies. They have numerous materials for dealing with travel, school, and eating out in addition to a dedicated website for kids and teens dealing with specific topics related to those age groups and compliance issues.

The Food Allergen Labeling and Consumer Protection Act took effect in January 1, 2006. The new labeling law requires simple terms and plain language to be used to indicate the presence of the top eight food allergens in packaged foods. It would either identify an allergen, for example, casein, in a product with the words "contains milk" or declare it immediately after the term such as "albumin (egg)." These ingredients are to be listed even if they are present in colors, flavors, or even spice blends. This new law should help with identification of safe foods for allergic individuals.

Nutritional Issues

Teaching the parent how to replace, for example, egg in the diet by providing an alternate source of nutrients is essential. It is also important to provide appropriate substitutions so that egg-free baked goods with appropriate texture and taste can be prepared. Palatability of these products determines the degree of compliance to the elimination diet. Cookbooks from FAAN and other resources are available with recipes and substitution guidelines that do contain any milk, egg, soy, wheat, peanuts, or tree nuts.

When one food or a food group is eliminated from the diet, alternative sources of nutrients that are lost through the elimination diet need to be identified. For example, if the allergy is to milk, which is a major contributor to the diet, all dairy products need to be avoided. Hence, calcium, phosphorus, riboflavin, pantothenic acid, vitamin B_{12}, vitamin A, and vitamin D need to be supplied from other sources.

| TABLE 7.9 | How To Read A Label |

HOW TO READ A LABEL FOR A MILK-FREE DIET
Avoid foods that contain milk or any of these ingredients:

artificial butter flavor
butter, butter fat, butter oil
buttermilk
casein (*casein hydrolysate*)
caseinates (*in all forms*)
cheese
cream
cottage cheese
curds
custard
ghee
half & half
lactalbumin, lactalbumin phosphate
lactoferrin
lactulose
milk (*in all forms including condensed, derivative, dry, evaporated, goat's milk and milk from other animals, low-fat, malted, milkfat, non-fat, powder, protein, skimmed, solids, whole*)
nisin
nougat
pudding
recaldent
rennet casein
sour cream, sour cream solids
sour milk solids
whey (*in all forms*)
yogurt

May indicate the presence of milk protein:

carmel candies
chocolate
flavorings (*including natural and artificial*)
high protein flour
lactic acid started culture
lactose
luncheon meat, hot dogs, sausages
margarine
non-dairy products

HOW TO READ A LABEL for an EGG-FREE DIET
Avoid foods that contain eggs or any of these ingredients:
albumin (*also spelled as* albumen)
egg (*dried, powdered, solids, white, yolk*)
eggnog
lysozyme
mayonnaise
meringue (*meringue powder*)
surimi

May indicate the presence of egg protein:

flavoring (*including natural and artificial*)
lecithin
macaroni
marzipan
marshmallows
nougat
pasta

HOW TO READ A LABEL for a PEANUT-FREE DIET
Avoid foods that contain peanuts or any of these ingredients:

artificial nuts
beer nuts
cold pressed, expelled, or extruded peanut oil
goobers
ground nuts
mixed nuts
monkey nuts
nutmeat
nut pieces
peanut
peanut butter
peanut flour

May indicate the presence of peanut protein:

African, Asian (*especially Chinese, Indian, Indonesian, Thai, and Vietnamese*), and Mexican dishes
baked goods (*pastries, cookies, etc.*)
candy (*including chocolate candy*)
chili
egg rolls
enchilada sauce
flavoring (*including natural and artificial*)
marzipan
mole sauce
nougat

- Mandelonas are peanuts soaked in almond flavoring.
- Studies show most allergic individuals can surely eat peanut oil (*not* cold pressed, expelled, or extruded peanut oil).
- Arachis oil is peanut oil.
- Experts advise patients allergic to peanuts to avoid tree nuts as well.
- A study showed that unlike other legumes, there is a strong possibility of cross reaction between peanuts and lupine.
- Sunflower seeds are often produced on equipment shared with peanuts.

HOW TO READ A LABEL for a WHEAT-FREE DIET
Avoid foods that contain wheat or any of these ingredients:
bran
bread crumbs
bulgur
club wheat
couscous
cracker meal
durum
einkorn
emmer
farina
flour (*all purpose, bread, cake, durum, enriched, graham, high gluten, high protein, instant, pastry, self-rising, soft wheat, steel ground, stone ground, whole wheat*)
gluten
kamut
matzoh, matzoh meal (*also spelled as matzo*)
pasta
seitan
semolina
spelt
triticale

TABLE 7.9 How To Read A Label (continued)

vital gluten
wheat (*bran, germ, gluten, malt, sprouts*)
wheat grass
whole wheat berries

May indicate the presence of wheat protein:
flavoring (*including natural and artificial*)
hydrolyzed protein
soy sauce
starch (*gelatinized starch, modified starch, modified food starch, vegetable starch, wheat starch*)
surimi

HOW TO READ A LABEL for a SOY-FREE DIET
Avoid foods that contain soy or any of these ingredients:
edamame
hydrolyzed soy protein
miso
natto
shoyu sauce
soy (*soy albumin, soy fiber, soy flour, soy grits, soy milk, soy nuts, soy sprouts*)
soya
soybean (*curd, granules*)
soy protein (*concentrate, isolate*)
soy sauce
Tamari
Tempeh
textured vegetable protein (*TVP*)
tofu

May indicate the presence of soy protein:
Asian cuisine
flavoring (*including natural and artificial*)
vegetable broth
vegetable gum
vegetable starch

- Studies show most individuals allergic to soy may safely eat soybean oil.
- Most individuals allergic to soy can safely eat soy lecithin.

Check with your doctor if you have questions about these ingredients.

HOW TO READ A LABEL for a SHELLFISH-FREE DIET
Avoid foods that contain shellfish or any of these ingredients:
abalone
clams (*cherrystones, littleneck, pismo, quahog*)
cockle (*periwinkle, sea urchin*)
crab
crawfish (*crayfish, ecrevisse*)
lobster (*langouste, langoustine, scampo, coral, tomalley*)
mollusks
mussels
octopus
oysters
prawns
scallops
shrimp (*crevette*)
snails (*escargot*)
squid (*calamari*)

May indicate the presence of shellfish protein:
bouillabaisse
cuttlefish ink
fish stock
flavoring (*including natural and artificial*)
seafood flavoring (*such as crab or clam extract*)
surimi

Keep the following in mind:
- Any food served in a seafood restaurant may be cross contaminated with fish or shellfish.
- For some individuals, a reaction may occur from cooking odors or from handling fish or shellfish.
- Always carry medications and use them as soon as symptoms develop.

HOW TO READ A LABEL for a TREE NUT-FREE DIET
Avoid foods that contain nuts or any of these ingredients:
almonds
artificial nuts
beech nut
Brazil nuts
butternut
caponata
cashews
chestnuts
chinquapin
coconut
filberts/hazelnuts
gianduja (*a nut mixture found in some chocolate*)
ginko nut
hickory nuts
lichee/lychee nut
macadamia nuts
marzipan/almond paste
nan-gai nuts
natural nut extract (*i.e., almond, walnut*)
nougat
nut butters (*i.e., cashew butter*)
nut meal
nutmeat
nut oil
nut paste (*i.e., almond paste*)
nut pieces (*Mashuga Nuts®*)
pecans
pesto
pili nut
pine nuts (*also referred to as Indian, piñon, pinyon, pignoli, pigñolia, and pignon nuts*)
pistachios
praline
sheanut
walnuts

- Mandelonas are peanuts soaked in almond flavoring.
- Mortadella may contain pistachios.
- Natural and artificial flavoring may contain tree nuts.
- Experts advise patients allergic to tree nuts avoid peanuts as well.
- Talk to your doctor if you find other nuts not listed here.

It is rather difficult to obtain calcium from nondairy foods. There are, however, alternate milks (rice, soy, and potato) and juices (orange, apple, grape) that are enriched with calcium. Also, there are some milk-free calcium supplements available. Intake of other foods in the diet needs to be looked at to determine if adequate amounts of, for example, vitamin A are provided and, if necessary, to stress intake of foods high in vitamin A. Table 7.10 provides a listing of the problem nutrients in milk-, egg-, soy-, wheat-, and peanut-free diets (Mofidi, 2003). Obviously, the distribution of carbohydrates, protein, and fats is altered and needs to be addressed in an elimination diet. The RDA for age and gender can be used as a guide to provide the child with appropriate nutrition.

Manufacturers change product ingredients and production procedures frequently, where products that were safe may become unsafe and visa versa. Education of the family dealing with food allergies and specifically focusing on skills necessary to proceed with evaluating and identifying what is safe and what is not are critical for the management of food allergies. Thorough guidance, which may include providing information on label reading, brand identification, what to inquire when calling the manufacturers, restaurant dining, and recipe modification, is essential to ensure nutritional adequacy as well as management of symptoms.

Cross-Contamination

Another major source of hidden allergens is cross-contamination. Contact of one food with another even in trace amounts can pose a problem for a highly allergic child. Cross-contaminations can occur due to processing errors, where an ingredient is added to a batch of food by mistake, or due to processing on shared lines, where the equipment is not adequately cleaned. It also can occur when purchasing food items from bulk bins or at a deli counter, where, for example, the same slicer is used for cutting both meats and cheese, or from accidents in food preparation at home where the same knife is used for peanut butter and then simply wiped clean and used for jelly to make a sandwich. In the food industry the use of leftover products, or "rework," to the next batch of products is a common practice. For example, the addition of a small amount of cookie dough that has had the nuts filtered out to a new batch of chocolate chip cookies will add nut residues and possibly enough protein to elicit an allergic reaction in a nut-allergic child.

There are also nonedible sources of food allergens, such as milk or peanut products in pet foods, hacky sacks or bean bags filled with walnut shells, shampoos, cosmetics, or other body care products with a variety of food allergens (Bernhisel-Broadbent, 1999). Reviewing all ingredients and contacting the manufacturers regarding vague terms used on the labels is a requirement in allergen avoidance.

Oral Food Challenges

Oral food challenges are used to identify, confirm, or rule out a suspected allergy to food(s) in both IgE-mediated and non–IgE-mediated food allergies; oral food challenge remains the most accurate method for diagnosing food allergy (Bock et al., 1988; Sicherer, 1999; Mofidi & Bock, 2005). It can also be used to determine if clinical reactivity to a food is lost. When several foods are in question as possible causal foods and elimination of those foods from the diet resulted in resolution of symptoms, an oral food challenge to each food is warranted. An oral food challenge can also be used for complaints that are not typically associated with food allergy (headache, behavior, etc.). Food challenge in a child with a recent history of severe anaphylaxis to an isolated ingestion with positive specific IgE antibody to the particular food is contraindicated, although a physician-supervised follow-up challenge to determine resolution of the allergy may be indicated in some settings.

Several types of food challenges can be used depending on the history, results of IgE tests, and resources available to the physician. Food challenges can be open (parent and physician are aware of the challenge content), single blind (parent is unaware but the physician is aware of the challenge content), or a double-blind placebo-controlled food challenge (neither parent nor the physician is aware of the challenge

> **Oral food challenges:** A procedure during which the patient eats or drinks the suspected food allergen gradually in small portions over a given period of time under a physician's supervision.

TABLE 7.10	Problem Nutrients in an Allergen-Restricted Diet
Allergen	**Nutrients**
Milk	Vitamin A, vitamin D, riboflavin, pantothenic acid, cyanocobalamin, calcium, and phosphorus
Egg	Cyanocobalamin, riboflavin, pantothenic acid, biotin, and selenium
Soy	Thiamin, riboflavin, pyridoxine, folate, calcium, phosphorus, magnesium, iron, and zinc
Wheat	Thiamin, riboflavin, niacin, iron, and folate if fortified
Peanut	Vitamin E, niacin, magnesium, manganese, and chromium

contents) (Sicherer, 1999; Mofidi & Bock, 2005). The double-blind placebo-controlled food challenge is considered the "gold standard" for the diagnosis of food allergy (Sampson, 2004a; Sicherer & Teuber, 2004). In a clinic setting, use of double-blind placebo-controlled food challenges is recommended because bias in the diagnosis of allergy to a particular food is removed from all parties; however, it is very labor intensive. The advantage of an open challenge is that it is quick and easy and a good screening tool.

Food challenges are generally performed in a fasting state with gradually increasing amounts of the food given with the dose and the timing individualized to the child's history for a total of 60 to 90 minutes (Sicherer, 1999; Mofidi & Bock, 2005). The child is evaluated for the development of symptoms throughout the challenge. Medical supervision and immediate access to emergency medications, including epinephrine, antihistamines, steroids, and inhaled beta agonists, in addition to equipment for cardiopulmonary resuscitation are required because reactions can be severe (Bock et al., 1988; Sicherer, 1999; Sicherer & Teuber, 2004). Challenges are terminated when a reaction becomes apparent, followed by administration of emergency medication. Patients are also observed and monitored for delayed reactions.

Negative challenges are always followed by an open feeding of a normal serving size of the challenge food to rule out a false-negative challenge (Mofidi & Bock, 2005). If the child can tolerate this portion of the challenge without any symptoms, the specific food can be added back to the diet.

The selection of the food for food challenges is determined by the history and results of IgE tests. Foods that are identified by positive skin or blood tests without a significant history of a reaction or that are unlikely to provoke a reaction can be screened by open challenges. In IgE-mediated food allergies, a negative food challenge is definite proof that the patient is no longer sensitive to the particular food and allows the addition of the food to the diet (Mofidi & Bock, 2005). Suspected food allergens should be eliminated for 7 to 14 days before the food challenge in IgE-mediated disorders and up to 12 weeks in some gastrointestinal disorders. Before the challenge the child should be off antihistamines long enough to promote a normal histamine response (Sampson, 1999, 2004b).

Prevention of Food Allergies

Several studies have looked at and tried to generate reasonable recommendations for prevention of food allergies. Exclusive breast-feeding and introduction of solid foods after 4 to 6 months of age have been shown to be associated with decreased risk of atopic dermatitis and cow's milk allergy in infants with an atopic predisposition. If breast-feeding is not possible, extensively hydrolyzed formulas may potentially prevent atopic disease and food allergy (von Berg et al., 2003; Zeiger, 2003). Avoidance of highly allergenic foods such as peanuts has not been shown to have a consistent protective effect when consumed during pregnancy and/or lactation. Exclusive breast-feeding and/or use of extensively hydrolyzed formula in addition to delayed introduction of solids until 6 months has been suggested for infants with a positive family history of food allergies. In addition, delayed introduction of the highly allergenic foods such as peanuts, tree nuts, and seafood to 3 to 4 years of age has also been suggested (American Academy of Pediatrics, Committee on Nutrition, 2000).

Summary

Vegetarian diets can be healthful and nutritionally adequate for infants, children, and adolescents and can provide health and nutritional benefits. Key nutrients for vegetarian children and adolescents include protein, iron, zinc, calcium, vitamin D, vitamin B_{12}, and omega-3 fatty acids. A vegetarian diet can meet requirements for all these nutrients, although in some instances fortified foods or supplements can be especially useful in meeting recommendations. Dietetics professionals play key roles in counseling vegetarian children and adolescents and their families.

Health care practitioners may use existing nutrition and social programs as opportunities to promote evidenced-based strategies to prevent obesity in children. Because many nutrition and social programs have a narrow focus, population-based services are essential to help communities, schools, worksites, other organizations, and families to adopt healthy behaviors. Healthy eating among children cannot be addressed without addressing the family as a whole and the environment. As discussed earlier, almost 65% of adults are overweight or obese, and this is a risk factor for their children to become overweight. Indeed, childhood obesity is a major public health concern; however, preventive efforts must target the parents and caregivers, as well as the children. Improving family interaction through healthy eating practices and physical activity is essential to preventing childhood obesity. Healthy life-style behaviors can be taught in parenting classes, discussed during doctor's office visits, and presented at worksites, health fairs, parent–teacher organizations, and other sites. In addition, population-based services and partners can develop and implement policy and environmental interventions that make it convenient for families to include healthy eating practices and daily physical activity.

Food allergy is a simple term for a variety of immune-mediated adverse reactions to foods. The prevalence of food allergy has increased significantly over the last few years with increased awareness of the general public and the scientific community. An accurate diagnosis is extremely important to clarify the nature and cause of the reactions to determine effective measures of disease management. Elimination diets and oral food challenges are fundamental to not only identify but also to verify and rule out a suspected allergy to a food or several foods.

Dietary restrictions should be relevant to the observed symptoms, and unnecessary restrictions should be avoided in the interest of the patient's health. To date, the treatment of food allergy is directed at complete removal and avoidance of the offending food allergen. The success of this treatment depends on correct identification of the allergens with complete exclusion of those allergens from the diet, provision of an adequate diet, and recognition and prompt treatment of acute reactions. Education of the family dealing with food allergies and specifically focusing on mastering the skills necessary to proceed with evaluating and identifying what is safe and what is not is critical for the management of food allergies.

Issues to Debate

1. How would you advise a vegetarian family whose 12-year-old wants to begin eating meat?
2. Read the following two articles and discuss whether or not milk and dairy products are necessary for bone health in growing children and adolescents.
   - Lanou, A. J., Berkow, S. E., & Barnard, N. D. (2005). Calcium, dairy products, and bone health in children and young adults: A reevaluation of the evidence. *Pediatrics, 115*, 736–743.
   - Greer, F. R. (2005). Bone health: It's more than calcium intake. *Pediatrics, 115*, 792–794.
3. What suggestions could you make to the adolescent and the adolescent's nonvegetarian parents when the adolescent wants to be a vegetarian who will not eat dairy products, eggs, beans, tofu, or most vegetables?
4. Would it ever be appropriate to tell a vegetarian family that their children have to eat meat?

5. Physical activity and exercise are equally important as healthy eating in the pediatric population. How would you include physical activity as an intervention for children if you have limited training in this area?
6. What power (if any) does the government have to influence factors that impact childhood obesity?
7. Discuss how the media may promote childhood obesity and how it may be used to prevent this problem.
8. What should the health care practitioner consider when he or she plans or implements childhood obesity prevention interventions for families in clinic settings or special programs?
9. Discuss how a child with multiple food allergies can be nutritionally threatened.
10. How is a child with food allergies affected in school? What special provisions are necessary and are these really available?

Case Study: School-Aged Child With Nut Allergy

I have a client with a 6-year-old son with severe food allergies to peanut, dairy, egg, and soy. His mother is trying to find a margarine-like spread that does not have any of these foods as the ingredients. She has also been told that her son should avoid all tree nuts. The mother also said that someone told her that almonds would be safe because they are more related to apricots (fruit) versus the tree nut family.

1. How should the mother go about finding an appropriate margarine-like spread for her son?
2. Would almonds be safe to eat? What professional advice would you give this mother?
3. What other precautions should this mother take to ensure the safety of her son at school and other places away from the home?

Case Study: Overweight Vegetarian

Jacob is a 16-year-old lifelong lacto-ovo-vegetarian. His father has recently discovered he has elevated cholesterol. Jacob also has borderline high cholesterol and is about 20 pounds above ideal weight.

A typical intake for a day for Jacob includes the following:
- Breakfast: three scrambled eggs with melted cheese, three slices of toast with butter, and chocolate milk
- Lunch: three slices of cheese pizza, French fries, and a milkshake
- Dinner: A large serving of macaroni and cheese, two slices of bread and butter, whole milk, and a bowl of ice cream
- Snacks include potato chips, soft drinks, and candy bars

1. What are your concerns with Jacob's diet?
2. What modifications can you suggest?

Case Study: An Underweight Vegetarian

Mollie is a 15-year-old dedicated cross-country runner. During the season (now), she runs 50 to 60 miles weekly. She has been a lacto-ovo-vegetarian for the past 2 years. She doesn't drink much milk, however, because she is lactose intolerant.

Mollie's parents are concerned because she has unintentionally lost 5 lbs in the past month. Mollie is 5'5" and weights 105 lbs (BMI = 18). Mollie is concerned because she seems to get sick easily and doesn't have as much energy as she would like.

Mollie says she just doesn't have time to eat well. A typical day includes the following diet:
- Dry cereal with fruit for breakfast
- A veggie burger and fries for lunch
- A big salad with cheese cubes and beans and salad dressing along with a couple of rolls for dinner
- Snacks include air-popped popcorn and iced tea

Her estimated calorie requirement is 2,200 kcal, whereas her estimated intake is 1,500 kcal.

1. What can Mollie do to improve her diet?
2. How can she get extra food when she has no time to cook or prepare food?

Websites

American Dietetic Association and Dietitians of Canada Position Paper on Vegetarian Diets http:// www.eatright.org/cps/rde/xchg/ada/hs. xsl/advocacy_933_ENU_HTML.htm

American Dietetic Association: A New Food Guide for North American Vegetarians http:// www.eatright.org/cps/rde/xchg/ada/ hs.xsl/governance_5105_ENU_HTML.htm

Vegetarian Resource Group http://www.vrg.org/nutrition/pregnancy.htm; http://www.vrg.org/nutrition/teennutrition.htm; http://www.vrg.org/nutshell/kids.htm

Vegetarian Baby http://www.vegetarianbaby.com/

Vegetarian Society of the UK http://www.vegsoc.org/info/childre1.html

Vegetarian Nutrition Dietetic Practice Group http:// www.andrews.edu/NUFS/Vegan% 20Children.html

Professional Organizations

American Academy of Pediatricians www.aap.org; www.pediatrics.org

American Dietetic Association http://www.eatright.org

American Medical Association http://ama-assn.org

American Nurse Association http://www.ana.org

American Psychological Association http://www.apa.org

American Public Health Association http://www.apha.org

Society of Nutrition Education www.sne.org

Statistical or Surveillance Systems

Behavioral Risk Factor Surveillance System www.cdc.gov/brfss

Combined Health Information Database http://chid.nih.gov

Kaiser Family Foundation's State Health facts Online www.statehealthfacts.kff.org

Maternal and Child Health Data www.mchdata.net/

National Center for Health Statistics http://www.cdc.gov/nchs

Pediatric Nutrition Surveillance System http://www.cdc.gov/nccdphp/dnpa/PedNSS.htm

Statistics related to overweight or obesity summary fact sheet www.niddk.nih.gov/health/nutrit/ pubs/statobes.htm

Statistical Abstract of the United States: 2001 www.census.gov/statab/www

Youth Behavioral Risk Factor Surveillance System http://www.cdc.gov/HealthyYouth/yrbs/ index.htm

Policy and Environmental Interventions

Center for Nutrition Policy and Promotion http://www.usda.gov/cnpp

CSPI School Nutrition Kit http://www.cspinet.org/nutritionpolicy

NASBE—Fit, Healthy and Ready to Learn: A School Health Policy Guide http://www.nasbe.org

National Recreation and Park Association http://www.nrpa.org

The Community Tool Box http://ctb.ku.edu

Nutrition

Dietary Guidelines for Americans www.nal.usda.gov/fnic/dga

Food and Nutrition Information Center www.nal.usda.gov/fnic/dga

Healthcare of Atlanta www.choa.org

School Foods Tool Kit. A Guide to Improving School Foods and Beverages www.cspinet.org/schoolfoodkit/

Center of Science in the Public Interest Nutrition Policy Project www.cspinet.org/schoolfoods
Junior Master Gardner Program http://jmgkids.com
5–A-Day www.5Aday.com
1% or less Campaign—School Kit www.cspinet.org/kids
Dairy Council www.nationaldairycouncil.org
3-A-Day www.3aday.org

Exercise

Heart N' Parks Program http://www.nhlbi.nih.gov; http://www.nhlbi.nih.gov/health/prof/heart/obesity/hrt_n_pk/index.htm
National Association for Sports and Physical Education www.aahperd.org/naspe
P.E. 4 Life www.pe4Life.com
Take 10! http://www.take10.net
The President's Council on Physical Fitness and Sports www.fitness.gov
National Park and Recreation http://www.program@nrpa.org

Media

CDC, Youth Media Campaign http://www.cdc.gov/youthcampaign
TV Turnoff Network www.tvturnoff.org

Schools Resources

Action for Healthy Kids http://www/actionforhealthykids.org
Changing the Scene—Improving the School Nutrition Environment www.fns.usda.gov/tn
National Association of State Boards of Education http://www.nasbe.org/HealthySchools/States/state_Policy.html
Planet Health www.planethealth.com/ Carter, J., Wiecha, J., Peterson, K., Gortmaker, S. L. (2001). Planet Health: An interdisciplinary curriculum for teaching middle school nutrition and physical activity. Human Kinetics.
School Health Index for Physical Activity: Healthy Eating and a Tobacco-Free Lifestyle. A Self Assessment and Planning Tool http://apps.nccd.cdc.gov/shi
SPARK Program http://www.sparkpe.org
The Center for Health and Healthcare in Schools http://www.healthinschools.org/sh/obesity.asp

Community Resources

Active Community Environments http://www.cdc.gov/nccdphp/dnpa/aces.htm
Coalition for Healthier Cities and Communities www.healthycommunities.org

Community Service Block Grant http://www.acf.dhhs.gov/programs/ocs/csbg/index/htm
North Carolina Prevention Partners www.ncpreventionpartners.org
U.S. Task Force on Community Preventive Strategies http://www.thecommunityguide.org

Other Resources

APHA Food and Nutrition Section on Overweight in Childhood http://www.aphafoodandnutrition.org/overwt.html
Bright Futures http://www.brightfutures.org
Center for Disease Control and Prevention http://www.cdc.gov
Center for Science in the Public Interest www.cspinet.org
Cooperative State Research, Education, and Extension Service http://www.reeusda.gov
Evaluation and Logic Models http://www.cdc.gov/eval/index.htm
Federal Grant Information www.hhs.gov/grantsnet/
Healthy People 2010 http://www.healthypeople.gov
Maternal and Child Health Bureau http://www.mchb.hrsa.gov
National Institutes of Health http://www.nih.gov/health
U.S. Department of Health and Human Services http://www.hhs.gov
YMCA of the USA http://www.ymca.org

Allergy

Allergy, Asthma & Immunology Online www.allergy.mcg.edu
American Academy of Allergy, Asthma and Immunology www.aaaai.org
American College of Allergy, Asthma & Immunology www.acaai.org
American Dietetic Association www.eatright.org
American Partnership for Eosinophilic Disorders www.apfed.org
Anaphylaxis Canada www.anaphylaxis.ca
Asthma and Allergy Foundation of America www.aafa.org
Food Allergy & Anaphylaxis Network www.foodallergy.org
Food Allergy Initiative www.foodallergyinitiative.org
International Food Information Council Foundation www.ific.org
National Institute of Allergy & Infectious Diseases, National Institutes of Health www.niaid.nih.gov

National Jewish Medical and Research Center
http://www.nationaljewish.org/
The Allergy and Asthma Disease Management
Center www.aaaai.org/aadmc
MedicAlert Foundation www.MedicAlert.org
EpiPen & EpiPen, Jr. www.epipen.com
Twinject www.twinject.com

References

Pediatric Vegetarianism

Allen, L. H. (1998). Zinc and micronutrient supplements for children. *American Journal of Clinical Nutrition, 68*(Suppl.), 495S–498S.

Barr, S. I. (1999). Vegetarianism and menstrual cycle disturbances: Is there an association? *American Journal of Clinical Nutrition, 70*(Suppl.), 549S–554S.

Barr, S. I., & Chapman, G. E. (2002). Perceptions and practices of self-defined current vegetarian, former vegetarian, and non-vegetarian women. *Journal of the American Dietetic Association, 102*, 354–360.

Birch, E. E., Garfield, S., Hoffman, D. R., Uauy, R., & Birch, C. G. (2000). A randomized controlled trial of early dietary supply of long-chain polyunsaturated fatty acids and mental development in term infants. *Developmental Medicine and Child Neurology, 42*, 174–181.

Black, R. E., Williams, S. M., Jones, I. E., & Goulding, A. (2002). Children who avoid drinking cow milk have low dietary calcium intakes and poor bone health. *American Journal of Clinical Nutrition, 76*, 675–680.

Carvalho, N. F., Kenney, R. D., Carrington, P. H., & Hall, D. E. (2001). Severe nutritional deficiencies in toddlers resulting from health food milk alternatives. *Pediatrics, 107*, E46.

Centers for Disease Control and Prevention (CDC). (2003). Neurologic impairment in children associated with maternal dietary deficiency of cobalamin—Georgia, 2001. *Morbidity and Mortality Weekly Report, 52*, 61–64.

Conquer, J. A., & Holub, B. J. (1996). Supplementation with an algae source of docosahexaenoic acid increases (n-3) fatty acid status and alters selected risk factors for heart disease in vegetarian subjects. *Journal of Nutrition, 126*, 3032–3039.

Dagnelie, P. C., van Staveren, W. A., & van den Berg, H. (1991). Vitamin B-12 from algae appears not to be bioavailable. *American Journal of Clinical Nutrition, 53*, 695–697.

Dagnelie, P. C., van Staveren, W. A., van Klaveren, J. D., & Burema, J. (1988). Do children on macrobiotic diets show catch-up growth? *European Journal of Clinical Nutrition, 42*, 1007–1016.

Dagnelie, P. C., van Staveren, W. A., Vergote, F. J. V. R. A., Burema, J., Van't Hof, M. A., van Klaveren, J. D., et al. (1989a). Nutritional status of infants aged 4 to 18 months on macrobiotic diets and matched omnivorous control infants: A population-based mixed-longitudinal study. II. Growth and psychomotor development. *European Journal of Clinical Nutrition, 43*, 325–338.

Dagnelie, P. C., van Staveren, W. A., Vergote, F. J. R. V. A., Dingjan, P.G., van den Berg, H., & Hautvast, J. G. A. J. (1989b). Increased risk of vitamin B-12 and iron deficiency in infants on macrobiotic diets. *American Journal of Clinical Nutrition, 50*, 818–824.

Dagnelie, P. C., van Staveren, W. A., Verschuren, S. A. J. M., & Hautvast, J. G. A. J. (1989c). Nutritional status of infants aged 4 to 18 months on macrobiotic diets and matched omnivorous control infants: A population-based mixed longitudinal study. I. Weaning pattern, energy and nutrient intake. *European Journal of Clinical Nutrition, 43*, 311–323.

Dagnelie, P. C., Vergote, F. J. R. V. A., van Staveren, W. A., van den Berg, H., Dingjan, P. G., & Hautvast, J. G. A. J. (1990). High prevalence of rickets in infants on macrobiotic diets. *American Journal of Clinical Nutrition, 51*, 202–208.

Davis, B., & Kris-Etherton, P. (2003). Achieving optimal essential fatty acid status in vegetarians: Current knowledge and practical implications. *American Journal of Clinical Nutrition, 78*(Suppl.), 640S–646S.

Dhonukshe-Rutten, R. A., van Dusseldorp, M., Schneede, J., de Groot, L. C., & van Staveren, W. A. (2005). Low bone mineral density and bone mineral content are associated with low cobalamin status in adolescents. *European Journal of Nutrition, 44*, 341–347.

Dibba, B., Prentice, A., & Ceesay, M. (2000). Effect of calcium supplementation on bone mineral accretion in Gambian children accustomed to a low-calcium diet. *American Journal of Clinical Nutrition, 71*, 544–549.

Dobson, B., & Murtaugh, M. A. (2001). Position of the American Dietetic Association: Breaking the barriers to breastfeeding. *Journal of the American Dietetic Association, 101*, 1213–1220.

Donovan, U. M., & Gibson, R. S. (1995). Iron and zinc status of young women aged 14 to 19 years consuming vegetarian and omnivorous diets. *Journal of the American College of Nutrition, 14*, 463–472.

Donovan, U. M., & Gibson, R. S. (1996). Dietary intakes of adolescent females consuming vegetarian, semi-vegetarian, and omnivorous diets. *Journal of Adolescent Health, 18*, 292–300.

Ellis, R., Kelsay, J. L., Reynolds, R. D., Morris, E. R., Moser, P. B., & Frazier, C. (1987). Phytate:zinc and phytate x calcium:zinc millimolar ratios in self-selected diets of Americans, Asian Indians, and Nepalese. *Journal of the American Dietetic Association, 87*, 1043–1047.

Francois, C. A., Connor, S. L., Bolewicz, L. C., & Connor, W. E. (2003). Supplementing lactating women with flaxseed oil does not increase docosahexaenoic acid in their milk. *American Journal of Clinical Nutrition, 77*, 226–233.

Geppert, J., Kraft, V., Demmelmair, H., & Koletzko, B. (2005). Docosahexaenoic acid supplementation in vegetarians effectively increases omega-3 index: A randomized trial. *Lipids, 40*, 807–814.

Gibson, R. S., Yeudall, F., Drost, N., Mtitmunit, B., & Cullinan, T. (1998). Dietary interventions to prevent zinc deficiency. *American Journal of Clinical Nutrition, 68*(Suppl.), 484S–487S.

Hallberg, L., & Hulthen, L. (2000). Prediction of dietary iron absorption: An algorithm for calculating absorption and bioavailability of dietary iron. *American Journal of Clinical Nutrition, 71*, 1147–1160.

Heaney, R. P., Dowell, M. S., Rafferty, K., & Bierman, J. (2000). Bioavailability of the calcium in fortified soy imitation milk, with some observations on method. *American Journal of Clinical Nutrition, 71*, 1166–1169.

Heaney, R. P., Rafferty, K., & Bierman, J. (2005). Not all calcium-fortified beverages are equal. *Nutrition Today, 40*, 39–45.

Hebbelinck, M., & Clarys, P. (2001). Physical growth and development of vegetarian children and adolescents. In J. Sabate (Ed.), *Vegetarian Nutrition* (pp.173–193). Boca Raton, FL: CRC Press.

Hermann, W., & Geisel, J. (2002). Vegetarian lifestyle and monitoring vitamin B_{12} status. *Clinica Chimica Acta; International Journal of Clinical Chemistry, 26*, 47–59.

Holick, M. F. (2004). Sunlight and vitamin D for bone health and prevention of autoimmune diseases, cancers, and cardiovascular disease. *American Journal of Clinical Nutrition, 80*(6 Suppl.), 1678S–1688S.

Houghton, L. A., Green, T. J., Donovan, U. M., Gibson, R. S., Stephen, A. M., & O'Connor, D. L. (1997). Association between dietary fiber intake and the folate status of a group of female adolescents. *American Journal of Clinical Nutrition, 66*, 1414–1421.

Hunt, J. R. (2002). Moving toward a plant-based diet: Are iron and zinc at risk? *Nutrition Review, 60*, 127–134.

Hunt, J. R., Matthys, L. A., & Johnson, L. K. (1998). Zinc absorption, mineral balance, and blood lipids in women consuming controlled lacto-ovo vegetarian and omnivorous diets for 8 wk. *American Journal of Clinical Nutrition, 67*, 421–430.

Imataka, G., Mikami, T., Yamanouchi, H., Kano, K., & Eguchi, M. (2004). Vitamin D deficiency rickets due to soybean milk. *Journal of Paediatrics and Child Health, 40*, 154–155.

Institute of Medicine (IOM), Food and Nutrition Board. (1997). *Dietary Reference Intakes for Calcium, Phosphorus, Magnesium, Vitamin D, and Fluoride.* Washington, DC: National Academy Press.

Institute of Medicine (IOM), Food and Nutrition Board. (1998). *Dietary Reference Intakes for Thiamin, Riboflavin, Niacin, Vitamin B6, Folate, Vitamin B12, Pantothenic Acid, Biotin, and Choline.* Washington, DC: National Academy Press.

Institute of Medicine (IOM), Food and Nutrition Board. (2001). *Dietary Reference Intakes for Vitamin A, Vitamin K, Arsenic, Boron, Chromium, Copper, Iodine, Iron, Manganese, Molybdenum, Nickel, Silicon, Vanadium, and Zinc.* Washington, DC: National Academy Press.

Institute of Medicine (IOM), Food and Nutrition Board. (2002). *Dietary Reference Intakes for Energy, Carbohydrate, Fiber, Fat, Fatty Acids, Cholesterol, Protein, and Amino Acids.* Washington, DC: National Academy Press.

Janelle, K. C., & Barr, S. I. (1995). Nutrient intakes and eating behavior scores of vegetarian and nonvegetarian women. *Journal of the American Dietetic Association, 95*, 180–186, 189.

Kalkwarf, H. J., Khoury, J. C., & Lanphear, B. P. (2003). Milk intake during childhood and adolescence, adult bone density, and osteoporotic fractures in US women. *American Journal of Clinical Nutrition, 77*, 257–265.

Kissinger, D. G., & Sanchez, A. (1987). The association of dietary factors with the age of menarche. *Nutrition Research, 7*, 471–479.

Krajcovicova-Kudlackova, M., Simoncic, R., Babinska, K., & Bederova, A. (1995). Levels of lipid peroxidation and antioxidants in vegetarians. *European Journal Epidemiology, 111*, 207–211.

Krajcovicova-Kudlackova, M., Simoncic, R., Bederova, A., Grancicova, E., & Megalova, T. (1997a). Influence of vegetarian and mixed nutrition on selected haematological and biochemical parameters in children. *Die Nahrung, 41*, 311–314.

Krajcovicova-Kudlackova, M., Simoncic, R., Bederova, A., & Klvanova, J. (1997b). Plasma fatty acid profile and alternative nutrition. *Annals of Nutrition Metabolism, 41*, 365–370.

Larsson, C. L., & Johansson, G. K. (2002). Dietary intake and nutritional status of young vegans and omnivores in Sweden. *American Journal of Clinical Nutrition, 76*, 100–106.

Larsson, C. L., & Johansson, G. K. (2005). Young Swedish vegans have different sources of nutrients than young omnivores. *Journal of the American Dietetic Association, 105*, 1438–1441.

Larsson, C. L., Ronnlund, U., Johansson, G., & Dahlgren, L. (2003). Veganism as status passage: The process of becoming a vegan among youths in Sweden. *Appetite, 41*, 61–67.

Leung, S. S., Lee, R., Sung, S., Luo, H. Y., Kam, C. W., Yuen, M. P., et al. (2001). Growth and nutrition of Chinese vegetarian children in Hong Kong. *Journal of Paediatrics and Child Health, 37*, 247–253.

Licht, D. J., Berry, G. T., Brooks, D. G., & Younkin, D. P. (2001). Reversible subacute combined degeneration of the spinal cord in a 14-year-old due to a strict vegan diet. *Clinical Pediatrics, 40*, 413–415.

Louwman, M. W. J., van Dusseldorp, M., van de Vijver, F. J. R., Thomas, C. M., Schneede, J., Ueland, P. M., et al. (2000). Signs of impaired cognitive function in adolescents with marginal cobalamin status. *American Journal of Clinical Nutrition, 72*, 762–769.

Mangels, A. R., & Messina, V. (2001). Considerations in planning vegan diets. I. Infants. *Journal of the American Dietetic Association, 101*, 670–677.

Mangels, A. R., Messina, V., & Melina, V. (2003). Position of the American Dietetic Association and Dietitians of Canada: Vegetarian diets. *Journal of the American Dietetic Association, 103*, 748–765.

Martins, Y., Pliner, P., & O'Connor, R. (1999). Restrained eating among vegetarians: Does a vegetarian eating style mask concerns about weight? *Appetite, 32*, 145–154.

McCann, J. C., & Ames, B. N. (2005). Is docosahexaenoic acid, an n-3 long-chain polyunsaturated fatty acid, required for development of normal brain function? An overview of evidence from cognitive and behavioral tests in humans and animals. *American Journal of Clinical Nutrition, 82*, 281–295.

Messina, V., & Mangels, A. R. (2001). Considerations in planning vegan diets: Children. *Journal of the American Dietetic Association, 101*, 661–669.

Messina, V., Melina, V., & Mangels, A. R. (2003). A new food guide for North American vegetarians. *Journal of the American Dietetic Association, 103*, 771–775.

Messina, V. K., Mangels, R., & Messina, M. (2004). *The Dietitian's Guide to Vegetarian Diets* (2nd ed.). Boston: Jones and Bartlett Publishers.

Nathan, I., Hackett, A. F., & Kirby, S. (1996). The dietary intake of a group of vegetarian children aged 7–11 years compared with matched omnivores. *British Journal of Nutrition, 75*, 533–544.

Nathan, I., Hackett, A. F., & Kirby, S. (1997). A longitudinal study of the growth of matched pairs of vegetarian and omnivorous children, aged 7–11 years, in the north-west of England. *European Journal of Clinical Nutrition, 51*, 20–25.

Neumark-Sztainer, D., Story, M., Resnick, M. D., & Blum, R. W. (1997). Adolescent vegetarians: A behavioral profile of a school-based population in Minnesota. *Archives of Pediatric and Adolescent Medicine, 151*, 833–838.

Perry, C. L., McGuire, M. T., Newmark-Sztainer, D., & Story, M. (2001). Characteristics of vegetarian adolescents in a multiethnic urban population. *The Journal of Adolescent Health: Official Publication of the Society for Adolescent Medicine, 29*, 406–416.

Perry, C. L., McGuire, M. T., Neumark-Sztainer, D., & Story, M. (2002). Adolescent vegetarians. How well do their dietary patterns meet the Healthy People 2010 objectives? *Archives of Pediatric and Adolescent Medicine, 156*, 431–437.

Roberts, I. F., West, R. J., Ogilvie, D., & Dillon, M. J. (1979). Malnutrition in infants receiving cult diets: A form of child abuse. *British Medical Journal, 1*, 296–298.

Rosell, M. S., Lloyd-Wright, Z., Appleby, P. N., Sanders, T. A., Allen, N. E., & Key, T. J. (2005). Long-chain n-3 polyunsaturated fatty acids in plasma in British meat-eating, vegetarian, and vegan men. *American Journal of Clinical Nutrition, 82*, 327–334.

Sabaté, J., Linsted, K. D., Harris, R. D., & Johnston, P. K. (1990). Anthropometric parameters of schoolchildren with different life-styles. *American Journal of Diseases of Children, 144*, 1159–1163.

Sabaté, J., Linsted, K. D., Harris, R. D., & Sanchez, A. (1991). Attained height of lacto-ovo vegetarian children and adolescents. *European Journal of Clinical Nutrition, 45*, 51–58.

Sabaté, J., Llorca, C., & Sanchez, A. (1992). Lower height of lacto-ovovegetarian girls at preadolescence: An indicator of physical maturation today? *Journal of the American Dietetic Association, 92*, 1263–1264.

Sanders, T. A. B. (1988). Growth and development of British vegan children. *American Journal of Clinical Nutrition, 48*, 822–825.

Sanders, T. A. B. (1995). Vegetarian diets and children. *Pediatric Clinics of North America, 42*, 955–965.

Sanders, T. A. B., & Manning, J. (1992). The growth and development of vegan children. *Journal of Human Nutrition and Dietetics: The Official Journal of the British Dietetic Association, 5*, 11–21.

Sanders, T. A. B., & Reddy, S. (1992). The influence of a vegetarian diet on the fatty acid composition of human milk and the essential fatty acid status of the infant. *Journal of Pediatrics, 120*, S71–S77.

Sandstrom, B. (2001). Micronutrient interactions: Effects on absorption and bioavailability. *British Journal of Nutrition, 85*(Suppl. 2), S181–S185.

SanGiovanni, J. P., Parra-Cabrera, S., Colditz, G. A., Berkey, C. S., & Dwyer, J. T. (2000). Meta-analysis of dietary essential fatty acids and long-chain polyunsaturated fatty acids as they relate to visual resolution acuity in healthy preterm infants. *Pediatrics, 105*, 1292–1298.

Scott, M. (2003). Nutrition for the full-term infant. In N. Nevin-Folino (Ed.), *Pediatric Manual of Clinical Dietetics* (2nd ed., pp. 55–71). Chicago: American Dietetic Association.

Stepaniak, J., & Melina, V. (2003). *Raising Vegetarian Children*. Chicago: Contemporary Books.

Thane, C. W., & Bates, C. J. (2000). Dietary intakes and nutrient status of vegetarian preschool children from a British national survey. *Journal of Human Nutrition and Dietetics: The Official Journal of the British Dietetic Association, 13*, 149–162.

Thane, C. W., Bates, C. J., & Prentice, A. (2003). Risk factors for low iron intake and poor iron status in a national sample of British young people aged 4–18 years. *Public Health Nutrition, 6*, 485–496.

Truesdell, D. D., & Acosta, P. B. (1985). Feeding the vegan infant and child. *Journal of the American Dietetic Association, 85*, 837–840.

Uauy, R., Peirano, P., Hoffman, D., Mena, P., Birch, D., & Birch, E. (1996). Role of essential fatty acids in the function of the developing nervous system. *Lipids, 31*, S167–S176.

van den Berg, H., Dagnelie, P. C., & van Staveren, W. A. (1988). Vitamin B12 and seaweed. *Lancet, 1*, 242–243.

van Dusseldorp, M., Arts, I. C. W., Bergsma, J. S., de Jong, N., Dagnelie, P. C., & van Staveren, W.A . (1996). Catch-up growth in children fed a macrobiotic diet in early childhood. *Journal of Nutrition, 126*, 2977–2983.

Vegetarian Resource Group. (2001, Jan/Feb). How many teens are vegetarian? How many kids don't eat meat? *Vegetarian Journal*.

Watanabe, F., Katsura, H., Takenaka, S., Fujita, T., Abe, K., Tamura, Y., et al. (1999). Pseudovitamin B (12) is the predominant cobalamide of an algal health food, Spirulina tablets. *Journal of Agricultural and Food Chemistry, 47*, 4736–4741.

Weaver, C. M., & Plawecki, K. L. (1994). Dietary calcium: Adequacy of a vegetarian diet. *American Journal of Clinical Nutrition, 59*(Suppl.), 1238S–1241S.

Worsley, A., & Skrzypiec, G. (1998). Teenage vegetarianism: Prevalence, social and cognitive contexts. *Appetite, 30*, 151–170.

Young, V. R., & Pellett, P. L. (1994). Plant proteins in relation to human protein and amino acid nutrition. *American Journal of Clinical Nutrition, 59*, 1203S–1212S.

Childhood Obesity

Alaimo, K., Olson, C. M., & Frongillo, Jr., E. A. (2001). Low family income and food insufficiency in relation to overweight in US children. Is there a paradox? *Archives of Pediatric and Adolescent Medicine, 155*, 1161–1167.

Allison, D. B., & Faith, M. S. (2000). Genetic and environmental influences on human body weight: Implications for the behavior therapist. *Nutrition Today, 35*, 18–21.

American Dietetic Association. (2002). Position paper. The role of dietetics professionals in health promotion and disease prevention. *Journal of the American Dietetic Association, 102*, 1680–1687.

American Dietetic Association, Society for Nutrition Education, and the American School Food Service Association. (2003). Position paper. Nutrition services: An essential component of comprehensive school health programs. *Journal of the American Dietetic Association, 103*, 505–514.

Andersen, R. E., Crespo, C. J., Bartlett, S. J., Cheskin, L. J., & Pratt, M. (1998). Relationship of physical activity and television watching with body weight and level of fatness among children: Results from the Third National Health and Nutrition Examination Survey. *Journal of the American Medical Association, 279*, 938–942.

Armstrong, J., & Reilly, J. J. (2002). Breastfeeding and lowering the risk of childhood obesity. Child Health Information Team. *Lancet, 359*, 2003–2004.

Augustin, L. S., Franceschi, S., Jenkins, D. J. A., Kendall, C. W. C., & La Vecchia, C. (2002). Glycemic index in chronic disease: A review. *European Journal Clinical Nutrition, 56*, 1049–1071.

Berenson, G. S. (2002). Childhood risk factors predict adult risk associated with subclinical cardiovascular disease: The Bogalusa Heart Study. *American Journal of Cardiology, 90*(Suppl.), 3L–7L.

Birch, L. L., & Fischer, J. O. (1998). Development of eating behaviors among children and adolescents. *Pediatrics, 101*, 539–547.

Booth, S. L., Sallis, J. F., Ritenbaugh, C., Hill, J. O., Birch, L. L., Frank, L. D., et al. (Working Group II). (2001). Environmental and societal factors affect food choice and physical activity: Rationale, influences, and leverage points. *Nutrition Reviews, 59*(3, part 2), S21–S39.

Borzekowski, D. L. G., & Robinson, T. N. (2001). The 30-second effect: an experiment revealing the impact of television commercials on food preferences of preschoolers. *Journal of the American Dietetic Association, 101*, 42–46.

Bowman, S. A., Gortmaker, S. L., Ebbeling, C. B., Pereira, M. A., & Ludwig, D. S. (2004). Effects of fast-food consumption on energy intake and diet quality among children in a national household survey. *Pediatrics, 113*, 112–118.

Briefel, R. R., & Johnson, C. L. (2004). Secular trends in dietary intake in the United States. *Annual Review of Nutrition, 24*, 401–431.

Buechner, J. (2001). *Stress-free Feeding Curriculum and Video*. Atlanta, GA: Children's Healthcare of Atlanta, Inc.

Burgenson, C. R., Wechsler, H., Brener, N. D., Young, J. C., & Spain, C. G. (2001). Physical education and activity: Results from the School Health Policies and Programs Study 2000. *Journal of School Health, 71*, 279–293.

Centers for Disease Control and Prevention (CDC). (n.d.-a). KidsWalk-to-School. Nutrition and physical activity. Retrieved June 30, 2007, from http://www.cdc.gov/nccdphp/dnpa/kidswalk/

Centers for Disease Control and Prevention (CDC). (2003). Resource guide for nutrition and physical activity interventions to prevent obesity and other chronic disease. Retrieved June 30, 2007 from http://www.cdc.gov/nccdphp/dnpa/obesity/resource_guide.htm

Conner, W. E. (2000). Importance of n-3 fatty acids in health and disease. *American Journal of Clinical Nutrition, 71*, 171S–175S.

Crawford, P., Gosliner, W., Anderson, C., Strode, P., Becerra-Jones, Y., Samuels, S., et al. (2004). Counseling Latina mothers of preschool children about weight issues: Suggestions for a new framework. *Journal of American Dietetic Association, 104*, 87–394.

Dietz, W. H. (2001). Breastfeeding may help prevent overweight children. *Journal of the American Medical Association, 285*, 2506–2507.

Dietz, W. H. (2004). Overweight in childhood and adolescence. *New England Journal of Medicine, 350*, 855–857.

Dowda, M., Ainsworth, B. E., Addy, C. L., Saunders, R., & Riner, W. (2001). Environmental influences, physical activity, and weight status in 8- to 16-year-olds. *Archives of Pediatric Adolescent Medicine, 155*, 711–717.

Drewnowski, A., & Specter, S. E. (2004). Poverty and obesity: The role of energy density and energy costs. *American Journal of Clinical Nutrition, 79*, 6–16.

Ellis, K. J., Abrams, S. A., & Wong, W. W. (1999). Monitoring childhood obesity: Assessment of weight/height^2 index. *American Journal of Epidemiology, 150*, 939–946.

Erickson, S. J., Robinson, T. N., Haydel, K. F., & Killen, J. D. (2000). Are overweight children unhappy? *Archives of Pediatric and Adolescent Medicine, 154*, 931–935.

Fischer, J. O., & Birch, L. L. (1999). Restricting access to palatable foods affects children's behavioral response, food selection, and intake. *American Journal of Clinical Nutrition, 69*, 1264–1272.

Freedman, D. S., Khan, L. K., Dietz, W. H., Srinivasan, S. R., & Berenson, G. S. (2001). Relationship of childhood obesity to coronary heart disease risk factors in adulthood: The Bogalusa Heart Study. *Pediatrics, 108*, 712–718.

Frumkin, H. (2002). Urban sprawl and public health. *Public Health Reports, 117*, 201–217.

Gibson, D. (2004). Long-term Food Stamp Program participation is differently related to overweight in young girls and boys. *Journal of Nutrition, 134*, 372–379.

Gortmaker, S. L., Must, A., Sobol, A. M., Peterson, K., Colditz, G. A., & Dietz, W. H. (1996). Television viewing as a cause of increasing obesity among children in the United States, 1986–1990. *Archives of Pediatric and Adolescent Medicine, 150*, 356–362.

Harnack, L., Stang, J., & Story, M. (1999). Soft drink consumption among US children and adolescents: Nutritional consequences. *Journal of the American Dietetic Association, 99*, 436–441.

Hassink, S. (2003). Problems in childhood obesity. *Primary Care Office Practice, 30*, 357–374.

Hill, J. O., & Trowbridge, F. L. (1998). Childhood obesity: Future directions and research priorities. *Pediatrics, 101*(Suppl.), 570–574.

Hill, J. O., Wyatt, H. R., Reed, G. W., & Peters, J. C. (2003). Obesity and the environment: Where do we go from here? *Science, 299*, 853–855.

Johnson, S. L. (2000). Improving preschoolers' self-regulation of energy intake. *Pediatrics, 106*, 1429–1435.

Johnson, S. L., & Birch, L. L. (1994). Parents' adiposity and children's eating style. *Pediatrics, 94*, 653–661.

Jones, S. J., Jahns, L., Laraia, B. A., & Haughton, B. (2003). Lower risk of overweight in school-aged food insures girls who participate in food assistance. *Archives of Pediatric and Adolescent Medicine, 157*, 780–784.

Kaiser Family Foundation. (n.d.). Kids & media @ the new millenium: A Kaiser Family Foundation report. Retrieved June 30, 2007, from http://www.kff.org

Kurtzweil, P. (1996). Taking the fat out of food. *FDA Consumer Magazine*, online version, USDA. Retrieved June 30, 2007, from http://www.fda.gov/fdac/features/696_fat.html

Ludwig, D. S., Peterson, K. E., & Gortmaker, S. L. (2001). Relation between consumption of sugar-sweetened drinks and childhood obesity: A prospective, observational analysis. *Lancet, 357*, 505–508.

McBean, L. D., & Miller, G. D. (1999). Enhancing the nutrition of America's youth. *Journal of the American College of Nutrition, 18*, 563–571.

Munoz, K. A., Krebs-Smith, S. M., Ballard-Barbash, R., & Cleveland, L. E. (1997). Food intakes of US children and adolescents compared with recommendations. *Pediatrics, 100*, 323–329.

National Center for Health Statistics. (1999). Prevalence of overweight and obesity among adults. Retrieved June 4, 2007 from www.cdc.gov/nchs/products/pubs/pubd/hestats/obese/obse99.htm

Nelson, J. A., Chiasson, M. A., & Ford, V. (2004). Overweight children in a New York City WIC population. *American Journal of Public Health, 94*, 458–462.

Nicklas, T. A., Baranowski, T., Cullen, K. W., & Berenson, G. (2001). Eating patterns, dietary quality, and obesity. *Journal of the American College of Nutrition, 20*, 599–608.

Ogden, C. L., Carroll, M. D., Curtin, L. R., McDowell, M. A., Tabak, C. J., & Flegal, K. M. (2006). Prevalence of overweight and obesity in the United States, 1999–2004. *Journal of the American Medical Association, 295*, 1549–1555.

Ogden, C. L., Flegal, K. M., Carroll, M. D., & Johnson, C. L. (2002). Prevalence and trends in overweight among US children and adolescents, 1999–2000. *Journal of the American Medical Association, 288*, 1728–1732.

O'Keefe, J. H., & Cordain, L. (2004). Cardiovascular disease resulting from a diet and lifestyle at odds with our Paleolithic genome: How to become a 21st century hunter-gatherer. *Mayo Clinical Proceedings, 79*, 101–108.

Paeratakul, S., Ferdinand, D. P., Champagne, C. M., Ryan, D. H., & Bray, G. A. (2003). Fast-food consumption among US adults and children: Dietary and nutrient intake profile. *Journal of the American Dietetic Association, 103*, 1332–1338.

Raman, R. P. (2002). Obesity and health risks. *Journal of the American College of Nutrition, 21*, 134S–139S.

Roberts, S. B. (2000). High-glycemic index foods, hunger and obesity: Is there a connection? *Nutrition Reviews, 58*, 163–169.

Robinson, T. N., Hammer, L. D., Killen, J. D., Kraemer, H. C., Wilson, D. M., Hayward, C., et al. (1993). Does television viewing increase obesity and reduce physical activity? Cross-sectional and longitudinal analyses among adolescent girls. *Pediatrics, 91*, 273–280.

Satter, E. (1987). *How to Get Kids to Eat...But Not Too Much.* Palo Alto, CA: Bull Publishing.

Satter, E. (1999). *Secrets of Feeding a Healthy Family.* Madison, WI: Kelcy Press.

Satter, E. (2000). *Child of Mine: Feeding with Love and Good Sense.* Palo Alto, CA: Bull Publishing.

Serdula, M. K., Ivery, D., Coates, R. J., Freedman, D. S., Williamson, D. F., & Byers, T. (1993). Do obese children become obese adults? A review of literature. *Preventive Medicine, 65*, 167–177.

Simopoulos, A. P. (1999). Evolutionary aspects of omega-3 fatty acids in the food supply. *Prostaglandins, Leukotrienes, and Essential Fatty Acids, 60*, 421–429.

Simopoulos, A. P. (2002). The importance of the ratio of omega-6/omega-3 fatty acids. *Biomedical Pharmacotherapy, 56*, 365–379.

Steinbeck, K. S. (2001). The importance of physical activity in the prevention of overweight and obesity in childhood: A review and an option. *Obesity Reviews, 2*, 117–130.

Strauss, R. S., & Pollack, H. A. (2001). Epidemic increase in overweight children, 1986–1998. *Journal of the American Medical Association, 286*, 2845–2848.

Taylor, R. W., Jones, I. E., Williams, S. M., & Goulding, A. (2002). Body fat percentages measured by dual-energy x-ray absorptiometry corresponding to recently recommended body mass index cutoffs for overweight and obesity in children and adolescents aged 3–18 y. *American Journal of Clinical Nutrition, 76*, 1416–1421.

TV Turnoff Network. (n.d.). Retrieved June 30, 2007, from www.tvturnoff.org

U.S. Department of Health and Human Services. (2000). *Healthy People 2010* (2nd ed.). *With Understanding and Improving Health and Objectives for Improving Health* (2 vols.). Washington, DC: U.S. Government Printing Office.

Warren, J. M., Henry, C. J., & Simonite, V. (2003). Low glycemic index breakfasts and reduced food intake in preadolescent children. *Pediatrics, 112*, e414.

Food Allergies

American Academy of Pediatrics, Committee on Nutrition. (2000). Hypoallergenic infant formulas. *Pediatrics, 106*, 346–349.

Bernhisel-Broadbent, J. (1999). Diagnosis and management of food hypersensitivity. *Immunology and Allergy Clinics of North America, 19*, 463–477.

Beyer, K., Ellman-Grunther, L., Jarvinen, K. M., Wood, R. A., Hourihane, J., and Sampson, H. A. (2003). Measurement of peptide-specific IgE as an additional tool in identifying patients with clinical reactivity to peanuts. *Journal of Allergy and Clinical Immunology, 112*, 202–207.

Beyer, K., Jarvinen, K. M., Bardina, L., Mishoe, M., Turjanmaa, K., Niggemann, B., et al. (2005). IgE-binding peptides coupled to a commercial matrix as a diagnostic instrument for persistent cow's milk allergy. *Journal of Allergy and Clinical Immunology, 116*, 704–705.

Beyer, K., & Teuber, S. S. (2005). Food allergy diagnostics: Scientific and unproven procedures. *Current Opinion in Allergy and Clinical Immunology, 5*, 261–266.

Bock, S. A. (2000). Evaluation of IgE-mediated food hypersensitivities. *Journal of Pediatric Gastroenterology and Nutrition, 30*, S20–S27.

Bock, S. A., Sampson, H. A., Atkins, F. M., Zeiger, R. S., Lehrer, S., Sachs, M., et al. (1988). Double-blind, placebo-controlled food challenge (DBPCFC) as an office procedure: A manual. *Journal of Allergy and Clinical Immunology, 82*, 986–997.

Eigenmann, P. A., Sicherer, S. H., Borowski, T. A., Cohen, B. A., & Sampson, H. A. (1998). Prevalence of IgE-mediated food allergy among children with atopic dermatitis. *Pediatrics, 101*, E8.

Jones, R. B., Robins, G. G., & Howdle, P. D. (2006). Advances in celiac disease. *Current Opinion in Gastroenterology, 22*, 117–123.

Justinich, C. J. (2000). Update in gastrointestinal allergic disease. *Current Opinion in Pediatrics, 12*, 456–459.

Justinich, C. J., Katz, A., Gurbindo, C., Lepage, G., Chad, Z., Bouthillier, L., et al. (1996). Elemental diet improves steroid-dependent eosinophilic gastroenteritis and reverses growth failure. *Journal of Pediatric Gastroenterology and Nutrition, 23*, 81–85.

Kelly, K. J. (2000). Eosinophilic gastroenteritis. *Journal of Pediatric Gastroenterology and Nutrition, 30*, S28–S35.

Kelly, K. J., Lazenby, A. J., Rowe, P. C., Yarley, J. H., Perman, J. A., & Sampson, H. A. (1995). Eosinophilic esophagitis attributed to gastroesophageal reflux: Improvement with an amino acid-based formula. *Gastroenterology, 109*, 1503–1512.

Liacouras, C. A. (2003). Eosinophilic esophagitis in children and adults. *Journal of Pediatric Gastroenterology and Nutrition, 37*, S23–S28.

Liacouras, C. A. (2006). Eosinophilic esophagitis: treatment in 2005. *Current Opinion in Gastroenterology, 22*, 147–152.

Liacouras, C. A., Spergel, J. M., Ruchelli, E., Verma, R., Mascarenhas, M., Semeao, E., et al. (2005). Eosinophilic esophagitis: A 10-year experience in 381 children. *Clinical Gastroenterology and Hepatology, 3*, 1198–1206.

Liacouras, C. A., Wenner, W. J., Brown, K., & Ruchelli, E. (1998). Primary eosinophilic esophagitis in children: Successful treatment with oral corticosteroids. *Journal of Pediatric Gastroenterology and Nutrition, 26*, 380–385.

Markowitz, J. E., Spergel, J. M., Ruchelli, E., & Liacorous, C. A. (2003). Elemental diet is an effective treatment for eosinophilic esophagitis in children and adolescents. *American Journal of Gastroenterology, 98*, 777–782.

Mofidi, S. (2003). Nutritional management of pediatric food hypersensitivity. *Pediatrics, 111*, 1645–1653.

Mofidi, S., & Bock, S. A. (Eds.). (2005). *A Health Professional's Guide to Food Challenges*. Fairfax, VA: The Food Allergy and Anaphylaxis Network.

Munoz-Furlong, A. (2003). Daily coping strategies for patients and their families. *Pediatrics, 111*, 1654–1661.

Niggemann, B., Reibel, S., & Wahn, U. (2000). The atopy patch test (APT)—a useful tool for the diagnosis of food allergy in children with atopic dermatitis. *Allergy, 55*, 281–285.

Noel, R. J., Putnam, P. E., Collins, M. H., Assa'ad, A. H., Guajardo, J. R., Jameson, S. C., et al. (2004a). Clinical and immunopathologic effects of swallowed fluticasone for eosinophilic esophagitis. *Clinical Gastroenterology and Hepatology: The Official Clinical Practice Journal of the American Gastroenterological Association, 2*, 568–575.

Noel, R. J., Putnam, P. E., and Rothenberg, M. E. (2004b). Eosinophilic esophagitis. *New England Journal of Medicine, 351*, 940–941.

Nowak-Wegrzyn, A., Sampson, H. A., Wood, R. A., & Sicherer, S. H. (2003). Food protein-induced enterocolitis syndrome caused by solid food proteins. *Pediatrics, 111*, 829–835.

Orenstein, S. R., Shalaby, T. M., Di Lorenzo, C., Putnam, P. E., Sigurdsson, L., Mousa, H., et al. (2000). The spectrum of pediatric eosinophilic esophagitis beyond infancy: A clinical series of 30 children. *American Journal of Gastroenterology, 95*, 1422–1430.

Ortolani, C., Bruijnzeel-Koomen, C., Bengtsson, U., Bindslev-Jensen, C., Bjorksten, B., Host, A., et al. (1999). Position paper: Controversial aspects of adverse reactions to food. *Allergy, 54*, 27–45.

Ortolani, C., Ispano, M., Pastorello, E. A., Ansaloni, R., & Magri, G. C. (1989). Comparison of results of skin prick tests with fresh foods and commercial food extracts and RAST in 100 patients with oral allergy syndrome. *Journal of Allergy and Clinical Immunology, 83*, 683–690.

Ortolani, C., Ispano, M., Pastorello, E. A., Bigi, A., & Ansaloni, R. (1988). The oral allergy syndrome. *Annals of Allergy, 61*, 47–52.

Ortolani, C., Pastorello, E., Farioli, L., Ispano, M., Pravettoni, V., Berti, C., et al. (1993). IgE-mediated allergy from vegetable allergens. *Annals of Allergy, 71*, 470–476.

Potter, J. W., Saeian, K., Staff, D., Massey, B. T., Komorowski, R. A., Shaker, R., et al. (2004). Eosinophilic esophagitis in adults: An emerging problem with unique esophageal features. *Gastrointestinal Endoscopy, 59*, 355–361.

Roehr, C. C., Reibel, S., Zeigert, M., Sommerfeld, C., Wahn, U., & Niggeman, B. (2001). Atopy patch tests, together with determination of specific IgE levels, reduce the need for oral food challenges in children with atopic dermatitis. *Journal of Allergy and Clinical Immunology, 107*, 548–553.

Rothenberg, M. E. (2004). Eosinophilic gastrointestinal disorders. *Journal of Allergy and Clinical Immunology, 113*, 11–28.

Rothenberg, M. E., Mishra, A., Collins, M. H., & Putnam, P. E. (2001). Pathogenesis and clinical features of eosinophilic esophagitis. *Journal of Allergy and Clinical Immunology, 108*, 891–894.

Sampson, H. A. (1999). Food allergy. Part 2: Diagnosis and management. *Journal of Allergy and Clinical Immunology, 103*, 981–989.

Sampson, H. A. (2001). Utility of food-specific IgE concentrations in predicting symptomatic food allergy. *Journal of Allergy and Clinical Immunology, 107*, 891–896.

Sampson, H. A. (2003). Food allergy. *Journal of Allergy and Clinical Immunology, 111*, S540–S547.

Sampson, H. A. (2004a). Food-induced anaphylaxis. *Novartis Foundation Symposium, 257*, 161–171.

Sampson, H. A. (2004b). Update on food allergy. *Journal of Allergy and Clinical Immunology, 113*, 805–819.

Sampson, H. A., & Anderson, J. A. (2000). Summary and recommendations: Classification of gastrointestinal manifestations due to immunologic reactions to foods in infants and young children. *Journal of Pediatric Gastroenterology and Nutrition, 30*, S87–S94.

Sampson, H. A., & Ho, D. G. (1997). Clinical aspects of allergic disease: Relationship between food-specific IgE concentrations and the risk of positive food challenges in children and adolescents. *Journal of Allergy and Clinical Immunology, 100*, 444–451.

Sampson, H. A., Munoz-Furlong, A., Campbell, R. L., Adkinson, N. F. Jr., Bock, S. A., Branum, A., et al. (2006). Second symposium on the definition and management of anaphylaxis: Summary report—Second National Institute of Allergy and Infectious Disease/Food Allergy and Anaphylaxis Network symposium. *Annals of Emergency Medicine, 47*, 373–380.

Sampson, H. A., Sicherer, S. H., & Birnbaum, A. H. (2001). American Gastroenterological Association Practice Guidelines—AGA technical review of the evaluation of food allergy in gastrointestinal disorders. *Gastroenterology, 120*, 1026–1040.

Sicherer, S. H. (1999). Food allergy: When and how to perform oral food challenges. *Pediatric Allergy and Immunology, 10*, 226–234.

Sicherer, S. H. (2000). Food protein-induced enterocolitis syndrome: Clinical perspectives. *Journal of Pediatric Gastroenterology and Nutrition, 30*, S45–S49.

Sicherer, S. H. (2002). Food allergy. *Lancet, 360*, 701–710.

Sicherer, S. H., Munoz-Furlong, A., & Sampson, H.A. (2003). Prevalence of peanut and tree nut allergy in the United States determined by means of a random digit dial telephone survey: A 5-year follow-up study. *Journal of Allergy and Clinical Immunology, 112*, 1203–1207.

Sicherer, S. H., Munoz-Furlong, A., & Sampson, H. A. (2004). Prevalence of seafood allergy in the United States determined by a random telephone survey. *Journal of Allergy and Clinical Immunology, 114*, 159–165.

Sicherer, S. H., & Sampson, H. A. (2006). Food allergy. *Journal of Allergy and Clinical Immunology, 117*, S470–S475.

Sicherer, S. H., & Teuber, S. (2004). Current approach to the diagnosis and management of adverse reactions to foods. *Journal of Allergy and Clinical Immunology, 114*, 1146–1150.

Spergel, J. M., Andrews, T., Brown-Whitehorn, T. F., Beausoleil, J. L., & Liacouras, C. A. (2005). Treatment of eosinophilic esophagitis with specific food elimination diet directed by a combination of skin prick and patch tests. *Annals of Allergy, Asthma and Immunology, 95*, 336–343.

Sporik, R., Hill, D. J., & Hosking, C. S. (2000). Specificity of allergen skin testing in predicting positive open food challenges to milk, egg, and peanut in children. *Clinical and Experimental Allergy, 30*, 1540–1546.

Steinman, H. A. (1996). "Hidden" allergens in food. *Journal of Allergy and Clinical Immunology, 98, 241–250.*

*Terr, A. I., & Salvaggio, J. E. (1996). Contro*versial concepts in allergy and clinical immunology. In C. W. Bierman, D. S. Pearlman, G. G. Shapiro, & W. W. Busse (Eds.), Allergy, Asthma, and Immunology from Infancy to Adulthood (pp. 749–760). Philadelphia: W. B. Saunders.

von Berg, A., Koletzko, S., Grubl, A., Filipiak-Pittroff, B., Wichmann, H. E., Bauer, C. P., et al. (2003*). The effect of hydrolyzed cow's milk formula* for allergy prevention in the first year of life: The German Infant Nutritional Intervention Study, a randomized doub*le-blind trial.* Journal of Allergy and Clinical Immunology, 111, 533–540.

Zeiger, R. S. (2003). Food allergen avoidance in the prevention of food allergy in infants and children. Pediatrics, 111, 1662–1671.

Special Section: Celiac Disease

Anne R. Lee, MSEd, RD

Reader Objectives

After studying this special section and reflecting on the contents, you should be able to

1. Identify safe foods and grains within the gluten-free dietary pattern.
2. Understand and complete an in-depth nutritional assessment of an individual with celiac disease.
3. Understand and identify the different modes of presentation of celiac disease.
4. Know where to obtain accurate information on celiac disease and the gluten-free dietary pattern.

Celiac Disease/Gluten Enteropathy

To begin a discussion of celiac disease we must first understand what gluten is. Gluten is often used as the generic term for the storage protein in wheat, rye, and barley. It is the specific amino acid sequence in wheat (gliadin), rye (secalin), and barley (hordein) that renders these grains toxic for individuals with celiac disease. The specific amino acid sequence in these three grains triggers the immune response in an individual with celiac disease. Different grains have different protein sequences, thus rendering them as either toxic or safe. Oats do not share the same protein sequence and therefore are chemically safe. They have been considered a questionable grain because of frequent cross-contamination from wheat during the harvesting, milling, and processing (Kasarda, 1997, 2000, 2001). Several companies are beginning to grow, process, and mill uncontaminated oats. In some studies the inclusion of oats was linked to acceptance of the gluten-free diet with no negative affect on the intestinal biopsy. The toxic grains are wheat (and all its derivatives), rye, and barley. See Table 7.11 for the fundamentals of a gluten-free diet and Table 7.12 for gluten-free starch alternatives.

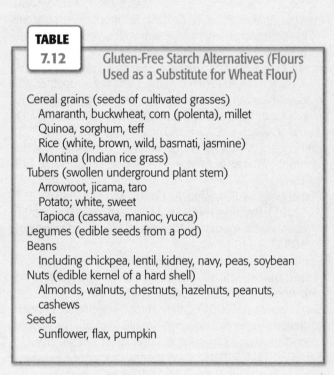

TABLE 7.12	Gluten-Free Starch Alternatives (Flours Used as a Substitute for Wheat Flour)

Cereal grains (seeds of cultivated grasses)
    Amaranth, buckwheat, corn (polenta), millet
    Quinoa, sorghum, teff
    Rice (white, brown, wild, basmati, jasmine)
    Montina (Indian rice grass)
Tubers (swollen underground plant stem)
    Arrowroot, jicama, taro
    Potato; white, sweet
    Tapioca (cassava, manioc, yucca)
Legumes (edible seeds from a pod)
Beans
    Including chickpea, lentil, kidney, navy, peas, soybean
Nuts (edible kernel of a hard shell)
    Almonds, walnuts, chestnuts, hazelnuts, peanuts, cashews
Seeds
    Sunflower, flax, pumpkin

Physiologic Description of Celiac Disease

Presentation

Individuals with celiac disease or gluten enteropathy react to the specific protein sequences found in wheat, rye, and barley. It is the specific amino acid sequence that triggers the immune response. In an individual with celiac disease, when gluten is ingested the digestive process fails and a toxic fragment of gliadin remains. It is this 33 amino acid molecule that appears to be the cause for the inflammatory response (Shan et al., 2002). This protein sequence enters the intestinal mucosa and cannot be broken down by either digestive or pancreatic enzymes. It then enters the lamina propria, which causes the release of the T-cells. The presence of the T-cells in the lamina propria triggers the activation of cytokines, the production of the an-

TABLE 7.11	Fundamentals of the Gluten-Free Diet

Safe Grains	Toxic Grains
Amaranth	Wheat (includes spelt, kamut, semolina, triticale)
Millet	Rye
Quinoa	Barley (including malt)
Corn sorghum	
Teff	
Oats	

tibodies, and the inflammation response (Alaedini & Green, 2005). The resulting villous atrophy and inflammation of the mucosa lead to malabsorption.

Classic presentation is the malnourished individual with diarrhea, bloated belly, weight loss, abdominal pain, wasting, malabsorption, and failure to thrive (grow). However, not all individuals have symptoms. In clinical practice Green and colleagues (2001) showed that celiac disease is being diagnosed in many individuals who are seeking treatment for other conditions that are actually secondary to their celiac disease. Often, individuals present with anemia, osteoporosis, peripheral neuropathy, fatigue, or even screening of first-degree relatives (Murray, 1999). Celiac disease has now been categorized into four main classes according to the National Institutes of Health Consensus Conference (2004).

Prevalence

Historically, it was thought that celiac disease was a rare disease affecting only children. It was also commonly thought that children grew out of celiac disease. In Europe the prevalence was thought to be 1 in 100 to 250, whereas in the United States it was very rare, at 1 in 1,000. Now the research indicates that celiac disease is as common in the United States as it is in Europe, with rates of 1 in 133. These numbers are similar to the current findings in Europe. We are now realizing that celiac disease is found not just in those of Northern European ancestry. Celiac disease is also found in Africa, the Middle East, Asia, New Zealand, and Australia (Shan et al., 2002).

Diagnosis

Typically in the United States, there is a long lag time between the initial onset of symptoms and diagnosis of celiac disease, averaging 11 years (Green & Jabri, 2003). The delay in diagnosis is not believed to be due to patients not seeking health care (Shan et al., 2002), but rather because celiac disease is thought by the medical community to be a rare disorder. The diagnostic process consists of serologic testing for antibody markers and the genotype; if those are positive, endoscopic biopsy is performed. Endoscopic biopsy is considered the "gold standard" because of the characteristic histologic features of celiac disease. These biopsies are graded according to a scale developed by Marsh (1992), ranging from Marsh I, which indicates only blunting of the villi, to Marsh IV, which indicates total villous atrophy with hyperplasia of the crypts and increased intraepithelial lymphocyte count (Shan et al., 2002).

Treatment

Regardless of the severity of the intestinal damage or lack of intestinal symptoms, the only treatment for celiac disease is strict adherence to a gluten-free diet for life. Although this treatment may sound simple, it requires diligence to maintain a gluten-free diet. The obvious sources of gluten are found in wheat, rye, and barley and their derivatives. There are also hidden sources of gluten in many of the foods we commonly eat. It takes only one-eighth of a teaspoon of flour to cause visible damage to the intestinal mucosa (Semrad, 2004), but with a strict gluten-free diet the intestine will recover. However, the long-term effect of repeated small doses of gluten remains unknown. One case reported the effects of repeated ingestion of a piece of a communion wafer, which caused sustained elevated antibody levels as well as intestinal damage on an otherwise strict gluten-free diet (Biagi et al., 2004).

Noncompliance has serious consequences. Untreated celiac disease is associated with increased mortality rates of 1.9 to 3.8 compared with the normal population (Green, Rostami, & Marsh, 2005). Increased incidence of infertility, osteoporosis, peripheral neuropathy, lymphomas, and cancers of the small bowel and esophagus are associated with untreated celiac disease. Of note, however, is the protective effect of the gluten-free diet. One group of patients followed for 5 years had no increased mortality compared with control subjects (Green et al., 2005).

Hidden Sources of Gluten

It is important to remember that a gluten-free diet affects the starch and grain portion of a meal plan. The other food groups offer many naturally gluten-free options, which should be emphasized for a nutritionally balanced intake. However, many foods are considered to be questionable. Wheat flour and malt from barley are common ingredients in medications and in foods such as soups, gravies, soy sauce, seasonings, processed or packaged foods, and even cake icings. The list of ingredients must be checked thoroughly; if the ingredient list is not clear, the manufacturer must be contacted before the food can be considered safe to eat.

The Food Allergen Labeling and Consumer Protection Act passed by Congress in 2004 requires food manufacturers to clearly state if a product contains any of the eight major food allergens, in which wheat is one. The law went into effect in 2006, and new labels now must state whether wheat is an ingredient. However, the law does not cover barley and rye.

The U.S. Food and Drug Administration proposed new rules for gluten-free labeling in January 2007. The use of the term "gluten-free" provides both manufacturers and patients a clear definition of a food's safety from all sources of gluten.

Safe Foods

The traditional cornerstone foods of the gluten-free diet are rice, corn, and potato. Any foods derived from wheat, rye, and barley were historically believed to be toxic. Foods such as vinegars, distilled alcohol, spices, and many ancient or alternative grains are safe. Grains such as quinoa and millet are not related to wheat, rye, or barley, and they do not share the same protein sequence and therefore are safe. These grains provide texture, fiber, iron, B complex vitamins, and many minerals to a gluten-free diet. The usual staples of the gluten-free diet—rice, corn, and potato—do not provide adequate amounts of nutrients (Thompson, 1997, 2000). Special dietary products are not required to be fortified or enriched as are their wheat-based counterparts.

Nutritional Assessment

As our understanding of gluten intolerance unfolds, the medical nutrition therapy we use must also continue to evolve. The standard assessments, including weight and laboratory data, are the cornerstone of the nutritional evaluation of an individual with celiac disease. However, for a complete assessment of an individual with celiac disease we need to look beyond the basics. One must be aware of the need for nutritional supplementation, the various modes of presentation, and the social and emotional components of the gluten-free life-style to fully assess and educate these individuals.

Nutrition counseling of an individual with celiac disease must be all-inclusive. The nutrition care plan should include an in-depth nutritional assessment that includes a diet history and/or a 3-day intake record, height, weight, BMI, review of medical and family history, review of symptoms, review of laboratory data, and other tests (Table 7.13). Of equal importance is a review of eating and shopping behaviors, a social and emotional assessment, and an in-depth education component (Lee, 2003).

For the individual with celiac disease, special attention should be placed on laboratory data. With damage to the small intestine, malabsorption is common. Therefore iron, calcium, electrolytes, and albumin should be closely monitored. Other tests to perform are thyroid function, bone density, and calcium absorption.

The last component of the nutrition care plan is education. This component is probably the most intense in terms of time and depth of information. Although instructing a patient on a gluten-free diet is enmeshed in the social aspects of a gluten-free life-style, we need to be mindful of information overload and individual readiness to learn. Instruction on the gluten-free life-style should be broken up into at least two sessions. The first session should focus on survival skills, any nutritional deficiencies, shopping for gluten-free products, and social issues. The second session should focus on alternate grains, exercise, and general health maintenance (Lee, 2003). School and social issues should be reviewed at each session because these have been reported to be the areas most negatively impacted by the gluten-free life-style (Green et al., 2001; Lee & Green, 2004).

Noncompliance and Complications

Green found that some individuals would "intentionally cheat" on their diet during social situations, dining out, parties, and other functions outside the home. Only 68% of individuals reported following the diet "all the time," and 30% reported following the diet "most of the time" (Green et al., 2001). Although this adherence rate may be viewed as positive among other diet regimes, the consequences of nonadherence for the individual with celiac disease are grave: increased risks of infertility, peripheral neuropathies, bone loss, lymphomas, and cancers of the small bowel and esophagus (Green & Jabri, 2003).

In a subsequent study it was found that both males and females reported a high rate of compliance (98% of males and females). However, when asked about where they intentionally went off the diet, a surprising number admitted to dietary indiscretion. Males reported intentionally going off the diet at social activities 81% of the time, 82% at restaurants, and 58% with friends. Females reported 88% intentional noncompliance to the diet at social

Label Reading

Additives to avoid:
- Wheat starch
- Modified food starch (from wheat)
- Malt, malt flavoring
- Malt vinegar
- Hydrolyzed vegetable or plant protein
- Soy sauce

Safe additives:
- Citric acid
- Maltodextrin
- Dextrin
- Vinegar
- Mono- and diglycerides
- Artificial colors and flavors
- Natural colors and flavors
- MSG (monosodium glutamate)
- Carmel color

| TABLE |
| 7.13 |

Nutrition Care Plan for Celiac Disease or Gluten-Sensitive Enteropathy

Tools	Assessment	Interventions
Diet history/food record	Look for adequate • Calories • Protein • Calcium • Iron • B Complex • Fruits/vegetables • Iron Eating and shopping behaviors • Cultural/religious preferences • Cooking experience • Willingness/time to cook • Use of prepared vs. whole foods • Eating at restaurants vs. home • Favorite foods/preferences	General diet recommendations ✓ 1–2 g protein/kg body weight ✓ 35–40 calories/kg body weight ✓ Possibly low fiber at first, gradually increasing fiber content ✓ Possibly lactose free ✓ Possibly fat restricted ✓ Use food record and suggest ways to correct nutrient deficits. Include recipe modification and snacks as ways to increase nutrient intake. ✓ Add fruits and vegetables if intake is inadequate

Physical	• Height, weight, BMI, growth chart for children
	• Skin, hair, and nails
		General recommendation
		✓ Calcium supplement
		  ➢ Children 500 mg/day
		  ➢ Adults 1,000/1,500 mg/day

Test/labs	• Bone density/endoscopy results
	• Any other tests
	• Albumin, cholesterol, high-density and low-density lipoproteins
	• Hemoglobin, hematocrit, iron, transferrin, TIBC, B_{12}
	• Na, K^+, Ca^+
	• Skin, hair, and nails
		✓ Multivitamin if needed
		  ➢ Children standard 1/day
		  ➢ Adults 18–55
		  ➢ Male standard 1/day
		  ➢ Female prenatal w/moderate vitamin A content
		  ➢ If ≥56 senior formula
		✓ Iron supplementation if needed
		✓ Modify diet for any other medical conditions i.e., diabetes, hypertension

Medical	• Family history • Associated symptoms or related illnesses. • Medications/supplements	✓ Check medications for possible gluten or food–medication interactions
Social/emotional assessment	• Query response to diagnosis and diet • Family support • Literacy level	✓ Referral to social services if needed ✓ Positive reinforcement of health benefits of gluten-free diet ✓ Include family in nutrition education
Symptoms review	• Bloating/gas • Diarrhea • Constipation	✓ Trial of lactose-free diet ✓ If lactose free, highlight nondairy sources of calcium and stress adequate protein ✓ Use lactose enzyme tablets or drops when using dairy products ✓ Use soluble fiber from fruits, vegetables, and grains to resolve diarrhea/constipation ✓ Encourage adequate fluid intake ✓ Use 3 small meals and 3 snacks pattern; include protein at each ✓ If fat tolerance is diminished, digestive or pancreatic enzymes may be beneficial

activities, 88% in restaurants, and 67% with friends. When queried as to the reason they were noncompliant in those settings, 73% reported that the diet was too restrictive. Other reasons reported for noncompliance included the following: the diet is uncomfortable in social settings (69%), too difficult (68%), tasteless (45%), and too expensive (33%) (Lee et al., in press).

Celiac Disease in Pediatrics

The pediatric presentation of celiac disease covers a wide spectrum of symptoms and related illnesses. To define the range of *potential presenta*tions in this population, we use the National Institutes of Health criteria as our benchmarks (National Institutes of Health Consensus Conference, 2004):

- *Classic symptoms:* Classic symptoms are usually seen starting between 6 and 24 months of age. These symptoms usually coincide with the introduction of gluten into the diet. Infants and young children typically present with impaired growth, chronic diarrhea, abdominal distention, muscle wasting and hypotonia, poor appetite, and unhappy behavior (Fasano & Catassi, 2005). Within weeks to months of starting to ingest gluten, weight gain velocity decreases, and finally weight loss can be observed. A celiac crisis, characterized by explosive watery diarrhea, marked abdominal distention, dehydration, electrolyte imbalance, hypotension, and lethargy, was more commonly described at the beginning of the century but now it is rarely observed. This classic form of celiac disease is a common presentation internationally.

- *Nonclassic symptoms:* Currently, there is a general trend of delayed onset of symptomatic celiac disease involving older children, usually ages 5 to 7 years. These children tend to experience unusual intestinal complaints such as recurrent abdominal pain, nausea, vomiting, bloating, and constipation. These children could also present with no gastrointestinal complaints but rather with short stature, pubertal delay, iron deficiency anemia, dental enamel defects, and abnormalities in liver function tests. Dermatitis herpetiformis, a blistering skin manifestation of celiac disease, is rarely seen in the pediatric population (Fasano & Catassi, 2005).

- *Silent presentation:* Silent presentation refers to those patients who otherwise appear healthy and asymptomatic except for the typical gluten sensitive intestinal enteropathy. Significant numbers of silent cases have been reported from population screenings in both the at-risk group (those with family members with celiac disease and those with insulin-dependent diabetes) and as the general population (Fasano & Catassi, 2005).

- *Potential celiac disease:* These individuals have positive antibody serologies and/or the genetic markers (HLA DQ2 or DQ8) but a normal or minimally abnormal mucosal architecture at the intestinal biopsy. These individuals are at risk of developing typical celiac disease later in life (Fasano & Catassi, 2005).

A recent study on feeding practices in the United States found differences in presentation and symptoms due to infant feeding practices. Those children who were exclusively breast-fed reported fewer symptoms and presented with symptoms later (D'Amico et al., 2005). Introduction of wheat after 6 months also delayed onset of symptoms. This finding is in sharp contrast to what was discovered in Sweden. The unusual celiac epidemic in Sweden does highlight the influence of environmental factors. In the 1980s there was a dramatic threefold increase in the number of diagnosed cases. In reviewing the many levels of factors that play a role in the development of celiac disease, it appeared that breast-feeding as well as the timing of gluten introduction did have an impact on both the severity and presentation time of symptoms. The epidemic was linked to a decrease in breast-feeding at the same time as a later but larger introduction of gluten-containing foods in the infant's diet.

In the celiac adolescent population an increased association was also found with depression and behavioral disorders. A 31% prevalence of lifetime major depressive disorder was found. It was also suggested that treatment with a gluten-free diet and early diagnosis may decrease the vulnerability to depression (Pynnonen et al., 2004).

Quality of Life in the Pediatric Population with Celiac Disease

Travel, social occasions, school and college, or sleepaway camp are all areas of special concerns to children with celiac disease. Elementary and middle school years are all about learning to be social and interact in a group. Compliance to a gluten-free diet makes this a very difficult task for children with celiac disease. Not only must their food be gluten free, it also cannot be mixed with the other meals and snacks because of cross-contamination issues. In addition to the hazards of meal and snack time, the classroom itself poses several threats to these children. Many art supplies contain gluten, and many projects requiring glue and other materials are usually performed at the child's desk. This seemingly simple task renders the child's own desk contaminated, and therefore it must be cleaned before the child has his or her snack or lunch at the same table or desk. (See the Sidebar for a list of classroom products that may contain wheat.) Also, careful hand washing avoids any potential trace ingestion: Remember, it only takes one-eighth of a teaspoon of flour to cause intestinal damage (Semrad, 2004).

Potential Gluten-Containing Classroom Supplies
Crayons
Glue
Stickers
Paint
Play dough
Paper mache

Another area of concerns for teens is leaving the safety of their home and going away to college. The prospect of entering that semi–adult world of college is daunting enough on its own. Now the adolescent with celiac disease must also maneuver the dining services to make sure they are able to obtain a safe, uncontaminated, gluten-free meal.

The pediatric population presents a special concern in the area of quality of life for two reasons. First, childhood and adolescence are often difficult years to maneuver unscathed, even without the added burden of a chronic disease. Second, the lack of comprehensive studies in this age group leaves us with incomplete data on the quality of life and social implications of a rigid life-style over an extended period of time. However, there are several resources specifically targeted for this population group (see Sidebar on National Support Groups). In addition, several fact sheets and handouts have been developed to help navigate social situations while maintaining a strict gluten-free life-style.

Conclusion

Celiac disease is a common autoimmune disorder. Individual presentation varies from asymptomatic to the extraintestinal skin manifestation of dermatitis herpetiformis to severe wasting and malnutrition. Regardless of presentation, the only treatment is following a strict gluten-free diet for life. Because the dietary regime requires strict adherence in a wheat-laden world, quality of life is affected. Though the overall quality of life of individuals improves with the gluten-free diet, the social impact of the diet and diagnosis on the quality of life remains an issue.

Important questions remain in the treatment and care of individuals with celiac disease. Further research is needed in the areas of long-term health risks in the pediatric population, the benefits associated with vitamin and mineral supplementation, and the appropriate levels of nutrient supplementation. The questions of what constitutes an acceptable amount of gluten ingestion as well as the long-term effects of a naturally gluten-free versus a wheat starch–based gluten-free diet need to be evaluated. Probably the most pressing question remains: do we treat the child with potential or latent celiac disease? Only further research will help answer these queries.

National Support Groups

Teen Support Group, Celiac Disease Center, Columbia University, www.celiacdiseasecenter.org

American Celiac Disease Alliance (ACDA), 4331 E. Baseline Rd., Suite B 105–216, Gilbert, AZ 85234. Website: www.americanceliac.org

Celiac Disease Foundation (CDF), 13251 Ventura Blvd., Suite 1, Studio City, CA 91604. Phone: 818-990-2354, Website: http:// www.celiac.org/

The Gluten Intolerance Group of North America (GIG), 15110 10th Ave. SW, Suite A, Seattle, WA 98166. Phone: 206-246-6652, Website: http:// www.gluten.net/

Celiac Sprue Association/United States of America (CSA), P.O. Box 31700, Omaha, NE 68131. Phone: 402-558-0600, Website: http:// www.csaceliacs.org/

Magazines

Gluten-Free Living. A magazine for people with celiac disease. Ann Whelan, Editor/Publisher, 19A Broadway, Hawthorne, NY 10532. Phone: 914-741-5420, Website: www.glutenfreeliving.com

Sully's Living Without. A magazine for people with food allergies, intolerances, and sensitivities, including celiac disease. P.O. Box 2126, Northbrook, IL 60065. Phone: 847-480-8810, Website: www. livingwithout.com

Websites

www.celiac.org, Celiac Disease and Gluten-Free Diet Support Page. This website contains information on a variety of issues pertaining to celiac disease.

http://www.eatright.org/, American Dietetic Association. This website contains a searchable database for nutrition-related topics.

www.gluten/freedrugs.com, Gluten-Free Drugs. This website contains listings of gluten-free medications alphabetically and by therapeutic category.

Celiac Disease and Religious Issues

Shemura Oat Matzos, Rabbie E. Kestenbaum, 22 Eagle Lodge, Golders Green, London NW 11 8BD, England. Web site: www.ubaccess.com/oatmatzos.html. Phone: +44 208 455 9476.

Low-Gluten Communion Wafers Congregation of Benedictine, Sisters of Perpetual Adoration, Alter Breads Department, 31970 State Highway P, Clyde, Missouri 64432. Website article: www.catholic review.org/articles2/Newlowglutenhostsafeforce liacdiseasesuffers.htm. Phone: 800-223-2772.

Celiac Disease Center at Columbia University, Columbia University College of Physicians and Surgeons, New York-Presbyterian Hospital, 161 Fort Washington Ave., New York, NY 10032, (212) 305-5590, www.cealiacdiseasecenter.org

Celiac Center, Beth Israel Deaconess Medical Center, Harvard Medical School, 330 Brookline Ave., Boston, MA 02215, (617) 667-7000, www.bidmc.harvard.edu

Celiac Disease Program, The University of Chicago, 5839 S. Maryland Ave., MC 4065, Chicago, IL 60637, (773) 702-7593, www.uchospitals.edu/specialities/celiac

Celiac Disease Research Center, Wm. K. Medical Research Center for Celiac Disease, UCSD Medical Center, 200 W. Arbor Drive, #8825, San Diego, CA 92103-8825, http://celiaccenter.ucsd.edu/

Center for Celiac Research, University of Maryland School of Medicine, 22 S. Greene St., Box 140, Baltimore, MD 21201, (401) 706-8021, www.celiaccenter.org

Celiac Disease Research Program and Celiac Disease Clinic, Division of Gastroenterology and Hepatology May Clinic, 200 First St., SW, Rochester, MN 55905, (507) 284-2511, www.mayoclinic.com

Question:

If a child is symptomatic yet has been categorized in the potential celiac disease category, how do you treat them?

Case Study: Celiac Disease

Patient J (age 12) presents to Pediatric Nutrition, Gastroenterology and Hepatology clinic for his annual check on his reflux disease. He presents with reflux, weight gain, and constipation. These symptoms have returned after a short hiatus during the summer months. His usual routine at home, school, and during the summer was reviewed. It detailed the usual diet mix of fast foods, school lunch program, and some home-cooked meals. The exception was during the summer months when he visited his grandmother in Jamaica where he consumed a traditional diet.

Lab data:

Ht: 5' 2"

Wt: 134 lb.

Albumin: 4.4

WBC: 5.0

RBC: 4.22

HGB: 12.3

HCT: 37.4

1. Should this patient be screened for celiac disease?
2. If so, what tests or clinical pathways would you follow?
3. What were the factors that influenced the change *in symptoms during the summer months?*

References

Alaedini, A., & Green, P. (2005). Narrative review: Celiac disease. Understanding a complex autoimmune disorder. *Annals of Internal Medicine, 142,* 289–298.

Biagi, F., Campanella, J., Martucci, S., Pezzimenti, D., Ciclitira, P., Ellis, H., et al. (2004). A milligram of gluten a day keeps the mucosal recovery away: A case report. *Nutrition Reviews, 62,* 360–363.

D'Amico, M., Holmes, J., Stavropoulos, S., Frederick, M., Levy, J., DeFelice, A., et al. (2005). Presentation of pediatric celiac disease in the United States: Prominent effect of breastfeeding. *Clinical Pediatrics, 44*, 249–258.

Fasano, A., & Catassi, C. (2005). Coeliac disease in children. Best Practice & Research Clinical. *Gastroenterology, 19*, 467–478.

Green, P. H., & Jabri, B. (2003). Coeliac disease. *Lancet, 362*, 383–391.

Green, P. H., Rostami, K., & Marsh, M. N. (2005). Diagnosis of coeliac disease. *Best Practice & Research. Clinical Gastroenterology, 19*, 389–400.

Green, P. H. R., Stavropoulos, S., Pangagi, S., Goldstein, S., McMahon, D. J., Absan, H., et al. (2001). Characteristics of adult celiac disease in the USA: Results of a national survey. *American Journal of Gastroenterology, 96*, 126–131.

Kasarda, D. (1997). Gluten and gliadin: Precipitating factors in celiac disease. In M. Maki, P. Collin, & J. K. Visakorpi (Eds.), *Coeliac Disease* (Proceedings of the 7th International Symposium on Coeliac Disease, 1996, Tampere, Finland, pp. 195–212). Tampere, Finland: Coeliac Disease Study Group.

Kasarda, D. (2000). Celiac disease. In *The Cambridge World History of Food* (vol. 1, pp. 1008–1022). Cambridge, UK: Cambridge University Press.

Kasarda, D. (2001). Grains in relation to celiac disease. *Cereal World, 46*, 209–210.

Lee, A. R. (2003). Nutritional assessment and care of celiac disease. *American Dietetic Association Clinical Connections, 24*, 1–8.

Lee, A. R., Diamond, B., Ng, D., & Green, P. H. R. (in press). Quality of life of individuals with celiac disease in the United States.

Lee, A. R., & Green, H. R. (2004). Impact on quality of life in patients with celiac disease in the United States. Proceedings of the 11th International Symposium, Belfast, Ireland.

Marsh, M. N. (1992). Gluten, major histocompatibility complex, and the small intestine. A molecular and immunobiologic approach to the spectrum of gluten sensitivity ("celiac sprue"). *Gastroenterology, 102*, 330–354.

Murray, J. (1999). The widening spectrum of celiac disease. *American Journal of Clinical Nutrition, 69*, 354–365.

National Institutes of Health Consensus Conference. (2004). Development statement: Celiac disease. Retrieved November, 2004, from http://consensus.nih.gov/cons/118/118celiacPDF.pdf

Pynnonen, P., Isometsa, E., Aronen, E., Verkasalo, M., Savilahti, E., & Aalberg, V. (2004). Mental disorders in adolescents with celiac disease. *Psychosomatics, 45*, 325–335.

Semrad, C. (2004). How much gluten is too much? Paper presented at the Annual Patient Education Day 2004. Celiac Disease Center, Columbia University, New York City, October 23, 2004.

Shan, L., Molberg, O., Parrot, I., Hausch, F., Filiz, F., Gray, G. M., et al. (2002). Structural basis for gluten intolerance in celiac sprue. *Science, 297*, 2275–2279.

Thompson, T. (1997). Do oats belong in a gluten-free diet? *Journal of the American Dietetic Association, 97*, 1417–1423.

Thompson, T. (2000). Folate, iron, and dietary fiber content of the gluten free diet. *Journal of the American Dietetic Association, 100*, 1389–1393.

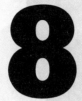

CHAPTER

8

Special Topics in Preadolescence and Adolescent Nutrition: Dietary Guidelines for Athletes, Pediatric Diabetes, and Disordered Eating

Pamela S. Hinton, PhD, and Karen Chapman-Novakofski, RD, LDN, PhD

CHAPTER OUTLINE

Reader Objectives

After studying this chapter and reflecting on the contents, you should be able to

1. Determine fuel utilization during exercise.
2. Describe optimal nutrition before, during, and after an endurance competition.
3. Describe the consequences of chronic undernutrition and how they differ between males and females.
4. Recognize the prevalence and incidence for pediatric diabetes in the United States.
5. Understand the pathogenesis of types 1 and 2 diabetes in children.
6. Identify risk factors for types 1 and 2 diabetes in children.
7. Recognize conditions associated with pediatric diabetes.
8. Understand management principles to achieve optimal glycemic goals.
9. Describe the similarities and differences among the three eating disorders defined by the American Psychiatric Association.
10. Know the medical consequences of eating disorders.
11. Describe effective treatment for eating disorders, including recommendations for nutrition interventions.
12. Know the prevalence, etiology, and recommended treatment practices for eating disorders in special populations.
13. Identify childhood eating disorders and explain how they differ from anorexia nervosa and bulimia nervosa.

Dietary Guidelines for Athletes

Pamela S. Hinton, PhD

Energy

Total energy expenditure is the sum of resting energy expenditure, dietary-induced thermogenesis, and physical activity and varies with gender, age, and body size. Typically, physical activity accounts for 10% to 15% of total energy expenditure, but athletes in strenuous training programs or who participate in endurance sports may increase total energy expenditure by two- to threefold due to physical activity. For example, cyclists competing in stage races such as the Tour de France may expend up to 8,000 kcal/day (Saris, van Erp-Baart, Brouns, Westerterp, & ten Hoor, 1989). The Institute of Medicine recently published formulas for estimated energy requirement based on gender, age, weight, height, and physical activity (Table 8.1).

Accurately determining energy needs from prediction equations is difficult. Interindividual variation in resting energy expenditure is large, and energy expended during physical activity varies with exercise duration and intensity. Tables of **metabolic equivalent** values for various activities can be used to estimate energy expenditure in physical activity and activities of daily living (Ainsworth, Jacobs, Leon, Richardson, & Montoye, 1993).

Even if we have an estimate of how many calories are needed to be in energy balance, the error associated with evaluating dietary intake is largely due to over- or under-reporting, various methods of food preparation, and accuracy of food composition tables. Changes in body weight and/or composition

Metabolic equivalent: The ratio of the work metabolic rate to the resting metabolic rate. One metabolic equivalent is defined as 1 kcal/kg/h or 3.5 mL O_2 consumed/kg/min.

may be the best way for athletes to self-monitor their energy balance over time.

Carbohydrate

Dietary carbohydrates (sugar and starch) have a **metabolizable energy** density of 4 kcal/g and are readily digested and absorbed. During exercise, glucose is the preferred substrate for ATP production. For this reason, and to replenish hepatic and muscle glycogen, athletes should consume 60% to 75% of their energy from carbohydrate. It is recommended that endurance athletes consume from 6 to 10 g carbohydrate/kg body weight (BW) (American Dietetic Association, Dietitians of Canada, and the American College of Sports Medicine, 2000). This recommendation assumes that an athlete is not over- or underweight. For example, an athlete weighing 70 kg needs between 420 and 720 g carbohydrate/day (which is 1,680 to 2,880 kcal carbohydrate). To equate grams of carbohydrate to foods, a serving from the grains, breads, and cereals group contains approximately 15 g of carbohydrate. A serving is one slice of bread, 1 ounce of cereal, or ½ cup of cooked rice or pasta (U.S. Department of Health and Human Services [DHHS]). This recommendation applies only to athletes who are regularly depleting their glycogen stores (i.e., 2 to 3 hours of aerobic exercise a day 5 to 7 days a week).

There are several reasons for the emphasis on dietary carbohydrates, especially for athletes. First, the central nervous system and red blood cells have a high glucose requirement. Red blood cells do not have mitochondria so they cannot oxidize fat; ATP must be produced from glycolysis and anaerobic metabolism of pyruvate to lactate. Second, dietary carbohydrates are needed to replenish liver and muscle glycogen stores. Inadequate carbohydrate intake necessitates gluconeogenesis from dietary or endogenous amino acids because fat cannot be used to make glucose.

Glucose is by far the most abundant dietary monosaccharide; the most prevalent dietary disaccharides are sucrose (glucose + fructose), more commonly referred to as table

Metabolizable energy: Gross energy in a food minus the energy lost in feces, urine, and combustible gases. The metabolizable energies for protein and carbohydrate are 4 kcal/g and the metabolizable energy for fat is 9 kcal/g.

TABLE 8.1	Institute of Medicine Equations for Estimating Energy Requirements in Healthy Adults

Males
EER = 662 − 9.53 × age (yr) + PA × [5.91 × weight (kg) + 539.6 × height (m)]
Females
EER = 354 − 6.91 × age (yr) + PA × [9.36 × weight (kg) + 726 × height (m)]
PA = 1.25 if you are "active" and 1.48 if you are "very active"

EER, estimate energy requirement; PA, physical activity.

From Food and Nutrition Board (2003).

sugar; lactose (glucose + galactose), which is milk sugar; and maltose (glucose + glucose). The mono- and disaccharides fall into the category of "sugars" and are sometimes referred to as "simple carbohydrates." The term "complex carbohydrate" is used to describe carbohydrates that are glucose polymers. Short chains of glucose molecules linked together, such as maltodextrin or dextrose, are used by the food industry as sweeteners. These are also the "complex carbohydrates" added to sports drinks. The most complex carbohydrate molecules are the polysaccharides, which typically contain 10,000 to 1,000,000 glucose molecules. Polysaccharides comprise the starches that are present in grains, legumes, and some vegetables.

Carbohydrates differ not only in their complexity, but also in their effect on blood sugar (Foster-Powell, Holt, & Brand-Miller, 2002). The effect of carbohydrates on blood sugar is important for overall health, fueling muscle during exercise, and replenishing glycogen stores after exercise. The effect of a food on blood glucose concentrations depends on the type and amount of carbohydrate in the food and on how quickly that carbohydrate can be digested and absorbed. Some foods cause a rapid increase in blood glucose concentrations, whereas others produce a slower and more prolonged rise. The glycemic index (GI) is used to quantify the effect of a food on blood glucose and to make comparisons among foods. The GI is defined as the increase in blood glucose concentration above baseline during the 2 hours after eating a test food relative to the response to glucose for an equivalent amount of carbohydrate. The glycemic response to glucose is set at 100, and the GI for all other foods is less than 100.

> **● Learning Point** Foods that have rapidly digestible carbohydrate and contain glucose have the highest glycemic indices. For example, Gatorade® has a GI of 80.

The actual GIs of foods may vary from the published values because they are affected by multiple factors. The physical form of the food alters the GI. Breaking down the food matrix increases the GI. For example, the GI of potatoes is increased by 25% if the potatoes are mashed. And, thin linguini has a GI of 87, but thick linguini is lower, at 68. The ripeness of fruit also has an effect on the GI because as a fruit ripens the starch is converted into sugar. Under-ripe bananas have a GI of 30 versus 50 for a ripe banana. Food processing and cooking methods also alter the GI. Heating, moisturizing, and pressing foods make the starch easier to digest, increasing the GI. For example, raw carrots have a GI of 20, and peeling and boiling them increases the GI to 40.

The GI of a food assumes that only that food has been eaten. However, most humans do not eat single foods but eat meals and snacks composed of several foods. Protein and fat do not cause an increase in blood glucose; only foods containing carbohydrate have this effect. However, the GI of a food eaten alone is different from the same food eaten as part of a mixed meal of carbohydrate, protein, and fat. For example, a plain French baguette has a GI of 95; bread with butter has a GI of 60. Meals that are high in soluble fiber or have a high acid content also lower the GI because the rate of gastric emptying is decreased, slowing the increase in blood glucose.

Glycemic load is the net effect of a food on blood glucose concentrations. Glycemic load depends not just on the GI of that food, but on how much of it is eaten. For example, jelly beans have a GI of 80, but eating only five jelly beans causes a much smaller increase in blood glucose than eating a handful of peanut M&Ms®, which have a GI of 30.

Despite these limitations, the concept of GI still has some practical value for athletes. Even if the GI of a food cannot be accurately determined when it consumed as part of a meal, foods can be categorized as generally high or low GI. For example, a dinner of whole wheat fettuccine with chunky tomato sauce and sautéed vegetables has a lower GI than Spaghettios because of the whole grain flour, size of the pasta, greater acidity of the tomato sauce, and the fiber in the vegetables.

For overall health, most dietary carbohydrate should come from unrefined whole grains, legumes, and fresh fruits and vegetables (Murphy & Johnson, 2003). Unrefined grains are superior to refined varieties because they provide more fiber and vitamins. Unrefined grains also have lower GIs, which may reduce the risk of non–insulin-dependent (type 2) diabetes. High GI foods may contribute to insulin resistance because the rapid increase in blood glucose levels after eating these foods stimulates a greater insulin response than lower GI foods. Although somewhat controversial, there is evidence that high GI foods contribute to elevated blood triglycerides (fats), which is a risk factor for heart disease.

Protein

Dietary protein has a metabolizable energy density of 4 kcal/g. Protein in meat, dairy products, eggs, and legumes is digested into amino acids, which are used to repair or build new tissues. If energy or carbohydrate intake is insufficient, amino acids from dietary protein or catabolism of endogenous protein are used for gluconeogenesis in the liver. Athletes have slightly higher protein requirements (1.2 to 1.7 g/kg BW) than nonathletes (0.8 g/kg BW) (American Dietetic Association, et al., 2000; Wolfe, 2000). Endurance athletes should consume 1.2 to 1.4 g protein/kg BW to maintain lean body mass and strength-trained athletes 1.6 to 1.7 g/kg to maximize muscle hypertrophy. Athletes who follow vegetarian diets have greater protein requirements (1.3 to 1.8 g/kg BW) because of the lower quality of plant-derived proteins. A 70-kg athlete who participates in a team sport like basketball or soccer needs 84 to 98 g protein/day.

● **Learning Point** To put grams of protein into food terms, a serving from the protein food group is equivalent to ~20 g. A serving from this group is 2 to 3 ounces cooked meat, 1 cup of cooked beans, ¼ cup of peanut butter, or ⅔ cup of nuts. Excess dietary protein is metabolized to glucose and fatty acids and stored as glycogen and triglycerides in adipose tissue.

Fat

Dietary fat has a metabolizable energy density of 9 kcal/g, making it a more concentrated source of energy than carbohydrate or protein. For this reason, and because of the association between diets high in fat and cardiovascular disease, some female athletes restrict their fat intake. However, dietary fat plays an essential role in maintaining health. It is needed for absorption of the fat-soluble vitamins (vitamins A, D, E, and K), and vegetable oils are excellent sources of the antioxidant, vitamin E. Fatty acids are incorporated into cell membranes and are required for normal immune function. It is recommended that athletes consume moderate amounts of fat (20% to 25% of energy) and no less than 15% of their total energy from dietary fat, preferably polyunsaturated fats (American Dietetic Association, et al., 2000). As an example, if an athlete needs 3,000 calories per day, at least 450 of those calories should be from fat. This would be equivalent to 50 g of fat (i.e., 300 calories divided by 9 calories per gram of fat). The easiest way to change the amount of dietary fat is to increase or decrease the amount of fat added to foods, like butter or cream cheese on bagels, dressing on salads, mayonnaise on sandwiches, and oil in cooking. One tablespoon of butter, cream cheese, dressing, or oil contains about 10 g of fat and 100 calories.

Athletes should make an effort to consume fats from different sources to ensure they consume adequate amounts of the essential fatty acids. Omega-3 fatty acids are more likely to be missing from the typical U.S. diet, whereas omega-6 fatty acids are plentiful in the food supply. Dietary sources of omega-3 fatty acids include fatty fish, walnuts, flaxseed, and canola oil. Eicosapentaenoic acid and docosahexaenoic acid are the most common omega-3 fatty acids in the diet; purified eicosapentaenoic acid and docosahexaenoic acid also are sold as dietary supplements. Regular consumption of omega-3 fatty acids may reduce the risk of developing cardiovascular disease by lowering serum cholesterol and triglycerides and by reducing inflammation in the lining of the blood vessels (Connor, 2000; James, Gibson, & Cleland, 2000).

Omega-3 fatty acids alter cell metabolism by activating genes that are needed for cellular transport and use of fat. Omega-3 fatty acids promote the cellular uptake of fat by increasing the activity of lipoprotein lipase (Park & Harris, 2003) and by increasing the amount of fatty acid binding protein, which carries fatty acids across the cell membrane into the cells. Omega-3 fatty acids also facilitate production of energy from fat due to increased hepatic carnitine palmitoyltransferase-2 activity (Ukropec et al., 2003) and accelerated transport of fatty acids into the mitochondria (Raastad, Hostmark, & Stromme, 1997).

● **Learning Point** There is no direct evidence that omega-3 fatty acids improve athletic performance in humans. In one study of highly trained soccer players, 10 weeks of omega-3 supplementation in the form of fish oil had no effect on maximal aerobic power, anaerobic power, or running performance (Raastad et al., 1997).

Regardless of whether or not omega-3 fatty acids improve performance, they are needed to optimize health and may reduce the risk of osteoporosis (Watkins, Li, Lippman, & Seifert, 2001), rheumatoid arthritis, asthma, cancer, and heart disease (Connor, 2000). According to the Food and Nutrition Board of the Institute of Medicine (2003), adult males should consume 1.6 g/day and adult females 1.1 g/day. Four ounces of cold water fish, such as salmon, swordfish, or bluefish, contain about 1.5 g omega-3 fatty acids. One ounce of walnuts or flaxseeds (or 1 tablespoon of the oil) has about 2 g of omega-3 fatty acids.

Vitamins and Minerals

Athletes often believe their vitamin and mineral needs are significantly higher than those of the typical nonathlete, so they consume micronutrients in excess of the Recommended Daily Allowances (RDAs). What athletes do not realize is that RDAs are set above the mean requirement for the general population, so there is a "safety factor" built into them. For example, the RDA for iron for women ages 19 to 50 years is 18 mg/day, whereas the mean requirement is 8 mg/day (Food and Nutrition Board, Institute of Medicine, 2001). Athletes may require more of some nutrients than nonathletes because of increased nutrient excretion, metabolic waste production, and tissue synthesis and repair. However, the increment is small relative to the safety factor.

> ● **Learning Point** Most athletes meet their nutrient needs if they consume the RDAs, which usually can be achieved by eating a varied and balanced diet. The exceptions are athletes who restrict their food intake and vegetarian and vegan athletes. Iron, zinc, and calcium are the most common inadequate nutrient intakes in these populations.

Iron

In the general population of adults in the United States, 3% to 5% of women are anemic and 11% to 13% are iron deficient; less than 1% of men are iron deficient (Looker, Dallman, Carroll, Gunter, & Johnson, 1997). The reasons for the relatively high prevalence of iron deficiency in women are increased iron losses in menstrual blood flow and lower dietary iron intake. Endurance athletes, regardless of gender, are more likely to become iron deficient than nonathletes. A recent study of recreationally competitive runners, cyclists, and triathletes found 36% of women and 6% of men to be iron deficient but not anemic (Sinclair & Hinton, 2005). The increased prevalence of iron deficiency in endurance athletes is because of greater iron losses, primarily via sweat and occult gastrointestinal bleeding.

Iron plays a critical role in oxidative metabolism. Hemoglobin and myoglobin bind dioxygen via the porphyrin ring of heme. Hemoglobin carries oxygen from the environment to the tissues; myoglobin transfers oxygen from erythrocytes to muscle cells. The electron transport chain depends on heme-containing cytochromes (a, a_3, b, b_5, c, c_1) and on non-

heme iron–sulfur enzymes (NADH dehydrogenase, succinate dehydrogenase, and ubiquinone-cytochrome c reductase).

Iron deficiency is a degenerative condition that progresses through three stages (Food and Nutrition Board, Institute of Medicine, 2001): depleted iron stores but functional iron is unchanged, early functional iron deficiency without anemia, and iron deficiency anemia. The clinical indicators used to assess each stage of iron deficiency are shown in Table 8.2. The clinical signs and symptoms of iron depletion are determined by the severity of the deficiency. Early functional iron deficiency reduces endurance capacity and energetic efficiency during submaximal work in young women (Hinton, Giordano, Brownlie, & Haas, 2000; Brownlie, Utermohlen, Hinton, Giordano, Haas, 2002; Brownlie, Utermohlen, Hinton, & Haas, 2004; Brutsaert et al., 2003). Based on animal studies, this deficit is due to decreased activity of iron-containing oxidative enzymes and cytochromes (Finch et al., 1976; Davies et al., 1984; Willis, Brooks, Henderson, & Dallman, 1987). The hallmark symptoms of anemia are fatigue, lack of energy, and apathy. Anemia impairs maximal work performance (maximal oxygen consumption) by reducing oxygen delivery to the body (Celsing, Ekblom, Sylven, Everett, & Astrand, 1988).

Daily basal iron losses are small compared with total body iron (0.9 to 1.2 mg iron/day): 0.6 mg/day are lost from the gastrointestinal tract, mostly in sloughed mucosal cells; 0.08 mg/day are lost in urine; and 0.2 to 0.3 mg/day are lost through the skin. Menstruating women require an additional 0.6 to 0.7 mg/day to account for menstrual blood loss. The estimated average requirement for iron was set to maintain the functional iron pool with minimal iron stores (i.e., serum ferritin > 15 µg/L) using factorial mod-

TABLE 8.2 Laboratory Measurements Commonly Used in the Evaluation of Iron Status

Stage of Iron Deficiency	Indicator	Diagnostic Range
Depleted stores	Stainable bone marrow iron	Absent
	Total iron binding capacity	>400 µg/dL
	Serum ferritin concentration	<12 µg/L
Early functional iron deficiency	Transferrin saturation	<16%
	Free erythrocyte protoporphyrin	>70 µg/dL erythrocyte
	Serum transferrin receptor	>8.5 mg/L
Iron deficiency anemia	Hemoglobin concentration	<130 g/L male <20 g/L female
	Mean cell volume	<80 fL

From Food and Nutrition Board (2003).

eling of basal and menstrual iron losses and iron accretion (Food and Nutrition Board, Institute of Medicine, 2001).

Increased iron losses and low dietary intake are associated with increased risk of iron deficiency. Blood donation results in a loss of 200 to 250 mg iron/0.5 L of blood. Intense endurance exercise increases whole body iron turnover and iron losses. The increased loss via the gastrointestinal tract, hematuria, and hemoglobinuria may elevate the estimated average requirement for athletes by 30% to 70% (Food and Nutrition Board, Institute of Medicine, 2001). Because of lower bioavailability of non-heme iron compared with heme iron, vegetarians have an iron requirement that is 1.8 times that of individuals who consume a mixed diet.

To avoid becoming iron deficient, endurance athletes, especially women, should pay attention to how much iron they consume and to the source of iron in their diet. The current daily recommended intake for women ages 18 to 50 years is 18 mg iron/day. This is difficult to achieve through diet alone because the amount of iron in the United States' food supply is about 6 mg per 1,000 calories. Iron from plant sources is non-heme iron, which is poorly absorbed. For example, a 1 cup serving of raw spinach contains 6 mg of iron, but only 2% to 15%, or 0.1 to 0.6 mg of that, is absorbed in the small intestine. In contrast, animal sources of iron (i.e., meat) contain heme iron that has a higher bioavailability. A 3-ounce serving of steak contains 4 mg of iron, up to 50% of which is absorbed in the intestine for an actual intake of 2 mg iron. Thus women who follow a vegetarian diet must be especially careful to consume enough iron.

Supplemental ferrous iron is available in complexes with sulfate, succinate, citrate, lactate, fumarate, and gluconate. Iron supplements should be taken with ascorbic acid to enhance absorption. Hematocrit and hemoglobin respond to supplemental iron after about 2 weeks; it may take up to 12 months to replete iron stores. Unlike most other minerals, iron cannot be actively excreted from the body, so the potential for toxicity is high. Iron supplements only should be used under medical supervision.

Calcium

Calcium also is a mineral that is likely to be lacking in the diets of athletes, particularly vegans and women. Studies of the diets of athletes have repeatedly shown that many women do not meet the rec-

ommended intake of 1,000 mg calcium/day, primarily because they do not consume three to four servings of dairy products. Women who are concerned about their body weight or about cardiovascular disease may avoid dairy products because they believe they are high in fat (Leachman Slawson et al., 2001; Turner & Bass, 2001).

Inadequate calcium intake contributes to loss of bone mineral and/or failure to maximize bone mineral density during skeletal growth, which increases the risk of osteoporosis. Low dietary calcium and/or vitamin D consumption causes mobilization of calcium from bone to maintain the concentration of calcium in blood, allowing muscle contraction and nerve impulse transmission to continue uninterrupted.

Individuals who are lactose intolerant because they do not have adequate amounts of lactase cannot consume dairy products. Recently, food manufacturers have begun fortifying other foods with calcium, and women can now choose calcium-fortified orange juice, breakfast cereal, and soy milk as alternatives to dairy products.

Calcium also is available in dietary supplements. Calcium derived from oyster shells, coral, bone meal, or dolomite is poorly absorbed because of poor solubility in the intestine. The best types of supplemental calcium are calcium carbonate or calcium citrate; both are available in chewable tablets or soft chews. Some chewable antacid tablets contain calcium carbonate and are cheaper than most other calcium supplements.

> ● **Learning Point** There is no advantage to taking more than 1,200 mg calcium/day (DHHS, n.d.).

Fluid and Electrolytes

Dehydration due to an imbalance between fluid loss and intake is the most common cause of heat-related illness in athletes (Convertino et al., 1996). Athletes may lose water at a rate of 0.5 to 1.5 L/h and up to 6% to 10% of their body weight. Water is lost from all fluid compartments, resulting in decreased sweating and impaired heat dissipation. The decline in blood volume decreases blood pressure and cardiac output. Heart rate increases 3 to 5 beats/min for every 1% of body weight lost to compensate for decreased stroke volume. Skin blood flow also is decreased, further reducing the ability to decrease body temperature. Symptoms of heat-related illness are headache, nausea, dizziness, apathy, confusion, exhaustion, and chills. Performance declines markedly because of decreased muscle perfusion. Paradoxically, gastric emptying is slowed, impairing fluid absorption and restoration of fluid balance. The risk of heat-related illness is increased by exercise in hot and humid environments, diuretics use, and older age.

A disproportionate amount of fluid lost in sweat is from the extracellular fluid compartment, the fluid outside of the cells, including the blood plasma. The average concentration of sodium in sweat is 1,150 mg/L but can vary greatly (450 to 2,300 mg/L) (Convertino et al., 1996). Assuming a sweat rate of 1.5 L/h, an athlete with sweat of average saltiness would lose about 1,700 mg sodium/h. Excessive sweating, combined with consumption of plain water in copious amounts (e.g., 10 L in 4 hours), results in a sodium deficit, referred to as **dilutional hyponatremia.** The symptoms of hyponatremia are disorientation, confusion, seizure, and coma. This condition is quite rare and most often occurs in marathon and ultramarathon type events lasting longer than 3 hours and in individuals who ingest large volumes of fluid without electrolytes.

Dilutional hyponatremia: Low blood sodium concentrations; in athletes typically resulting from sodium losses in sweat and excessive consumption of plain water during exercise.

Because potassium is located in the intracellular fluid, much smaller amounts are lost in sweat compared with sodium. The average potassium concentration in sweat is about 350 mg/L, so the quantity lost in sweat is negligible compared with the total amount of potassium in the body (180,000 mg for a typical adult male). The Institute of Medicine recommends a daily potassium intake of 4,700 mg/day, which can easily be achieved by consuming fresh fruits and vegetables (Food and Nutrition Board, Institute of Medicine, 2005).

Like potassium, the amount of magnesium lost in sweat is minimal. This is because most of the magnesium in the body is part of the bone mineral matrix or in the intracellular fluid of muscle cells. It is not necessary to replace magnesium while exercising, but it is important to consume adequate amounts of magnesium in the diet. The recommended intake is about 300 mg daily for adult females and about 400 mg daily for adult males (Food and Nutrition

● **Learning Point** Magnesium supplements should be used with caution. Because magnesium and calcium are chemically similar, magnesium can interfere with intestinal absorption of calcium and with calcium's function in the body. For example, magnesium can block calcium binding to muscle cells and inhibit normal muscle contraction.

Board, Institute of Medicine, 1997). Nuts, legumes, whole grains, green leafy vegetables, and chocolate are good food sources of magnesium.

Preexercise Hydration

The first step in preventing dehydration is adequate hydration before exercise or competition. Ensure euhydration by drinking fluid volumes that produce colorless urine in the 24 hours before competition. Glycerol ingestion induces hyperhydration (Anderson, Cotter, Garnham, Casley, & Febbraio, 2001); however, the performance benefit of overhydration while competing in hot and humid conditions can be attributed to the volume of fluid consumed and not to glycerol, per se (Marino, Kay, & Cannon, 2003). The day of the event, consumption of 16 ounces of fluid 2 to 3 hours before the start allows time for excretion of excess water in urine before the competition begins.

Hydration During Exercise

Ideally, athletes should drink 8 to 12 ounces of fluid every 15 to 20 minutes during exercise. If a training session or competition exceeds 1 hour, a commercial fluid replacement beverage that contains carbohydrates and sodium is superior to plain water. Exogenous carbohydrate maintains blood glucose concentrations, so glycogenolysis is delayed. Sodium increases the palatability of the beverage and enhances fluid consumption; replacing some of the sodium lost in sweat reduces the risk of hyponatremia. The recommended concentration of sodium in a fluid replacement beverage is 500 to 700 mg/L (Convertino et al., 1996). Most sports drinks contain sodium, although the amount varies from 300 to 650 mg/L. An alternative to commercial fluid replacement beverages is easily prepared by adding ¼ to ½ teaspoon of salt to 1 L (32 ounces) of water, which is equivalent to about 600 and 1,200 mg sodium/L. Salt (sodium chloride) tablets are available, but 8 ounces of fluid (250 mL) must be consumed with every 200 mg of sodium so that the concentration of sodium in blood does not rise too rapidly. Salt tablets are more effective and better tolerated (they may cause gastrointestinal problems in some people) if they are crushed and mixed with water.

The fluid that is consumed must be emptied from the stomach and absorbed from the intestine to be of any benefit. The rate of gastric emptying can reach 1 L/h and is maximized when gastric volume is high

(> 600 mL), solutions are hypotonic, and the carbohydrate concentration is 4% to 8% (Convertino et al., 1996). The rate of fluid absorption is negatively affected by high intensity exercise (> 80% maximal oxygen consumption), carbohydrate concentrations that exceed 8%, and dehydration (> 4% BW) (Convertino et al., 1996).

Postexercise Hydration

Rehydration after exercise is important because most athletes do not consume enough fluids during exercise to replenish the fluid lost in sweat and respiration. In general, an athlete should consume 24 ounces of fluid for every pound of weight lost during an exercise session (Convertino et al., 1996). Excess fluid consumption offsets "obligatory urine losses" that occur when a large volume of water is consumed within a short period of time. Obligatory urine losses can be minimized by drinking a beverage that contains sodium (Shirreffs & Maughan, 1998) and by eating foods that are high in sodium after exercise, such as pretzels, pickles, pizza, cheese, tomato sauce, soy sauce, and ketchup.

Nutrition During Exercise

During prolonged exercise, depletion of glycogen stores is associated with the onset of fatigue (Costill et al., 1988; Sherman, Doyle, Lamb, & Strauss, 1993). By consuming carbohydrate (glucose) during exercise, the onset of fatigue may be delayed by providing the body with an alternate glucose supply, which spares muscle glycogen (Couture, Massicotte, Lavoie, Hillaire-Marcel, & Peronnet, 2002). The recommended carbohydrate intake during exercise is 30 to 60 g carbohydrate/h. Drinking 16 to 32 ounces of a 4% to 8% carbohydrate commercial fluid replacement beverage every hour meets this guideline. The potential for erosion of dental enamel is partially negated by increasing the pH and calcium concentration of the sports drink (Venables et al., 2005). Solutions that have a carbohydrate concentration greater than 8% slow gastric emptying and those that exceed 10% cause a net efflux of water from the intestine, contributing to dehydration. Energy gels contain about 25 g carbohydrate per packet and can be used if consumed with water to avoid gastrointestinal distress. Note that the recommendation for carbohydrate consumption during exercise maintains blood glucose concentrations but does not replenish energy used during exercise.

Sports Beverages

Sports beverages or gels contain either simple sugars or short-chain complex carbohydrates that are rapidly digested into monosaccharides. The significant difference among products is what simple sugars they contain or result from enzymatic hydrolysis in the small intestine. Glucose and galactose are absorbed quickly against a concentration gradient, using Na^+/glucose cotransporters on the mucosal side of the enterocytes. This is an energy-consuming process because the intracellular concentration of Na^+ must be maintained via a serosal Na^+/K^+ ATPase. Glucose and galactose are transported out of the enterocyte into the blood via GLUT (glucose-lactate-uptake-transporters) at the serosal surface. Galactose, however, must be converted into glucose in the liver before it can be used to generate ATP, so a sports beverage with galactose does not increase the energy available to the muscle as quickly as a glucose-only beverage.

Fructose is absorbed by GLUT5 transporters, and its rate of absorption is slower than that of glucose and galactose. Fructose is phosphorylated to fructose-1 phosphate in cells. Most fructose is metabolized in the liver to glyceraldehyde and dihydroxyacetone phosphate. These intermediates can proceed through glycolysis to pyruvate and can be used in fatty acid synthesis or in gluconeogenesis. Aldolase B is the rate-limiting enzyme in fructose metabolism and has a much lower affinity for fructose-1 phosphate than for fructose-1,6 bisphosphate. As a result the aldolase B reaction proceeds very slowly and fructose-1 phosphate tends to accumulate in the liver after ingestion of a large amount of fructose. Other tissues also can metabolize fructose but do so at a rate that is even slower than the rate of hepatic metabolism. In extrahepatic tissues fructose must be phosphorylated by hexokinase to fructose-6 phosphate. The affinity of hexokinase is much greater for glucose than it is for fructose, so the phosphorylation of fructose proceeds very slowly. Because of the way it is metabolized, fructose is not an optimal carbohydrate source during exercise.

Use of dietary carbohydrate for energy during exercise is limited by the rate of absorption (i.e., how fast the sugar molecule gets across the intestine into the bloodstream). One way to increase the speed at which glucose is absorbed is to add a small amount of fructose (or sucrose) to the sports beverage. This strategy works because glucose and fructose are absorbed by different pathways (Jentjens, Achten, & Jeukendrup, 2004; Jentjens, Moseley, Waring, Harding, & Jeukendrup, 2004; Jentjens, Venables, & Jeukendrup, 2004). However, the fructose content should not exceed 2% to 3% because ingesting large amounts of fructose could overwhelm the absorptive capability of the intestine. Fructose that is not absorbed and remains in the gut can cause diarrhea, bloating, and intestinal cramps.

Some athletes drink soda pop as a carbohydrate replacement beverage during endurance events. A 12-ounce can of cola provides about 150 calories as sugar. Soda pop is not the optimal choice during exercise. The concentration of carbohydrate in soda pop is about 11%. Once the sugar concentration of the beverage exceeds 8%, gastric emptying is slowed, meaning it takes longer for the sugar to reach the bloodstream. This also has negative implications for rehydration during exercise. Most sodas are sweetened with high fructose corn syrup that is 55% fructose and 45% glucose by weight. When combined with glucose, small amounts of fructose (2% to 3%, i.e., 2 to 3 g fructose/100 mL) enhance fluid absorption. However, the concentration of fructose in soda pop sweetened with high fructose corn syrup is about 6.5%. This amount of fructose decreases the rate of fluid and carbohydrate absorption. To make matters worse, the fructose stays in the intestine and may cause gastrointestinal distress. The optimal rehydration solution not only contains glucose to maintain blood sugar, but contains sodium as well. A beverage that has 50 to 70 mg sodium/100 mL enhances fluid retention, increases voluntary fluid intake due to enhanced taste, and prevents low blood sodium levels. The concentration of sodium in cola is much less than this recommendation—about 10 mg sodium/100 mL.

Performance benefits have been demonstrated for consumption of sports beverages containing 4% to 8% carbohydrate during endurance exercise. Two recent studies demonstrated an additional benefit when protein was added to the carbohydrate-containing fluid replacement

Nutrition After Exercise

After exercise, elevating blood glucose levels quickly is beneficial to replenish glycogen stores, so high GI foods are recommended. Athletes should aim to consume 1.5 g carbohydrate/kg BW in the first 30 minutes after exercise and again every 2 hours for 4 to 6 hours after exercise (American Dietetic Association et al., 2000). Insulin secretion is needed for glycogen synthesis. Insulin increases glucose uptake into the muscle via GLUT4 and stimulates glycogen synthase. Therefore after exercise the greater insulin secretion associated with high GI foods is advantageous. For maximal glycogen repletion, it is the GI of a carbohydrate, rather than whether it is simple or complex, that is important. There are some complex carbohydrates that are also high GI—synthetic sweeteners like maltodextrin for example. In contrast, most complex carbohydrates in fruits, vegetables, grains, and legumes are lower on the GI scale.

High GI foods that are consumed in the proximal postexercise period are not converted into fatty acids and stored in adipose tissue. After exercise, skeletal muscle uses fatty acids, not glucose, for energy so that the glucose is available for glycogen storage (Wolfe, Klein, Carraro, & Weber, 1990). This diversion of glucose toward glycogen synthesis and away from lipogenesis occurs because acetyl-CoA carboxylase and glycerol-3-phosphate acyltransferase are inhibited by AMPK phosphorylase (Rasmussen, Hancock, & Winder, 1998; Hildebrandt, Pilegaard, & Neufer, 2003; Ruderman et al., 2003). At the same time, the rate of fatty acid release from adipose into the blood is increased to supply the muscles. There also is an increase in fatty acid transport into the mitochondria of skeletal muscle for beta-oxidation to produce ATP. The rate of glucose transport into muscle also increases after exercise. The net result is that there is more glucose getting into the muscle where it is used in glycogen synthesis.

The effect of protein on glycogen repletion is equivocal due to differences in study design. Studies that compare isoenergetic postexercise carbohydrate with carbohydrate plus protein usually conclude that there is no advantage to adding protein (Jentjens, van Loon, Mann, Wagenmakers, & Jeukendrup, 2001). Studies that compare treatments that are equivalent in carbohydrate but differ in protein and, therefore, energy content generally find that carbohydrate plus protein is superior to carbohydrate alone (Ivy et al., 2002; Williams, Raven, Fogt, & Ivy, 2003). Other factors affecting the conclusion are the dose and timing of the supplements after exercise. Studies providing large amounts of carbohydrate every 30 minutes during recovery from exercise maximized glycogen repletion compared with studies with less frequent feedings. If glycogen repletion is maximized with carbohydrate alone, then it is not possible for protein to enhance the response. Studies that found added protein increased glycogen synthesis after exercise could not attribute the difference to increased insulin levels, so the mechanism of the effect remains unknown (Ivy et al., 2002).

The best dietary strategy to optimize replacement of IMTG (intramuscular lipid storage) stores without compromising glycogen repletion is somewhat controversial. High carbohydrate diets, regardless of fat intake, seem to interfere with the restoration of intramuscular fat stores to preexercise levels (Johnson et al., 2003; van Loon et al., 2003). One study of highly trained cyclists found that intramuscular fat stores were replenished after 48 hours of a diet providing 39% of energy as fat and 49% as carbohydrate, but an isoenergetic low fat diet providing 24% of energy as fat and 62% as carbohydrate was ineffective. However, there is a tremendous downside to consuming inadequate carbohydrates after exercise. Glycogen stores are then not repleted, and it is well established that preexercise glycogen levels are strongly associated with time to fatigue during endurance exercise.

● **Learning Point** The best practical recommendation is to consume carbohydrates immediately after exercise and then a mixed diet containing carbohydrate, protein, and fat thereafter.

Exercise increases the rates of protein breakdown and synthesis in skeletal muscle, and with adequate nutrition it has an anabolic effect on skeletal muscle (i.e., it results in a net increase in protein synthesis). Carbohydrate consumed after exercise is beneficial because it reduces the rate of protein degradation (Borsheim, Aarsland, & Wolfe, 2004; Borsheim, Cree, et al., 2004). However, to increase protein synthesis and achieve a net increase in muscle mass, it is important to consume protein after exercise. Studies have shown that consuming about 0.2 g protein/kg BW per hour during the first 2 to 3 hours after exercise results in net protein synthesis (Tipton, Borsheim, Wolf, Sanford, & Wolfe, 2003; Tipton, Ferrando, Phillips, Doyle, & Wolfe, 1999; Borsheim, Tipton, Wolf, & Wolfe, 2002).

Alcohol, Coffee, Soda, and Other Vices

Alcohol

Ethanol is metabolized in the liver to acetate and acetaldehyde. ATP can be generated from beta-oxidation of acetate. Acetate (like fatty acids) cannot be used to make glucose, so alcohol cannot be used to replenish glycogen stores. Dietary carbohydrate consumed with ethanol can be used in glycogen synthesis. This was shown in a study of well-trained cyclists who exercised for 2 hours to deplete their glycogen stores and then consumed one of three test meals to look at the effects of alcohol ingestion on glycogen synthesis in muscle (Burke et al., 2003). The three test meals were carbohydrate, providing 7 g carbohydrate and 24 kcal per kg BW; alcohol, providing 1 g carbohydrate, 1.5 g alcohol, and 24 kcal per kg BW; and carbohydrate + alcohol, providing 7 g carbohydrate, 1.5 g alcohol, and 34 kcal per kg BW. The alcohol, equivalent to about 10 drinks, was consumed in the first 3 hours after exercise. Muscle biopsies of the quadriceps muscle were taken 8 and 24 hours after exercise. Although both groups that consumed alcohol had lower blood glucose levels, at 8 and 24 hours after exercise, than the CHO group, muscle glycogen was lower only in the alcohol group.

The acute effects of alcohol ingestion on performance are mostly negative and are dose dependent. Psychomotor function is impaired, and small to moderate doses of alcohol (2 to 4 ounces of alcohol) slow reaction time; interfere with eye–hand coordination, accuracy, and balance; and make performing gross motor skills more difficult. Alcohol causes vasodilation of blood vessels and loss of body heat, increasing the risk of hypothermia when exercising in the cold. Alcohol lowers blood glucose and decreases glucose uptake by skeletal muscle, so an athlete experiences earlier onset of fatigue.

Caffeine

Caffeine is a mild stimulant; it interferes with the binding of adenosine, a neurotransmitter with calming effects, to its receptor. Hence, the stimulatory effects on many systems of the body are neural activity in parts of the brain, heart rate and blood pressure, water excretion by the kidneys, and secretion of the "stress hormones" adrenaline and cortisol by the adrenal gland. There is considerable evidence from scientific studies that caffeine improves athletic performance in sprints and in endurance events. Enhanced alertness and reaction time contribute to improvements in sprinting. During endurance events, caffeine improves performance by stimulating the release of fatty acids into the blood due to increased activity of hormone sensitive lipase. This allows increased utilization of fat rather than glucose, so muscle glycogen is not depleted as rapidly and the onset of fatigue is delayed. The effects of caffeine on lipolysis are mediated, at least in part, via the sympathetic nervous system, as evidenced by partial abrogation of the caffeine effect with pharmacologic beta-adrenergic blockade (Van Baak & Saris, 2000). Caffeine also may improve performance during submaximal exercise through other mechanisms. Time to fatigue during performance of submaximal isometric contractions was increased with caffeine (6 mg/kg BW) due to maintenance of force output and not because of altered firing rates (Acheson et al., 2004).

Caffeine is metabolized rapidly by the body; peak blood levels occur 30 minutes after oral ingestion, and the half-life of caffeine is 4 hours. For this reason caffeine should be consumed within 1 hour of an athletic event to have an effect on performance. An effective dose is 2 to 9 mg caffeine/kg BW, and no additional benefit is derived from higher doses. The caffeine content of coffee varies significantly; an 8-ounce cup may contain 100 to 300 mg. Drinking 1 to 2 cups of coffee should not produce the adverse effects of excess caffeine consumption, such as anxiety, jitteriness, heart arrhythmias, dehydration, and dry mouth.

Athletes may develop a tolerance to caffeine, but the variation in individual response to the drug is large—some people develop tolerance and others remain responsive (Lovallo et al., 2004). The rate at which tolerance to caffeine develops and the magnitude of the effect varies with the physiologic response (Watson, Deary, & Kerr, 2002). For example, 400 to 500 mg of caffeine (2 to 3 cups of regular coffee) a day for 7 days results in complete tolerance of its sleep-disrupting effects. Regular consumption of caffeine, however, does not eliminate the hypertensive response. Caffeine was removed from the World Anti-Doping Agency's "Prohibited List" in 2005 (World Anti-Doping Agency, 2005).

Soda Pop

Endurance athletes abstain from carbonated beverages because they believe the carbon dioxide interferes with oxygen use. In reality, the potential negative effect of drinking carbonated beverages has nothing to do with oxygen transport or blood pH but with hydration. Most of the CO_2 in blood arises as a waste product of cellular metabolism. This carbon dioxide is dissolved in blood and carried as carbonic acid and bicarbonate to the lungs where it is expired. When blood concentrations of CO_2 are high, the body responds by breathing more deeply and frequently to expire the excess CO_2.

The CO_2 in carbonated beverages has no effect on the amount of CO_2 in blood or on the acid-base balance of the blood. This is because the CO_2 that is in soda never gets into the circulation. Most of the carbonation is lost before it is even swallowed. The increased temperature of the mouth versus the environment causes a large amount of the dissolved gas to come out of solution. The physical process of swallowing also reduces the amount of CO_2 in solution. Any CO_2 that does make it to the stomach is released from the body via the mouth (sometimes audibly) as a "belch." This is because the low pH (acid) in the stomach also makes the CO_2 less soluble. Because a carbonated beverage helps create a sensation of fullness in the stomach that is out of proportion to the amount consumed, voluntary fluid intake may be reduced (Lambert, Bleiler, Chang, Johnson, & Gisolfi, 1993).

The main source of dietary phosphoric acid is soda pop. Because of the association between soda consumption and increased risk of bone fractures, the constituents of soda (caffeine, phosphoric acid, citric acid, and fructose) have been scrutinized for their potential to cause calcium loss from bone. Anyone who has ever soaked a bone in vinegar would agree that phosphoric acid probably causes a loss of calcium and a weakening of the bones. However, what is observed in the test tube is not always what happens in the body, which has the ability to maintain constant internal conditions, including acidity of the blood.

Heaney and Rafferty (2001) compared the effects of caffeine, phosphoric acid, and citric acid (consumed in soda) on calcium excretion in the urine. Subjects consumed 20 ounces of either caffeinated cola (Coke, containing caffeine and phosphoric acid), noncaffeinated cola (Coke-Free, phosphoric acid only), caffeinated noncola (Mt. Dew, caffeine and citric acid), or noncaffeinated noncola (Sprite, citric acid only). Neither phosphoric acid nor citric acid increased calcium loss. Consumption of the caffeinated sodas caused an increase in calcium excretion, but the effect was small (6 to 14 mg) compared with the recommended daily calcium intake (1,000 mg).

When the kidney's ability to excrete acid is compromised, as in chronic renal failure, and the body is exposed to very high acid loads, then appreciable amounts of calcium may be lost from bone. However, in a healthy individual the acid load that results from the phosphoric acid in 20 ounces of soda is very small (4.5 to 5.0 mEq), which is much less than the acid load produced during normal metabolism of food (50 to 100 mEq). Consuming seven 12-ounce colas per day only produces an acid load of about 20 mEq, which is well within the excretory capacity of the kidney.

Body Composition

Body weight and composition influence an athlete's performance because body size and relative muscle mass affect strength, speed, and appearance. Body fat increases body weight without increasing strength, thereby reducing the power to body weight ratio. In sports that require moving the body over long distances or against the gravitational force, such as running and cycling, a high power to weight ratio is advantageous. In "appearance" sports such as gymnastics, figure skating, diving, and dance, a lean physique also is desirable. However, being too lean can negatively affect performance and overall physical and psychological health. The physical risks associated with excessive leanness are over-training syndrome, frequent illness and injury, and loss of bone mass. Unrealistic body weight or composition goals can lead to increased body dissatisfaction, disordered eating, and negative affect.

In setting body weight goals, athletes must consider gender, body composition, genetics, and overall physical and mental health. Five percent to 10% body fat may be appropriate for an elite male athlete, but the healthy range for a female athlete is 12% to 28%. Athletes may be classified as overweight based on standard height and weight tables when in fact they are lean, simply because they have more muscle mass than the "reference" man or woman. Each person has a set-point weight, which is largely determined by genetics, that the body maintains over time. Muscle mass, like body weight, is highly regulated (Keesey & Corbett, 1984). Attempts to achieve a body weight or muscle mass above or below the set-point range result in metabolic adaptations to maintain the set point (Loucks, 2004).

Guidelines to Increase Muscle Mass

With adequate energy and protein intake, resistance training causes an increase in muscle mass. Protein turnover in skeletal muscle is increased for up to 48 hours after resistance exercise. Exercise reduces nitrogen losses during fasting by suppressing protein breakdown, although protein balance remains negative. Consuming a mixture of carbohydrates and amino acids before or immediately after resistance training results in net protein synthesis. Mammalian target of rapamycin (mTOR) is a kinase that stimulates protein synthesis via transcription and translation of messenger RNAs coding translation

proteins, ribosome biosynthesis, and cell proliferation; mTOR also inhibits autophagy. Growth factors, insulin, and amino acids activate mTOR (Deldicque, Theisen, & Francaux, 2005). Resistance exercise activates mTOR, whereas endurance exercise inhibits mTOR activity due to activation of AMPK by AMP (Atherton et al., 2005). This finding has practical applications for athletes who engage in endurance and strength training. Protein synthesis in response to resistance training can be maximized by allowing adequate recovery after endurance exercise in conjunction with dietary carbohydrate and protein.

A reasonable rate of weight gain is 0.5 kg/wk. This requires an additional 500 kcal/day, in addition to the energy required to maintain current body weight. To increase skeletal muscle mass, additional amino acids are required. Athletes who are involved in strenuous resistance training should consume 1.6 to 1.7 g protein/kg BW. Protein in food can be scored based on how closely the proportion of amino acids it contains matches the amino acid composition of muscle protein, correcting for digestibility of the protein. Proteins that are high quality have the right mix of amino acids and receive a score of 1.00, whereas proteins that are missing in an essential amino acid or are poorly digested receive a lower score. Typically, protein from animal sources like meat (0.9) and egg whites (1.0) is high quality, and protein from plant sources like beans (0.6) and wheat (0.4) is lower quality. For this reason vegetarians need to combine plant sources of protein so they get all the essential amino acids. Examples of complementary foods are beans and rice, peanut butter and wheat bread, and tofu and rice. Because of the lower protein quality of plant-based foods, vegetarian athletes should consume 1.6 to 1.7 g protein/kg BW; this is higher than the recommendation for nonvegetarians of 1.2 to 1.4 g/kg BW.

Weight Cycling

The information of the effects of weight cycling in athletes is limited. There is a positive association between "yo-yo dieting" and heart disease in populations with other risk factors for cardiovascular disease, such as smoking, excessive weight and **obesity**, and lack of physical activity (Petersmarck et al., 1999). Weight cycling in conjunction with ad libitum consumption

Obesity: Category of body weight above overweight; for children, a body mass index for age and gender percentile is used.

Low Intensity Exercise Is Better for Burning Fat

Energy balance is where the rubber hits the road when it comes to weight loss. Although it is true that a greater proportion of the energy comes from fat oxidation during low intensity exercise, the total energy used is less (if the duration is constant) during low versus high intensity exercise. It follows, then, that the absolute amount of fat oxidized is less during low versus high intensity activities. For example, riding at 10 mph uses 6 kcal/kg/h and 80% of those kilocalories come from fat. One hour of cycling at 10 mph uses a total of 600 kcal, and 480 of those kilocalories are from fat. Contrast that with riding at 18 mph, which uses 12 kcal/kg/h but only 50% of the energy from fat. At the faster speed the total energy cost is 1,200 kcal, and 600 kcal come from fat.

Low-Carbohydrate Diets Increase Weight Loss

Low-carbohydrate high-protein weight loss diets have increased in popularity recently, even among athletes. These diets restrict carbohydrate intake to 30 to 120 g/day. The RDA for carbohydrate was determined based on the carbohydrate requirement of the brain. For healthy adults the RDA is 130 g of carbohydrate per day (Food and Nutrition Board, Institute of Medicine, 2003).

Skeletal muscle can use fat for energy at rest or during exercise of low intensity. As exercise intensity increases, skeletal muscle relies increasingly on carbohydrate for energy. The primary source of carbohydrate during exercise is what is stored in the muscle as glycogen. Athletes need more carbohydrate than the brain's minimum requirement to replete their muscle and liver glycogen stores. Training and performance will decline significantly on a low-carbohydrate diet.

These diets are popular because, by design, they promote rapid weight loss. During the first 24 to 48 hours of a low-carbohydrate diet, glycogen stores that remain are used to fuel the brain. When glycogen is broken down, the water that is part of the glycogen is released and excreted in the urine. This water loss can be 3 to 4 pounds. With continued inadequate carbohydrate intake, catabolism of skeletal muscle ensues and the amino acids that make up muscle proteins are used in gluconeogenesis. Muscle is about 73% water. So catabolism of skeletal muscle results in a significant change in body weight due to the loss of body water. The number on the scale may drop rapidly on this diet, but losing water and not body fat will do nothing to enhance performance.

of a high-fat diet increases transcription of lipogenic genes in adipose tissue: fatty acid synthase, acetyl CoA carboxylase, malic enzyme, pyruvate kinase, and lipoprotein lipase (Sea et al., 2000). The body weight changes that occur in athletes who are relatively lean, nonsmoking, and active are very different from the weight fluctuations in people who start out overweight or obese. Athletes may experience in and out of season fluctuations in body weight, but even then most athletes stay within the normal range of weight for height. In the general population weight cycling is prevalent among people who are overweight and have repeatedly tried and failed to maintain a lower body weight. As a result, it is difficult to separate the effects of weight cycling from the effects of being overweight with regard to a person's overall risk of cardiovascular disease. Studies that found a relationship between weight cycling and risk factors for heart disease or type 2 diabetes saw that relationship disappear when they factored in the effects of being overweight or obese (Petersmarck et al., 1999). The metabolic benefits of endurance training on risk factors for cardiovascular disease (triglycerides, total cholesterol, low-density and high-density lipoproteins, insulin, LPL—lipoprotein lipase—activity) do not persist with detraining (Petibois, Cassaigne, Gin, & Deleris, 2004).

Most of the information that exists on the health effects of weight cycling in athletes comes from wrestlers. During their competitive season wrestlers restrict their food intake and exercise to "make weight," often losing 5% to 10% of their normal weight. Several studies examined how body composition and metabolic rate change as wrestlers lose and regain weight (Steen, Oppliger, & Brownell, 1988; Melby, Schmidt, & Corrigan, 1990; McCargar & Crawford, 1992). Although the results are equivocal, resting metabolic rate decreases during the weight loss phase. Thyroid hormone levels also decrease during weight loss, suggesting that the brain perceives an energy shortage and sends out signals for the body to conserve energy (Loucks et al., 1992). Once the competitive season is over and wrestlers are no longer in a chronic energy deficit, metabolic rate returns to normal.

Eating Disorders and the Female Athlete Triad

In an effort to achieve or maintain an unrealistically low body weight or percentage of body fat, some athletes restrict their food intake so severely that endocrine function is disrupted. The hypothalamus senses the energy deficit, and the secretion of gonadotropin-releasing hormone, thyrotropin-releasing hormone, corticotropin-releasing hormone, and growth hormone-releasing hormone are altered at different thresholds of energy availability (Loucks et al., 1992; Laughlin & Yen, 1996; Loucks & Verdun, 1998; Loucks, 2004). As a result secretion of luteinizing hormone, follicle-stimulating hormone, thyroid-stimulating hormone, and growth hormone (GH) are abnormal and production of reproductive hormones, thyroid hormone, and insulin-like growth factor I (IGF-I) are reduced (Laughlin & Yen, 1996; Waters, Qualls, Dorin, Veldhuis, & Baumgartner, 2001; Rickenlund, Thoren, Carlstrom, von Schoultz, & Hirschberg, 2004).

The sex hormones are decreased in both men (testosterone) and women (estrogen and progesterone). Women experience irregular (**oligomenorrhea**) or absent menstrual cycles (**amenorrhea**); men may notice a decline in sex drive. Thyroid hormone (triiodothyronine) is decreased in both genders, resulting in the signs and symptoms of decreased metabolic rate, such as **bradycardia**, hypotension, slowed respiration rate, and delayed reflexes. GH secretion is increased, but because of the energy-deficient state, the liver and other tissues are resistant to GH. As a consequence, hepatic production of IGF-I is decreased. In addition, the secretion of adrenocorticotropic hormone is increased, and serum cortisol concentrations are elevated.

Oligomenorrhea: Irregular or infrequent menstruation in menarchal females; cycles occur at an interval of 35 days or greater, resulting in four to nine cycles per year.

Amenorrhea: Absence of three consecutive menstrual cycles in a menarchal female.

Bradycardia: Abnormally slow heart rate (<60 beats/min) that does not meet the body's metabolic demands.

Each of these hormonal changes has a negative impact on bone mineral content and density. Bone turnover becomes uncoupled when energy availability is 10 to 20 kcal/kg lean body mass per day (Ihle & Loucks, 2004). Hypoestrogenemia and hypercortisolemia accelerate bone resorption. Bone formation is slowed with low testosterone, thyroid hormone, and IGF-I. Osteopenia, osteoporosis, and fractures are consequences of chronic low energy intake. Measurable loss of bone mineral density is evident after missing only six consecutive menstrual cycles. Loss of bone mass is insidious because it is irreversible and often proceeds undetected for long periods of time (Keen & Drinkwater, 1997). In women, the constellation of disordered eating, amenorrhea, and osteopenia/osteoporosis has been labeled "the female triad" by the American College of Sports Medicine (Yeager, Agostini, Nattiv, & Drinkwater, 1993; Otis, Drinkwater, Johnson, Loucks, & Wilmore, 1997).

There are other negative consequences of chronic low energy availability. Protein turnover is slowed, making athletes more susceptible to injury, illness, and over-training syndrome. In response to inadequate energy intake from the diet, the body has to rely on other energy sources. The body uses energy that is stored body fat and breaks down muscle, converting the protein into glucose. Proteolysis of skeletal muscle results in a loss of strength and power, with negative effects on performance.

Childhood Through Adolescence

Children and adolescents have higher energy and protein needs per kilogram of body weight than adults to support growth. Growth is relatively constant at a rate of approximately 5 to 6 cm and 2.5 kg/yr from age 4 until puberty. At puberty, androgens, estrogens, GH, and IGF-I cause increases in bone mineral, muscle mass, and sex-specific deposition of body fat (Rogol, 2000). The RDA for protein is 0.95 g/kg BW for children ages 9 to 13 years and 0.85 g/kg BW for teenagers, compared with 0.8 g/kg BW for adults (Food and Nutrition Board, Institute of Medicine, 2003). Greater than 90% of peak bone mass is acquired by age 18 years, and bone mass doubles between the onset of puberty and young adulthood. Thus children and adolescents require more calcium than adults; the adequate intake for calcium is 1,300 mg/day for ages 9 to 18 years (Food and Nutrition Board, Institute of Medicine, 1997). Iron and zinc needs also are increased during adolescence to support an increase in skeletal muscle mass and an expansion in red blood cell number (Food and Nutrition Board, Institute of Medicine, 2001).

Special Focus on Children and Adolescents

Weight-bearing physical activity has a greater effect on bone mass in children and adolescents compared with adults. The effects of exercise on growth and development are closely related to the energy drain created by the physical activity. Growth and sexual maturation can be delayed by intense physical training before puberty. Weight and height growth velocities can be decreased in elite female athletes and menarche delayed 1 to 2 years compared with a population reference menarchal age of 13.0 years. Delayed menarche and hypoestrogenism compromise acquisition of bone mass and bone mineral. Exercise duration and training intensity were negatively associated with bone mass density (BMD) in elite female adolescent gymnasts, and the younger the athlete started training, the greater the effect on bone (Markou et al., 2004). A cross-sectional study of 5,461 girls aged 11 to 17 years found that girls who participated in at least 16 hours of exercise per week were at greater risk for stress fractures than those who participated in less than 4 hours per week. Each hour per week spent running, performing gymnastics, or cheerleading also increased the risk of stress fracture (Loud, Gordon, Micheli, & Field, 2005). Some catch-up growth may be possible if an athlete's training load is reduced. Because there are few longitudinal growth studies that follow athletes before the onset of training, it is difficult to determine the effects of slowed growth and delayed maturation on adult body size.

Normal growth and development in males are less affected by training than in females. This may be, in large part, due to selection bias. Physical maturity is an asset in most male sports where strength and power confer a competitive advantage. Wrestlers are unique because of the ubiquitous practice of losing weight through dietary restriction and excessive exercise to compete in lower competitive weight classes. Growth velocity is slowed during the season and catch-up growth occurs during the off season. It is not clear if the short stature of wrestlers is due to growth restriction, selection bias, or a combination (Rogol, Clark, & Roemmich, 2000).

Children and adolescents also are more susceptible to heat-related illnesses because of a greater impairment of thermal regulation with dehydration (Bar-Or, 2001). Until puberty, children and adolescents sweat less than adults. In addition, children have a greater surface area to body weight ratio than adults and therefore receive greater exposure to solar radiation. Similar to adult athletes, children and adolescents do not consume adequate fluids during exercise to remain euhydrated. Provision of a flavored carbohydrate–electrolyte drink increases fluid consumption and reduces voluntary dehydration in children (Rivera-Brown, Gutierrez, Gutierrez, Frontera, & Bar-Or, 1999).

Oral contraceptives agents (OCAs) have benefits for female athletes: timing of the menstrual cycle around important competitions, reduced risk of iron deficiency anemia due to decreased blood loss via menstrual bleeding, and reduced loss of bone mass in estrogen-deficient athletes with amenorrhea (Bennell, White, & Crossley, 1999). Despite these potential benefits, plus the obvious one of birth control, many athletes (and their coaches) worry that taking the pill will cause weight gain, decrease aerobic capacity, and negatively affect fuel metabolism. However, there is very little evidence to support these fears (Bonen, Haynes, & Graham, 1991; Bryner, Toffle, Ullrich, & Yeater, 1996; Casazza, Suh, Miller, Navazio, & Brooks, 2002; Jankowski, Ben-Ezra, Gozansky, & Scheaffer, 2004). Only a few studies have investigated the effects of oral contraceptives

on athletic performance and only a fraction of these used highly trained athletes as subjects. It is important to recognize that the effects of OCAs in trained women may differ from those observed in sedentary women.

A recent study of endurance-trained athletes and sedentary control subjects examined the effects of 10 months of OCA treatment (both estrogen and progesterone) on body weight and composition, aerobic capacity (maximal oxygen consumption), muscular strength, and bone mineral density. Half of the athletes were regularly menstruating and the other half were either oligomenorrheic (cycles at intervals > 6 weeks) or amenorrheic (absence of menstrual cycles for at least 3 consecutive months) (Rickenlund, Carlstrom, et al., 2004). The women with irregular menstrual cycles gained weight (body weight increase from 124 to 128 pounds, on average) and increased their percentage of body fat (from 17% to 20%, on average) after OCA treatment. Despite this increase in body weight, relative maximal oxygen consumption did not change with OCA treatment (56.7 vs. 55.6 mL/kg/min). The bone mineral density of the women with oligomenorrhea and amenorrhea significantly increased with OCAs, and the improvement in BMD was greatest in individuals with the lowest initial BMD. Ten months of OCAs did not alter body weight, body composition, aerobic capacity, strength, or bone mineral density in the regularly menstruating women or in the sedentary control subjects.

Dietary Supplements As Ergogenic Aids

Supplement Labeling and Performance Claims

The laws regarding supplements put the burden of investigating the benefits and harms of dietary supplements on the consumer. Because of the way dietary supplements are regulated, at least in the United States, manufacturers may put essentially any performance-related claim on the label, even if it is unsubstantiated. Unlike food and drugs, the U.S. Food and Drug Administration does not monitor supplements for ingredient content or purity. In other words, the ingredients on the label may or may not be present and additional compounds not listed on the label may be included. For example, small amounts of anabolic steroids have been found in supplements that claim to increase muscle mass. Many supplements that are evaluated by consumer protection groups are found to contain much less of the active ingredient than what is listed on the label. Both practices are illegal, but without quality control of the supplement industry they take place nonetheless. Therefore safety of dietary supplements is a concern. Between 1995 and 1999 there were 2,500 adverse events reported to the U.S. Food and Drug Administration by consumers, health care professionals, and poison control centers. It is estimated that this represents only 1% of the actual adverse events. A good source of reliable information on dietary supplements is from the National Center for Complementary and Alternative Medicine of the National Institutes of Health (www.nccam.nih.gov/health). Information on whether a supplement contains what is on the ingredient list can be found at www.ConsumerLabs.com.

Placebo Effect

The power of the mind cannot be underestimated. If an athlete believes that a supplement is going to help his or her performance, it probably will. However, if the ergogenic effects of that supplement were studied in a double-blind placebo-controlled trial (meaning subjects randomly receive the supplement or an identical-looking placebo treatment and neither the subjects nor the investigators knows who gets what), a significant difference between the supplement and placebo may not be detected.

Dietary supplements range from the conventional (multivitamins) to the everyday (caffeine), exotic (Chinese herbs), weird (caterpillar fungus), disgusting (pituitary extract), and dangerous (ephedra). In general, supplements taken to correct a nutrient deficiency will benefit the deficient individual. With a few exceptions, there is little evidence from double-blind placebo-controlled studies to support the use of dietary supplements to enhance athletic performance. A search of PubMed, a database of peer-reviewed journal articles, using the phrase "supplements and sports" returned over 500 entries, with most of these studies finding no effect of supplements on performance.

Even among the few supplements where a performance-enhancing effect has been repeatedly demonstrated, the magnitude of the effect is relatively small compared with the sum of the improvements that could be obtained from increased training or better equipment (Jeukendrup & Martin, 2001).

Vitamin and Mineral Supplements

Consuming excessive amounts of any nutrient (even water) can have detrimental effects. Vitamin and mineral excesses produce negative health consequences. Potential toxicity is greater for fat-soluble vitamins than for water-soluble vitamins because excess fat-soluble vitamins are stored in the liver and body fat, accumulating to toxic levels over time. For example, consuming just three to four times the RDA for vitamin A results in toxicity symptoms of loss of appetite, hair loss, and bone and muscle pain. Excess vitamin D causes calcification of the organs, high blood pressure, and kidney dysfunction. Large doses of water-soluble vitamins also can be harmful. For example, vitamin C normally acts as an antioxidant, preventing damage to the cell membrane by reacting with harmful molecules. However, at high levels (>50 times the RDA), vitamin C can act as a pro-oxidant, reacting with iron or copper to generate compounds that can cause cell damage. Megadoses of vitamin B_6 can cause degeneration of nerves, resulting in unsteady gait, numbness in the extremities, and impaired tendon reflexes. Consuming more than the RDA for iron can result in iron toxicity. Because iron is a pro-oxidant, it damages cell membranes and can ultimately result in loss of organ function.

Consuming too much of one nutrient often creates a deficiency of another. This can happen in several ways. If two or more nutrients are absorbed by the same pathway (i.e., transport proteins) in the intestine, then there is competition among those nutrients for absorption. For example, zinc, copper, and iron are absorbed by the same pathway. So if large amounts of one of these minerals are consumed, that mineral monopolizes the transport system and less of the other two minerals is absorbed. If two nutrients have similar chemical properties, they can interfere with each other's function in biochemical reactions. For example, calcium and magnesium are similar chemically but have opposing actions on blood clot formation. Calcium is needed for the clotting process. At high doses, magnesium substitutes for calcium, inhibiting blood clot formation. Similarly, at very high doses, vitamin E interferes with the actions of vitamin K.

Consuming supplemental vitamins and minerals in excess of needs is a waste of money. Absorption and excretion of vitamins and minerals are highly regulated. In general, the more the body needs, the more is absorbed from the intestine. By limiting nutrient absorption to what is needed, the chances of toxicity are reduced. Likewise, if the vitamin or mineral is already adequate, then the excess that is consumed is either stored or excreted. However, these built-in safety mechanisms of absorption and excretion can be overwhelmed if nutrients are consumed in large amounts.

Creatine

Creatine is a nitrogen-containing compound that is made in the liver and kidneys from the amino acids arginine and glycine. About 1 to 2 g of creatine is synthesized in the human body per day, and the typical diet provides another 1 to 2 g/day from meat and fish. Skeletal muscle contains most of the body's creatine, but there is an upper limit to the amount of creatine that the muscle will retain. Any excess creatine consumed in the diet or from supplements is excreted by the kidneys. For this reason, individuals who consume adequate amounts of creatine in their diet are less likely to derive any benefit from taking additional creatine than vegetarians whose diets are lacking creatine. The effects of creatine supplementation on oxygen consumption during exercise depends on the exercise intensity, fitness of the subjects, and the proportions of type I and type II muscle fibers (which is related to cardiovascular fitness but also influenced by genetics) (Wyss & Kaddurah-Daouk, 2000; Jones, Carter, Pringle, & Campbell, 2002).

In individuals who respond to supplementation, the amount of creatine in skeletal muscle typically increases 15% to 20% and body weight increases 1 to 3 kg during the first 5 to 7 days of supplementation. Creatine is not anabolic; it does not stimulate muscle protein synthesis or muscle growth. The rapid weight gain associated with creatine supplementation is due to water retention in the muscle cells. When the muscle cells take in more creatine, they also have to retain more water to maintain the correct intracellular fluid pressure. The extra water not only decreases the power to weight ratio (by increasing weight and not power), but it may impair muscle function and cause muscle stiffness and cramping. Because body water will shift from the blood to the muscle cells, sweating and thermoregulation may be impaired. Athletes who supplement with creatine must be especially careful not to become dehydrated—they should consume copious fluids and refrain from strenuous exercise, especially in the heat.

Creatine is used by skeletal muscle to make phosphocreatine. During maximal anaerobic efforts, phosphocreatine allows the muscle to generate large amounts of ATP very rapidly. However, there is only enough phosphocreatine to last 30 seconds. The idea behind "creatine loading" is that by increasing the amount of creatine in the muscle, there will be more phosphocreatine on hand to generate ATP. If there is more ATP available for use during maximal anaerobic efforts, then the muscle will have more energy and performance will improve. Creatine supplementation has been shown to improve performance in repeated cycling sprints and maximal weight lifting efforts. In other words, creatine does not increase maximal power or strength but allows an individual to achieve his or her maximum potential during repetitive tests separated by short rest intervals. Creatine does not increase endurance performance because ATP is derived from aerobic metabolism of glucose and fat and not from phosphocreatine. There is not enough evidence supporting an ergogenic effect of creatine on endurance performance to endorse its use for that purpose; this position is consistent with that published by the American College of Sports Medicine (Terjung et al., 2000).

Glutamine

Glutamine is a conditionally essential amino acid, meaning that under normal circumstances the body can make what it needs. Skeletal muscle is the most significant source of glutamine in the body. When muscle is broken down in response to the stress hormone cortisol, glutamine is released from the muscle into the blood. During times of extraordinary stress, such as severe trauma, burns, or sepsis, the body's demand for glutamine exceeds its ability to make the amino acid and it becomes essential (Castell, 2003). In clinical studies of critically ill patients, providing supplemental glutamine improved patient outcome and survival. This is in large part because cells of the immune system use glutamine for energy. During times of stress, the immune system is activated, requiring more energy. Although not nearly as stressful as a burn injury or sepsis, exhaustive exercise (e.g., running a marathon) causes a short-term (< 12 hours) decrease in blood glutamine concentrations. Over-training syndrome also produces a decrease in blood glutamine concentrations (Halson, Lancaster, Jeukendrup, & Gleeson, 2003).

Because athletes competing in endurance events often experience a mild decrease in immune function and an increase in upper respiratory tract infections after the event, the effect of glutamine supplementation on immune response has been studied in endurance athletes (Krzywkowski, Petersen, Ostrowski, Kristensen, et al., 2001; Krzywkowski, Petersen, Ostrowski, Link-Amster, et al., 2001; Krieger, Crowe, & Blank, 2004). One study found that runners who consumed glutamine immediately and 2 hours after a marathon had fewer self-reported upper respiratory tract infections in the week after the race. Consuming glutamine for 3 to 4 weeks before competition also reduced self-reported infections in marathon runners and triathletes. However, numerous other studies investigating the mechanism behind the beneficial effect of glutamine found no effect of glutamine supplementation on immune cell function.

It should be noted that glutamine is not stable in solution and exposure to ultraviolet light degrades it as well. The effective dose (0.1 g glutamine/kg BW) should not be exceeded. Amino acids compete with each other for absorption in the intestine and consuming an excess of one amino acid can create a deficiency of another. Excessive protein consumption unnecessarily stresses the kidneys, and excess amino acids that are not used in protein synthesis will be stored as adipose tissue.

Other Supplements

Nitric oxide is made in the body from L-arginine and oxygen. This gaseous signal molecule plays an important role in many physiologic processes, including smooth muscle contraction, immune function, and nervous system activity. Because nitric oxide is a potent vasodilator, it plays an important role in oxygen use during exercise. Exercise stimulates nitric oxide production in blood vessels that perfuse skeletal muscle and causes increased blood flow to the working muscle (Krzywkowski, Petersen, Ostrowski, Kristensen, et al., 2001; Krzywkowski, Petersen, Ostrowski, Link-Amster, et al., 2001; Miyauchi et al., 2003). Interestingly, nitric oxide decreases mitochondrial oxygen consumption by inhibiting several key enzymes involved in synthesis of ATP (Stamler & Meissner, 2001). The net result is that nitric oxide release acts to increase the oxygen available to muscle by increasing delivery and decreasing the rate at which it is used. Because nitric oxide is a gas, it is not commercially available in supplement form. Dietary supplements that claim to increase nitric oxide levels contain arginine.

Cordyceps sinensis, also known as Chinese caterpillar fungus, was popularized by the sudden success of the Chinese female distance runners in the early 1990s. When Wang Junxia shattered the world record in the 10,000 m, her coach attributed her performance to a diet of turtle blood and caterpillar fungus. Needless to say, the success and running careers of the Chinese women were short-lived. Cordyceps is a black fungus that is a parasite for several species of caterpillar. The fungus kills the caterpillar and uses it for nutrients as it grows. Because cordyceps in nature is rare, a strain (Cs-4) that contains the active components is now cultivated for commercial purposes (Zhu, Halpern, & Jones, 1998a,b). Other than the success of the Chinese runners, there is very little evidence to support the claim that cordyceps improves performance. In fact, two recent studies of trained male cyclists found no effect of cordyceps supplementation on maximal oxygen consumption, **ventilatory threshold**, or performance compared with placebo (Parcell, Smith, Schulthies, Myrer, & Fellingham, 2004).

Ventilatory threshold: The workload or exercise intensity that causes the first rise in the ventilatory equivalent of oxygen without a concurrent rise in the ventilatory equivalent of carbon dioxide; occurs near the lactate threshold.

Sports during Pregnancy, Lactation, and Menopause

Pregnancy and Sports

The American College of Obstetrics and Gynecology recommends that all women with uncomplicated pregnancies participate in moderate physical activity for at least 30 minutes most, if not all, days of the week (American College of Obstetricians and Gynecologists, 2002). Regular exercise has been shown to reduce the occurrence of physical complaints during pregnancy, to improve mood, and to shorten delivery time (Clapp, 2000). Women who are accustomed to exercising at high intensity and female athletes may continue to train vigorously during pregnancy, but they should be aware that some of the physiologic changes associated with pregnancy may require them to back off the intensity or modify the type of activity. Resting metabolic rate is increased during pregnancy, meaning the body requires more oxygen at rest. As the uterus grows during the second and third trimesters, it puts pressure on the diaphragm, increasing the work required to breathe. Because the body requires more oxygen and has to work harder to obtain that oxygen, less oxygen is available for exercise. For this reason, maximal workload may be reduced and exercise may feel more difficult at a given intensity during pregnancy. Another consequence of the elevated metabolic rate is an increased susceptibility to overheating and dehydration. There is some evidence that maternal overheating (core temperature above 39.2°C) during the first trimester may increase the risk of birth defects. Therefore pregnant women should avoid exercising in hot humid weather and consume adequate fluids in the event of fever. The weight gain associated with pregnancy changes a woman's center of gravity, which may preclude activities that require balance to avoid abdominal trauma.

Pregnant women require an additional 300 kcal/day for growth of the fetus and maternal tissues (Food and Nutrition Board, Institute of Medicine, 2003). Inadequate energy consumption during pregnancy results in a low birth weight infant, which increases the chances of neonatal complications. Hormones produced by the placenta (human placental lactogen, estrogen, progesterone) cause changes in maternal metabolism such that the mother preferentially uses fat for energy, which allows glucose to be used by the fetus. These metabolic changes cause pregnant women to have lower fasting glucose levels and to use more glucose during exercise than nonpregnant women. Therefore adequate carbohydrate consumption especially is important during exercise.

Lactation

The American Academy of Pediatrics (2005) recommends that infants be breast-fed for at least 12 months. Breast-feeding not only benefits the infant but is advantageous for the mother as well. Exercise during lactation enhances cardiovascular fitness, decreases postpartum weight retention, improves postprandial insulin response, and increases high density lipoprotein (Larson-Meyer, 2002). Lactating women may exercise without any adverse effect on milk volume or composition, infant feeding, or growth. Maximal, but not submaximal, exercise increases the concentration of lactic acid in breast milk for 0.5 to 1.0 hours after exercise. Whether the increased lactic acid concentration reduces milk consumption is controversial. Wright and colleagues (2002) in a well-controlled study suggested that the increase in lactic acid has no effect on milk consumption.

Menopause

Menopause is defined as the absence of regular menstrual cycles for 12 consecutive months. Typically, women experience menstrual cycle irregularity before cycles stop completely; changes in cycle length and frequency are common. During this perimenopausal period, estrogen concentrations also may be highly variable, and after 3 months of missed periods, estrogen declines significantly. Menopause, like puberty, is a time of hormonally driven changes in body shape and composition. During middle age, women gain an average of 0.5 kg (~1 lb.) per year, and menopause does not seem to increase this rate of weight gain. Women lose muscle mass and increase fat mass during menopause, but these changes seem to be due to a decrease in physical activity as women get older rather than an inevitable consequence of menopause. Even if total body fat does not increase after menopause, there is a shift in body fat distribution from the hips and thighs to the abdomen. In other words, the "pears" start to look more and more like "apples."

It is the accumulation of fat around the internal organs located in the abdomen that probably causes changes in fat and glucose metabolism. Postmenopausal women have higher total cholesterol, low-density lipoprotein (bad) cholesterol, and triglycerides (fat) and lower high-density lipoprotein (good) concentrations in blood than premenopausal women. These changes explain why the risk of cardiovascular disease increases in women after menopause. Women, especially those who gain abdominal fat, after menopause may become insulin resistant. These changes in body composition and metabolism result not only from the direct effects of lower estrogen, but also from estrogen-mediated changes in other hormones. GH and IGF-I exert anabolic effects on bone and muscle, and GH increases fat use as an energy source by stimulating release of fatty acids from body fat stores. Hypoestrogenemia reduces pulsatile release of GH, consequently lowering IGF-I secretion.

Exercise counteracts many of the unfavorable metabolic changes that occur after menopause by reducing weight gain, increasing fat utilization, maintaining skeletal muscle mass, improving cholesterol and triglycerides, and increasing the body's response to insulin. Strength training helps to prevent the decline in muscle mass and offsets the decline in metabolic rate. Strength training with weights also benefits the skeleton by stimulating bone growth because of the mechanical stress placed on the skeleton.

Adequate calcium intake is especially important for postmenopausal women. In addition to dairy products, some vegetables, fish with bones, and fortified foods (e.g., orange juice, cereal) are good sources of calcium. During the first 5 to 7 years of menopause women lose up to 20% of their skeletal mass (DHHS, n.d.). Consuming 1,200 mg calcium/day may minimize that loss.

Pediatric Diabetes

Karen Chapman-Novakofski, RD, LDN, PhD

Incidence and Prevalence

Type 1 diabetes: Diabetes due to a lack of endogenous insulin.

More than 150,000 children have **type 1 diabetes** in the United States, with 10,000 to 15,000 new cases diagnosed each year (Centers for Disease Control and Prevention, 2005). The incidence of type 1 diabetes peaks in children both between 5 and 7 years of age and at puberty (Haller, Atkinson, & Schatz, 2005). Incidence rates vary considerably among countries, with a low incidence in China, Venezuela, and India at 0.1 per 100,000 and a high incidence in Sardinia and Finland at 50 cases per 100,000 persons per year. The United States has an incidence rate of approximately 16 per 100,000/year (LaPorte & Chang, 1995; Karvonen et al., 2000).

Until recently, children and adolescents diagnosed with diabetes were assumed to have type 1 of an autoimmune etiology. Currently, children are also being diagnosed with **type 2 diabetes,** ranging from 8% to 45% of cases reported (American Diabetes Association, 2000). There is some discrepancy in diagnosis, with one report from Chicago suggesting that 24% of African-American and Hispanic-American adolescents diagnosed with type 1 diabetes may instead have type 2 diabetes (Keenan et al., 1999). The incidence is higher among older children, those who are obese, and minorities (Aye & Levitsky 2003).

Type 2 diabetes: Diabetes due to ineffective or low levels of insulin.

A report concerning national reference values for hemoglobin A_{Ic} levels among individuals aged 5 to 24 years concluded that, in general, higher hemoglobin A_{Ic} values were found in those aged 10 to 14 years old, in those who were overweight, in those with parental history of diabetes, and in those with a blood glucose level greater than 126 mg/dL. These differences were small and usually represented hemoglobin A_{Ic} levels within a normal range, but these values may reflect differences in metabolism (Saaddine et al., 2002).

Diagnosis of Diabetes in Children

The diagnosis of diabetes in children does not differ from that of adults. Symptoms of diabetes plus a random (nonfasting) blood glucose level of 200 mg/dL or greater, fasting plasma glucose level of 126 mg/dL or greater, or a 2-hour plasma glucose level of 200 mg/dL or greater during an oral glucose tolerance test are all diagnostic of diabetes. However, these criteria should be repeated on a different day to confirm results (American Diabetes Association, 2005).

Pathogenesis of Type 1 Diabetes in Children

The classic model for type 1 diabetes is the genetically susceptible child exposed to an environmental trigger that results in pancreatic beta cell autoimmunity and eventual self-destruction (Eisenbarth, 1986). The autoimmunity is specific to the pancreatic beta cells, but the mechanisms have yet to be identified. Typically, it is believed that symptoms do not occur until 80% to 90% of the beta cells have been destroyed, although more recent evidence suggests that symptoms may present themselves when only 40% to 50% have been destroyed (Haller et al., 2005).

● **Learning Point** The classic symptoms of type 1 diabetes are polyuria, polydipsia, polyphagia, and weight loss, with children often brought to the hospital with diabetic ketoacidosis.

Type 1 diabetes is a complex disease despite responding to genetic influences. Although having a first-degree family member with type 1 diabetes increases the risk of developing the condition, 85% of those diagnosed with type 1 diabetes have no family history of the disease (Hamalainen & Knip, 2002). Clearly, environmental influences are also important. Among those environmental factors, both viral and nonviral agents have been suggested. Prenatal rubella, maternal enterovirus infection, and common childhood diseases such as mumps, chickenpox, measles, and rotavirus have possible associations with autoimmunity and type 1 diabetes (Haller et al., 2005). Although there seems to be a protective effect of breast-feeding, the early introduction of cow's milk as a potential environmental trigger remains controversial (Bell, Grochoski, & Clarke, 2006). A role of possible allergens such as soy and wheat has been suggested but requires additional research (Norris et al., 2003; Ziegler, Schmid, Huber, Hummel, & Bonifacio, 2003). Many other perinatal factors have been proposed, including maternal–child blood group incompatibility, maternal preeclampsia, and maternal age (Haller et al., 2005). Additional research is needed to define the role of these factors in the pathogenesis of type 1 diabetes.

Type 1 diabetes is at times further classified as type 1A, which is classic type 1 diabetes, and type 1B, which is diabetes with no known etiology. In type 1B there is no evidence of autoimmunity (Botero & Wolfsdorf, 2005).

Pathogenesis of Insulin Resistance in Children

Insulin resistance is characterized by **hyperinsulinemia.** The increased levels of insulin attempt to compensate for a declining peripheral sensitivity to insulin to maintain blood glucose levels within a normal range. The hyperinsulinemia is often accompanied by an increase in pancreatic islet cell size and beta cell mass (Artz & Freemark, 2004). Insulin resistance may be defined as the inability of circulating insulin levels to promote peripheral glucose disposal and to suppress hepatic glucose production. Fasting insulin levels greater than 15 μU/mL, or post–oral glucose tolerance test peak insulin levels greater than 150 μU/mL, or post–oral glucose tolerance test insulin levels at 120 minutes of greater than 75 μU/mL indicate insulin resistance (Reaven et al., 1993).

Hyperinsulinemia: Blood levels of insulin above the normal range.

Insulin resistance often manifests during puberty, although diagnosis of type 2 diabetes may occur in later years. The peak reduction in insulin sensitivity occurs at Tanner stage III, with a recovery by Tanner stage V. Theories explaining this transient decline in insulin sensitivity include changes in body fat, sex hormone changes, or variation in GH (Goran, Ball, & Cruz, 2003).

Although not all cases of hyperinsulinemia progress to impaired fasting glucose, or "prediabetes," hyperinsulinemia is a significant risk factor for impaired fasting glucose. With impaired fasting glucose there is a dysregulation of basal insulin secretion, most notably with a loss of first phase glucose-dependent insulin secretion and an increase in the circulating ratio of proinsulin to insulin (Bergman, Finegood, & Kahn, 2002). Insulin resistance may progress to type 2 diabetes in children and is usually associated with obesity.

Other Diabetes Classifications in Children

Maturity onset diabetes of the young only occurs in a small subset of these children (Botero & Wolfsdorf, 2005). Cases of maturity onset diabetes of the young reflect a genetic defect that affects insulin secretion but not insulin action. Many other types of diabetes classification exist but are rare in children (American Diabetes Association, 2006).

Risk Factors for Diabetes

Genetics plays a significant role in the development of diabetes, with a higher incidence of diabetes in those with a family history of the disease. Genetic predisposition seems to be an important factor in determining when hyperinsulinemia occurs and when it progresses to diabetes. However, many pathways lead to insulin resistance, most notably many molecular pathways involved in energy homeostasis, lipid metabolism, insulin receptor signaling pathways, cytokine regulation, hormone-binding protein regulation, and protease regulators (Ten & Maclaren, 2004). Genetic involvement in any of these pathways, or a combination of these pathways, could lead to a predisposition to diabetes.

In addition to genetics, the development of diabetes is influenced by a number of factors associated with the incidence of diabetes. Infants who are small for gestational age are at increased risk of developing diabetes (Barker, 2000). This is particularly true when small for gestational age infants undergo rapid postnatal weight gain, leading to obesity (Wilkin et al., 2002). Large for gestational age infants are also at higher risk for insulin resistance, as are infants from mothers with gestational diabetes or type 1 diabetes (Sobngwi et al., 2003).

The environmental factors associated with increased incidence of pediatric diabetes focus on obesity development. Obesity develops when caloric intake exceeds caloric output in the form of physical activity. Few studies in children have examined the role of macronutrients and their respective contribution to obesity and insulin resistance. In adults, the reports concerning the relative importance of dietary fat are conflicting (Steyn et al., 2004). Longitudinal studies in children have not shown a significant relationship between macronutrient distribution and body composition or weight gain (Maffeis, Talamini, & Tato, 1998; Magarey, Daniels, Boulton, & Cockington, 2001). In fact, most studies fail to show a relationship between energy intake and obesity, although this may be due to inaccurate reporting, the difficulty of discerning relatively small increases in caloric intake in short time frames, and the limitations of cross-sectional studies (Rodriguez & Moreno, 2006).

Additional dietary factors that have been explored in relation to obesity include meal patterns, meal frequency, family dining frequency, snacking frequency, beverage consumption, fast food consumption, and portion sizes. None of these factors has been found to have a significant influence on obesity development, although each may play a role for the individual child (Marr, 2004; Ello-Martin, Ledikwe, & Rolls, 2005; Rodriguez & Moreno, 2006; Taveras et al., 2005; Jeffery, Baxter, McGuire, & Linde, 2006). Children tend to eat foods that are accessible and in the quantities served, which if food is highly accessible and in large quantities may contribute to increasing body weight.

Studies in adults have shown that increased physical activity can reduce the risk of type 2 diabetes, reducing insulin resistance and improving glucose tolerance. Fewer studies have been conducted in children, but those that have been done also support the finding that greater physical activity is related to an improved metabolic profile (Ku, Gower, Hunter, & Goran, 2000; Nassis et al., 2005). It is likely that a combination of higher caloric intake and lower physical activity contributes to the development of obesity in children. Central adiposity seems to be more influential on fasting insulin, whereas increased total body fat decreases insulin sensitivity (Goran et al., 2003).

Leptin is a peptide hormone secreted from adipose tissue that has a role in regulating food intake and energy expenditure. Preliminary studies in children with diabetes have found lower leptin levels at the time of diagnosis and before insulin therapy that rise with subsequent insulin regulation (Soliman et al., 2002).

Associated Clinical Conditions

Youth with type 2 diabetes may present with **acanthosis nigricans,** a velvety skin texture often found in intertriginous areas such as skin folds of the groin, axilla, and breasts as well as the nape of the neck. Acanthosis nigricans that is not associated with cancer may occur neonatally, in childhood, or in adults. The skin condition is often associated with obesity and is more prevalent in the African-American population (Hermanns-Lê, Scheen, & Pierard, 2004). Obese patients with acanthosis nigricans have been found to have hyperinsulinemia. Acanthosis nigricans has been reported to be closely associated with insulin resistance in Native American children as well (Copeland et al., 2006).

The mechanism by which hyperinsulinemia may cause acanthosis nigricans is complex and not completely understood. The process probably involves excess insulin binding to IGF receptors that increase fibroblast and keratinocyte proliferation. This increase may lead to subsequent defects in the skin tissue (Hermanns-Lê et al., 2004).

Polycystic ovarian syndrome is also associated with type 2 diabetes in young women. The diagnosis is

> **Acanthosis nigricans:** A velvety skin texture often found in skin fold areas that is often associated with obesity and type 2 diabetes.

> **Polycystic ovarian syndrome:** A clinical syndrome in women consisting of two of the following three conditions: oligo- or anovulation, hyperandrogenism, and polycystic ovaries.

difficult because polycystic ovarian syndrome is a clinical syndrome, but generally the presence of two of the following three conditions is diagnostic: oligo- or anovulation, hyperandrogenism, and polycystic ovaries (PCOS Consensus Workshop Group, 2004; Meurer, Kroll, Jamieson, & Yousefi, 2006). Usually manifested during adolescence, polycystic ovarian syndrome may originate in intrauterine development and has a strong genetic component (Xita & Tsatsoulis, 2006). Weight loss through life-style modification is recommended for improvement in insulin sensitivity and decreasing androgens. Oral contraceptives for managing menses and cyproterone acetate, an antiandrogen medication, for decreasing androgen levels may be beneficial. Indications for these and other oral hypoglycemic agents depend on the age of the child and the clinical severity (Evangelia, Erasmia, & Dimitrios, 2006).

Management

There are not as yet evidence-based guidelines for pediatric diabetes. However, the overall management goal in pediatric diabetes is similar to that for adults: near normalization of blood glucose levels for the prevention of complications and improvement in health. Glycemic goals and ways to achieve these goals differ for children because of emotional and physical issues. As always, glycemic goals must be individualized to reflect physical, emotional, health, and cultural needs of the individual. The benefits of achieving lower **glycemic control** should be weighed against the possibility of hypoglycemia in the child. In general, the guidelines in **Table 8.3** provide a framework. Self-monitoring of blood glucose is advisable, especially necessary if the child is taking insulin. In addition, urinary ketone measurement is recommended if the child has a fever

Glycemic control: Maintaining blood glucose within the target range.

or is vomiting, if the blood glucose continues to rise in an ill child, if the child becomes unusually drowsy or has stomach pains, or if overnight insulin insufficiency is suspected (International Society for Pediatric and Adolescent Diabetes, 2000).

Medical nutrition therapy is an important factor in achieving both glycemic control and normal growth and development. Macronutrient distribution is based on adult recommendations but should be tailored to meet individual needs. Total calories should be balanced between needs for growth and prevention of obesity. The Dietary Reference Intakes listed in **Table 8.4** are guidelines for estimating caloric needs (Institute of Medicine, 2005).

Initial education for the child with type 1 diabetes and his or her family may be in the medical center. Topics discussed are generally "survival strategies," such as how to store and inject insulin. After hospitalization in the case of the child with type 1 diabetes and certainly for the child with type 2 diabetes, outpatient education should be multidisciplinary and similar to that for adults. For the child with type 1 diabetes, carbohydrate counting education is essential for both the child and caregiver(s) if continuous subcutaneous insulin infusion or basal-bolus insulin regimens are to be successful. Insulin therapies need to be accompanied by self-management of blood glucose training and home glucose monitoring. Usually, families are taught "correction factors" to treat elevated blood glucose levels. A common correction factor can be estimated by dividing 1,600 by the total daily dose of insulin. The result approximates the glucose lowering effect of additional insulin. For example, a child normally taking 27 units of insulin each day would have a correction factor of $1,600/27 = 60$, meaning that the child should take an additional 1 unit of a rapid-acting insulin for every 60 mg/dL glucose above the target range (Haller et al., 2005).

For the child with type 2 diabetes, body weight reduction must be a goal without compromising normal growth and development. Increased physical activity with healthy eating patterns and amounts are preferable to very restricted diets. The scientific literature supporting particular interventions for overweight and obese youth are lacking. Multicomponent

TABLE 8.3	Blood Glucose and Hemoglobin A_{Ic} Goals for Children With Type 1 Diabetes		
	Blood Glucose Goal Range (mg/dl)		
	Before Meals	**Bedtime/Night Time**	**Hemoglobin A_{Ic} (%)**
Toddlers less than 6 years	100–180	110–200	7.7–8.5
Ages 6–12 years	90–180	100–180	<8.0
Ages 13–19 years	90–130	90–150	<7.5

Copyright ©American Diabetes Association. (2005). From *Diabetes Care*, 28, S4–S36. Reprinted with permission from The American Diabetes Association.

TABLE

8.4 Estimated Energy Requirements for Children and Adolescents

3–8 years

Boys $88.5 - (61.9 \times \text{age [yr]}) + PA \times (26.7 \times \text{weight [kg]} + 903 \times \text{height [m]}) + 20\ kcal$

Girls $135.3 - (30.8 \times \text{age [yr]}) + PA \times (10.0 \times \text{weight [kg]} + 934 \times \text{height [m]}) + 20\ kcal$

9–18 years

Boys $88.5 - (61.9 \times \text{age [yr]}) + PA \times (26.7 \times \text{weight [kg]} + 903 \times \text{height [m]}) + 25\ kcal$

Girls $135.3 - (30.8 \times \text{age [yr]}) + PA \times (10.0 \times \text{weight [kg]} + 934 \times \text{height [m]}) + 25\ kcal$

PA = physical activity coefficient:
1.0 if sedentary
1.13 if low active
1.26 if active
1.42 if very active
Source: From Institute of Medicine (2005).

The Role of Exercise

Exercise is an important part of a healthy life-style. National guidelines suggest that adolescents engage in physical activity for a minimum of 60 minutes most days (U.S. Department of Agriculture, Department of Health and Human Services, 2005). Increasing the amount of moderate to vigorous physical activity is supported by evidence-based data for disease prevention in youth (Strong et al., 2005). However, few intervention studies have been conducted on the effects of physical activity on prevention or treatment of chronic disease in youth (Cruz et al., 2005).

For the child with type 2 diabetes, regular physical activity may help to achieve a healthier body weight. For the child with type 1 diabetes, care should be taken to prevent hypoglycemia (U.S. Department of Health and Human Services, National Diabetes Education Program, 2006). Hypoglycemia may occur after prolonged moderate intensity aerobic exercise, as might occur in an after-school program, and may require more carbohydrate than a traditional 15 g for treatment (Diabetes Research in Children Network Study Group, 2006). Children on continuous subcutaneous insulin infusion may need to use a variety of

interventions for families of children aged 5 to 12 years and school-based interventions for older children are recommended for treating obesity (American Dietetic Association, 2006). If life-style modifications are not successful, medication may be prescribed. Currently, only insulin and metformin are approved by the U.S. Food and Drug Administration for children with type 2 diabetes (Botero & Wolfsdorf, 2005). Metformin is an oral hypoglycemic agent whose main site of action is the liver, where it decreases hepatic gluconeogenesis and increases hepatic glucose uptake. Because metformin does not affect insulin levels, the risk of hypoglycemia is minimized. Preliminary stud-

ies suggest that metformin may be beneficial in hyperinsulinemic euglycemic adolescents in reducing body weight and insulin levels, thereby possibly reducing the risk of subsequent diabetes development (Artz & Freemark, 2004).

The child with diabetes should be routinely screened for complications. Developing nephropathy should be monitored once the child is 10 years old and has had diabetes for 5 years. A random spot urine analyzed for the microalbumin-to-creatinine ratio is recommended. Blood pressure should be monitored and treated if persistently elevated, as should blood lipid levels. Regular ophthalmologic care should begin once the child with diabetes is 10 years old and has had diabetes for at least 3 years (American Diabetes Association, 2005).

As with adults, diabetes self-management education is essential for optimal care. However, in pediatric diabetes care, additional supportive measures are usually required to manage social issues of adolescents and the subsequent effect on glycemic control and general health (Berry, Urban, & Grey, 2006).

strategies depending on the physical activity. The pump can be removed for intense exercise such as in organized sports, but it must be recognized that blood glucose may drop due to the intense exercise or rise due to the excitement of the game. There may also be a risk of nocturnal hypoglycemia after an eventful full day of physical activity such as a soccer or basketball tournament. For prolonged although evenly exerted activities such as biking or hiking, the pump may be set at half the usual rate of infusion, although this should also be individually calibrated (Tamborlane, Fredrickson, & Ahern, 2003).

To reach national guidelines of physical activity for youth in general, families, schools, after-school programs, and youth sports and recreation programs should all be involved at the individual and community level. To promote physical activity in youth, media campaigns and the communities' structural environment should be engaged (Centers for Disease Control and Prevention, n.d.). Although the American Diabetes Association (1999) and the American College of Sports Medicine (Pollock et al., 2000) recommend a combination of both strength training and aerobic exercise for those adults with diabetes, guidelines for youth are yet to be disseminated.

Disordered Eating

Pamela Hinton, PhD

Eating disorders are psychiatric disorders with significant medical and psychosocial complications affecting about 5 million Americans, primarily adolescent girls and young women. Three eating disorders have been identified by the American Psychiatric Association, anorexia nervosa (AN), bulimia nervosa (BN), and eating disorder not otherwise specified (EDNOS); the diagnostic criteria are outlined in the *Diagnostic and Statistical Manual of Mental Disorders* (American Psychiatric Association, 2000). Although behaviorally distinct, with AN characterized by severe dietary restriction and BN by binge eating and compensatory purging behaviors, the eating disorders share an excessive importance of body weight and shape to self-concept and self-esteem. Eating disorder diagnoses are mutually exclusive; however, an individual may meet diagnostic criteria for more than one disorder during the course of their illness.

Anorexia Nervosa

AN is characterized by a relentless pursuit of thinness (Table 8.5). Individuals with AN may achieve very low body weights via severe restriction of the amount and types of food eaten and compulsive and excessive exercise. Patients with binge eating–purging subtype of AN occasionally use self-induced vomiting, laxatives, or diuretics to control their body weight. AN is a progressive condition, in that the standard for "thin" is lowered over time and patients are never satisfied with their body weight or shape. As weight loss progresses, impaired cognitive function, depression, anxiety, and social isolation worsen. Academic and work performance and personal re-

lationships are often sacrificed to spend time exercising or to avoid social situations that require eating.

Bulimia Nervosa

Individuals with BN also desire thinness, but their chronic dieting is interspersed with recurrent episodes of binge eating, followed by compensatory purging behaviors (e.g., self-induced vomiting) to "undo" the effects of the binge (Table 8.6). As a result most patients with BN are of normal body weight. Feelings of guilt, shame, depression, anxiety, and negative ego-syntonicity increase in parallel with the frequency of binge–purge cycles. Poor impulse regulation often manifests as substance misuse and abuse and self-harming behavior in patients with BN. For some individuals BN also is a progressive condition with the need to binge–purge interfering with academic or work performance and relationships and characterized by stealing.

Eating Disorder Not Otherwise Specified

EDNOS diagnoses should not imply a less serious condition or one that is not worthy of intervention. Typically, EDNOS is nearly identical to AN or BN

TABLE 8.5	Diagnostic Criteria for Anorexia Nervosa	
Criterion	**Description**	
A	Refusal to maintain body weight at or above a minimally normal weight for age and height.	
B	Intense fear of gaining weight or becoming fat, even though underweight.	
C	Disturbance in the way in which one's body weight or shape is experienced, undue influence of body weight or shape on self-evaluation, or denial of the seriousness of the current low body weight.	
D	In postmenarchal females, amenorrhea, i.e., the absence of at least three consecutive menstrual cycles. (A woman is considered to have amenorrhea if her periods occur only after hormone [e.g., estrogen] administration.)	
AN subtypes		
Restricting type	During the current episode of anorexia nervosa, the person has not regularly engaged in binge eating or purging behavior (i.e., self-induced vomiting or the misuse of laxative, diuretics, or enemas).	
Binge eating– purging type	During the current episode of anorexia nervosa, the person has regularly engaged in binge eating or purging behaviors (i.e., self-induced vomiting or the misuse of laxative, diuretics, or enemas).	

From U.S. Department of Health and Human Services, National Institute of Mental Health (2001).

| | TABLE 8.6 | Diagnostic Criteria for Bulimia Nervosa |

Criterion	Description
A	Recurrent episodes of binge eating. An episode of binge eating is characterized by both of the following: 1. Eating, in a discrete period of time (e.g., within any 2-hour period), an amount of food that is definitely larger than most people would eat during a similar period of time and under similar circumstances. 2. A sense of lack of control over eating during the episode (e.g., a feeling that one cannot stop eating or control what or how much one is eating).
B	Recurrent inappropriate compensatory behavior to prevent weight gain, such as self-induced vomiting; misuse of laxatives, diuretics, enemas, or other medications; fasting; or excessive exercise.
C	The binge eating and inappropriate compensatory behaviors both occur, on average, at least twice a week for 3 months.
D	Self-evaluation is unduly influenced by body shape and weight.
E	The disturbance does not occur exclusively during episodes of anorexia nervosa.
BN subtypes Purging type	During the current episode of bulimia nervosa, the person has regularly engaged in self-induced vomiting or the misuse of laxatives, diuretics, or enemas.
Nonpurging type	During the current episode of bulimia nervosa, the person has used other inappropriate compensatory behaviors, such as fasting or excessive exercise, but has not regularly engaged in self-induced vomiting or the misuse of laxatives, diuretics, or enemas.

From U.S. Department of Health and Human Services, National Institute of Mental Health (2001).

but without meeting all the diagnostic criteria for either AN or BN (Henig, 2004). All the criteria for AN are met except

- The individual has regular menses.
- The individual's current weight is in the normal range.

All the criteria for BN are met except

- Binge eating and inappropriate compensatory mechanisms occur at a frequency of less than twice a week or for a duration of less than 3 months
- Regular use of inappropriate compensatory behavior by an individual of normal body weight after eating small amounts of food
- Chewing and spitting out, but not swallowing, large amounts of food
- Purging disorder
- Binge eating disorder

For example, an individual may meet all the diagnostic criteria for AN except amenorrhea. As in AN and BN, undue influence of body weight or shape on self-worth is the core psychopathology of most individuals who receive an EDNOS diagnosis. Binge eating disorder (BED) is a subtype of EDNOS, de-

fined by criteria that are for research purposes only (Table 8.7).

Psychiatric Comorbidity

Psychiatric comorbidity is high among individuals with eating disorders (Becker, Grinspoon, Klibanski, & Herzog, 1999; American Psychiatric Association, 2000; Fairburn & Harrison, 2003), but as demonstrated in the Minnesota Starvation Study, starvation causes significant changes in mood, personality, and cognition and behavior (Keys, Brozek, Henschel, Mickelsen, & Taylor, 1950). Thus it is sometimes difficult to differentiate between primary and secondary psychological disturbances. Depression is common in both AN and BN, but affect improves significantly with refeeding and reduction in binge–purge symptomology. Obsessive-compulsive disorder and anxiety disorders are common among individuals with eating disorders, but the obsessions (thoughts), compulsions (behaviors), and fears often are related to the eating disorder. A significant proportion of individuals with eating disorders also suffer from personality disorders, and cotreatment of personality

Psychiatric comorbidity: Presence of additional mental disorders, e.g., substance abuse or personality disorder.

TABLE 8.7	Research Criteria for Binge Eating	

Criterion	Description

A	Recurrent episodes of binge eating characterized by both of the following:
	  a. Eating, in a discrete period of time, an amount of food that is definitely larger than most people would eat during a similar period of time under similar circumstances. Not continual snacking or grazing. Objective definition of quantity.
	  b. A sense of lack of control over eating during the episode.

B	Binge eating episodes are associated with three or more of the following:
	  a. Eating much more rapidly than usual
	  b. Eating until uncomfortably full
	  c. Eating large amounts when not feeling physically hungry
	  d. Eating alone because embarrassed about quantity
	  e. Feeling disgusted with oneself, depressed, or very guilty after overeating

C	Marked distress regarding binge eating is present due to loss of control, implication for weight and health
D	Binge eating occurs, on average, at least 2 days a week for 6 months
E	Binge eating is not associated with the regular use of inappropriate compensatory behaviors and does not occur exclusively during the course of anorexia nervosa

From U.S. Department of Health and Human Services, National Institute of Mental Health (2001).

disorders may preclude recovery from eating disorders. Cluster B (Antisocial, Borderline, Histrionic, Narcissistic) personality disorders are more common in individuals with BN; patients with AN are more likely to have Cluster C personality disorders (Avoidant, Dependent, Obsessive-Compulsive). Self-harming behaviors, substance misuse and abuse, and suicide are present at higher rates in patients with eating disorders compared with the general population. If psychology comorbidity is present, it is important to treat all pathologies; otherwise, diminution of the eating disorder may exacerbate symptoms of the remaining disorders.

Etiology and Course of Eating Disorders

Eating disorders have multifactorial etiologies. Sociocultural, genetic, family, and personality factors predispose an individual to engage in behavioral risk factors, which are dieting and excessive exercise, which universally precede a clinical eating disorder. Negative life events, role transitions, developmental milestones, sexual and physical abuse, and criticism of physical appearance often precipitate the progression from dieting to eating disorder (American Psychiatric Association, 2000; Fairburn & Harrison, 2003).

Based on physical and behavioral criteria, about 50% of individuals diagnosed with AN and BN achieve full recovery, which is usually defined based on physical and behavioral criteria (i.e., normal body weight, regular menses, and normalization of eating patterns). An additional 30% of eating disorder patients partially recover; for the remaining 20% of affected individuals the eating disorder becomes chronic. Protection, control, and positive social reinforcement are benefits that eating disorder individuals derive from their disorder, thus contributing to the chronicity of the conditions. AN has the highest mortality rate of any psychiatric illness; the adjusted mortality rate ranges from 1.2% to 12.8% and the suicide rate is 56.9% (Agras et al., 2004).

The single most important positive prognostic factor is a short interval between onset of the eating disorder and intervention; thus less severe weight loss and symptomology also are positive prognostic indicators (American Psychiatric Association, 2000; Fairburn & Harrison, 2003; Agras et al., 2004). Younger age at onset of the eating disorder also is associated with increased likelihood of recovery. Recovery is very difficult after the eating disorder has become **ego-syntonic** and the behaviors entrenched. Psychiatric comorbidity, high vomiting frequency, self-harming behaviors, and substance abuse disorders are negative prognostic indicators (Fairburn & Harrison, 2003).

Ego-syntonic: Consistent with self-concept.

Epidemiology

Eating disorders are disorders of Western societies, although there are isolated reports of self-imposed starvation of adolescents from non-Western societies. Food refusal and thinness have little meaning where food is scarce and malnutrition is endemic.

Eating disorders are more common in whites than in other ethnic and racial minorities, and 90% of individuals with AN and BN are female. The disparity between whites and African-Americans is less for BED than for AN and BN. The onset of AN typically occurs during adolescence, compared with young adulthood for BN and middle age for BED. Worldwide, the estimated prevalence of AN is 0.7% in teenage girls and that of BN is 1% to 2% in females aged 16 to 35 years. The estimated combined prevalence of AN and BN in the United States is 3% among young women and an additional 3% have EDNOS, affecting about 5 million Americans (Becker et al., 1999). The incidence of AN is 19 females and 2 males per 100,000 per year compared with 29 females and 1 male for BN (Fairburn & Harrison, 2003). Approximately 40% of patients with BED are male.

It is thought that the incidence of both AN and BN has increased in the recent past. However, it is very difficult to accurately determine the frequency of eating disorders in the general population (Agras et al., 2004). Because of the reluctance to seek treatment, many eating disorders go undiagnosed in the community. In addition, there is bias in access to treatment, which in turn biases the reported prevalence of eating disorders among different ethnic and racial groups and between the genders. There is very little epidemiologic data regarding EDNOS, although these atypical eating disorders seem to primarily affect adolescents and young adult women (Fairburn & Bohn, 2005).

Medical Consequences of Eating Disorders

Routine laboratory tests include measurements of serum electrolytes, glucose, blood urea nitrogen, creatinine, and a complete blood count (American Psychiatric Association, 2000; American Dietetics Association, 2001). However, normal laboratory findings are common in patients with eating disorders. Additional laboratory tests, such as serum calcium, magnesium, and phosphorus, liver function tests, electrocardiogram, bone density assessment, estradiol or testosterone levels, are warranted if the patient exhibits signs and symptoms of malnutrition (American Psychiatric Association, 2000; Fairburn & Harrison, 2003).

Most of the medical complications of AN are due to inadequate energy intake and thus are reversed upon refeeding (American Psychiatric Association, 2000; Fairburn & Harrison, 2003). The exception is loss of bone mineral density, which may persist after restoration of body weight (Heer, Mika, Grzella, Heussen, & Herpertz-Dahlmann, 2004). Fifty percent of women with AN have BMD that is more than 2 standard deviations below the average value for young adult women (Becker et al., 1999). Physical signs and symptoms and clinical abnormalities associated with AN are presented in Table 8.8.

Apparently, low energy availability is sensed in the brain; leptin and ghrelin (De Souza, Leidy, O'Donnell, Lasley, & Williams, 2004) may be signals from the periphery to the brain of energy status. Hypothalamic release of thyrotropin-releasing hormone and gonadotropin-releasing hormone are suppressed, resulting in decreased production of thyroid hormone (triiodothyronine, thyroxine), estrogen, and progesterone. In contrast, hypothalamic secretion of growth hormone-releasing hormone and corticotropin-releasing hormone are elevated and, subsequently, so are GH and cortisol. Although GH secretion is increased, the liver and extrahepatic tissues become GH resistant and systemic and local production of IGF-I is decreased. These hormonal alterations produce many of the physical signs and symptoms associated with AN:

- Low triiodothyronine results in cold intolerance, bradycardia, **orthostatic hypotension**, **acrocyanosis**, and delayed reflexes.
- Low estradiol causes anovulatory amenorrhea, loss of BMD, hypertriglyceridemia and hypercholesterolemia, elevated adhesion molecule expression, and impaired flow-mediated dilation.
- GH resistance and low IGF-I results in muscle atrophy, loss of BMD, stunting in growing adolescents, and, possibly, **leucopenia**.
- Hypercortisolemia may contribute to loss of muscle mass and BMD as well as to immune modulation.

Growth of fine downy hair (**lanugo**), dry skin, brittle hair, and electrocardiographic abnormalities, usually prolongation of the Q-T interval (Swenne, 2000), are characteristic signs of malnutrition.

Orthostatic hypotension: A sudden fall in blood pressure that occurs when a person assumes a standing position, causing dizziness, lightheadedness, blurred vision, and syncope.

Acrocyanosis: Blueness of the extremities (the hands and feet), caused by narrowing (constriction) of small arterioles (tiny arteries) toward the end of the arms and legs.

Leucopenia: A decrease in the number of white blood cells circulating within the blood.

Lanugo: Downy, very fine, soft, and usually unpigmented hair.

TABLE

8.8 Medical Consequences of Eating Disorders

Physical symptoms
  Cold intolerance
  Gastrointestinal complaints
  Dizziness
  Amenorrhea
  Poor sleep with early morning waking
  Apathy, poor concentration
  Muscle pain
  Weakness, lassitude

Physical signs
  Emaciation; stunted growth and failure/regression of secondary sex characteristics
  Dry skin
  Lanugo
  Orange discoloration of palms and soles with hypercarotenemia
  Swelling of parotid and submandibular glands (vomiting)
  Erosion of inner surface of front teeth (perimylolysis, due to vomiting)
  Scarring on dorsum of hand (Russell's sign, due to self-induced vomiting)
  Esophagitis, gastroesophageal reflux, erythema of pharynx
  Cold hands and feet, hypothermia, acrocyanosis
  Bradycardia, orthostatic hypotension, cardiac arrhythmias
  Edema
  Muscle weakness
  Cognitive impairment, depressed irritable mood

Abnormalities on physical investigation
  Endocrine
    Low luteinizing hormone, follicle-stimulating hormone, estradiol
    Low triiodothyronine, thyroxine in normal range, normal thyroid-stimulating hormone
    Mild hypercortisolemia
    Elevated GH
    Hypoglycemia
    Low leptin
  Cardiovascular
    Electrocardiographic abnormalities (especially prolonged Q-T interval)
  Gastrointestinal
    Delayed gastric emptying
    Decreased colonic motility
    Acute gastric dilation
  Hematologic
    Moderate normocytic normochromic anemia
    Mild leucopenia with relative lymphocytosis
    Thrombocytopenia
  Other metabolic abnormalities
    Hypercholesterolemia
    Hypercarotenemia
    Hypophosphatemia
    Dehydration
    Electrolyte disturbance: metabolic alkalosis and hypokalemia (vomiting); metabolic acidosis, hypokalemia and hyponatremia (laxative abuse)
  Other abnormalities
    Osteopenia and osteoporosis
    Enlarged cerebral ventricles and external cerebrospinal fluid spaces

From U.S. Department of Health and Human Services, National Institute of Mental Health (2001).

The focus of eating disorder treatment should be correcting the self-imposed starvation rather than correcting hormone abnormalities via replacement therapy (Fairburn & Harrison, 2003). However, because of the irreversible nature of the loss of BMD, use of anabolic and antiresorptive pharmacologic interventions may be warranted to treat osteopenia and osteoporosis (Miller et al., 2004). There is limited evidence that the combination of rhIGF-I and estradiol may ameliorate loss of BMD during AN (Grinspoon, Miller, Herzog, Clemmons, & Klibanski, 2003; Grinspoon, Friedman, 2003; Grinspoon, Miller, Herzog, Grieco, & Klibanski, 2004).

The primary medical complications of BN result from electrolyte and fluid imbalances due to self-induced vomiting and laxative and diuretic misuse. Frequent vomiting results in metabolic alkalosis and hypokalemia; laxative misuse creates metabolic acidosis, hypokalemia, and hyponatremia. Electrolyte abnormalities cause cardiac arrhythmias, which are potentially life-threatening in severely underweight individuals. Peripheral edema and dehydration also result from electrolyte imbalances. Chronic laxative use creates colonic dependence; constipation results when laxative use is stopped because of decreased intestinal motility. Physical symptoms resulting from self-induced vomiting include callous on the dorsum of the hand (Russell's sign), swelling of the submandibular and parotid glands, and erosion of dental enamel on the occlusal and lingual surfaces of the teeth.

Individuals with EDNOS experience medical complications of AN and BN, depending on the nature of their disordered eating behaviors. A diagnosis of EDNOS does not mean that physical health is not jeopardized. Patients with BED are typically overweight and at risk for chronic diseases associated with excess adiposity.

Treatment

Unfortunately, treatment of eating disorders, especially AN, is often dictated by insurance reimbursement rather than need or long-term efficacy. Treatment of AN is costly: Approximately 50% of patients require hospitalization, 50% are prescribed pharmacotherapy, and all require outpatient therapy. In the United States, short-term hospitalization to achieve nutritional stabilization or avert a medical crisis is the norm. However, in other countries, long-term hospitalization with weight restoration and psychotherapy is the standard (Agras et al., 2004).

Treatment Goals

Ideally, treatment should achieve three objectives (American Dietetic Association, 2001; Fairburn & Harrison, 2003). First, effective management of eating disorders fosters motivation to change disordered eating behaviors. The second goal is normalization of body weight, which not only improves physical health but also facilitates improvements in mood and responsiveness to psychotherapy. Patients with AN cannot respond to serotonin reuptake inhibitors during semistarvation because serotonin production is impaired by malnutrition. The third treatment goal is to help patients accord body weight and shape an appropriate level of significance in their self-evaluation, to reduce disordered eating and exercise patterns, and to improve psychosocial functioning. In the case of chronic eating disorders that are resistant to treatment, the goal of therapy is to minimize the negative physical, social, and emotional consequences of the eating disorder.

Eating disorder treatment programs generally use a multidisciplinary treatment team to achieve these therapeutic goals (American Psychiatric Association, 2000; Stewart & Williamson, 2004). A physician oversees the treatment plan and monitors the physical health of the patient. Psychotherapy, by a psychologist, psychiatrist, psychiatric nurse, or social worker trained in eating disorders, helps the patient address unresolved emotional issues, dysfunctional cognitive styles, problematic relationships, and psychiatric comorbidity. A nutritionist or registered dietitian with eating disorder expertise counsels the patient regarding healthful diet and modification of eating habits (American Dietetic Association, 2001).

Inpatient Treatment

Outpatient therapy is preferable to inpatient whenever possible because of the high monetary cost of hospitalization and to the perception by the patient that inpatient treatment is punitive (Agras et al., 2004; Stewart & Williamson, 2004). It sometimes is helpful to the patient to refer to "food as medicine." However, there are circumstances that necessitate inpatient treatment: significant medical risk, very low body weight ($<75\%$ ideal body weight), dehydration, electrolyte disturbances, cardiac dysrhythmia, physiologic instability, arrested growth, acute medical complications of malnutrition (**syncope**, seizures, cardiac failure, pancreatitis), acute psychiatric emergencies (suicidal ideation, self-harming behaviors), uncontrollable binge eating and purging, substance abuse, and circumstances that interfere with treatment (dysfunctional family, abusive relationship). Some patients requiring inpatient treatment may need 24-hour care because of their extreme medical instability (Becker et al., 1999; American Psychiatric Association, 2000; Fairburn & Harrison, 2003; Stewart & Williamson, 2004). Although body weight often is the primary admission criterion, it should not be the single determinant of inpatient treatment. Individuals with eating disorders are adept at artificially elevating their body weight to avoid hospitalization via hyperhydration, which can result in acute hyponatremia. The rate of readmission is relatively high: Approximately 20% of individuals treated in hospital settings will be admitted a second time (Stewart & Williamson, 2004).

Syncope: Temporary loss of consciousness.

Outpatient Treatment

Outpatient therapy for eating disorders may be associated with an eating disorder treatment program or may be physician monitoring of body weight and physical health, psychotherapy, and nutritional counseling. Outpatient day-care facilities are an alternative to inpatient treatment and also serve as a transition from inpatient care (American Psychiatric Association, 2000).

Therapeutic Alliance

Successful treatment of eating disorders depends on the relationship between the treatment team and the affected individual (Stewart & Williamson, 2004), referred to as the **therapeutic alliance**. Unconditional positive regard, genuineness, warmth, and empathy foster a positive relationship. Validation of the patient's feelings and thoughts by the treatment team increases the patient's self-trust. The treatment plan always should encourage the patient's sense of responsibility and autonomy.

> **Therapeutic alliance:**
> Cooperation between the patient and the therapist to engage in treatment; dependent on good rapport between patient and therapist.

Medical Nutrition Therapy

Weight Gain Goal

Although low body weight is only a symptom of underlying psychopathology, it is the focus of nutritional interventions. Because body weight often is used as the criterion for admission to or release from inpatient treatment programs and because low body weight is associated with increased morbidity and mortality, it frequently is monitored. The perceived focus on weight gain and measurement of body weight can cause significant distress for eating disordered individuals because of their intense fear of becoming fat. In addition, patients may believe the cause of their eating disorder is going to be ignored and go untreated if they perceive the primary treatment focus is restoration of body weight. Because the eating disorder often arises out of an unmet need to be "taken seriously," patients need reassurance that they will continue to receive the psychological treatment and therapeutic support they need even if they gain weight.

To minimize the distress associated with determination of body weight, patients are often weighed with their back to the scale. It also is helpful to focus on improving overall health during refeeding and weight restoration. Monitoring clinical signs and symptoms associated with malnutrition can provide the patient empirical evidence that they are becoming "healthy" rather than "fat."

Target body weight usually is determined as 92% of ideal body weight, 90% of previous highest weight, and weight at which menstruation resumes (Stewart & Williamson, 2004). Often, patients are initially not told their target body weight or the energy prescription required to achieve their goal weight.

Refeeding

The desired rate of weight gain is 1 to 2 pounds per week in outpatient therapy and 2 to 3 pounds for inpatient treatment (American Dietetic Association, 2001). Paradoxically, initial weight gain often is difficult for patients with AN. Although resting metabolic rate is suppressed even when expressed relative to lean body mass in AN, there is evidence that patients become hypermetabolic during refeeding (de Zwaan, Aslam, & Mitchell, 2002). Up to 70 to 100 kcal/kg BW a day may be needed for individuals with AN to gain weight (American Psychiatric Association, 2000). However, because of the risk of refeeding syndrome, energy intake should be increased gradually, that is, by about 200 kcal/day for 1 week (American Dietetic Association, 2001). Refeeding syndrome is characterized by hypophosphatemia (Fisher, Simpser, & Schneider, 2000), hypomagnesemia (Birmingham, Puddicombe, & Hlynsky, 2004), hypokalemia, glucose intolerance, pancreatitis (Morris, Stephenson, Herring, & Marti, 2004), gastrointestinal dysfunction, cardiac arrhythmias, and congestive heart failure. Fluid retention and edema are common and complicate accurate determination of changes in body cell mass. The risk of refeeding syndrome is greater with enteral and parenteral tube feeding.

The goal is to first achieve an energy intake of 2,500 kcal/day for 1 week, regardless of weight changes. This is followed by an incremental increase over an additional week to 3,500 kcal/day. At this point energy intake is adjusted to achieve a rate of weight gain of at least 2 pounds per week. If the patient does not gain a minimum of 2 pounds per week after 2 weeks of inpatient therapy, bed rest or nasogastric tube feeding may be implemented (Stewart & Williamson, 2004).

Micronutrient Deficiencies

Surprisingly, vitamin and mineral inadequacies are uncommon in patients with eating disorders, possibly due to decreased requirements (American Dietetic Association, 2001). Poor intakes of iron, zinc, and calcium are frequently reported in AN. There also is evidence of poor folate and vitamin B_{12} status, as evidenced by low red blood cell folate in patients with AN. Abnormalities in carotenoid metabolism result in elevated serum carotene concentrations. To minimize loss of bone mineral, it is important to ensure that patients with eating disorders consume adequate calcium and vitamin D (American Dietetic Association, 2001).

Normalization of Eating and Exercise Patterns

A goal of medical nutrition therapy is to enable the patient to eat regular meals that meet nutrient needs and include a variety of foods (American Dietetic Association, 2001). In addition, individuals recovering from eating disorders need to learn to be sensitive to hunger and satiety cues. This often involves learning to "trust" one's body, that is, that eating when hungry will not lead to excessive weight gain. Individuals with eating disorders often believe their bodies are somehow defective and different, that they will become obese if they eat like "normal people." Normalization of eating patterns often requires giving up "forbidden" foods and idiosyncratic rituals around food preparation and eating. It is unrealistic to expect an individual recovering from an eating disorder to give up all their disordered eating behaviors at once. Change seems possible if it is incremental.

Patients with BN often present wanting to lose weight. Key to recovery from BN is the recognition that weight loss cannot be achieved by "dieting" and that dieting initiates the binge eating–purging cycle. Individuals recovering from BN must learn that eating regular meals will not "make them fat" but will, in fact, facilitate weight control by minimizing binge eating. Nutritionists should assist patients with BN in structuring their eating patterns to three regular meals and one to three snacks per day. Initially, energy intake should be determined by hunger, because hunger is positively associated with binge eating and purging. Normalization of eating patterns and cessation of vomiting and laxative abuse may cause significant fluid retention and edema, which may be troubling to patients. Chronic laxative users benefit from a high-fiber diet and adequate fluid intake to minimize constipation (American Dietetic Association, 2001).

Individuals recovering from eating disorders should be educated on benefits of exercise in addition to weight control, and they should be encouraged to view exercise as pleasurable rather than compulsory. Trying new activities or sports may foster adoption of this positive view of physical activity. As with hunger and satiety, individuals with eating disorders often ignore feelings of fatigue and pain, exercising when sick or injured. They should be encouraged to "listen" to their bodies and to have an integrated view of their bodies, rather than viewing the body as something to be mastered or controlled.

Psychotherapy

A variety of psychological treatments has been used in the treatment of eating disorders: psychodynamic, interpersonal, cognitive behavioral (CBT), cognitive analytical, behavioral, and family psychotherapy (Fairburn & Harrison, 2003). There are very few controlled outpatient treatment studies comparing modes of psychotherapy for AN. The existing data are limited by small sample sizes, high rates of attrition, lack of standardized treatment protocols, and variation in outcome variables. In early onset AN, family therapy appears to be effective, and thus it is used in treatment of adolescents with eating disorders. There is some support for modest efficacy of psychodynamic therapy, cognitive analytical therapy, and CBT in AN (Becker et al., 1999; Agras et al., 2004).

The evidence in support of the efficacy of CBT for BN is strong. CBT is short-term (20 weekly sessions), structured, and manual-based therapy that focuses on changing dysfunctional cognitive styles that lead to disordered eating and exercise behaviors. About one-third to one-half of patients who participate in CBT experience significant and sustained improvements in bulimic behaviors. Interpersonal therapy, which focuses on problematic relationships, was shown to be as effective as CBT in two short-term trials (Becker et al., 1999; Agras et al., 2004).

Psychotropic Medications

Antidepressants are the most common pharmacologic intervention for eating disorders (Becker et al., 1999; Fairburn & Harrison, 2003). Patients with AN and BN often experience significant depressive symptoms, and there is increased prevalence of depression in families of eating disordered individuals. Recently, genetic linkage studies examined the association between variants of the serotonin receptor gene and AN. There is limited evidence that one variation of a serotonin receptor gene (5-HTR2A) is associated with AN (Kaye, Frank, Bailer, & Henry, 2005; Kaye, Frank, Bailer, Henry, Meltzer, 2005; Klump & Gobrogge, 2005). Serotonin reuptake inhibitors increase the availability of serotonin within the brain. These antidepressants significantly improve mood and bulimic symptoms acutely, but the positive effect is not sustained. Furthermore, antidepressants are neither as effective as CBT nor do they consistently augment the effects of CBT. There is no empirical evidence supporting the use of antidepressants in treatment of AN, especially during semistarvation. Serotonin synthesis is sensitive to nutritional status, rendering serotonin reuptake inhibitors ineffective in malnourished individuals.

Fluoxetine may prevent relapse in weight-restored individuals with AN (Becker et al., 1999).

Special Populations

Males

Eating disorders are less common in men than in women. It is estimated that the ratio of male to female cases of AN is 1:6 and for BN, 1:20. However, the true gender ratio is unknown, because eating disorders are more likely to go undiagnosed in men than in women. Eating disorders are more common in homosexual compared with heterosexual males because of the increased social value of thinness in the homosexual community. Except in certain subcultures (e.g., homosexual community, wrestlers, and jockeys) there is no positive reinforcement of thinness for males. In males with eating disorders, the etiology of the eating disturbance is more likely to be related to improving athletic performance, avoiding medical disease, and escaping peer teasing. There are subtle differences in the body dissatisfaction experienced between the genders. Women with AN are preoccupied with body weight, and men generally are dissatisfied with their body shape or size, rather than weight per se. Males with AN experience the same medical complications as females, including a decline in testosterone and loss of bone mineral density. Limited evidence has shown that treatment outcome is improved if therapy is limited to all-male patients and the treatment team includes some male members. Strength training, in combination with nutrition counseling, improves body dissatisfaction in males who are concerned with their body shape or size (Andersen, 1999).

Pregnancy

Although fertility is reduced in women with AN, ovulation may still occur in some individuals. Women with eating disorders have increased complications during pregnancy and are more likely to have a low birth weight infant and to deliver prematurely (Helgstrand & Andersen, 2005; Kouba, Hallstrom, Lindholm, & Hirschberg, 2005). BN is associated with increased risk of miscarriage. Prenatal death is more common in infants born to mothers with AN (Becker et al., 1999; Fairburn & Harrison, 2003; Kouba et al., 2005). Pregnancy is a time when women are receptive to making significant life-style changes to increase their chances of delivering a healthy baby. Women with eating disorders experience a decrease in the severity of their illness during pregnancy. Unfortunately, the symptoms often recur after delivery when the developing infant is no longer in jeopardy (Rocco et al., 2005).

Athletes

As discussed previously, athletes may be at an increased risk for eating disorders than nonathletes. Some studies have reported increased body dissatisfaction, drive for thinness, and disordered eating in athletes compared with nonathletes. Other investigations, however, found that athletes have a more positive body image than nonathletes and are not at greater risk for eating disorder than nonathletes. The prevalence of eating disorders may vary with the nature of the sport; endurance and aesthetic sports have higher rates of eating disorders than sports where body weight, composition, and appearance do not play a central role in performance (Goodman, 2005; Sanford et al., 2005).

When counseling athletes with eating disorders, it is important that the nutritionist be trained in sports nutrition. Athletes discredit diet and exercise recommendations that are not made by a professional who understands sports. Athletes often believe they are "special" and have unique nutrient requirements. This is especially important regarding exercise counseling. For example, an athlete who has been participating in rigorous training will be highly critical of any suggestion that 20 to 30 minutes of moderate exercise 5 days per week is "normal" or adequate. When the health of an athlete is compromised, the team physician may determine that participation in organized practice and competition is contingent on maintenance of a minimal weight or percent of body fat or on behavioral criteria. Athletes may be reluctant to admit to an eating disorder and to seek help because they fear losing their scholarship and disappointing their coach and teammates. Some coaches facilitate intervention and treatment, whereas others resist, believing their authority has been overstepped. It is helpful if sports medicine professionals and coaches view eating disorders in athletes as they would any other injury or illness that requires treatment and physician release before return to practice and competition (Goodman, 2005).

Insulin-Dependent Diabetes Mellitus

There is limited evidence that insulin-dependent diabetes mellitus increases the risk for eating disorders. It has been hypothesized that dietary interventions and weight gain associated with insulin treatment are etiologic factors (Verrotti, Catino, De Luca, Morgese, & Chiarelli, 1999). Individuals with insulin-dependent diabetes mellitus may not comply with insulin therapy to prevent weight gain. Poor glycemic control is associated with rapid progression of complications from diabetes and should be considered a warning sign of eating disorder.

Childhood Eating Disorders

Disordered eating is problematic in pediatric and adolescent populations. Neither the American Psychiatric Association nor the World Health Organization provides diagnostic criteria for the classification of problematic eating in children. However, clinicians and researchers have defined several types of disordered eating in children based on psychological and behavioral characteristics (Watkins, 2002).

Pervasive refusal syndrome is characterized by refusal to eat, drink, talk, walk, and perform self-care (Lask, 2004). Social withdrawal and resistance to treatment are remarkable and further aggravate a serious and potentially life-threatening condition. The average age at onset is 8 to 16 years, and far more girls are affected than boys. Affected children are usually high achievers with high self-expectations, fear of failure, and difficulty dealing with failure to achieve personal standards. There is limited evidence that family violence and sexual abuse also are causal factors. The onset of pervasive refusal syndrome is usually acute. Illness and injury are the most common precipitating factors. Treatment is multidisciplinary, and hospitalization in a child psychiatric unit usually is required. The goal of medical nutrition therapy is to reverse dehydration and electrolyte imbalances and to improve energy intake and nutritional status. Nasogastric tube feedings are almost always needed; resistance to the nasogastric tube feeding is not uncommon. Because affected children are immobile, they must be moved frequently to prevent bedsores and infections. Passive stretching and hydrotherapy prevent muscle stiffness and contractions. Psychotherapy, which often involves nonverbal communication, helps patients identify and express emotions and deal with concerns about returning to normal life. Family therapy may help resolve dysfunctional family interactions. Recovery from pervasive refusal syndrome is slow, typically requiring 1 year after identification and entering treatment, but most children have a complete recovery.

> **● Learning Point** The goal of medical nutrition therapy is to reverse dehydration and electrolyte imbalances and to improve energy intake and nutritional status.

Children with *food avoidance emotional disorder* present with symptoms similar to AN, depression, or anxiety disorders. Although the apparent lack of appetite and inadequate food intake result from negative affect, these children are not preoccupied with body weight or shape.

Children with *functional dysphagia and food phobias* are fearful of certain foods or textures, usually lumpy or solid foods. Their fears are rooted in beliefs that the food is poisonous or will make them gag, choke, or vomit. The origin of the phobia may be a traumatic event or a misplaced association between the food and expected negative consequence of eating the feared food.

Another type of disordered eating in children is *selective eating* or *extreme faddism*. It is normal for preschool children to go on "food jags" where they will consume only five or six acceptable foods. During this phase children resist trying new foods and may gag if forced to eat a novel food. It is thought that children with selective eating have not progressed beyond the preschool stage characterized by food faddism. Because affected children consume their preferred foods they are usually of normal height and weight. This problem, which is most common in children ages 7 to 11 years, improves with increased social interaction.

Summary

Children and adolescents have higher energy and protein needs per kilogram of body weight than adults to support growth. Because of this fact, nutrition during athletic performance must be properly planned and supported by diet. At puberty, androgens, estrogens, GH, and IGF-I cause increases in bone mineral, muscle mass, and sex-specific deposition of body fat. The RDA for protein is 0.95 g/kg BW for children aged 9 to 13 and 0.85 g/kg BW for teenagers, compared with 0.8 g/kg BW for adults. Greater than 90% of peak bone mass is acquired by age 18 years, and bone mass doubles between the onset of puberty and young adulthood. Thus children and adolescents require more calcium than adults; the adequate intake for calcium is 1,300 mg/day for ages 9 to 18 years. Iron and zinc needs also are increased during adolescence to support an increase in skeletal muscle mass and an expansion in red blood cell number.

Both the prevalence and severity of subsequent complications place type 1 and type 2 diabetes as significant diseases among the pediatric population.

Whereas type 1 diabetes pathogenesis is autoimmune dysfunction that is believed to be triggered by environmental factors, type 2 diabetes focuses on obesity development. Associated with type 2 diabetes in youth is acanthosis nigricans and in young or adolescent females, polycystic ovarian syndrome.

Treatment for both type 1 and type 2 diabetes in youth involves appropriate calories for achieving and maintaining a healthy weight while preventing obesity and allowing for growth. Adolescence can be difficult emotionally for children without a chronic disease; for those with diabetes the transition to adulthood can be especially challenging. The health care team needs to work with the family and child not only to achieve glycemic control, but also to maintain a healthy social and psychological environment.

Eating disorders are psychiatric disorders with significant medical and psychosocial complications, affecting about 5 million Americans—primarily adolescent girls and young women. Three eating disorders have been identified by the American Psychiatric Association: AN, BN, and EDNOS. Although behaviorally distinct, with AN characterized by severe dietary restriction and BN by binge eating and compensatory purging behaviors, the eating disorders share an excessive importance of body weight and shape to self-concept and self-esteem. Eating disorder diagnoses are mutually exclusive; however, an individual may meet diagnostic criteria for more than one disorder during the course of their illness. Treatment is multidisciplinary, and hospitalization in a psychiatric unit usually is required. The goal of medical nutrition therapy is to reverse dehydration and electrolyte imbalances and to improve energy intake and nutritional status.

Issues to Debate

1. Should coaches and schools be responsible for the proper nutrition of their child athletes?
2. Although several lawsuits and media attention have focused on the role of the fast food industry on the increasing obesity prevalence in the United States, others have professed that individuals have a right to eat where and what they want. With a strong link between obesity and type 2 diabetes, should children of parents who are obese and have type 2 diabetes receive health warnings about places to eat or particular foods they should avoid? Is it the business world, the community, the parents, or the child themself who should be responsible for eating patterns?
3. Adolescents with type 1 diabetes take insulin and monitor their blood glucose. However, it is not uncommon to experience some episodes of hypoglycemia. Should these young adults be allowed to take driver's education? Is having blood glucose levels checked before driving an invasion of privacy?
4. Knowing the medical consequences of eating disorders, should children be placed in a medical facility against their will for treatment?

Website Resources

American Diabetes Association www.diabetes.org
American Dietetic Association www.eatright.org
International Society for Pediatric and Adolescent Diabetes www.diabetesguidelines.com/health/dwk/pro/guidelines/ispad/ispad.asp
Juvenile Diabetes Research Foundation International www.jdrf.org/
National Diabetes Education Program www.ndep.nih.gov/diabetes/youth/youth.htm

References

Dietary Guidelines for Athletes

Acheson, K. J., Gremaud, G., Meirim, I., Montigon, F., Krebs, Y., Fay, L. B., et al. (2004). Metabolic effects of caffeine in humans: Lipid oxidation or futile cycling? *American Journal of Clinical Nutrition, 79*, 40–46.

Ainsworth, B. E., Jacobs, D. R., Jr., Leon, A. S., Richardson, M. T., & Montoye, H. J. (1993). Assessment of the accuracy of physical activity questionnaire occupational data. *Journal of Occupational Medicine, 35*, 1017–1027.

American Academy of Pediatrics. (2005). Breastfeeding and the use of human milk. *Pediatrics, 115*, 496–450.

American College of Obstetricians and Gynecologists. (2002). ACOG committee opinion. Exercise during pregnancy and the postpartum period. *International Journal of Gynaecology and Obstetrics, 77*, 79–81.

American Dietetic Association, Dietitians of Canada, and the American College of Sports Medicine. (2000). Position paper: Nutrition and athletic performance. *Journal of the American Dietetic Association, 100*, 1543–1556.

Anderson, M. J., Cotter, J. D., Garnham, A. P., Casley, D. J., & Febbraio, M. A. (2001). Effect of glycerol-induced hyperhydration on thermoregulation and metabolism during exercise in heat. *International Journal of Sport Nutrition and Exercise Metabolism, 11*, 315–333.

Atherton, P. J., Babraj, J., Smith, K., Singh, J., Rennie, M. J., & Wackerhage, H. (2005). Selective activation of AMPK-PGC-1alpha or PKB-TSC2-mTOR signaling can explain specific adaptive responses to endurance or resistance training-like electrical muscle stimulation. *The FASEB Journal: Official Publication of the Federation of American Societies for Experimental Biology, 19*, 786–788.

Bar-Or, O. (2001). Nutritional considerations for the child athlete. *Canadian Journal of Applied Physiology = Revue Canadienne de Physiologie Appliquée, 26*(Suppl.), S186–S191.

Bennell, K., White, S., & Crossley, K. (1999). The oral contraceptive pill: A revolution for sportswomen? *British Journal of Sports Medicine, 33*, 231–238.

Bonen, A., Haynes, F. W., & Graham, T. E. (1991). Substrate and hormonal responses to exercise in women using oral contraceptives. *Journal of Applied Physiology, 70*, 1917–1927.

Borsheim, E., Aarsland, A., & Wolfe, R. R. (2004). Effect of an amino acid, protein, and carbohydrate mixture on net muscle protein balance after resistance exercise. *International Journal of Sport Nutrition and Exercise Metabolism, 14*, 255–271.

Borsheim, E., Cree, M. G., Tipton, K. D., Elliott, T. A., Aarsland, A., & Wolfe, R. R. (2004). Effect of carbohydrate intake on net muscle protein synthesis during recovery from resistance exercise. *Journal of Applied Physiology, 96*, 674–678.

Borsheim, E., Tipton, K. D., Wolf, S. E., & Wolfe, R. R. (2002). Essential amino acids and muscle protein recovery from resistance exercise. *American Journal of Physiology. Endocrinology and Metabolism, 283*, E648–E657.

Brownlie, T., Utermohlen, V., Hinton, P. S., Giordano, C., & Haas, J. D. (2002). Marginal iron deficiency without anemia impairs aerobic adaptation among previously untrained women. *American Journal of Clinical Nutrition, 75*, 734–742.

Brownlie, T., Utermohlen, V., Hinton, P. S., & Haas, J. D. (2004). Tissue iron deficiency without anemia impairs adaptation in endurance capacity after aerobic training in previously untrained women. *American Journal of Clinical Nutrition, 79*, 437–443.

Brutsaert, T. D., Hernandez-Cordero, S., Rivera, J., Viola, T., Hughes, G., & Haas, J. D. (2003). Iron supplementation improves progressive fatigue resistance during dynamic knee extensor exercise in iron-depleted, nonanemic women. *American Journal of Clinical Nutrition, 77*, 441–448.

Bryner, R. W., Toffle, R. C., Ullrich, I. H., & Yeater, R. A. (1996). Effect of low dose oral contraceptives on exercise performance. *British Journal of Sports Medicine, 30*, 36–40.

Burke, L. M., Collier, G. R., Broad, E. M., Davis, P. G., Martin, D. T., Sanigorski, A. J., et al. (2003). Effect of alcohol intake on muscle glycogen storage after prolonged exercise. *Journal of Applied Physiology, 95*, 983–990.

Casazza, G. A., Suh, S. H., Miller, B. F., Navazio, F. M., & Brooks, G. A. (2002). Effects of oral contraceptives on peak exercise capacity. *Journal of Applied Physiology, 93*, 1698–1702.

Castell, L. (2003). Glutamine supplementation in vitro and in vivo, in exercise and in immunodepression. *Sports Medicine, 33*, 323–345.

Celsing, F., Ekblom, B., Sylven, C., Everett, J., & Astrand, P. O. (1988). Effects of chronic iron deficiency anaemia on myoglobin content, enzyme activity, and capillary density in the human skeletal muscle. *Acta Medica Scandinavica, 223*, 451–457.

Clapp, J. F., 3rd. (2000). Exercise during pregnancy. A clinical update. *Clinical Sports Medicine, 19*, 273–286.

Connor, W. E. (2000). Importance of n-3 fatty acids in health and disease. *American Journal of Clinical Nutrition, 71* (1 Suppl.), 171S–175S.

Convertino, V. A., Armstrong, L. E., Coyle, E. F., Mack, G. W., Sawka, M. N., Senay, L. C., Jr., et al. (1996). American College of Sports Medicine position stand. Exercise and fluid replacement. *Medicine and Science in Sports and Exercise, 28*, i–vii.

Costill, D. L., Flynn, M. G., Kirwan, J. P., Houmard, J. A., Mitchell, J. B., Thomas, R., et al. (1988). Effects of repeated days of intensified training on muscle glycogen and swimming performance. *Medicine and Science in Sports and Exercise, 20*, 249–254.

Couture, S., Massicotte, D., Lavoie, C., Hillaire-Marcel, C., & Peronnet, F. (2002). Oral [(13)C] glucose and endogenous energy substrate oxidation during prolonged treadmill running. *Journal of Applied Physiology, 92*, 1255–1260.

Davies, K. J., Donovan, C. M., Refino, C. J., Brooks, G. A., Packer, L., & Dallman, P. R. (1984). Distinguishing effects of anemia and muscle iron deficiency on exercise bioenergetics in the rat. *American Journal of Physiology, 246*(6 Pt. 1), E535–E543.

Deldicque, L., Theisen, D., & Francaux, M. (2005). Regulation of mTOR by amino acids and resistance exercise in skeletal muscle. *European Journal of Applied Physiology, 94*, 1–10.

Finch, C. A., Miller, L. R., Inamdar, A. R., Person, R., Seiler, K., & Mackler, B. (1976). Iron deficiency in the rat. Physiological and biochemical studies of muscle dysfunction. *Journal of Clinical Investigations, 58*, 447–453.

Food and Nutrition Board, Institute of Medicine. (1997). Dietary reference intakes for calcium, phosphorous, magnesium, vitamin D, and fluoride.

Food and Nutrition Board, Institute of Medicine. (2001). Dietary reference intakes for vitamin A, vitamin K, Arsenic, boron, chromium, copper, iodine, iron, manganese, nickel, silicon, vanadium, and zinc.

Food and Nutrition Board, Institute of Medicine. (2003). Dietary reference intakes for energy, carbohydrate, fiber, fat, protein and amino acids.

Food and Nutrition Board, Institute of Medicine. (2005). Dietary reference intakes for water, potassium, sodium, chloride, and sulfate. Washington, DC: National Academy of Sciences. Foster-Powell, K., Holt, S. H., & Brand-Miller,

J. C. (2002). International table of glycemic index and glycemic load values: 2002. *American Journal of Clinical Nutrition, 76*, 5–56.

Halson, S. L., Lancaster, G. I., Jeukendrup, A. E., & Gleeson, M. (2003). Immunological responses to overreaching in cyclists. *Medicine and Science in Sports and Exercise, 35*, 854–861.

Heaney, R. P., & Rafferty, K. (2001). Carbonated beverages and urinary calcium excretion. *American Journal of Clinical Nutrition, 74*, 343–347.

Hildebrandt, A. L., Pilegaard, H., & Neufer, P. D. (2003). Differential transcriptional activation of select metabolic genes in response to variations in exercise intensity and duration. *American Journal of Physiology. Endocrinology and Metabolism, 285*, E1021–E1027.

Hinton, P. S., Giordano, C., Brownlie, T., & Haas, J. D. (2000). Iron supplementation improves endurance after training in iron-depleted, nonanemic women. *Journal of Applied Physiology, 88*, 1103–1111.

Ihle, R., & Loucks, A. B. (2004). Dose-response relationships between energy availability and bone turnover in young exercising women. *Journal of Bone and Mineral Research: The Official Journal of the American Society for Bone and Mineral Research, 19*, 1231–1240.

Ivy, J. L., Goforth, H. W., Jr., Damon, B. M., McCauley, T. R., Parsons, E. C., & Price, T. B. (2002). Early postexercise muscle glycogen recovery is enhanced with a carbohydrate-protein supplement. *Journal of Applied Physiology, 93*, 1337–1344.

Ivy, J. L., Res, P. T., Sprague, R. C., & Widzer, M. O. (2003). Effect of a carbohydrate-protein supplement on endurance performance during exercise of varying intensity. *International Journal of Sport Nutrition and Exercise Metabolism, 13*, 382–395.

James, M. J., Gibson, R. A., & Cleland, L. G. (2000). Dietary polyunsaturated fatty acids and inflammatory mediator production. *American Journal of Clinical Nutrition, 71*(1 Suppl.), 343S–348S.

Jankowski, C. M., Ben-Ezra, V., Gozansky, W. S., & Scheaffer, S. E. (2004). Effects of oral contraceptives on glucoregulatory responses to exercise. *Metabolism, 53*, 348–352.

Jentjens, R. L., Achten, J., & Jeukendrup, A. E. (2004). High oxidation rates from combined carbohydrates ingested during exercise. *Medicine and Science in Sports and Exercise, 36*, 1551–1558.

Jentjens, R. L., Moseley, L., Waring, R. H., Harding, L. K., & Jeukendrup, A. E. (2004). Oxidation of combined ingestion of glucose and fructose during exercise. *Journal of Applied Physiology, 96*, 1277–1284.

Jentjens, R. L., van Loon, L. J., Mann, C. H., Wagenmakers, A. J., & Jeukendrup, A. E. (2001). Addition of protein and amino acids to carbohydrates does not enhance postexercise muscle glycogen synthesis. *Journal of Applied Physiology, 91*, 839–846.

Jentjens, R. L., Venables, M. C., & Jeukendrup, A. E. (2004). Oxidation of exogenous glucose, sucrose, and maltose during prolonged cycling exercise. *Journal of Applied Physiology, 96*, 1285–1291.

Jeukendrup, A. E., & Martin, J. (2001). Improving cycling performance: How should we spend our time and money? *Sports Medicine, 31*, 559–569.

Johnson, N. A., Stannard, S. R., Mehalski, K., Trenell, M. I., Sachinwalla, T., Thompson, C. H., et al. (2003). Intramyocellular triacylglycerol in prolonged cycling with high- and low-carbohydrate availability. *Journal of Applied Physiology, 94*, 1365–1372.

Jones, A. M., Carter, H., Pringle, J. S., & Campbell, I. T. (2002). Effect of creatine supplementation on oxygen uptake kinetics during submaximal cycle exercise. *Journal of Applied Physiology, 92*, 2571–2577.

Keen, A. D., & Drinkwater, B. L. (1997). Irreversible bone loss in former amenorrheic athletes. *Osteoporosis International: A Journal established as result of cooperation between the European Foundation for Osteoporosis and the National Osteoporosis Foundation of the USA, 7*, 311–315.

Keesey, R. E., & Corbett, S. W. (1984). Metabolic defense of the body weight set-point. *Research Publications-Association for Research in Nervous and Mental Disease, 62*, 87–96.

Krieger, J. W., Crowe, M., & Blank, S. E. (2004). Chronic glutamine supplementation increases nasal but not salivary IgA during 9 days of interval training. *Journal of Applied Physiology, 97*, 585–591.

Krzywkowski, K., Petersen, E. W., Ostrowski, K., Kristensen, J. H., Boza, J., & Pedersen, B. K. (2001). Effect of glutamine supplementation on exercise-induced changes in lymphocyte function. *American Journal of Physiology. Cell Physiology, 281*, C1259–C1265.

Krzywkowski, K., Petersen, E. W., Ostrowski, K., Link-Amster, H., Boza, J., Halkjaer-Kristensen, J., et al. (2001b). Effect of glutamine and protein supplementation on exercise-induced decreases in salivary IgA. *Journal of Applied Physiology, 91*, 832–838.

Lambert, G. P., Bleiler, T. L., Chang, R. T., Johnson, A. K., & Gisolfi, C. V. (1993). Effects of carbonated and noncarbonated beverages at specific intervals during treadmill running in the heat. *International Journal of Sport Nutrition, 3*, 177–193.

Larson-Meyer, D. E. (2002). Effect of postpartum exercise on mothers and their offspring: A review of the literature. *Obesity Research, 10*, 841–853.

Laughlin, G. A., & Yen, S. S. (1996). Nutritional and endocrine-metabolic aberrations in amenorrheic athletes. *The Journal of Clinical Endocrinology and Metabolism, 81*, 4301–4309.

Leachman Slawson, D., McClanahan, B. S., Clemens, L. H., Ward, K. D., Klesges, R. C., Vukadinovich, C. M., et al. (2001). Food sources of calcium in a sample of African-

American and Euro-American collegiate athletes. *International Journal of Sport Nutrition and Exercise Metabolism, 11,* 199–208.

Looker, A. C., Dallman, P. R., Carroll, M. D., Gunter, E. W., & Johnson, C. L. (1997). Prevalence of iron deficiency in the United States. *Journal of the American Medical Association, 277,* 973–976.

Loucks, A. B. (2004). Energy balance and body composition in sports and exercise. *Journal of Sports Science, 22,* 1–14.

Loucks, A. B., Laughlin, G. A., Mortola, J. F., Girton, L., Nelson, J. C., & Yen, S. S. (1992). Hypothalamic-pituitary-thyroidal function in eumenorrheic and amenorrheic athletes. *The Journal of Clinical Endocrinology and Metabolism, 75,* 514–518.

Loucks, A. B., & Verdun, M. (1998). Slow restoration of LH pulsatility by refeeding in energetically disrupted women. *American Journal of Physiology, 275*(4 Pt. 2), R1218–R1226.

Loud, K. J., Gordon, C. M., Micheli, L. J., & Field, A. E. (2005). Correlates of stress fractures among preadolescent and adolescent girls. *Pediatrics, 115,* e399–e406.

Lovallo, W. R., Wilson, M. F., Vincent, A. S., Sung, B. H., McKey, B. S., & Whitsett, T. L. (2004). Blood pressure response to caffeine shows incomplete tolerance after short-term regular consumption. *Hypertension, 43,* 760–765.

Marino, F. E., Kay, D., & Cannon, J. (2003). Glycerol hyperhydration fails to improve endurance performance and thermoregulation in humans in a warm humid environment. *Pflügers Archiv: European Journal of Physiology, 446,* 455–462.

Markou, K. B., Mylonas, P., Theodoropoulou, A., Kontogiannis, A., Leglise, M., Vagenakis, A. G., et al. (2004). The influence of intensive physical exercise on bone acquisition in adolescent elite female and male artistic gymnasts. *The Journal of Clinical Endocrinology and Metabolism, 89,* 4383–4387.

McCargar, L. J., & Crawford, S. M. (1992). Metabolic and anthropometric changes with weight cycling in wrestlers. *Medicine and Science in Sports and Exercise, 24,* 1270–1275.

Melby, C. L., Schmidt, W. D., & Corrigan, D. (1990). Resting metabolic rate in weight-cycling collegiate wrestlers compared with physically active, noncycling control subjects. *American Journal of Clinical Nutrition, 52,* 409–414.

Miyauchi, T., Maeda, S., Iemitsu, M., Kobayashi, T., Kumagai, Y., Yamaguchi, I., et al. (2003). Exercise causes a tissue-specific change of NO production in the kidney and lung. *Journal of Applied Physiology, 94,* 60–68.

Murphy, S. P., & Johnson, R. K. (2003). The scientific basis of recent US guidance on sugars intake. *American Journal of Clinical Nutrition, 78,* 827S–833S.

Otis, C. L., Drinkwater, B., Johnson, M., Loucks, A., & Wilmore, J. (1997). American College of Sports Medicine position stand. The female athlete triad. *Medicine and Science in Sports and Exercise, 29,* i–ix.

Parcell, A. C., Smith, J. M., Schulthies, S. S., Myrer, J. W., & Fellingham, G. (2004). Cordyceps sinensis (CordyMax Cs-4) supplementation does not improve endurance exercise performance. *Internation Journal of Sport Nutrition and Exercise Metabolism, 14,* 236–242.

Park, Y., & Harris, W. S. (2003). Omega-3 fatty acid supplementation accelerates chylomicron triglyceride clearance. *Journal of Lipid Research, 44,* 455–463.

Petersmarck, K. A., Teitelbaum, H. S., Bond, J. T., Bianchi, L., Hoerr, S. M., & Sowers, M. F. (1999). The effect of weight cycling on blood lipids and blood pressure in the Multiple Risk Factor Intervention Trial Special Intervention Group. *International Journal of Obesity and Related Metabolic Disorders, 23,* 1246–1255.

Petibois, C., Cassaigne, A., Gin, H., & Deleris, G. (2004). Lipid profile disorders induced by long-term cessation of physical activity in previously highly endurance-trained subjects. *The Journal of Clinical Endocrinology and Metabolism, 89,* 3377–3384.

Rasmussen, B. B., Hancock, C. R., & Winder, W. W. (1998). Postexercise recovery of skeletal muscle malonyl-CoA, acetyl-CoA carboxylase, and AMP-activated protein kinase. *Journal of Applied Physiology, 85,* 1629–1634.

Rickenlund, A., Carlstrom, K., Ekblom, B., Brismar, T. B., Von Schoultz, B., & Hirschberg, A. L. (2004). Effects of oral contraceptives on body composition and physical performance in female athletes. *The Journal of Clinical Endocrinology and Metabolism, 89,* 4364–4370.

Rickenlund, A., Thoren, M., Carlstrom, K., von Schoultz, B., & Hirschberg, A. L. (2004). Diurnal profiles of testosterone and pituitary hormones suggest different mechanisms for menstrual disturbances in endurance athletes. *The Journal of Clinical Endocrinology and Metabolism, 89,* 702–707.

Rivera-Brown, A. M., Gutierrez, R., Gutierrez, J. C., Frontera, W. R., & Bar-Or, O. (1999). Drink composition, voluntary drinking, and fluid balance in exercising, trained, heat-acclimatized boys. *Journal of Applied Physiology, 86,* 78–84.

Rogol, A. D. (2000). Sex steroid and growth hormone supplementation to enhance performance in adolescent athletes. *Current Opinion on Pediatrics, 12,* 382–387.

Rogol, A. D., Clark, P. A., & Roemmich, J. N. (2000). Growth and pubertal development in children and adolescents: Effects of diet and physical activity. *American Journal of Clinical Nutrition, 72*(2 Suppl.), 521S–528S.

Ruderman, N. B., Park, H., Kaushik, V. K., Dean, D., Constant, S., Prentki, M., et al. (2003). AMPK as a metabolic switch in rat muscle, liver and adipose tissue after exercise. *Acta Physiologica Scandinavica, 178,* 435–442.

Saris, W. H., van Erp-Baart, M. A., Brouns, F., Westerterp, K. R., & ten Hoor, F. (1989). Study on food intake and energy expenditure during extreme sustained exercise: The Tour de France. *International Journal of Sports Medicine, 10*(Suppl 1.), S26–S31.

Saunders, M. J., Kane, M. D., & Todd, M. K. (2004). Effects of a carbohydrate-protein beverage on cycling endurance and muscle damage. *Medicine and Science in Sports and Exercise, 36*, 1233–1238.

Sea, M. M., Fong, W. P., Huang, Y., & Chen, Z. Y. (2000). Weight cycling-induced alteration in fatty acid metabolism. *American Journal of Physiology. Regulatory, Integrative and Comparative Physiology, 279*, R1145–R1155.

Sherman, W. M., Doyle, J. A., Lamb, D. R., & Strauss, R. H. (1993). Dietary carbohydrate, muscle glycogen, and exercise performance during 7 d of training. *American Journal of Clinical Nutrition, 57*, 27–31.

Shirreffs, S. M., & Maughan, R. J. (1998). Volume repletion after exercise-induced volume depletion in humans: Replacement of water and sodium losses. *American Journal of Physiology, 274*(5 Pt. 2), F868–F875.

Sinclair, L. M., & Hinton, P. S. (2005). Prevalence of iron deficiency with and without anemia in recreationally active men and women. *Journal of the American Dietetic Association, 105*, 975–978.

Stamler, J. S., & Meissner, G. (2001). Physiology of nitric oxide in skeletal muscle. *Physiology Review, 81*, 209–237.

Steen, S. N., Oppliger, R. A., & Brownell, K. D. (1988). Metabolic effects of repeated weight loss and regain in adolescent wrestlers. *Journal of the American Medical Association, 260*, 47–50.

Terjung, R. L., Clarkson, P., Eichner, E. R., Greenhaff, P. L., Hespel, P. J., Israel, R. G., et al. (2000). American College of Sports Medicine roundtable. The physiological and health effects of oral creatine supplementation. *Medicine and Science in Sports and Exercise, 32*, 706–717.

Tipton, K. D., Borsheim, E., Wolf, S. E., Sanford, A. P., & Wolfe, R. R. (2003). Acute response of net muscle protein balance reflects 24-h balance after exercise and amino acid ingestion. *American Journal of Physiology. Endocrinology and Metabolism, 284*, E76–E89.

Tipton, K. D., Ferrando, A. A., Phillips, S. M., Doyle, D., Jr., & Wolfe, R. R. (1999). Postexercise net protein synthesis in human muscle from orally administered amino acids. *American Journal of Physiology, 276*(4 Pt. 1), E628–E634.

Turner, L. W., & Bass, M. A. (2001). Osteoporosis knowledge, attitudes, and behaviors of female collegiate athletes. *International Journal of Sport Nutrition and Exercise Metabolism, 11*, 482–489.

Ukropec, J., Reseland, J. E., Gasperikova, D., Demcakova, E., Madsen, L., Berge, R. K., et al. (2003). The hypotriglyceridemic effect of dietary n-3 FA is associated with increased beta-oxidation and reduced leptin expression. *Lipids, 38*, 1023–1029.

U.S. Department of Health and Human Services (DHHS). Technical report to USDA and HHS.

U.S. Department of Health and Human Services (DHHS). (n.d.). *Bone Health and Osteoporosis: A Report of the Surgeon General.* Washington, DC: Office of the Surgeon General.

Van Baak, M. A., & Saris, W. H. (2000). The effect of caffeine on endurance performance after nonselective beta-adrenergic blockade. *Medicine and Science in Sports and Exercise, 32*, 499–503.

van Loon, L. J., Schrauwen-Hinderling, V. B., Koopman, R., Wagenmakers, A. J., Hesselink, M. K., Schaart, G., et al. (2003). Influence of prolonged endurance cycling and recovery diet on intramuscular triglyceride content in trained males. *American Journal of Physiology. Endocrinology and Metabolism, 285*, E804–E811.

Venables, M. C., Shaw, L., Jeukendrup, A. E., Roedig-Penman, A., Finke, M., Newcombe, R. G., et al. (2005). Erosive effect of a new sports drink on dental enamel during exercise. *Medicine and Science in Sports and Exercise, 37*, 39–44.

Waters, D. L., Qualls, C. R., Dorin, R., Veldhuis, J. D., & Baumgartner, R. N. (2001). Increased pulsatility, process irregularity, and nocturnal trough concentrations of growth hormone in amenorrheic compared to eumenorrheic athletes. *The Journal of Clinical Endocrinology and Metabolism, 86*, 1013–1019.

Watkins, B. A., Li, Y., Lippman, H. E., & Seifert, M. F. (2001). Omega-3 polyunsaturated fatty acids and skeletal health. *Experimental Biology and Medicine, 226*, 485–497.

Watson, J., Deary, I., & Kerr, D. (2002). Central and peripheral effects of sustained caffeine use: Tolerance is incomplete. *British Journal of Clinical Pharmacology, 54*, 400–406.

Williams, M. B., Raven, P. B., Fogt, D. L., & Ivy, J. L. (2003). Effects of recovery beverages on glycogen restoration and endurance exercise performance. *Journal of Strength and Conditioning Research/National Strength & Conditioning Association, 17*, 12–19.

Willis, W. T., Brooks, G. A., Henderson, S. A., & Dallman, P. R. (1987). Effects of iron deficiency and training on mitochondrial enzymes in skeletal muscle. *Journal of Applied Physiology, 62*, 2442–2446.

Wolfe, R. R. (2000). Protein supplements and exercise. *American Journal of Clinical Nutrition, 72*(2 Suppl.), 551S–557S.

Wolfe, R. R., Klein, S., Carraro, F., & Weber, J. M. (1990). Role of triglyceride-fatty acid cycle in controlling fat metabolism in humans during and after exercise. *American Journal of Physiology, 258*(2 Pt. 1), E382–E389.

World Anti-Doping Agency. (2005). The Prohibited List. World Anti-Doping Code. Montreal, Canada: Author.

Wright, K. S., Quinn, T. J., & Carey, G. B. (2002). Infant acceptance of breast milk after maternal exercise. *Pediatrics, 109*, 585–589.

Wyss, M., & Kaddurah-Daouk, R. (2000). Creatine and creatinine metabolism. *Physiology Review, 80*, 1107–1213.

Yeager, K. K., Agostini, R., Nattiv, A., & Drinkwater, B. (1993). The female athlete triad: Disordered eating, amenorrhea, osteoporosis. *Medicine and Science in Sports and Exercise, 25*, 775–777.

Zhu, J. S., Halpern, G. M., & Jones, K. (1998a). The scientific rediscovery of an ancient Chinese herbal medicine: Cordyceps sinensis. Part I. *Journal of Aternative and Complementary Medicine (New York, N.Y.), 4*, 289–303.

Zhu, J. S., Halpern, G. M., & Jones, K. (1998b). The scientific rediscovery of a precious ancient Chinese herbal regimen: Cordyceps sinensis. Part II. *Journal of Aternative and Complementary Medicine (New York, N.Y.), 4*, 429–457.

Pediatric Diabetes

American Diabetes Association. (1999). Diabetes mellitus and exercise. *Diabetes Care,* (Suppl.), S49–S53.

American Diabetes Association. (2000). Type 2 diabetes in children and adolescents. *Pediatrics, 105*, 671–680.

American Diabetes Association. (2005). Standards of medical care. *Diabetes Care, 28* (Suppl. 1), S4–S36.

American Diabetes Association. (2006). Diagnosis and classification of diabetes mellitus. *Diabetes Care, 29* (Suppl. 1), S43–S48.

American Dietetic Association. (2006). Position of the American Dietetic Association: Individual-, family-, school-, and community-based interventions for pediatric overweight. *Journal of the American Dietetic Association, 106*, 925–945.

Artz, E., & Freemark, M. (2004). The pathogenesis of insulin resistance in children: metabolic complications and the roles of diet, exercise and pharmacotherapy in the prevention of type 2 diabetes. *Pediatric Endocrinology Reviews, 1*, 296–309.

Artz, E., Haqq, A., & Freemark, M. (2005). Hormonal and metabolic consequences of childhood obesity. *Endocrinology and Metabolism Clinics of North America, 34*, 643–658.

Aye, T., & Levitsky, L. L. (2003). Type 2 diabetes: An epidemic disease in childhood. *Current Opinion in Pediatrics, 15*, 411–415.

Barker, D. J. (2000). In utero programming of cardiovascular disease. *Theriogenology, 53*, 555–574.

Bell, S. J., Grochoski, G. T., & Clarke, A. J. (2006). Health implications of milk containing ß-casein with the A2 genetic variant. *Critical Reviews in Food Science and Nutrition, 46*, 93–100.

Bergman, R. N., Finegood, D. T., & Kahn, S. E. (2002). The evolution of beta cell dysfunction and insulin resistance in type 2 diabetes. *European Journal of Clinical Investigations, 32*, 35–45.

Berry, D., Urban, A., & Grey, M. (2006). Management of type 2 diabetes in youth (part 2). *Journal of Pediatric Health Care, 20*, 88–97.

Botero, D., & Wolfsdorf, J. I. (2005). Diabetes mellitus in children and adolescents. *Archives of Medical Research, 36*, 281–290.

Centers for Disease Control and Prevention. (2005). Diabetes projects. Retrieved June 28, 2006, from www.cdc.gov/diabetes/projects/cda2.htm

Centers for Disease Control and Prevention. (n.d.). National Center for Chronic Disease Prevention and Health Promotion. Healthy youth! Physical activity, promoting better health. Retrieved July 3, 2006, from http://www.cdc.gov/healthyyouth/physicalactivity/promoting_health/

Copeland, K., Pankratz, K., Cathey, V., Immohotichey, P., Maddox, J., Felton, B., et al. (2006). Acanthosis nigricans, insulin resistance (HOMA) and dyslipidemia among Native American children. *The Journal of the Oklahoma State Medical Association, 99*, 19–24.

Cruz, M. L., Shaibi, G. Q., Weigensberg, M. J., Spruijt-Metz, D., Ball, G. D., & Goran, M. I. (2005). Pediatric obesity and insulin resistance: Chronic disease risk and implications for treatment and prevention beyond body weight modification. *Annual Reviews of Nutrition, 25*, 435–468.

Diabetes Research in Children Network Study Group. (2006). The effects of aerobic exercise on glucose and counterregulatory hormone concentrations in children with type 1 diabetes. *Diabetes Care, 29*, 20–25.

Ello-Martin, J. A., Ledikwe, J. H., & Rolls, B. J. (2005). The influence of food portion size and energy density on energy intake: implications for weight management. *American Journal of Clinical Nutrition, 82* (1 Suppl.), 236S–241S.

Eisenbarth, G. S. (1986). Type 1 diabetes mellitus: A chronic autoimmune disease. *New England Journal of Medicine, 314*, 1360–1368.

Evangelia, Z., Erasmia, K., & Dimitrios, L. (2006). Treatment options of polycystic ovary syndrome in adolescence. *Pediatric Endocrinology Reviews: PER, 3* (Suppl. 1), 208–213.

Fagot-Campagna, A., Pettitt, D. J., Engelgau, M. M., Burrows, N. R., Geiss, L. S., Valdez, R., et al. (2000). Type 2 diabetes among North American children and adolescents: An epidemiologic review and a public health perspective. *Journal of Pediatrics, 136*, 664–672.

Goran, M. I., Ball, G. D., & Cruz, M. L. (2003). Obesity and risk of type 2 diabetes and cardiovascular disease in children and adolescents. *The Journal of Clinical Endocrinology and Metabolism, 88*, 1417–1427.

Haller, M. J., Atkinson, M. A., & Schatz, D. (2005). Type 1 diabetes mellitus: etiology, presentation, and management. *Pediatric Clinics of North America, 52*, 1553–1578.

Hamalainen, A. M. & Knip, M. (2002). Autoimmunity and familial risk of type 1 diabetes. *Current Diabetes Reports, 2*, 347–353.

Hermanns-Lê, T., Scheen, A., & Pierard, G. E. (2004). Acanthosis nigricans associated with insulin resistance: Pathophysiology and management. *American Journal of Clinical Dermatology, 5*, 199–203.

Institute of Medicine. (2005). Panel on Micronutrients, Subcommittees on Upper Reference Levels of Nutrients and of Interpretation and Use of Dietary Reference Intakes, and the Standing Committee on the Scientific Evaluation of Dietary Reference Intakes. Dietary reference intakes for energy, carbohydrates, fiber, fat, protein, and amino acids (macronutrients). Washington, DC: National Academy Press.

International Society for Pediatric and Adolescent Diabetes. (2000). Consensus guidelines for the management of type 1 diabetes mellitus in children and adolescents. Retrieved July 6, 2006, from http://www.diabetesguidelines.com/health/dwk/pro/guidelines/ispad/ispad.asp

Jeffery, R. W., Baxter, J., McGuire, M., & Linde, J. (2006). Are fast food restaurants an environmental risk factor for obesity? Retrieved July 10, 2006, from http://www.ijbnpa.org/content/3/1/2

Karvonen, M., Viik-Kajander, M., Moltchanova, E., Libman, I., LaPorte, R., & Tuomilehto, J. (2000). Incidence of childhood type 1 diabetes worldwide: Diabetes Mondiale (DiaMond) Project Group. *Diabetes Care, 23*, 1516–1526.

Keenan, H., Lipton, R., Zierold, K., Patel, A., Stolte, K., & Chambers, E. (1999). What proportion of diabetes in minority young people is actually type 2? *American Journal of Epidemiology, 149* (Suppl. 2), 11.

Kitagawa, T., Owada, M., Urakami, T., & Yamauchi, K. (1998). Increased incidence of non-insulin dependent diabetes mellitus among Japanese schoolchildren correlates with an increased intake of animal protein and fat. *Clinical Pediatrics, 37*, 111–115.

Ku, C. Y., Gower, B. A., Hunter, G. R., & Goran, M. I. (2000). Racial differences in insulin secretion and sensitivity in prepubertal children: Role of physical fitness and physical activity. *Obesity Research, 8*, 506–515.

LaPorte, R. E. M. M., & Chang, Y.-F. (1995). *Prevalence and Incidence of Insulin-Dependent Diabetes.* Bethesda, MD: National Institutes of Health.

Maffeis, C., Talamini, G., & Tato, L. (1998). Influence of diet, physical activity and parents' obesity on children's adiposity: a four-year longitudinal study. *International Journal of Obesity and Related Metabolic Disorders, 22*, 758–764.

Magarey, A. M., Daniels, L. A., Boulton, T. J., & Cockington, R. A. (2001). Does fat intake predict adiposity in healthy children and adolescents aged 2–15 y? A longitudinal analysis. *European Journal of Clinical Nutrition, 55*, 471–481.

Marr, L. (2004). Soft drinks, childhood overweight, and the role of nutrition educators: Let's base our solutions on reality and sound science. *Journal of Nutrition Education and Behavior, 36*, 258–265.

Meurer, L. N., Kroll, A. P., Jamieson, B., & Yousefi, P. (2006). Clinical inquiries. What is the best way to diagnose polycystic ovarian syndrome? *Journal of Family Practice, 55*, 351–352, 354.

Nassis, G. P., Papantakou, K., Skenderi, K., Triandafillopoulou, M., Kavouras, S. A., Yannakoulia, M., et al. (2005). Aerobic exercise training improves insulin sensitivity without changes in body weight, body fat, adiponectin, and inflammatory markers in overweight and obese girls. *Metabolism, 54*, 1472–1479.

Norris, J. M., Barriga, K., Klingensmith, G., Hoffman, M., Eisenbarth, G. S., Erlich, H. A., et al. (2003). Timing of initial cereal exposure in infancy and risk of islet autoimmunity. *Journal of the American Medical Association, 290*, 1713–1720.

PCOS Consensus Workshop Group. (2004). Revised 2003 consensus on diagnostic criteria and long-term health risks related to polycystic ovary syndrome (PCOS). *Human Reproduction, 19*, 41–47.

Pollock, M. L., Franklin, B. A., Balady, G. J., Chaitman, B. L., Fleg, J. L., Fletcher, B., et al. (2000). Resistance exercise in individuals with and without cardiovascular disease: Benefits, rationale, safety, and prescription. An advisory from the Committee on Exercise, Rehabilitation, and Prevention, Council on Clinical Cardiology, and American Heart Association. Position paper endorsed by the American College of Sports Medicine. *Circulation, 101*, 828–833.

Reaven, G. M., Chen, Y. D., Hollenbeck, C. B., Sheu, W. H., Ostrega, D., & Polonsky, K. S. (1993). Plasma insulin, C-peptide, and proinsulin concentrations in obese and nonobese individuals with varying degrees of glucose intolerance. *The Journal of Clinical Endocrinology and Metabolism, 76*, 44–48.

Rodriguez, G., & Moreno, L. A. (2006). Is dietary intake able to explain differences in body fatness in children and adolescents? *Nutrition, Metabolism, and Cardiovascular Diseases: NMCD, 16*, 294–301.

Saaddine, J. B., Fagot-Campagna, A., Rolka, D., Narayan, K. M., Geiss, L., Eberhardt, M., et al. (2002). Distribution of HbA(1c) levels for children and young adults in the U.S.: Third National Health and Nutrition Examination Survey. *Diabetes Care, 25*, 1326–1330.

Sobngwi, E., Boudou, P., Mauvais-Jarvis, F., Leblanc, H., Velho, G., Vexiau, P., et al. (2003). Effect of a diabetic environment in utero on predisposition to type 2 diabetes. *Lancet, 361*, 1861–1865.

Soliman, A. T., Omar, M., Assem, H. M., Nasr, I. S., Rizk, M. M., El Matary, W., et al. (2002). Serum leptin concentrations in children with type 1 diabetes mellitus: Relationship to body mass index, insulin dose, and glycemic control. *Metabolism, 51*, 292–296.

Steyn, N. P., Mann, J., Bennett, P. H., Temple, N., Zimmet, P., Tuomilehto, J., et al. (2004). Diet, nutrition and the prevention of type 2 diabetes. *Public Health Nutrition, 7*, 147–165.

Strong, W. B., Malina, R. M., Blimkie, C. J., Daniels, S. R., Dishman, R. K., Gutin, B., et al. (2005). Evidence based physical activity for school-age youth. *Journal of Pediatrics, 146*, 732–737.

Tamborlane, W., Fredrickson, L. P., & Ahern, J. H. (2003). Insulin pump therapy in childhood diabetes mellitus. *Treatments in Endocrinology, 2*, 11–21.

Taveras, E. M., Rifas-Shiman, S. L., Berkey, C. S., Rockett, H. R., Field, A. E., Frazier, A. L., et al. (2005). Family dinner and adolescent overweight. *Obesity Research, 13*, 900–906.

Ten, S., & Maclaren, N. (2004). Insulin resistance syndrome in children. *The Journal of Clinical Endocrinology and Metabolism, 89*, 2526–2539.

U.S. Department of Agriculture, Department of Health and Human Services. (2005). Dietary guidelines for Americans. Retrieved July 3, 2006, from http://www.healthierus.gov/dietaryguidelines/

U.S. Department of Health and Human Services, National Diabetes Education Program. (2006). Overview of diabetes in children and adolescents. Retrieved July 3, 2006, from http://ndep.nih.gov/diabetes/pubs/Youth_FactSheet.pdf

Wilkin, T. J., Metcalf, B. S., Murphy, M. J., Kirkby, J., Jeffery, A. N., & Voss, L. D. (2002). The relative contributions of birth weight, weight change, and current weight to insulin resistance in contemporary 5-year-olds: The Early Bird Study. *Diabetes, 51*, 3468–3472.

Williams, D. E., Cadwell, B. L., Cheng, Y. J., Cowie, C. C., Gregg, E. W., Geiss, L. S., et al. (2005). Prevalence of impaired fasting glucose and its relationship with cardiovascular disease risk factors in US adolescents, 1999–2000. *Pediatrics, 116*, 1122–1126.

Xita, N., & Tsatsoulis, A. (2006). Review: Fetal programming of polycystic ovary syndrome by androgen excess: Evidence from experimental, clinical, and genetic association studies. *The Journal of Clinical Endocrinology and Metabolism, 91*, 1660–1666.

Ziegler, A. G., Schmid, S., Huber, D., Hummel, M., & Bonifacio, E. (2003). Early infant feeding and risk of developing type 1 diabetes-associated autoantibodies. *Journal of the American Medical Association, 290*, 1721–1728.

Disordered Eating

Agras, W. S., Brandt, H. A., Bulik, C. M., Dolan-Sewell, R., Fairburn, C. G., Halmi, K. A., et al. (2004). Report of the National Institutes of Health workshop on overcoming barriers to treatment research in anorexia nervosa. *International Journal of Eating Disorders, 35*, 509–521.

American Dietetic Association. (2001). Position paper: Nutrition intervention in the treatment of anorexia nervosa, bulimia nervosa, and eating disorders not otherwise specified (EDNOS). *Journal of the American Dietetic Association, 101*, 810–819.

American Psychiatric Association. (2000). *Diagnostic and Statistical Manual of Mental Disorders* (4th ed., text revision). Washington, DC: American Psychiatric Association.

Andersen, A. E. (1999). Gender-related aspects of eating disorders: A guide to practice. *Journal of Gender Specific Medicine, 2*, 47–54.

Becker, A. E., Grinspoon, S. K., Klibanski, A., & Herzog, D. B. (1999). Eating disorders. *New England Journal of Medicine, 340*, 1092–1098.

Birmingham, C. L., Puddicombe, D., & Hlynsky, J. (2004). Hypomagnesemia during refeeding in anorexia nervosa. *Eating and Weight Disorders: EWD, 9*, 236–237.

De Souza, M. J., Leidy, H. J., O'Donnell, E., Lasley, B., & Williams, N. I. (2004). Fasting ghrelin levels in physically active women: Relationship with menstrual disturbances and metabolic hormones. *The Journal of Clinical Endocrinology and Metabolism, 89*, 3536–3542.

de Zwaan, M., Aslam, Z., & Mitchell, J. E. (2002). Research on energy expenditure in individuals with eating disorders: A review. *International Journal of Eating Disorders, 32*, 127–134.

Fairburn, C. G., & Bohn, K. (2005). Eating disorder NOS (EDNOS): An example of the troublesome "not otherwise specified" (NOS) category in DSM-IV. *Behaviour Research and Therapy, 43*, 691–701.

Fairburn, C. G., & Harrison, P. J. (2003). Eating disorders. *Lancet, 361*, 407–416.

Fisher, M., Simpser, E., & Schneider, M. (2000). Hypophosphatemia secondary to oral refeeding in anorexia nervosa. *International Journal of Eating Disorders, 28*, 181–187.

Goodman, L. R. (2005). The female athlete and menstrual function. *Current Opinion in Obstetrics and Gynecology, 17*, 466–470.

Grinspoon, S., Miller, K., Herzog, D., Clemmons, D., & Klibanski, A. (2003). Effects of recombinant human insulin-like growth factor (IGF)-I and estrogen administration on IGF-I, IGF binding protein (IGFBP)-2, and IGFBP-3 in anorexia nervosa: A randomized-controlled study. *The Journal of Clinical Endocrinology and Metabolism, 88*, 1142–1149.

Grinspoon, S., Miller, K. K., Herzog, D. B., Grieco, K. A., & Klibanski, A. (2004). Effects of estrogen and recombinant human insulin-like growth factor-I on ghrelin secretion in severe undernutrition. *The Journal of Clinical Endocrinology and Metabolism, 89*, 3988–3993.

Grinspoon, S. K., Friedman, A. J., Miller, K. K., Lippman, J., Olson, W. H., & Warren, M. P. (2003). Effects of a triphasic combination oral contraceptive containing norgestimate/ethinyl estradiol on biochemical markers of bone metabolism in young women with osteopenia secondary to hypothalamic amenorrhea. *The Journal of Clinical Endocrinology and Metabolism, 88*, 3651–3656.

Heer, M., Mika, C., Grzella, I., Heussen, N., & Herpertz-Dahlmann, B. (2004). Bone turnover during inpatient nutritional therapy and outpatient follow-up in patients with anorexia nervosa compared with that in healthy control subjects. *American Journal of Clinical Nutrition, 80*, 774–781.

Helgstrand, S., & Andersen, A. M. (2005). Maternal underweight and the risk of spontaneous abortion. *Acta Obstetricia Et Gynecologica Scandinavica, 84*, 1197–1201.

Henig, R. M. (2004, November 30). Sorry. Your Eating Disorder Doesn't Meet Our Criteria. *New York Times*.

Kaye, W. H., Frank, G. K., Bailer, U. F., & Henry, S. E. (2005). Neurobiology of anorexia nervosa: Clinical implications of alterations of the function of serotonin and other neuronal systems. *International Journal of Eating Disorders, 37* (Suppl.), S15–S19; discussion S20–S11.

Kaye, W. H., Frank, G. K., Bailer, U. F., Henry, S. E., Meltzer, C. C., Price, J. C., et al. (2005). Serotonin alterations in anorexia and bulimia nervosa: New insights from imaging studies. *Physiology & Behavior, 85*, 73–81.

Keys, A., Brozek, J., Henschel, A., Mickelsen, O., & Taylor, H. L. (1950). *The Biology of Human Starvation I-II*. Minneapolis, MN: University of Minnesota Press.

Klump, K. L., & Gobrogge, K. L. (2005). A review and primer of molecular genetic studies of anorexia nervosa. *International Journal of Eating Disorders, 37* (Suppl.), S43–S48; discussion S87–S49.

Kouba, S., Hallstrom, T., Lindholm, C., & Hirschberg, A. L. (2005). Pregnancy and neonatal outcomes in women with eating disorders. *Obstetrics and Gynecology, 105,* 255–260.

Lask, B. (2004). Pervasive refusal syndrome. *Advances in Psychiatric Treatment, 10,* 153–159.

Miller, K. K., Grieco, K. A., Mulder, J., Grinspoon, S., Mickley, D., Yehezkel, R., et al. (2004). Effects of risedronate on bone density in anorexia nervosa. *The Journal of Clinical Endocrinology and Metabolism, 89,* 3903–3906.

Morris, L. G., Stephenson, K. E., Herring, S., & Marti, J. L. (2004). Recurrent acute pancreatitis in anorexia and bulimia. *JOP: Journal of the Pancreas, 5,* 231–234.

Rocco, P. L., Orbitello, B., Perini, L., Pera, V., Ciano, R. P., & Balestrieri, M. (2005). Effects of pregnancy on eating attitudes and disorders: A prospective study. *Journal of Psychosomatic Research, 59,* 175–179.

Sanford, T. C., Davidson, M. M., Yakushoko, O. F, Martens, M. P., Hinton, P. S., & Beck, N. C. (2005). Clinical and subclinical eating disorders: An examination of collegiate athletes. *Journal of Applied Sport Psychology, 17,* 79–86.

Stewart, T. M., & Williamson, D. A. (2004). Multidisciplinary treatment of eating disorders. Part 1. Structure and costs of treatment. *Behavior Modification, 28,* 812–830.

Swenne, I. (2000). Heart risk associated with weight loss in anorexia nervosa and eating disorders: Electrocardiographic changes during the early phase of refeeding. *Acta Paediatrica, 89,* 447–452.

Verrotti, A., Catino, M., De Luca, F. A., Morgese, G., & Chiarelli, F. (1999). Eating disorders in adolescents with type 1 diabetes mellitus. *Acta Diabetologica, 36,* 21–25.

Watkins, B. L. B. (2002). Eating disorders in school-aged children. *Child and Adolescent Psychiatric Clinics of North America, 11,* 185–199.

SECTION

2

Adult Evidence-Based Nutrition in the Life Cycle

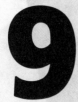

CHAPTER

9

Special Topics in Adult Nutrition: Chronic Disease Nutritional Assessment

Jennifer L. Bueche, PhD, RD, CDN

CHAPTER OUTLINE

After studying this chapter and reflecting on the contents, you should be able to

1. Outline the metabolic changes associated with the aging process and their impact on the nutritional requirements of adults throughout adulthood.

2. Refer to the Dietary Reference Intake to determine nutritional requirements for an individual or life stage group (specifically ages 19 to 30, 31 to 50, and 51 to 70).

3. Describe how to perform a nutritional assessment of an adult based on the American Dietetic Association Nutrition Care Process and Model.

4. Identify the chronic diseases in adulthood that are most related to diet, the resulting nutritional implications, and subsequent appropriate medical nutritional therapy.

5. Apply the American Dietetic Association Nutrition Care Process and Model to the case study provided.

6. Discuss the nutritional issues of epidemic proportion in the adult population and the recommended nutrition intervention.

This chapter begins by defining adulthood and outlining the metabolic changes associated with the aging process. This is important to understand because the maturation process greatly impacts the dietary recommendation and the nutritional requirements of adults throughout their life as they age. In 1997 the Recommended Daily Allowance (RDA) went through a major overhaul to incorporate not only prevention of disease but promotion of health. The Dietary Reference Intake (DRI) replaced the RDA and has been issued in stages since then (Appendix 2). This information is presented and discussed with regard to the life stage groups (i.e., ages 19 to 30, 31 to 50, and 51 to 70) that span most of the adult years. Next, this chapter reviews the components of the nutritional assessment process and introduces the new American Dietetic Association (ADA) Nutrition Care Process and Model. Given that this textbook is an evidence-based approach, for each of the chronic diseases presented, the research literature was reviewed to provide evidence-based practice guidelines as they exist related to the four steps in the nutrition care process (nutrition assessment, nutrition diagnosis, nutrition intervention, and/or nutrition monitoring) and evaluation for each particular chronic disease state. In addition, overweight/obesity and osteoporosis have been highlighted given their rise to epidemic proportions in the adult population.

Definition of Adulthood

Adulthood can span 60+ years depending on a person's genetic predisposition and the choices a person makes throughout his or her life, including how healthy he or she chooses to eat. Life expectancy in the United States is 77.6 years based on the latest data released in February 2005 by the National Center for Health Statistics, with women still living longer than men (80.1 years versus 74.8 years, respectively) (Kochanek, Murphy, Anderson, & Scott, 2004). Not surprising, given the obesity epidemic in this country and the ensuing health consequences, a potential decline in life expectancy has been predicted in the first half of this century (Olshansky et al., 2005). That is, for the first time in 1,000 years, children today will not live as long as their parents.

In this chapter the adult years are initially broken down into three phases, the *young* adult years, the *middle* adult years, and the *older* adult years, because they coincide with the life stage groups outlined by the DRI (i.e., ages 19 to 30, 31 to 50, and 51 to 70).

This makes presenting nutritional requirements across such a large span of years much easier to manage.

Young Adult Years (Ages 19 to 30)

- Typically, growth and maturation are completed by early adulthood, although some males can grow slightly after age 20 (Brown et al., 2005).
- At this point the focus shifts to maintaining health and physical fitness and avoiding weight gain. This may be particularly challenging for college students, especially freshman, given the requirement to purchase an "all you care to eat" dining plan, a lack of involvement in sports because of time constraints, and competing with the net average weight gain of 15 pounds (Kelly, 2003; Levitsky & Youn, 2004).
- Bone density continues to develop until ages 30 to 35.
- Muscle mass continues to grow as long as muscles are used.
- Young adults tend to be very involved in their careers. If they are married with children both parents are juggling the demands of work, family, and day care.
- There are many different definitions of "family." Reproduction may or may not be seen as a priority. According to the latest reports from the Centers for Disease Control and Prevention, in 1970 the average age for a first-time mother was about 21; today that age is 25 to 29 years (Martin et al., 2005).
- Women of reproductive age have special nutrition needs that must be addressed at each stage: before conception, prenatal, and postnatal/lactation.
- Alcohol intake accounts for 5% of calorie intake between ages 20 and 34 (Kant, 2000).
- The **prevalence** of selected chronic conditions for 18- to 24-year-olds based on the top five conditions were asthma (13.7%), chronic joint symptoms (11.1%), sinusitis (8.3%), hay fever (5.7%), and doctor's diagnosis of arthritis (3.5%) (National Center for Health Statistics, 1984–1995).

Prevalence: The percentage of a population that is affected with a particular disease at a given time.

Middle Adult Years (Ages 31 to 50)

- Beginning at about age 30, physiologic functions that impact mobility begin to decline at the rate of about 1% or more per year (Worthington-Roberts, 1996).

- Body composition begins to shift; weight may seem like it is harder to lose. Weight gain usually seen after age 40 in women and men goes hand in hand with hormonal changes and less exercise.
- Hormonal changes in men and women differ:
  - In men, testosterone levels begin to decline around ages 40 to 50, although sperm can fertilize eggs until much later. Decreased sperm production is linked to underweight status; malnutrition is linked to declining libido. National Health and Nutrition Examination Survey data show that as men age their calorie consumption decreases. Weight gain after 40 is more than likely due to less exercise.
  - In women, the reproductive cycle lasts approximately 40 years, with 13 menstrual cycles per year (minus those missed during pregnancy or for other reasons). Birth rates for women aged 35 to 39 are higher than they have ever been. The birth rate for women aged 40 to 44 has gone up more than 51% since 1990 (Martin et al., 2005).
- In 2002–2003 the prevalence of selected chronic conditions for 25- to 44-year-olds were as follows: chronic joint symptoms (17.9%), sinusitis (13.5%), asthma (9.9%), hay fever (9.5%), and doctor's diagnosis of arthritis (9.3%) (National Center for Health Statistics, 1984–1995). Comparing middle-aged adults to young adults, chronic joint symptoms replaced asthma as the top chronic health condition.

Older Adult Years (Ages 51 to 70)

- Typically, adults in this age group have more time to enjoy life with less responsibility in terms of raising children.
- Typically, there is more disposable income as careers are peaking.
- Many older adults enjoy the benefits of eating healthy and exercising. If they are not, it is more than likely because they are dealing with one or more chronic disease(s) (i.e., heart disease or diabetes).
- Muscle mass and strength decrease with age, but exercise can offset this decline (Chin et al., 2001). Lack of exercise results in lose of muscle mass, which in turn decreases overall lean

muscle mass, increases body fat, and decreases metabolic rates leading to weight gain.

- The immune system weakens with age and the ability to fight off infection becomes more and more difficult. This can be further compromised by an inadequate intake of nutrients or underlying chronic disease.
- Posture begins to deteriorate, which could be as a result of lack of exercise and poor muscle tone, bad habits, or bone loss.
- Major changes occur in the ability to taste and smell food. The senses are dulled; thus foods should have stronger smells and flavors to them so they will be more appealing.
- Saliva decreases, gastric secretions decline, and constipation, gas, and bloating can become more of a problem. Oftentimes the causes of these problems are incorrectly attributed to certain foods and the diet can become more and more restrictive as perceived intolerances increase.
- According to the latest National Health and Nutrition Examination Survey data, alcohol intake accounts for 3% of calorie intake between ages 51 and 64 (Kant, 2000).
- The prevalence of selected chronic conditions for 45- to 64-year-olds based on the top five conditions were chronic joint symptoms (33.7%), doctor's diagnosis of arthritis (29.5%), hypertension (29.5%), sinusitis (17.5%), and all types of heart disease (12.7%) (National Center for Health Statistics, 1984–1995).

Delaying the onset of disabilities caused by chronic disease in adulthood is referred to as compression of morbidity (Harvard Health Letter, 2002). Perhaps the overall goal should not necessarily be the *number* of years lived but the number of *healthy good-quality* years lived.

Nutritional Requirements for the Adult

Combining the tools of nutrition assessment and nutrition research currently available, nutritional requirements for the adult can be determined with confidence. The current Food and Nutrition Board was formed in 1993 and has been working on the DRI, which has been released in stages throughout the last few years. The DRI has become the overarching framework that encompasses four sets of standards: estimated average requirements, RDA, adequate intakes, and tolerable intake levels (upper levels).

Energy

The standard used to express energy needs, called estimated energy requirements, refers to the average needs based on height, age, gender, and activity level to promote weight maintenance. Excess energy consumed is not excreted like most vitamins and minerals; thus it is not desirable to consume excess calories in any form (i.e., protein, carbohydrate, fat, and/or alcohol).

> ● **Learning Point** The DRI: Estimated Energy Requirements for Men and Women 30 Years of Age were released in 2002 by the Food and Nutrition Board and allow for adjustment in kilocalories based on age. For each year below age 30, add 7 kcal/day for women and 10 kcal/day for men. For each year above 30, subtract 7 kcal/day for women and 10 kcal/day for men.

It is estimated that energy needs decrease by 6% between the ages of 51 and 74 years, and they decline a further 6% after the age of 74 years (Gary & Fleury, 2002). The doubly labeled water method revolutionized the understanding of energy requirement and energy balance in humans because for the first time this method could be applied to humans and energy requirements and energy balance could be measured. The doubly labeled water method contains two stable isotopes, deuterium oxide and oxygen–18. After administering an oral dose of water labeled with both isotopes (thus the term doubly labeled water) the deuterium is eliminated from the body as water and the oxygen–18 is eliminated as water and carbon dioxide. Periodic sampling of body water (urine, saliva, and plasma) is taken. The two isotopes are measured for 10 to 14 days and the difference between the two elimination rates is the measure of carbon dioxide production. Carbon dioxide can then be equated to total energy expenditure (Schoeller, 1999).

It is interesting to note that National Health and Nutrition Examination Survey data on energy consumption indicates that older adults are often below the current RDA recommendation, with men ages 65 to 74 years consuming on average 1,800 kcal/day and women ages 65 to 74 years consuming on average between 1,300 and 1,600 kcal/day (Committee on Nutrition Services for Medicare Beneficiaries and Institute of Medicine, 2000).

Macronutrients

Protein recommendations are based on the RDA for protein (0.8 g protein/kg body weight) listed on the DRI based on a reference weight for each life stage group. The amount of protein recommended for women is the same for all three life stages (i.e., ages 19 to 30, 31 to 50, and 51 to 70) and is 46 g/day. For men the recommended amount of protein for all three life stages is 56 g/day.

The DRI for carbohydrate is based on the RDA, which is 130 g for both men and women for all three life stages. In people over age 65, fasting blood glucose rises to a mean of 140 mg/dL, resulting in an increased **incidence** of non–insulin-dependent diabetes, which can be attributed to age, obesity, and decreased physical activity level. Thus recommendations regarding amount and distribution of carbohydrate must be individualized at this point (Fonesa & Wall, 1995).

Incidence: Rate of occurrence.

The grams of fat per day are not determinable but rather are recommended in terms of acceptable macronutrient distribution ranges. The acceptable macronutrient distribution ranges for fat are 20% to 35% kcal energy/day, for carbohydrate are 45% 65% kcal energy/day, and for protein are 10% to 35% kcal energy/day. These recommendations meet the needs of nearly 98% of all *healthy* individuals of similar age and gender based on each life stage group.

Micronutrients

Most vitamin and mineral requirements for healthy people remain the same as they move throughout each life stage group. Micronutrient status changes with age for vitamin D, vitamin B_{12}, and calcium related to the decline in absorption, use, or activation of these nutrients. As people age they can become deficient in vitamin D for a number of reasons, such as their skin is less able to take up vitamin D from the blood, their skin is unable to make vitamin D when exposed to sunlight, they spend less time outdoors, and when outdoors they are more likely to protect themselves from the sun (Hanley & Davison, 2005). The adequate intake for vitamin D for adults aged 51 to 70 is 10 μg as compared with 5 μg for adults ages 19 to 30 and 31 to 50.

Calcium needs increase with increasing age for men and women to compensate for bone loss. Calcium recommendations increase by 200 mg/day for 51- to 70-year-olds. This increase compensates for the loss of ability to absorb calcium from the diet because of the loss of vitamin D receptors in the gut. Increased fiber reduces calcium absorption, as does gastrointestinal distress or inflammation. Vitamin B_{12} needs increase after the age of 50 because about 10% to 30% of older people may poorly absorb food-bound vitamin B_{12} because of reduced acid production by the stomach.

Almost one-third of all older individuals have been observed to have deficiencies of vitamins and trace elements (Russell, 1997). The need for iron is increased to 18 mg/day for women aged 19 to 50 years to make up for iron lost during menstrual blood loss. After menopause, iron requirements decrease to 8 mg/day because of the cessation of the menstrual cycle.

Water

Often overlooked as a nutrient, water should be considered one of the most important nutrients because you can only survive days without it compared with weeks or months without food (Mahan, 2004). The DRI recommendations are based on adequate intakes for generally healthy individuals who are adequately hydrated. It is well known that water requirements vary from individual to individual. Water recommendations take into consideration water from all sources, including all beverages and food. The water content of many foods is quite high (i.e., an apple is 84% water). Moisture in foods can contribute 20% of the total water intake. For healthy men the recommendation of 3.7 L/day of water is the same for all three life stage groups. For healthy women the recommendation of 2.7 L/day of water is the same for all three life stage groups. No upper level has been set for water because of a lack of suitable data; however, caution is warranted in consuming levels above the recommended intakes. The RDA for an adult is approximately 1 mL water/kcal expended as long as kilocalorie needs are met (Food and Nutrition Board, National Research Council, & National Academy of Sciences, 1989).

Two other methods exist for determining water requirements in the clinical setting. The first method estimates fluid requirements starting with 100 mL/kg for the first 10 kg of body weight. For the second 10 kg of body weight another 50 mL/kg of water is added. For the remaining body weight 20 mL/kg is used if the person is less than 50 years old and 15 mL/kg is used if the person is older than 50 years. The second method is expressed in mL/kg based on age: 40 mL/kg, 15 to 30 years old; 35 mL/kg, 25 to 55 years old; 30 mL/kg, 44 to 65 years old; and 25 mL/kg, more than 65 years old.

Fiber

Fiber recommendations based on the average daily dietary fiber recommendations for 2002 (adequate intake) are 25 g for women (ages 19 to 50) and 38 g for men (ages 19 to 50) or 14 g of dietary fiber per 1,000 kcal. For women and men ages 51 to 70, average daily dietary fiber recommendations for 2002 (adequate intake) are 21 g and 28 g of fiber, respectively, per day. Daily median intakes are 12.1 to 13.8 g for women and 16.5 to 19.5 for men (Brown et al., 2005).

Nutritional Assessment in Chronic Disease

Relationship between nutrition and overall health and the prevention of chronic disease has been well documented (Public Health Service, 1988; Food and Nutrition Board, Committee on Diet and Health, & National Research Council, 1989). In the adult years nutrition plays an important role in maintaining wellness and reducing risk of chronic disease. According to the *Healthy People 2010* report issued by the U.S. Department of Health and Human Services, nutrition is one of the many factors affecting health and longevity of older people. This is especially true for older people who are minorities and of low income (U.S. Department of Health and Human Services, 2000). It is estimated that up to 60% of older people admitted to the hospital have protein energy malnutrition on admission or their nutritional status becomes compromised while hospitalized (Gallagher-Allred, Voss, Finn, & McCamish, 1996; Berry & Braunschwig, 1998; Gary & Fleury, 2002).

The physiologic changes in the adult and the assessment of energy expenditure in adults with chronic disease, two important knowledge and skill areas, are reviewed first before the discussion of nutrition assessment in chronic disease; that section follows below.

Physiologic Changes in the Adult: Nutritional Implications

Eighty-five percent of older adults have one or more nutrition-related problem (ADA, 2000). The most common are obesity, diabetes, cardiovascular disease, hypertension, arthritis, osteoporosis, and malnutrition. Many of these disorders put people at nutritional risk. Two major metabolic changes occur as people age. There is a decrease in lean body mass, with a 10% decrease in lean body mass from ages 25 to 60 years, another 10% decrease from ages 60 to 75 years, and another 20% to 25% decrease after age 75 (Chin et al., 2001). Basal metabolic rate also decreases with age and in response to the decrease in lean muscle mass and increase in adipose tissues. The challenge then becomes to make sure that nutrient needs are met with declining kilocalorie needs while maintaining weight. Table 9.1 summarizes the numerous physiologic changes experienced by adults as they

TABLE 9.1 Physiologic Changes Experienced With Aging

Decline in dental health
Reduced thirst sensation
Fall in gastrointestinal function
Changes in liver, gallbladder, and pancreatic function
Decline in kidney function
Reduced immune function
Reduced lung function
Reduced hearing and vision
Reduced cardiovascular health

age. These physiologic changes individually or cumulatively over time could negatively impact overall nutritional health.

RDAs and related standards apply only to healthy people, but many older people may not be healthy, especially those with a chronic disease. In addition, many older people take medications that may negatively impact specific nutrients. The use of a supplement to help meet vitamin D, vitamin B_{12}, and calcium needs may be beneficial for older people who require such a low energy intake that they are not able to consume enough nutrient-dense foods to meet their requirements. Certain conditions that are more prevalent with age increase the need for specific vitamins and minerals. Some examples include decrease in immune function (increased need for vitamin B_6, vitamin E, and zinc), increased gastric pH (increases need for vitamin B_{12}, folic acid, calcium, iron, and zinc), and increase in oxidative stress (increases need for beta-carotene, vitamin C, and vitamin E) (Wardlaw, Hampl, & DiSilvestro, 2004). In fact, because of these conditions a balanced multivitamin and mineral supplement is recommended for all older adults by many nutrition experts.

Assessment of Energy Needs in Adults With Chronic Disease

The assessment of energy needs can be measured in a number of ways. Indirect calorimetry is a method for estimating energy production by measuring O_2 consumption and CO_2 production at a specific point in time, accurately determining resting metabolic rate (Mahan, 2004). Devices such as the Douglas bag or metabolic cart are the most useful at measuring resting metabolic rate. Indirect calorimetry data such as the respiratory quotient tell clinicians the net substrate oxidation of fat, carbohydrate, and protein, allowing for precise changes in nutrition support

when necessary (Brandi & Calafa, 1997). New technology allows the production of smaller handheld versions of the larger, costly, less accessible models. Indirect calorimetry, although still used, is not used as a routine assessment of energy expenditure in clinical dietetic practice. Assessment of energy needs is most often determined by using energy prediction equations because they are practical and their accuracy rate is enough to provide a starting point in which adjustments (increases or decreases) can be made based on the patient's metabolic response to total kilocalories and diet composition provided. The following equations are currently used in clinical practice to determine energy needs:

- Harris-Benedict equation: Harris and Benedict conducted a study in which 239 subjects (aged 15 to 74 years) had their basal metabolic rates measured. By today's standards these measurements would be referred to as resting metabolic rates. The Harris-Benedict equation was derived from this study and is still used today. It is well known, however, that the Harris-Benedict equation can overestimate energy needs by as much as 20% to 30%, with an accuracy rate of 69% (Frankenfield, Roth-Yousey, & Compher, 2005).
- Mifflin-St. Jeor equation: Body composition has changed a great deal since 1919 when the Harris-Benedict equation first was derived. The Mifflin-St. Jeor equation was developed in 1990 and has been shown to report resting metabolic rate 82% of the time in nonobese adults. The Mifflin-St. Jeor equation has an overestimation error of 15% and an underestimation error of 18%. Once resting metabolic rate is calculated it is then multiplied by activity or injury and stress factors to determine the total energy required.
- Ireton-Jones equation: The Ireton-Jones equation provides estimated energy expenditure for hospitalized and critically ill patients who are

TABLE 9.2 Harris-Benedict Equation

Men: BEE=66.47+13.75 (wt in kg)+5 (ht in cm)
− 6.76 (age in yr)
Women: BEE=655.1+9.56 (wt in kg)+1.85 (ht in cm)
− 4.68 (age in yr)

TABLE 9.3 Mifflin-St. Jeor Energy Estimation Formula

Males: RMR = (10 × wt [in kg]) + (6.25 × ht [in cm])
− (5 × age [in yr]) + 5

Females: RMR = (10 × wt [in kg]) + (6.25 × ht 9in cm])
− (5 × age [in yr]) − 161

Activity or injury and stress factors

Sedentary or weight maintenance	1.2
Light activity	1.3
Moderately active, infection, healing	1.5
Very active, extreme stress, burns	2.0

RMR, resting metabolic rate.

TABLE 9.4 Ireton-Jones Equation for Spontaneous and Ventilator Dependent Breather

EEE spontaneous breather

EEE(S) = 629 − 11(A) + 25W − (609 if obese)

EEE(S) = 629 − 11(A) + 25(W in kg) − (609 if obese)

EEE ventilator dependent

EEE(V) = 1,784 − 11(A) + 5(W) + 244(S) + 239(T)
+ 804(B)

EEE(V) = 1,784 − 11(A) + 5(W in kg) + 244 (if male)
+ 239 (if trauma) + 804 (if burn)

EEE(S), spontaneously breathing; EEE(V), ventilator dependent;
S, sex (male, 1; female, 0); T, trauma; A, age; W, weight; B, burn.

either breathing spontaneously or are ventilator dependent. This equation takes into account age, weight (kg), and gender. The equation adjusts for trauma, burns, and/or obesity. The obesity adjustment should be used when the patient weighs more than 130% of their ideal body weight or has a **body mass index** (**BMI**) above 27 (Ireton-Jones, 1997).

Body mass index (BMI): Calculated by dividing weight in kilograms by height in meters squared (BMI = kg/m²); shown in the research literature to be correlated with adiposity and increase risk of chronic disease.

Depending on the illness, calorie needs can rise substantially in the hospitalized patient. For this reason, it is critically important to assess the energy needs of each patient individually (Klipstein-Grobusch, Reilly, Potter, Edwards, & Roberts, 1995).

Nutritional Care Process and Model

Before the adoption of the ADA's final version of the Nutrition Care Process and Model, no standardized

nutrition care process existed. Dietetic professionals strongly supported a standardized nutrition care process for use by registered dietitians and dietetic technicians because this standardized process would in effect promote the dietetic professional as the unique provider of nutrition care and enhance the practice of dietetics by improving outcomes and showing the value of our services (Lacey, 2003).

The ADA Nutrition Care and Process Model is circular in shape and looks very much like a dart board with a central core and middle and outer rings (Figure 9.1). The central core depicts the relationships between patient/client/group and the dietetics professional. This central core sits inside a larger central core, called the nutrition care process, of which there are four steps: nutritional assessment, nutritional diagnosis, nutritional intervention, and nutrition monitoring and evaluation. Two outer rings surround the nutrition care process. The middle ring depicts the knowledge and skills that dietetic professionals bring to the process. The outer ring depicts the environmental factors that influence the process, such as the practice setting.

Two very important systems that are not considered part of the Nutrition Care and Process Model but are critically important are the screening and referral system and the outcomes management system. Nutritional screening is not required to be done by a dietetic professional (registered dietitians or dietetic technicians); however, the process depends on accurate and timely nutritional screening. It is critically important that the nutritional screening process be monitored and evaluated as part of the outcomes management system to ensure that those who are at nutritional risk are identified. The outcomes management system allows data to be collected and analyzed to determine where improvements need to be made to improve overall quality of nutritional care provided.

It is important to distinguish between *standardized process* and *standardized care*. The Nutritional Care Process and Model does not attempt to standardize care (i.e., all patients receive the same care). Nutritional care still must be individualized. What the Nutritional Care Process and Model does do is provide a framework or guide based on a series of connected steps or actions in which nutrition care is provided. In a nutshell, the Nutritional Care Process and Model can be defined as "a systematic problem-solving method that dietetics professionals use to critically think and make decisions to address nutrition related problems and provide safe and effective quality nutrition care" (Lacey, 2003).

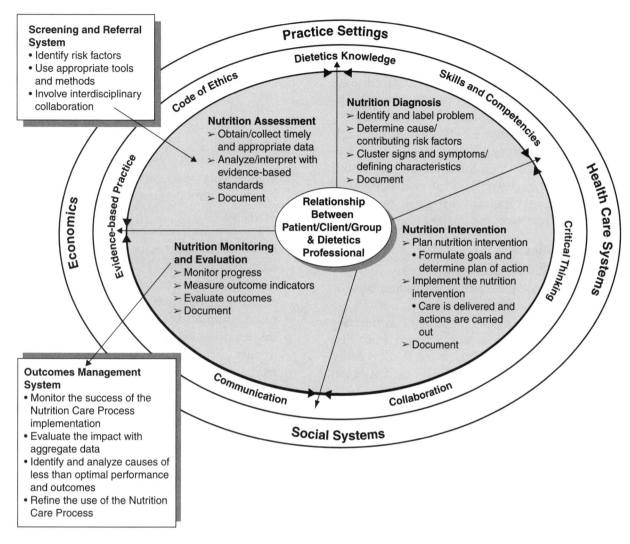

Screening and Referral System
- Identify risk factors
- Use appropriate tools and methods
- Involve interdisciplinary collaboration

Practice Settings

Dietetics Knowledge

Code of Ethics

Skills and Competencies

Economics

Evidence-based Practice

Health Care Systems

Critical Thinking

Nutrition Assessment
- Obtain/collect timely and appropriate data
- Analyze/interpret with evidence-based standards
- Document

Nutrition Diagnosis
- Identify and label problem
- Determine cause/contributing risk factors
- Cluster signs and symptoms/defining characteristics
- Document

Relationship Between Patient/Client/Group & Dietetics Professional

Nutrition Intervention
- Plan nutrition intervention
  - Formulate goals and determine plan of action
- Implement the nutrition intervention
  - Care is delivered and actions are carried out
- Document

Nutrition Monitoring and Evaluation
- Monitor progress
- Measure outcome indicators
- Evaluate outcomes
- Document

Outcomes Management System
- Monitor the success of the Nutrition Care Process implementation
- Evaluate the impact with aggregate data
- Identify and analyze causes of less than optimal performance and outcomes
- Refine the use of the Nutrition Care Process

Communication

Collaboration

Social Systems

Figure 9.1 ADA Nutrition Care Process and Model.

Reprinted with permission from Lacey et al. Nutrition Care Process and Model. *Journal of the American Dietetic Association*, 103, 1061–1072. © 2003 The American Dietetic Association.

There are four steps in the nutrition care process: (1) nutrition assessment, (2) nutrition diagnosis, (3) nutrition intervention, and (4) nutrition monitoring and evaluation. There is a difference between medical nutrition therapy and the nutrition care process. Medical nutrition therapy was redefined as part of the 2001 Medicare MNT benefit legislation as "nutritional diagnostic, therapy, and counseling services for the purpose of disease management, which are furnished by a registered dietitian or nutrition professional" (Smith, 2003). Medical nutrition therapy is only one type of nutrition care. The Nutritional Care Process and Model is broader in scope and guides nutrition education and other preventative nutrition services.

Evidence-based practice is needed to determine which practices support outcomes (Myers, Pritchett,

& Johnson, 2002). The government is looking to evidence-based practice as a way to improve the quality of medical care provided to patients while managing the rising costs of an overburdened nearly dysfunctional health care system (Smith, 2003). By applying evidence-based practice as a part of the Nutrition Care Process and Model, practitioners and educators can apply the best research knowledge to dietetics practice. Demonstrating the science behind dietary recommendation and validating nutritional assessment tools utilizing evidence-based analysis to further dietetics practice would strengthen the profession. The ADA has begun this process and has created evidence-based nutrition practice guidelines for numerous topic areas that can be accessed free by all ADA members through the ADA Evidence Analysis Library on the ADA website (www.eatright.org).

Nutritional Assessment in Chronic Diseases

In this section we review the following chronic diseases: cardiovascular disease (coronary heart disease and cerebrovascular disease), cancer, chronic obstructive pulmonary disease (COPD), diabetes, chronic kidney disease, and HIV/AIDS. For each chronic disease reviewed, disease-specific considerations are addressed when conducting a nutritional assessment. Evidence analysis for evidence-based practice is presented for each chronic disease based on a thorough review of the current literature.

Cardiovascular Disease

Cardiovascular disease affects more than 13 million Americans and is still the number one leading cause of death in the United States (Kochanek et al., 2004). Cardiovascular disease is a broad term that encompasses a number of conditions, such as coronary heart disease (often called heart disease), stroke, and any other conditions that affect the structure of function of the heart. If the heart does not receive adequate blood, the heart becomes starved of oxygen and the vital nutrients it needs to work properly. This could result in unstable angina (chest pain), damage to the heart muscle, and/or myocardial infarction; the severity and progression depends on the degree of blockage.

Symptoms are highly variable from person to person, more so when comparing symptoms for men versus women. Treatment for coronary artery disease involves an assessment of risk factors for determination of appropriate intervention as outlined by the latest report issued by the National Cholesterol Education Program (NCEP) Adult Treatment Panel III report recommendations (NCEP, 2001; National Heart, Lung, and Blood Institute & National Institutes of Health, 2002).

Nutritional Assessment in Coronary Heart Disease

Nutritional assessment should include the evaluation of the following:

- Excess weight for height: BMI > 25 (overweight), BMI > 30 (obese)
- Excess abdominal fat: waist circumference of 35 inches for females, 40 inches or more for males, or waist-to-hip ratio of less than 0.8 for women and less than 1.0 for men

> **Hypertension:** Systolic blood pressure above 140 mm Hg or diastolic blood pressure above 90 mm Hg.

  - Evidence of **hypertension** (blood pressure > 140/90 mm Hg)
  - Complete lipid profile, fasting preferred (total cholesterol, low-density lipoprotein and **high-density lipoprotein** cholesterol)
- Nonfasting total cholesterol, high-density lipoprotein if complete fasting lipid profile unavailable (proceed to lipoprotein profile if total cholesterol ≥ 200 mg/dL or high-density lipoprotein < 40 mg/dL)

> **High-density lipoproteins:** Often referred to as "good cholesterol," a lipoprotein that contains mostly protein with less cholesterol and triglyceride. High levels of high-density lipoproteins in the blood are associated with a decreased risk of coronary heart disease risk.

- Plasma apolipoprotein B (an atherogenic lipoprotein)
- **Homocysteine** levels
- Evidence of diabetes, fasting blood sugar levels

> **Homocysteine:** An amino acid that can be measured in the blood that has been shown to be an independent risk factor for cardiovascular disease.

- Evidence of atherogenic diet: evaluate dietary intake (saturated fat and trans fatty acid intake, omega-3 fatty acid intake; overall diet quality particularly with regard to intake of fruits, vegetables, and whole grains)
- Physical activity level
- Smoking, tobacco use
- Family history of premature coronary heart disease
- Gender
- Age (men ≥ 45 years, women ≥ 55 years)

Evidence Analysis for Evidence-Based Practice in Coronary Heart Disease

The original NCEP guidelines followed the recommendations of the American Heart Association's Step I and Step II diets (NCEP, 1988). The new NCEP guidelines released in 2002 are evidence-based guidelines that result in reduction of low-density lipoprotein cholesterol levels and reduced risk of coronary heart disease (National Heart, Lung, and Blood Institute, & National Institutes of Health, 2002). Therapeutic Lifestyle Changes diet lowers saturated fat and cholesterol intakes to levels of the previous Step II American Heart Association diet (Table 9.5). If lipid levels are not achieved initially, plant stanols/sterols (2 g/day) and viscous (soluble) fiber (10 to 25 g/day), known to have low-density lipoprotein lipid-lowering affects, may be added to the diet. The new NCEP Adult Treatment Panel III guidelines increase the emphasis on weight management and physical activity:

- Consume less than 200 mg of dietary cholesterol per day.
- Limit sodium intake to less than 2,400 mg a day.

TABLE 9.5	Therapeutic Lifestyle Changes Diet Guidelines	

Food Group	Number of Servings	Serving Size
Lean meat, fish, poultry, and dry beans	No more than 6 oz/day	6 ounces maximum per day lean meat, poultry, and fish ½ cup cooked dry peas or beans ½ cup tofu
Eggs	No more than four yolks a week	Two egg whites = 1 whole egg in recipes
Egg substitute/egg whites	Unlimited	
Low-fat milk, yogurt, and cheese	2–3	1 cup fat-free or 1% milk 1 cup nonfat or low-fat yogurt 1 ounce of low-fat or fat-free cheese (≤3 g of fat in 1 ounce)
Fats and oils	No more than 6–8	1 teaspoon soft margarine or vegetable oil 1 tablespoon salad dressing 1 ounce nuts
Fruits	2–4	1 piece of fruit ½ cup diced fruit ¾ cup juice
Vegetables	3–5	1 cup leafy or raw ½ cup cooked ¾ cup juice
Breads, cereals, pasta, rice, and other grains	6–11	1 slice of bread ½ bun, bagel, or muffin 1 ounce dry cereal ½ cup cooked cereal, potatoes, pasta, rice, or other grains
Sweets and snacks	Now and then	

Adapted from the National Cholesterol Education Program (Adult Treatment Panel III). Serving sizes are based on the USDA's MyPyramid.

- Eat 25% to 35% or less of the day's total calories from fat.
- Consume less than 7% of day's total calories from saturated fat.
- Eat just enough calories to achieve or maintain a healthy weight and reduce your blood cholesterol levels.
- The recommendations for cholesterol and sodium are the same for everyone on the Therapeutic Lifestyle Changes diet, regardless of caloric intake.
- The recommendations for saturated fat and total fat are based on the percentage of calories consumed and vary with intake.

Cholesterol-lowering medications may be necessary if diet alone does not adequately lower levels.

Cerebrovascular disease, or stroke, strikes about 700,000 Americans each year with most surviving, increasing the number of stroke survivors to close to 5 million who are managing their health today (http://www.webmd.com/ diseases_and _conditions/ stroke.htm). There are two types of stroke: ischemic or hemorrhagic based on cause. An ischemic stroke is caused by a blood clot that blocks the supply of blood to the brain. Most often this is due to atherosclerosis, which is caused by high blood pressure, diabetes, high cholesterol, or a combination of the three. Blood flow can also be interrupted by low blood pressure (hypotension), which may be a result of a heart attack, blood loss, or a severe infection. Clots can also break free as a result of procedure or surgery and cause a stroke. A hemorrhagic stroke is the result of bleeding in or around the brain as a result most often of a ruptured blood vessel or uncontrolled blood pressure.

Nutritional Assessment in Cerebrovascular Disease

Generally, the nutritional assessment here is the same as that for coronary heart disease except that a patient's functional status needs to be determined, especially as it relates to his or her ability to meet nutritional needs orally. Table 9.6 shows the recommended intakes of total fat and saturated fat.

Evidence Analysis for Evidence-Based Practice in Cerebrovascular Disease

Given the fact that evidence has already been presented above for the treatment of coronary heart disease (with the underlying cause of atherosclerosis), the focus here is on the evidence available to support

TABLE 9.6	Maximum Daily Intake of Fat and Saturated Fatty Acid							
	Calorie Level							
	1,600	1,800	2,000	2,200	2,400	2,600	2,800	3,000
Total fat, g	44–62	50–70	56–78	61–86	67–93	72–101	78–109	83–117
Saturated fat, g	12	14	16	17	19	20	22	23

Recommended intake of total fat 25% to 35% and saturated fat < 7%.
From the National Cholesterol Education Program (Adult Treatment Panel III).

prevention and control of hypertension, the other major underlying cause of strokes. The Trials of Hypertension Prevention and the Dietary Approaches to Stop Hypertension studies clearly demonstrated that dietary intervention prevented hypertension or lowered blood pressure in persons with high to normal blood pressure (Appel et al., 1997; Trials of Hypertension Prevention Collaborative Research Group, 1997). The Dietary Approaches to Stop Hypertension diet is used to prevent and control blood pressure and is based on a "heart healthy" diet with twice the average daily consumption of fruits and vegetables (available at http://www.nhlbi.nih.gov/health/public/heart/hbp/dash/new_dash.pdf).

Cancer

Cancer is a group of related diseases in which damage to the DNA of the cells causes uncontrolled growth and spread of abnormal cells. This abnormal cellular growth can have an effect on any one part of the body (breast, skin, lungs) or the whole body (**metastases**). Cancer is the second leading cause of death in the United States, with 1.2 million new cases diagnosed annually and nearly 9 million Americans with a history of cancer (Nutrition Screening Initiative, 2002; Kochanek et al., 2004). Given the fact that 35% of all cancers are diet related, cancer prevention depends to a large degree on the overall quality of diet and the ability to maintain a healthy weight.

Metastasis: Growth of malignant tissue that spreads to surrounding tissues or organs.

Nutritional Assessment

One of the most important markers of nutritional status is assessment of body weight, which can be represented by an unplanned weight loss or a BMI less than 22, a serum albumin less than 3.5, or a cholesterol level less than 150 mg/dL. The diet history is evaluated to determine adequacy of caloric intake and overall diet quality, especially with regard to protein and vitamin and mineral intake. Particular attention is paid to the use of vitamins and minerals and complementary and alternative therapies.

Evidence Analysis for Evidence-Based Practice

The main nutrition goal is to prevent or reverse nutrient deficiencies, to preserve lean body mass, to minimize nutrition-related side effects, and to maximize the quality of life. The role of nutrition is vitally important in the treatment of cancer patients. Much time is spent dealing with the common nutrition problems that occur as a result of the disease, treatment, or both. Common nutrition problems include anorexia/cachexia, nausea, vomiting, mucositis, esophagitis, xerostomia, dysgeusia, hypogeusia, diarrhea, and constipation. Recommendations for dealing with common nutrition problems are outlined in Table 9.7.

Nutritional recommendations for energy are highly variable and must be individualized. Protein requirements range from 1.2 to 2.0 with average protein requirements at 1.5 g/kg. Energy requirements are typically 25 to 30 kcal/kg or, if using an energy prediction equation, use an injury factor of 1.3 to 1.5 (Mahan, 2004). Patients with **cancer cachexia** exhibit a syndrome of irreversible weight loss, anorexia, asthenia, anemia, and abnormalities in protein, fat, and carbohydrate metabolism. This "wasting" is similar to what is experienced by patients with sepsis and inflammation (Mahan, 2004).

Cancer cachexia: Irreversible weight loss (body fat and muscle stores) that accompanies advanced cancer despite adequate nutritional intake.

Alterations occur in glucose, protein, and lipid metabolism because of the metabolic demands of the cancerous tumor(s). Tumors exert a constant demand for glucose and amino acids. To keep up with this constant need for glucose, gluconeogenesis and lipolysis occur at a high rate at the expense of skeletal muscle and adipose tissue as the fuel source. Catabolism can be so great that visceral organ and other body proteins (albumin) are affected.

TABLE 9.7 Strategies to Improve Intake in Cancer Patients

Strategies to address anorexia/cachexia:
- Identify factors contributing to poor appetite.
- Keep high calorie/high protein foods/liquids on hand for when appetite is good:
  - Milkshakes, Carnation Instant Breakfast, peanut butter, fruited yogurt
- Discourage intake of high-fiber foods that can cause early satiety.
- Appetite stimulant if anorexia is longstanding or other strategies fail to improve condition

Strategies to address nausea
- Sip liquids at frequent intervals separately from solid foods to maintain hydration.
- Discourage fasting because it may cause hypoglycemia and increase nausea.
- Cold or room temperature foods may be better tolerated.
- Avoid high-fat, high-fiber, spicy, or gas-producing foods that may be poorly tolerated.

Strategies to address vomiting:
- Encourage adequate fluids to prevent dehydration.
- Start with low-fat fluids and advance as tolerated.
- Introduce dry starchy foods first when advancing.
- Introduce high-fiber and high-fat foods last.
- Avoid eating 1½ to 2 hours pre- and posttreatment.

Strategies to Address Mucositis:
- Encourage good oral hygiene practices.
- Use oral baking soda rinse:
  - 1 mL of baking soda to 250 mL of water
- Soft, moist, semisolid, or blended foods may be tolerated better than rough/crisp foods.
- Discourage intake of known irritants:
  - Tart or acidic foods, spicy or salty foods, very hot or cold foods, tobacco, alcohol, and alcohol-based items
- Recommend dunking or moistening dry foods:
  - Order extra gravy on trays.
- Alter temperature and consistency to individual tolerances.
- Reinforce use of analgesics as prescribed before meals to reduce pain associated with eating.

Strategies to address esophagitis:
- Same as strategies for mucositis plus the following:
  - Suggest the use of local anesthetic and analgesic before meals.
  - In cases of peptic esophagitis, antireflux and antacid therapy may be helpful.
  - Recommend regular antacids before and 1 hour after meals and before bed.

Strategies to address thick saliva/mucus:
- Beverages or foods that are slightly tart or carbonated may help to thin secretions.
- If milk products are found to affect mucus try soy-based items (such as soy milk) for tolerance.
- Mucous production may be minimized if clear fluids are consumed after milk products.
- Limit caffeine, alcohol, and spicy foods.
- Encourage a mouth rinse throughout the day.

Strategies to address xerostomia:
- Increased liquid consumption may provide symptomatic relief; however, liquids have no lubricating properties.
- Encourage consumption of foods such as gravies, sauces, and salad dressings (Italian).
- Mint or tart sugar-free gum/candy may stimulate saliva production.
- Discourage commercial mouthwashes and alcohol because they contribute to dryness.
- Citric-acid-containing beverages such as lemonade, orange-flavored soft drinks, frozen juice bars, and sherbets may help increase secretions.
- Recommend sugar-free or diet products to reduce the risk of dental decay and mouth infection.

TABLE

9.7 Strategies to Improve Intake in Cancer Patients (continued)

Strategies to address dysgeusia:
- Determine specific taste or smell changes.
- Encourage fluids with meals to decrease unpleasant tastes.
- Reinforce proper oral care before and between meals.
- Tart foods can stimulate taste buds.
- Suggest mild-tasting foods such as biscuits, milk, pudding, and custards.
- If meat tastes bitter or metallic:
  - Serve meat cold or at room temperature.
  - Include meat in mixed dishes like casseroles.
  - Choose alternative protein sources from dairy group: cottage cheese, yogurt, custard.
  - Try tofu or eggs.
  - Marinate foods in pineapple or lime juice, vinegar, wine, or sweet and sour sauce.
  - Eat with plastic utensils in place of metal ones.
  - Cinnamon or sugar-free gum or mints may help mask the metallic taste.

Strategies to address hypogeusia:
- Reinforce proper oral care.
- Encourage experimenting with strong flavors and seasonings.
- Encourage liberal intake of "treats" or comfort foods.
- Emphasize a variety in colors and textures in a meal to encourage eating.

Strategies to address diarrhea:
- When appropriate use antidiarrheal agents as prescribed by physician first to avoid dietary limitations.
- Encourage energy-dense fluids to match output.
- Encourage potassium-rich foods.
- Try the following modifications one at a time to determine effectiveness:
  - Limit bowel stimulants (e.g., caffeine, alcohol, prunes).
  - Adjust fat intake as tolerated.
  - Restrict lactose.
  - Restrict fiber intake.
  - Limit gas-producing foods.
  - Limit foods or fluids that exacerbate symptoms (e.g., spices).

Strategies to address constipation:
- Encourage intake of naturally laxative foods such as prunes, rhubarb, papaya, and mango.
- Encourage physical activity as able.
- Advise the use of a bulk-forming laxative and reinforce the importance of adequate fluid intake.
- Daily use of stool softeners as necessary

Information adapted from the American Institute for Cancer Research (www.aicr.org)

Antitumor therapy, such as chemotherapy, radiation, surgery, or immunotherapy, can contribute to nutritional alterations in patients by interfering with their ability to ingest, digest, and absorb adequately. Ideally, early intervention is the key to minimize weight loss and to prevent or correct nutritional deficiencies as soon as possible and if at all possible.

Chronic Obstructive Pulmonary Disease

COPD is a slow progressive obstruction of the airways of the lung. COPD affects more than 16 million Americans and is the fourth leading cause of death (Nutrition Screening Initiative, 2002; Kochanek et al., 2004). There are two categories of patients with COPD. Type 1 or emphysema is seen in older patients who are thin and cachectic, with cor pulmonale that develops late in course. **Cor pulmonale** is a medical term used to describe enlargement and failure of the right side of the heart due to pulmonary hypertension from prolonged high blood pressure in the arteries or veins of the lungs. Type 2 or chronic bronchitis is seen in patients with normal weight or excessive weight and prominent hypoxemia in which cor pulmonale develops early in the course of the disease.

Nutritional Assessment

It is well known that the maintenance of a well-nourished nutritional state plays a key role in maintaining ventilatory muscle strength, improved immune response, and reduced risk of respiratory mortality (Whittaker, Ryan, Buckle, & Road, 1990; Rogers, Donahoe, & Constantino, 1992; Gray-Donald, Gibbson, Shapiro, Macklern, & Martin, 1996). Malnutrition, however, is common among patients with COPD (Schols, Mostert, Soester, Greve, & Wouters, 1989; Laaban et al., 1993). Given the degree of malnutrition in the COPD population, Thorsdottir and colleagues (2001) conducted a study to evaluate and develop a screening method for detecting malnutrition in patients with COPD based on previously published work by Elmore et al. (1994) and refinement of their previously published general screening tool (Thorsdottir, Eriksen, & Eysteinsdottir, 1999). Serum albumin, total lymphocyte count, BMI, and triceps skinfold thickness were sensitive measures in the identification of malnutrition. Triceps skinfold thickness and BMI were shown to be the best single parameters for detecting malnutrition, but neither one individually or together equaled the quality of the screening tool using the four-point criteria. Results of the study confirmed that patients with COPD are frequently malnourished and that the screening tool developed could identify 69% of malnourished patients.

In a study conducted by Soler-Cataluna et al. (2005), muscle mass depletion was estimated indirectly by determining the midarm muscle area (of the nondominant arm) and was determined to be a better predictor of mortality than BMI in COPD patients. This has important implications for nutritional screening given the obesity epidemic in this country because normal and overweight patients show muscle mass depletion (Schols et al., 1993). Adequacy of dietary intake and vitamins and minerals also needs to be addressed.

Evidence Analysis for Evidence-Based Practice

Identifying and correcting malnutrition is the main goal when working with patients with COPD. Energy needs must be increased to meet needs; however, this must be done in balance. A balanced protein-to-fat-to-carbohydrate ratio (15% to 20%:30% to 45%:40% to 55% of calories) is needed to preserve the respiratory quotient. Patients' nutritional needs should be assessed on an individual basis; however, a study conducted by Thorsdottir and Gunnarsdottir (2002) recommended energy intakes to be above 140% of basal energy expenditure and protein consumption to be at least 1.2 g/kg body weight to avoid protein losses, prevent weight loss, and prevent worsening nutritional status.

Deficiency in lung elasticity and respiratory muscle results in hypoproteinemia and in calcium, magnesium, phosphorus, vitamin K, and vitamin C deficiencies. Intakes based on DRI should be provided with magnesium and phosphorus levels monitored for patients receiving aggressive nutritional support. Increased vitamin D and vitamin K may be warranted based on results of **bone mineral density** tests, glucocorticoid medications, and adequacy of intake (Mahan, 2004). Lung function has been shown to be better when higher antioxidant levels are given (Hu & Cassano, 2000).

Diabetes

Diabetes is a serious chronic disease characterized by abnormalities in the metabolism of cholesterol, protein, and fat. The incidence of type 2 diabetes is tracking right along with the obesity epidemic and is fueling the diabetes epidemic (Cowie et al., 2003). Glucose intolerance or hyperglycemia is the common denominator and the body does not produce or respond to insulin. Insulin is a hormone produced by the B cells of the pancreas, and it is the key that "unlocks" the cells so that the cell can then utilize glucose as a fuel source. Diabetes affects 16 million people with more than 5 million undiagnosed; it is the sixth leading cause of death (Nutrition Screening Initiative, 2002; Kochanek et al., 2004). The three major forms of diabetes are type 1, type 2, and gestational diabetes, of which type 2 accounts for 90% to 95% of all cases.

Nutritional Assessment

A body weight assessment should be conducted (i.e., assessment of height, weight, BMI, and waist circumference). Waist circumference more than 40 inches for men and more than 35 inches for women has been shown to increase **insulin resistance** (Centers for Disease Control and Prevention, 2002). Blood pressure should be checked to determine whether a patient is hypertensive as well (at least 140/90 mm Hg). Laboratory work should be reviewed and evaluated based on the following: hemoglobin A_{Ic} or **glycosylated hemoglobin (HbA$_{Ic}$)**, fasting glucose, urinary glucose or ketones, blood urea nitrogen, creatine, potassium, sodium, alanine and aspartate aminotransferases, lactic acid dehydrogenase, and lipid profile. Clinical signs of malnutrition and poor control need to be recognized and addressed. Adequacy of intake and compliance needs to be assessed based on established goals individualized for each patient.

> **Insulin resistance:** An impaired biological response to either exogenous or endogenous insulin; plays a role in the etiology of type 2 diabetes.
>
> **Glycosylated hemoglobin (HbA$_{Ic}$):** A blood test that can reflect blood glucose control over a 3-month period. An A_{Ic} of 6% reflects an average plasma glucose level of about 120 mg/dL. In general, each 1% increase in A_{Ic} is a reflection of an increase in average glucose levels of about 30 mg/dL.

Evidence Analysis for Evidence-Based Practice

Although specific evidence-based nutrition principles and recommendations for the treatment and prevention of diabetes and related complications exist, they should be individualized based on each patient's usual intake and eating habits, metabolic profile, treatment goals, and desired outcomes (American Diabetes Association, 2002). The nutritional principles and recommendations are based on the following goals of medical nutrition therapy for diabetes as outlined in the 2002 American Diabetes Association Position Statement:

- Attain and maintain optimal metabolic outcomes including
  - Blood glucose levels in the normal range or as close to normal as is safely possible to prevent or reduce the risk of complications for diabetes.
  - A lipid and lipoprotein profile that reduces the risk for macrovascular disease.
  - Blood pressure levels that reduce the risk for vascular disease.
- Prevent and treat the chronic complications of diabetes. Modify nutrient intake and life-style as appropriate for the prevention and treatment of obesity, dyslipidemia, cardiovascular disease, hypertension, and nephropathy.

- Improve health through healthy food choices and physical activity.
- Address individual nutritional needs, taking into consideration personal, ethnic, and cultural preferences, and life-styles while respecting the individual's wishes and willingness to change.

In terms of specific dietary recommendations, evidence exists regarding the following:

- *Carbohydrates:* The total amount of carbohydrate in the meal or snack is more important than the source or type. Whole grains, fruits, vegetables, and low-fat milk are healthy choices. Sugar (sucrose) does not increase blood sugar levels any more than the same kilocalorie level of starch-containing food and as such does not need to be restricted in people with diabetes. If sucrose is consumed, it must be substituted for other carbohydrate sources. Nonnutritive sweeteners have been shown to be safe when consumed within the acceptable daily intake levels established by the U.S. Food and Drug Administration.
- *Protein:* There is no evidence to suggest that usual protein intakes (15% to 20%) need to be modified if renal function is not impaired.
- *Dietary fat:* Given the comorbidity of cardiovascular disease, a heart-healthy diet is warranted. Recommendations include less than 10% of total kilocalories from saturated fat and for individuals with low-density lipoprotein cholesterol more than 100 mg/dL it is recommended that saturated fat consumption be lowered to less than 7% of total kilocalories. The recommendation for total cholesterol intake is less than 300 mg/day. For individuals with low-density lipoprotein cholesterol more than 100 mg/dL cholesterol intake should be reduced to less than 200 mg/day.
- *Energy balance:* Weight loss, even modest weight loss, has been shown to improve insulin resistance and overall blood sugar control.
- *Micronutrients:* There is no clear evidence to support vitamin and mineral supplementation in people with diabetes unless they have known underlying vitamin and mineral deficiencies.
- *Alcohol:* The same guidelines apply to people with diabetes regarding alcohol intake based on the 2005 U.S. Dietary Guidelines. In addi-

tion to the fact that alcohol intake is limited to one drink for women and two drinks for men, to reduce the risk of hypoglycemia it is suggested that alcohol be consumed with food. (One drink is considered a 12 oz. beer, 5 oz. glass of wine, or 1.5 oz of 80 proof spirits.)

> **● Learning Point** Pregnancy and Lactation with Diabetes: Nutrition requirements during pregnancy and lactation are similar when compared with women who do not have diabetes. The major difference is the focus on appropriate weight gain, maintaining normoglycemia, and the absence of ketones. If weight gain is excessive, modest energy restriction may be appropriate.

- *Older adults with diabetes:* Older adults require less kilocalories to meet their nutritional needs, and they are more likely to be undernourished. Caution should be used when prescribing weight-loss diets in this population.

Chronic Kidney Disease

Chronic kidney disease is the inability of the kidney to function normally. The primary function of the kidney is to maintain homeostatic balance with respect to fluids, electrolytes, and organic solutes and to remove waste from the body through the production of urine. The kidney filters approximately 1,600 L of blood per day and produces 1 to 2 L of urine per day. Symptoms of chronic kidney disease include severe headache, **dyspnea**, failing vision, poor appetite, nausea and vomiting, abdominal pain, and mouth ulcers. Dialysis is postponed for as long as possible.

Dyspnea: Shortness of breath.

Nutritional Assessment

Nutritional assessment of the patient with chronic kidney disease is very similar to a standard nutritional assessment with some additional features based on the Kidney Dialysis Outcome Quality Initiative (K/DOQI) guidelines. In addition to evaluating the standard laboratory values available on admission, which would include albumin, the following laboratory values should be evaluated: serum prealbumin, predialysis serum creatinine, urea reduction ratio, serum bicarbonate, and lipid profile. The K/DOQI also recommends the use of the Subjective Global Assessment, a four-item seven-point scale, to monitor nutrition status changes and patients' anthropometric measurements using each patient as his or her own control.

Evidence Analysis for Evidence-Based Practice

Current clinical practice guidelines for nutritional care in chronic kidney disease are based on recommendations by the 2002 National Kidney Foundation K/QODI guidelines that can be accessed online (www.kidney.org/professionals/kdoqi). The guidelines are evidence-based with the rationale for each guideline explained and referenced based on extensive literature review evaluated for quality and strength (Beto, 2004).

More recently, under the 2003 K/DOQI guidelines, chronic kidney disease has been classified into five stages based on **glomerular filtration rate** upon which to diagnose and base care in a uniform manner (Beto, 2004). Stages 1 to 4 are predialysis, and stage 5 requires replacement therapy (dialysis) to sustain life. Dialysis therapies mimic the function of the kidneys to the extent possible, exchanging high levels of circulating products such as urea, phosphorus, and potassium that the kidney would normally remove using osmotic pressure to cross a barrier membrane to be removed from the body. There are two types of dialysis treatment: hemodialysis and peritoneal dialysis. Hemodialysis is artificial filtering of blood by a machine that requires permanent vein access through a fistula and the dialysis fluid similar to plasma. Peritoneal dialysis is artificial filtering of the blood by a hyperosmolar solution through the peritoneum.

Glomerular filtration rate: The quantity of glomerular filtrate formed per unit in all nephrons of both kidneys.

In clinical nutrition practice, intervention needs to be matched to the function of the kidney based on biochemical data and corresponding K/DOQI nutritional guidelines. This can be challenging because the function of the kidneys changes day to day and compliance to the diet can be difficult because of all the restrictions that must managed. The goals of nutritional intervention for stages 1 to 4 are to minimize tissue catabolism; maintain nutritional status, weight, appetite, electrolyte balance, and lean body mass; and postpone dialysis as long as possible. The specific nutrient recommendations based on K/DOQI guidelines for energy, protein, fat, and fluid are referenced in **Table 9.8**, and the nutrient guidelines for sodium, potassium, calcium, and phosphorus are referenced in **Table 9.9**.

HIV/AIDS

AIDS is a disease characterized by the transmission of a retrovirus called the human immunodeficiency virus by the exchange of bodily fluids through sexual contact, infected blood, contaminated needles,

TABLE 9.8 K/DOQI Nutritional Guidelines for Energy, Protein, Fat, and Fluid

Kidney Function	Energy (kcal/kg/day)	Protein (g/kg/day)	Fat (% total kcal)	Fluid (mL/day)
Normal kidney function	30–37	0.8	30–35	Unrestricted
Stage 1 to 4 chronic kidney disease	35 < 60 yr 30–35 ≥ 60 yr	0.6–0.75 50% HBV	*	Unrestricted with normal output
Stage 5 hemodialysis	35 < 60 yr 30–35 ≥ 60 yr	1.2 50% HBV	*	1,000 + urine output
Stage 5 peritoneal dialysis	35 < 60 yr 30–35 ≥ 60 yr Include kcal from dialysate	1.2–1.3 50% HBV	*	Monitored; 1,500–2,000
Transplant	30–35 initial 25–30 for maintenance	1.3–1.5 initial 1.0 for maintenance	*	Unrestricted unless indicated

*Patients at highest cardiovascular risk should follow NCEP Adult Treatment Panel III guidelines to the extent possible.

HBV, high biological value.

Source: National Kidney Foundation Kidney Dialysis Outcome Quality Initiative.

Pneumocystis carinii pneumonia, cytomegalovirus, or Kaposi's sarcoma (Gottlieb, Schanker, Saxon, Weisman, & Pozalski, 1981). HIV disease is currently the sixth leading cause of death for all races combined for the age group 25 to 44 years and ninth for the age group 45 to 64 years (Kochanek et al., 2004). AIDS is defined as an HIV infection with a CD4 cell count of 200 or less and the presence of at least one opportunistic infection, dementia, wasting syndrome, or malignant disease.

Nutritional Assessment

No nationally accepted standard of care for HIV/AIDS exists, but evidence does exist that medical nutrition therapy plays a critical role in increasing energy, protein, and micronutrient intake among HIV-positive and AIDS patients. In a joint position statement, the ADA and the Dietitians of Canada urged that nutrition referrals be made as soon as possible after the HIV-positive diagnosis to obtain the most benefit from medical

Opportunistic infection: Infection by an organism that would not ordinarily cause disease but because of an impaired immune response the organism becomes pathogenic.

or mother-to-child transmission. AIDS was first described by the Centers for Disease Control and Prevention in 1981 and included severe depression of cellular immunity accompanied by unusual **opportunistic infections** such as

TABLE 9.9 K/DOQI Nutritional Guidelines for Sodium, Potassium, Calcium, and Phosphorus

Kidney Function	Sodium (mg/day)	Potassium (mg/day)	Calcium (mg/day)	Phosphorus (mg/day)
Normal kidney function	Unrestricted	Unrestricted	Unrestricted	Unrestricted
Stage 1 to 4 chronic kidney disease	2,000	Based on lab values	1,200	Based on lab values
Stage 5 hemodialysis	2,000	2,000–3,000 (8–17 mg/kg/day)	≤2,000 from diet and medications	800–1,000
Stage 5 peritoneal dialysis	2,000	3,000–4,000 (8–17 mg/kg/day)	≤2,000 from diet and medications	800–1,000
Transplant	Unrestricted; monitor medication effect	Unrestricted; monitor medication effect	1,200	Unrestricted unless indicated

Source: National Kidney Foundation Kidney Dialysis Outcome Quality Initiative.

nutrition therapy (ADA and the Canadian Dietetic Association, 1994). In 1996 the ADA developed an HIV/AIDS medical nutrition therapy protocol that recommended a baseline nutritional assessment and nutrition self-management training to include follow-up assessment and training for the patients one to two times a year when asymptomatic and consultations two to six times a year when patients became symptomatic or converted to AIDS (Journal of the American Dietetic Association, 2004). The ADA nutritional assessment should be comprehensive and include an evaluation of weight in terms of percentage of usual weight. Anthropometric measurements are useful because many patients have multiple clinic visits and/or hospitalizations, making it possible to have numerous measurements over a period of time. Visceral protein (i.e., albumin, prealbumin) should be monitored to observe changes in visceral protein stores. Patients should be evaluated for **HIV wasting syndrome**, which is characterized by an unintentional loss of 10% body weight over 6 months, loss of 5% lean body mass within 6 months, body cell mass less than 35% and BMI less than 27 (men), body cell mass less than 23% and BMI less than 27 (women), and BMI less than 20 (Polsky, Kotler, & Steinhart, 2001).

HIV wasting syndrome: Catabolic condition; loss of body weight (body fat and muscle stores); very similar to cancer cachexia.

Evidence Analysis for Evidence-Based Practice

Studies indicate that weight determines outcome and mortality (Kotler, Tierney, Wang, & Pierson, 1989; Grunfeld & Feingold, 1992). Nutrient requirements need to be individualized for each patient and vary depending on health status. Keusch and Thea (1993) recommended when determining energy requirement using BEE × 1.3 for maintenance and BEE × 1.5 for weight gain. Additional kilocalories and protein need to be provided if fever is present, with energy requirements increasing by 13% and protein requirements increasing by 10% for every degree Celsius of temperature elevation above normal (Grunfeld & Feingold, 1992).

Nutritional Issues of Epidemic Proportion

Excessive Weight and Obesity

Excessive weight and obesity have reached epidemic proportions in the United States. The prevalence of obesity in the United States has increased at alarming rates in the last three decades (Kuczmarski, Fle-

gal, & Campbell, 1994). Excessive weight is defined as a BMI greater than 25 but less than 30. People who have a BMI of 30 or higher are considered obese. Consider the following obesity data; although not in line with young, middle, and older adults discussed earlier in the chapter, the data do differentiate between the first and second half of adulthood:

- Obesity data for 25- to 44-year-olds for 1999–2002 reported that 34.2% of adults in this age group were overweight and 28.5% were obese. Even more concerning was the 7.8% increase in the percentage of adults who were classified as obese when compared with the previous 10-year span (1988–1994). This increase in the number of obese adults contributed in part to the increase in the overall percentage of adults who were overweight or obese; 62.8% for overweight/obese up from 51.7% in 1988–1994 (Flegal, Carroll, Ogden, & Johnson, 2002; Hedley, Ogden, Carroll, Curtin, & Flegal, 2004).

- Obesity data for 45- to 64-year-olds for 1999–2002 reported that 35.7% of adults in this age group were overweight and 35.8% were obese. The increase in the percentage of adults in this age group who were overweight/obese was due to a 6.7% increase in the percentage of adults who were classified as obese. The overall percentage of adults who were overweight or obese was 71.5%, up from 65.5% in 1988–1994 (Flegal et al., 2002; Hedley et al., 2004).

Research in obesity has been extensive in the last two decades and has helped build our understanding of the genetic, psychological, metabolic, and environmental influences on body weight, which has served to increase our awareness of the complexities of weight management (ADA, 2002). The most-often-asked question is what is the cause? We live in an environment that is conducive to promoting obesity because of our sedentary life-style and the abundance of energy-dense foods (Wolf & Colditz, 1998; Allison, Fontaine, Manson, Steven, & Vanitallie, 1999). Data on weight-loss interventions do not produce long-term results and have a success rate of about 5% (National Institutes of Health & National Heart, Lung, and Blood Institute, 1998). What then is the role of the dietitian? The dietitian can play a critical role as a facilitator of change through the counseling process to help the patient formulate reasonable goals that can be met and sustained with a healthy eating approach. In terms of the nation as a whole, public policy must be changed and a battle must be waged on all fronts (i.e., the media, the food industry, etc.) if we are to win the war on obesity.

Osteoporosis

Osteoporosis, often called the "silent epidemic," is a disease that takes a lifetime to develop and consequently a lifetime to prevent. It is characterized by a decrease in bone mass and deterioration of bone tissue with no outward signs or symptoms until late in the disease when bones become much more fragile and are apt to break. Osteoporosis affects 10 million Americans annually, 80% of whom are women; women are four times more likely than men to develop osteoporosis (Kaunitz, 2000). However, men can develop osteoporosis; in fact, one-third of men by the age of 75 develop osteoporosis (Nutrition Screening Initiative, 2002). Osteoporosis leads to 1.5 million fractures every year in the United States, most commonly of the vertebrae. Visible signs of osteoporosis are altered posture caused by deformity of the spine, such as increased thoracis kyphosis (humpback) described as a "widow's hump," or postural slumping due to acute pain and loss of height as a result of vertebral collapse fractures.

Controllable measures an individual can take to avoid osteoporosis are to ensure adequate consumption of calories and to take in enough calcium to promote optimum bone development in the first three decades of life. As was mentioned earlier in the chapter, older adults need additional vitamin D and calcium as they age. Many young adults, especially women, do not consume an adequate amount of calcium and may benefit from calcium and vitamin D supplementation. Calcium and vitamin D supplementation may be beneficial for people who have a family history of osteoporosis or who are exhibiting early signs of osteoporosis. Weight-bearing exercise has been shown to be especially beneficial in helping to reduce the loss of bone mass that happens as a natural part of the aging process. More and more evidence supports the role of antiresorptive therapy, which includes hormonal therapy (estrogen replacement therapy during menopause), bisphosphate therapy (Fosamax or Actonel), selective estrogen receptor modulators (Evista), and calcitonin (Miacalcin), in reducing the incidence of osteoporosis (National Institutes of Health Consensus Development Panel on Osteoporosis Prevention, 2001; Nutrition Action Healthletter, 2002).

Summary

Although genetic predisposition determines longevity to a degree, each person can choose to live a longer healthier life by eating healthier and exercising. Nutrigenomics is a new and upcoming field that encompasses the study of nutrition and genetics. Thanks to the Human Genome Project, nutritional science is on the edge of a new frontier (Collins & McKusick, 2001). It may be possible someday to receive a nutrition prescription based on your genetic profile with nutrition recommendations that reflect the latest scientific evidence utilizing evidence-based analysis and practice guidelines. Nutrition experts have much work ahead of us if we are going to contribute to the impact of the obesity and osteoporosis epidemics in this country. At the same time we must pay close attention to what is fast becoming the next epidemic—type 2 diabetes. Although each person must take personal responsibility for the choices he or she makes, including food choices and how much to exercise, it is up to us as professionals to interpret the latest nutrition research and translate this information to the public and advocate for public policy that promotes an environment conducive to a healthier life.

Issues to Debate

1. What can the dietetics profession do to help people make better life-style choices?
2. How can some of these ideas be made a practical reality?
3. What is the responsibility of corporate America in keeping people healthy?

References

Allison, D. B., Fontaine, K. R., Manson, J. E., Steven, J., & Vanitallie, T. B. (1999). Annual deaths attributable to obesity in the United States. *Journal of the American Medical Association, 282,* 1530–1538.

American Diabetes Association. (2002). Position statement: Evidence-based nutrition principles and recommendations for the treatment and prevention of diabetes and related complications. *Journal of the American Dietetic Association, 102,* 109–120.

American Dietetic Association (ADA). (2000). ADA Reports: Position of the American Dietetic Association: Nutrition, aging and the continuum of care. *Journal of the American Dietetic Association, 100,* 580.

American Dietetic Association (ADA). (2002). Position of the American Dietetic Association: Weight management. *Journal of the American Dietetic Association, 102,* 1145–1155.

American Dietetic Association (ADA), & Canadian Dietetic Association. (1994). Nutrition intervention in the care of persons with human immunodeficiency virus infection. *Journal of the American Dietetic Association, 94,* 129–132.

Appel, L. J., Moore, T. J., Obarzanek, E., Vollmer, W. M., Svetkey, L. P., Sacks, F. M., et al. (1997). A clinical trial of the effects of dietary pattern on blood pressure. *New England Journal of Medicine, 336,* 1117-1124.

Berry, J. K., & Braunschwig, C. A. (1998). Nutritional Assessment of the critically ill patient. *Critical Care Nursing Quarterly, 21,* 33.

Beto, J. A., & Bansal, U. K. (2004). Medical nutrition therapy in chronic kidney failure; integrating clinical practice guidelines. *Journal of the American Dietetic Association, 104,* 404–409.

Brandi, L. S., & Calafa, M. (1997). Indirect calorimetry in critically ill patients: Clinical applications and practical advice. *Nutrition, 13,* 349–358.

Brown, J. E., Isaacs, J. S., Krinke, U. B., Murtaugh, M. A., Sharbaugh, C., Stang, J., et al. (2005). *Nutrition Through the Life Cycle* (2nd ed.). Belmont, CA: Thomson Wadsworth.

Centers for Disease Control and Prevention (CDC). (2002). Basics about overweight and obesity. Retrieved from www. cdc.gov/nccdphp/dnpa/obesity/basics.htm.

Chin, A., Paw, M. J., DeJong, N., Schouten, E. G., Hiddink, G. J., & Kok, F. J. (2001). Physical exercise and/or enriched foods for functional improvement in frail, independent living elderly: A randomized controlled trial. *Archives of Physical and Medical Rehabilitation, 82,* 811–817.

Collins, F. S., & McKusick, V. A. (2001). Implications of the Human Genome Project for medical science. *Journal of the American Medical Association, 285,* 540.

Committee on Nutrition Services for Medicare Beneficiaries and Institute of Medicine. (2000). *The Role of Nutrition in Maintaining Health in the Nation's Elderly.* Washington, DC.

Cowie, C. C., MMWR, & CDC Surveillance System. (2003). Diabetes rose slightly in the 1990s. In C. f. D. C. P. Release (Producer).

Elmore, M. F., Wagner, D. R., Knoll, D. M., Eizember, L., Oswall, M. A., Glowinski, E. A., et al. (1994). Developing an effective adult nutrition screening tool for a community hospital. *Journal of the American Dietetic Association, 94,* 1113–1118, 1121.

Flegal, K. M., Carroll, M. D., Ogden, C. L., & Johnson, C. L. (2002). Prevalence and trends in obesity among US adults, 1999–2000. *Journal of the American Medical Association, 288,* 1723–1727.

Fonesa, V., & Wall, J. (1995). Diet and diabetes in the elderly. *Clinical Geriatric Medicine, 11,* 613–624.

Food and Nutrition Board, Committee on Diet and Health, & National Research Council. (1989). *Diet and Health: Implications for Reducing Chronic Disease Risk.* Washington, DC: National Academy Press.

Food and Nutrition Board, National Research Council, & National Academy of Sciences. (1989). *Recommended Dietary Allowances.* Washington, DC: National Academy Press.

Frankenfield, D., Roth-Yousey, L., & Compher, C. (2005). Comparison of predictive equations for resting metabolic rate in healthy nonobese and obese adults: A systematic review. *Journal of the American Dietetic Association, 105,* 775–790.

Gallagher-Allred, C. R., Voss, A. C., Finn, S. C., & McCamish, M. A. (1996). Malnutrition and clinical outcomes: The case for medical nutrition therapy. *Journal of the American Dietetic Association, 96,* 361–367.

Gary, R., & Fleury, J. (2002). Nutritional status: Key to preventing decline in hospitalized older adults. *Topics in Geriatric Rehabilitation, 17,* 40–71.

Gottlieb, M. S., Schanker, H. M., Saxon, A., Weisman, J. D., & Pozalski, I. (1981). *Pneumocystis* pneumonia—Los Angeles. *Morbidity and Mortality Weekly Review, 30,* 250–252.

Gray-Donald, K., Gibbson, L., Shapiro, S. H., Macklern, P. T., & Martin, J. G. (1996). Nutritional status and mortality in chronic obstructive pulmonary disease. *American Journal of Respiratory and Critical Care Medicine, 153,* 961–966.

Grunfeld, C., & Feingold, K. R. (1992). Metabolic disturbances and wasting in the acquired immunodeficiency syndrome. *New England Journal of Medicine, 327,* 329–337.

Hanley, D. A., & Davison, K. S. (2005). Vitamin D insufficiency in North America. *Journal of Nutrition, 135,* 332–338.

Harvard Health Letter. (2002). Aging: Living to 100. What's the secret? *Harvard Health Letter, 27,* 1.

Hedley, A. A., Ogden, C. L., Carroll, M. D., Curtin, L. R., & Flegal, K. M. (2004). Overweight and obesity among US children, adolescents, and adults, 1999–2002. *Journal of the American Medical Association, 291,* 2847–2850.

Hu, G., & Cassano, P. (2000). Antioxidant nutrients and pulmonary function: The Third National Health and Nutrition Examination Survey. *American Journal of Epidemiology, 151,* 975.

Ireton-Jones, C. J. (1997). Why use predictive equations for energy expenditure assessment? *Journal of the American Dietetic Association, 9,* A44.

Journal of the American Dietetic Association. (2004). Position of the Amer Dietetic Assoc and Dietitians of Canada: Position paper. Nutrition Intervention in care of persons with HIV infection. *Journal of the American Dietetic Association, 104,* 1425–1441.

Kant, A. K. (2000). Consumption of energy-dense nutrient-poor foods by adult Americans: Nutritional and health implications. The third National Health and Nutrition

Examination Survey, 1984–1994. *American Journal of Clinical Nutrition, 72*, 929.

Kaunitz, A. M. (2000). Osteoporosis: The silent epidemic. *Jacksonville Medicine, 51*(5).

Kelly, K. (2003). The "freshman 15." *U.S. News and World Report, 135*, 54.

Keusch, G. T., & Thea, D. M. (1993). Malnutrition in AIDS. *Medical Clinics of North America, 77*, 795.

Klipstein-Grobusch, K., Reilly, J., Potter, J., Edwards, C., & Roberts, M. (1995). Energy intake and expenditure in elderly patients admitted to hospital with acute illness. *British Journal of Nutrition, 73*, 323–324.

Kochanek, K. D., Murphy, S. L., Anderson, R. N., & Scott, C. (2004). *Deaths: Final Data for 2002.* Hyattsville, MD: National Center for Health Statistics.

Kotler, D. P., Tierney, A. R., Wang, J., & Pierson, R. N. (1989). Magnitude of body cell mass depletion and the timing of death from wasting in AIDS. *American Journal of Clinical Nutrition, 50*, 444–447.

Kuczmarski, R. J., Flegal, K. M., & Campbell, S. M. (1994). Overweight prevalence and trends for children and adolescents: The National Health and Nutrition Examination Surveys, 1963 to 1991. *Journal of the American Medical Association, 149*, 1085–1092.

Laaban, J. P., Kouchakji, B., Dore, M. F., Orvoen-Frija, E., David, P., & Rochemaure, J. (1993). Nutritional status of patients with chronic obstructive pulmonary disease and acute respiratory failure. *Chest, 103*, 1362–1368.

Lacey, K. P. E. (2003). Nutrition Care Process and Model: ADA adopts road map to quality care and outcome management. *Journal of the American Dietetic Association, 103*, 1061–1072.

Levitsky, D. A., & Youn, T. (2004). The more food young adults are served, the more they overeat. *Journal of Nutrition, 134*, 2436–2550.

Mahan, L. E. (2004). *Krause's Food, Nutrition, and Diet Therapy* (11th ed.). Philadelphia: W. B. Saunders.

Martin, J. A., Hamilton, B. E., Sutton, P. D., Ventura, S. J., Menacker, F., & Munson, M. L. (2005). *Births: Final Data for 2003.* Hyattsville, MD: National Center for Health Statistics.

Myers, E. F., Pritchett, E., & Johnson, E. Q. (2002). Evidence-based practice guides vs protocols: What's the difference? *Journal of the American Dietetic Association, 101*, 1085–1090.

National Center for Health Statistics, (1984–1995). *Prevalence of Selected Conditions by Age and Sex: United States.* Retrieved January 12, 2006, from http://www.cdc.gov/nchc/agingact.htm.

National Cholesterol Education Program (NCEP). (1988). Report of the National Cholesterol Education Program Expert Panel on Detection, Education, and Treatment of High Blood Cholesterol in Adults. *Archives of Internal Medicine, 148*, 36–69.

National Cholesterol Education Program (NCEP). (2001). Executive summary of the third report of the National Cholesterol Education Program Expert Panel on Detection, Evaluation, and Treatment of High Blood Cholesterol in Adults (Adult Treatment Panel III). *Journal of the American Medical Association, 285*, 2486.

National Heart, Lung, and Blood Institute, & National Institutes of Health. (2002). *Third Report of the National Cholesterol Education Program Expert Panel on Detection, Evaluation and Treatment of High Cholesterol in Adults (Adult Treatment Panel III).* Washington, DC: National Institutes of Health.

National Institutes of Health, & National Heart, Lung, and Blood Institute. (1998). Clinical guidelines on the identification, evaluation and treatment of overweight and obesity in adults—The evidence report. *Obesity Research, 6*, 121.

National Institutes of Health Consensus Development Panel on Osteoporosis Prevention, Diagnosis, and Treatment. (2001). Osteoporosis prevention, diagnosis, and treatment. *Journal of the American Medical Association, 285*, 785.

Nutrition Action Healthletter. (2002). Bare bones: How to keep yours strong. *Nutrition Action Healthletter, 29*.

Nutrition Screening Initiative. (2002). *A Physician's Guide to Nutrition in Chronic Disease Management for Older Adults.* Retrieved February 25, 2006, from http://www.aafp.org/x16105.xml

Olshansky, S. J., Ludwig, D. S., Passaro, D. J., Allison, D. B., Hershow, R. C., Butler, R., et al. (2005). A potential decline in life expectancy in the United States in the 21st century. *New England Journal of Medicine, 352*, 1138–1146.

Polsky, B., Kotler, D., & Steinhart, C. (2001). HIV-associated wasting in the HAART era: Guidelines for assessment, diagnosis and treatment. *AIDS Patient Care and STDs, 15*, 411.

Public Health Service. (1988). *The Surgeon General's Report on Nutrition and Health: Summary and Recommendations.* Publ. No. 88-50211. Washington, DC: Department of Health and Human Service, Public Health Service.

Rogers, R. M., Donahoe, M., & Constantino, J. (1992). Physiologic effects of oral supplemental feeding in malnourished patients with chronic obstructive pulmonary disease. *The American Review of Respiratory Disease, 146*, 1511–1517.

Russell, R. (1997). New views on the RDAs for older adults. *Journal of the American Dietetic Association, 97*, 515–518.

Schoeller, D. A. (1999). Recent advances from application of doubly labeled water to measurement of human energy expenditure. *Journal of Nutrition, 129*, 1765–1768.

Schols, A. M. W. J., Mostert, R., Soester, P., Greve, L. H., & Wouters, E. M. F. (1989). Inventory of nutritional status in patients with COPD. *Chest, 96*, 247–249.

Schols, A. M. W. J., Soeters, P. B., Dingemans, A. M. C., Mostert, R., Frantzen, P. J., & Wouters, E. F. (1993). Prevalence and characteristics of nutritional depletion in patients with COPD eligible for pulmonary rehabiliation. *The American Review of Respiratory Disease, 147*, 1151–1156.

Smith, R. (2003). Expanding medical nutrition therapy: An argument for evidence-based practices. *Journal of the American Dietetic Association, 103*, 313–314.

Soler-Cataluna, J. J., Sanchez-Sanchez, L., Martinez-Garcia, M. A., Sanchez, P. R., Salcedo, E., & Navarro, M. (2005). Mid-arm muscle area is a better predictor of mortality than body mass index in COPD. *Chest, 128*, 2108–2115.

Thorsdottir, I., Gunnarsdottir, I, & Eriksen, B. (2001). Screening method evaluated by nutritional status measurements can be used to detect malnourishment in chronic obstructive pulmonary disease. *Journal of the American Dietetic Association, 101*, 648.

Thorsdottir, I., Eriksen, B., & Eysteinsdottir, S. (1999). Nutritional status at submission for dietetic services and screening for malnutrition at admission to hospital. *Clinical Nutrition, 18*, 15–21.

Thorsdottir, I., & Gunnarsdottir, I. (2002). Energy intake must be increased among recently hospitalized patients with chronic obstructive pulmonary disease to improve nutritional status. (Research and Professional Briefs). *Journal of the American Dietetic Association, 102*, 247.

Trials of Hypertension Prevention Collaborative Research Group. (1997). Effects of weight loss and sodium reduction intervention on blood pressure and hypertension incidence in overweight people with high-normal blood pressure. *Archives of Internal Medicine*, 157, 657.

U.S. Department of Health and Human Services. (2000). *Healthy People 2010* (2nd ed.). *With Understanding and Improving Health and Objectives for Improving Health.* Washington, DC: U.S. Government Printing Office.

Wardlaw, G. M., Hampl, J. S., & DiSilvestro, R. A. (2004). *Perspectives in Nutrition* (6th ed.). New York: McGraw Hill.

Whittaker, J. S., Ryan, C. F., Buckley, P. A., & Road, J. D. (1990). The effects of refeeding on peripheral and respiratory muscle function in malnourished chronic obstructive pulmonary disease patients. *The American Review of Respiratory Disease, 142*, 283–288.

Wolf, A. M., & Colditz, G. A. (1998). Current estimates of the economic cost of obesity in the United States. *Obesity Research, 6*, 97–106.

Worthington-Roberts, B. S. (1996). *Nutrition Throughout the Life Cycle* (3rd ed.). St. Louis: Mosby.

CHAPTER 10

Special Topics in Adults and Chronic Diseases: Nutrition and Public Health

Judith Sharlin, PhD, RD

CHAPTER OUTLINE

Reader Objectives

After studying this chapter and reflecting on the contents, you should be able to

1. Identify the primary causes of death and disability in adults in the United States.

2. Describe primary, secondary, and tertiary levels of health prevention and health promotion and their relationship to nutrition program planning.

3. Identify risk factors for chronic diseases and their implication for nutrition.

4. Describe the dietary risk factors associated with the leading chronic diseases.

5. Discuss the common features of the dietary guidelines issued by the major U.S. health organizations.

6. Compare different dietary interventions a public health nutritionist or dietitian offers to the community, family, or an individual at risk.

7. Recognize the mission and role of public health nutrition in preventing disease and promoting adult health.

8. Name some of the public health nutrition programs that exist today for maintaining adult health.

Preventing Disease and Promoting Health

Growing scientific evidence reveals that nutrition or dietary intake in adults contributes significantly to preventing illnesses and premature deaths in the United States (Frazao, 1999). Life expectancy has increased dramatically over the past 100 years, and today the average life expectancy is 77 years (U.S. Department of Health and Human Services [USDHHS], 2000a). Health and nutrition programs for adults aim at prevention and improving quality of life. However, chronic diseases account for 7 of every 10 deaths in the United States (USDHHS, 2004). The increasing cost of crisis medical care and the growing economic burden provide a cost-effective incentive for individuals and our nation to prevent chronic disease. Chronic diseases cost the United States 75% of the $1 trillion spent on health care annually (USDHHS, 2004). In spite of this, only 3% of the total annual health care expenditures in our nation were spent on prevention (Centers for Disease Control and Prevention [CDC], 1992). Nutrition interventions and policies target the factors related to adult health and aim to prevent chronic diseases that are the leading causes of death and disability.

Chronic Diseases: The Leading Causes of Death and Disability

To successfully create programs to promote health, longevity, and quality of life, we must examine the leading causes of death and disability. Data from the National Center for Health Statistics (NCHS) show that chronic diseases are the leading causes of death and disability (Table 10.1) (National Vital Statistics Report, 2003). Cardiovascular diseases and cancer account for more than half of all deaths in the United States (USDHHS, 2004).

● **Learning Point** More than 60% of chronic disease mortality can be attributed to life-style factors such as diet, which can be modified (Krauss et al., 2000).

A report on the health status of U.S. adults emphasized that increasing numbers of people still smoke, are physically inactive, and are overweight (NCHS, 2003). Mokdad and colleagues (2004) noted that about half of the deaths among U.S. adults in 2000 could have been prevented. These findings revealed that 400,000 deaths occur each year because of poor diet and physical inactivity. (This number was found to be 20% less in a subsequent study [Mokdad,

TABLE 10.1 Deaths and Percentage of Total Deaths for the 10 Leading Causes of Death: United States 2000–2001

Cause of death and year		Rank[1]	2001 Deaths	2001 Percent of total deaths	2000 Deaths	2000 Percent of total deaths
All causes		...	2,416,425	100.0	2,403,351	100.0
Diseases of the heart	(100–109,111,113, 120–151)	1	700,142	29.0	710,760	29.6
Malignant neoplasms	(C00–C97)	2	553,768	22.9	553,091	23.0
Cerebrovascular diseases	(160–169)	3	163,538	6.8	167,661	7.0
Chronic lower respiratory diseases	(J40–J47)	4	123,013	5.1	122,009	5.1
Accidents (unintentional injuries)	(V01–X59,Y85–Y86)	5	101,537	4.2	97,900	4.1
Diabetes mellitus	(E10–E14)	6	71,372	3.0	69,301	2.9
Influenza and pneumonia	(J10–J18)	7	62,034	2.6	65,313	2.7
Alzheimer's disease	(G30)	8	53,852	2.2	49,558	2.1
Nephritis, nephrotic syndrome, and nephrosis	(N00–N07,N17–N19, N25–N27)	9	39,480	1.6	37,251	1.5
Septicemia	(A40–A41)	10	32,238	1.3	31,224	1.3

...Category not applicable.
[1]Rank based on number of deaths.
Source: National Vital Statistics Report. (Nov. 7, 2003). Deaths and Leading Causes for 2001. Vol. 52, no. 9.

Marks, Stroup, & Gerberding, 2005].) It appears that the increasing trend of excessive weight and obesity will likely overtake tobacco as the leading preventable cause of mortality in the United States (Mokdad et al., 2004; USDHHS, 2002). Although mortality rates from heart disease, stroke, and cancer have declined, behavioral changes have led to an increased prevalence of obesity and diabetes (Koplan & Dietz, 1999; USDHHS, 2002). Dietary factors are now associated with 4 of the 10 leading causes of death: coronary heart disease (CHD), some types of cancer, stroke, and type 2 diabetes (NCHS, 1997). The Surgeon General's report in 1988 confirmed these findings: "For two out of three adult Americans who do not smoke and do not drink excessively, one personal choice seems to influence long-term health prospects more than any other, what we eat" (USDHHS, 1988).

Risk Factors and Chronic Disease

Chronic diseases, although prevalent and costly, are among the most preventable. Research has identified a Health Promotion and Preventive Action model for risk factors (Elo & Caltrop, 2002). In this model risk factor identification, reduction, modification, and education are related to human health and developmental stages (Elo & Caltrop, 2002). **Risk factors** can be defined as those specific characteristics associated with an increased chance of developing a chronic disease.

Risk factors: Specific characteristics associated with an increased chance of developing a chronic disease.

Risk factors that can be changed or modified, such as diet or physical activity, are those most commonly associated with life-style choices (Wimbush & Peters, 2000). There are four types of risk factors (USDHHS, 2000a):

1. Biological factors such as an individual's genetic makeup, family history, age, or gender
2. Environmental conditions, such as social and physical environment
3. Access to quality health care
4. Individual behavior and life-style factors such as smoking, exercise, and good eating habits

Healthy People 2010 (HP 2010) provides the most recent guidelines and recommendations for specific health objectives and goals for the nation (USDHHS, 2000a). HP 2010 reveals that individual biological behaviors and environmental factors are responsible for approximately 70% of all premature deaths (USDHHS, 2000a). Biological factors such as age or gender are not modifiable. However, the leading causes of death are associated with dietary factors, which are modifiable. The determinants of health illustrate how individual biology and behaviors influence health through the individual's social and physical environments (USDHHS, 2000a). Finally, health can be improved through policies and interventions with access to quality health care. Because the leading causes of illness and death in the United States, such as CHD, some types of cancer, stroke, type 2 diabetes, and atherosclerosis, are associated with dietary factors, we must address the concern that chronic diseases have resulted from dietary excesses and imbalance (USDHHS, 2000a). Furthermore, there is evidence that more intensive dietary counseling can lead to reduced intakes of dietary fat and cholesterol and increased fiber, fruit, and vegetable consumption (USDHHS, 2003b).

● **Learning Point** HP 2010 outlines 28 focus areas that include risk factors for chronic diseases and addresses nutrition and excessive weight, physical activity, tobacco use, cancer, diabetes, cardiovascular disease, and access to quality health care.

Prevention Strategies

Health promotion and disease prevention provide complementary interventions to change health risk factors. Prevention efforts in public heath, community, and worksite settings are divided into three levels: primary prevention (health promotion), secondary prevention (risk appraisal and reduction), and tertiary prevention (treatment and rehabilitation) (Shamansky & Clausen, 1980; Kaufman, 1990; American Dietetic Association [ADA], 1998).

Primary Prevention: Health Promotion

Primary prevention strategies, or health promotion, encourage health-enhancing behaviors by giving individuals, families, and communities ways to reduce risk factors associated with disease and injury (ADA, 1998). Risk factors include environmental, economic, social, and biological aspects.

Primary prevention strategies: Encourage health-enhancing behaviors by giving individuals, families, and communities ways to reduce risk factors associated with disease and injury.

Good examples of primary prevention strategies include nutrition and weight management classes in a community center for adults, environmental changes to provide nutritious choices in a school cafeteria vending machine, and local 5-A-Day for Better Health campaigns to increase the availability of fresh fruits and vegetables from farmers' markets (ADA,

1998). Primary prevention strategies seek to expand the positive potential of health (Brunner et al., 1997).

A **holistic approach,** embracing individual life-style factors, the environment, and economic, social, and political factors, can help communities and private sector partners achieve health promotion and disease prevention goals. Providing information, available on food labels and through health messages to the public, is one effective method. These messages encourage consumers to apply the U.S. Dietary Guidelines, the Food Guide Pyramid, Dietary Reference Intakes, and the Dietary Guidelines Alliance's It's All About You campaigns (U.S. Department of Agriculture [USDA] and USDHHS, 1992; Dietary Guidelines Alliance, 1996; USDA, 2000). Voluntary community and health organizations, the federal government, worksite programs, and schools can reach consumers daily to promote nutrition interventions.

> **Holistic approach:** Individual life-style factors, social and political issues, and access to quality health care.

The media remain an effective means of communicating nutrition issues to the public (ADA, 1996). Programs to promote physical activity and fitness, good nutrition, and smoking cessation must be broadly accessible. Worksite nutrition-centered health promotion and disease prevention programs provide opportunities to harness social support and influence (ADA, Office of Disease Prevention and Health Promotion, and USDHHS, 1993).

Motivations should be provided for food processors and vendors, restaurant chefs, and school and worksite cafeteria managers to prepare and serve foods lower in fat, calories, and sodium. Finally, legislation and regulations can be ratified to endorse more complete food and nutrition labeling. Food labels that provide short, unequivocal, positive messages aimed at a single behavior prove beneficial to consumers (Goldberg, 1992).

Secondary Prevention: Risk Appraisal and Risk Reduction

> **Secondary prevention:** Risk appraisal and screening to emphasize early detection and diagnosis of disease.

Secondary prevention includes risk appraisal and screening to emphasize early detection and diagnosis of disease (Shamansky & Clausen, 1980; JADA, 1998 ; Elo & Caltrop, 2002). Secondary prevention begins at the point where the pathology of a disease may occur. It encompasses diagnostic services that include screening, surveillance, and clinical examinations (Elo & Caltrop, 2002). Screening strategies include follow-up education, counseling, and health referral. One model for sec-

ondary prevention involving screening is a cholesterol screening program for early detection of cardiovascular problems, such as elevated blood pressure, elevated blood cholesterol, and high glucose levels (Sharlin, Posner, Gershoff, Zeitlin, & Berger, 1992). For people with an elevated blood cholesterol level, this means introducing "therapeutic life-style changes," such as reducing total and saturated fat in the diet, increasing physical activity, and reducing or maintaining a healthy weight. If this is not effective, or if low-density lipoprotein levels are abnormally high, drug therapy can be recommended by the physician.

Strategies in secondary prevention are aimed at self-care for people with chronic diseases. An example of a secondary prevention program involving self-care is an educational and awareness program to teach a woman with a history of gestational diabetes how to control her weight through diet and exercise (Shamansky & Clausen, 1980; ADA, 1998).

Tertiary Prevention: Treatment and Rehabilitation

> **Tertiary prevention:** Treatment and rehabilitation; reduction in the amount of disability caused by a disease to achieve the highest level of function.

Tertiary prevention involves treatment and rehabilitation and is defined as the reduction in the amount of disability caused by a disease to achieve the highest level of function (Pender, 1996). Examples of tertiary diseases include diabetes, kidney disease, and angina. The goal of treatment and rehabilitation is the prevention of further disability and any secondary conditions that might result from the initial health problem.

Examples of tertiary prevention programs include medical nutrition therapy (MNT) for people suffering from kidney disease, nutrition education about vitamin and mineral supplementation and feeding strategies to prevent further complications of wasting from HIV/AIDS, and cardiac rehabilitation through diet, exercise, and stress management. The ultimate goal of tertiary prevention is, through rehabilitation, to restore the individual to an "optimal" level of functioning, given the constraints of the disease (ADA, 1998).

Implications of the Prevention Levels

The prevention levels are useful concepts to help set objectives for public health programs concerned with adult health in communities, worksites, and other settings. Recent findings underscore the need to emphasize population-based prevention programs (Resnicow, Orlandi, Vaccaro, & Wynder, 1989; Wimbush & Peters, 2000). As discussed earlier, research points to a holistic approach that aims at health and prevention when using the level concept for public health programs. This approach is embraced in HP 2010 in terms of the nutrition and health objectives (USDHHS, 2000a). For each goal, the holistic approach involving individual life-style factors, environmental factors, social and political issues, and access to quality health care is addressed.

Public health endeavors focus on primary or secondary prevention. It is important to choose the appropriate prevention level when planning a public health program. This is illustrated with two different approaches for handling CHD risk factors: one intended to reduce the prevalence of high blood pressure and one to reduce obesity levels.

Almost all Americans have had their blood pressure measured sometime in their lives. Ninety percent of Americans had their blood pressure measured in the past two years and could state whether it was normal or abnormally high (USDHHS, CDC, & NCHS, 2003). Over 90% of Americans are aware of the relationship between hypertension and stroke and hypertension and heart disease (USDHHS & National Heart, Lung, and Blood Institute, 2004). Almost 70% of people with hypertension know about high blood pressure, yet the same percentage (70%) do not have their blood pressure under control (less than 140/90 mm Hg) (CDC, 2004a). Kannel et al. (1980) showed that systolic (higher number) blood pressure is a more important predictor of heart disease than diastolic blood pressure, especially in the elderly. In addition, ethnic disparities exist for prevalence rates of high blood pressure, and African-Americans in the United States have a greater prevalence of high blood pressure than do whites (CDC, 2004a). These data suggest that to reduce mortality from hypertension, secondary prevention strategies should be directed toward persons with hypertension (especially those with elevated systolic pressures), African-Americans, and the elderly. This would be more effective than primary prevention strategies aimed at increasing public awareness.

In contrast, many Americans are just beginning to be aware of the growing obesity epidemic and the significance of elevated body mass index (BMI) (30 and above) for the risk of death and illness (USDHHS, 2004). Americans understand the viability of lowering this risk factor associated with many chronic diseases. Extensive data exist to substantiate that making life-style changes such as engaging in regular physical activity and healthy eating could, at the very least, halt the continued growth of the obesity epidemic (USDHHS, 2004). Given the dramatic increases in overweight and obese U.S. adults between 1976–1980 and 1999–2000 (USDHHS, 2004), population-based efforts could be more efficient at reducing the obesity epidemic than efforts to identify those individuals at risk.

One primary prevention effort, called America on the Move (2004), is a national initiative dedicated to helping individuals and communities become more physically active and to eat more healthfully. The program creates and supports an "integrated grassroots network" at the state level to build communities that support individual behavior changes. In addition, America on the Move involves public and private partnerships at the national, state, and local levels. It publicizes small behavioral changes such as cutting 100 calories a day and taking 2,000 steps daily.

Health promotion and chronic disease prevention programs should focus on coalition building between community-based nutrition and health professionals, government, local businesses, health agencies, and insurers (ADA, 1998). In this rapidly changing healthcare environment, continued training and research in public health program development is crucial to provide evidence of the efficacy of health prevention and promotion.

All levels of prevention should be addressed when devising strategies for dietary behavior changes for chronic disease prevention. However, for some diseases, the nutrition strategy may prove similar at each prevention level. Weight reduction, for example, may prevent the onset of hypertension or may be part of the treatment for type 2 diabetes. In the case of other diseases, such as cancer, nutrition strategies might vary with the prevention level.

Dietary Guidelines for Disease Prevention

Various health organizations and government agencies have issued dietary guidelines and recommendations based on current scientific evidence. In 1989 the National Research Council published its report, *Diet and Health: Implications for Reducing Chronic Disease Risk*, providing evidence for the relationship between all major chronic conditions and diet (USDHHS, 2004). More recently, HP 2010 set forth a comprehensive health promotion and disease prevention program for the nation. HP 2010's comprehensive health agenda has two overarching goals: (1) to increase the quality and years of a healthy life and (2) to eliminate health disparities (USDHHS, 2000a). These goals embrace the dietary recom-

Visit www.health.gov for more information about the National Research Council's report, *Diet and Health: Implications for Reducing Chronic Disease Risk.*

mendations set forth by several government and health organizations.

In 2001 the U.S. Dietary Guidelines were assessed in terms of surveillance and research needs, especially related to risk for chronic diseases, such as cancer (American Institute of Cancer Research [AICR], 2001). In the same year, the revised Dietary Guidelines of the American Heart Association (AHA) gave greater emphasis to the diet as a whole and, specifically, to certain protective foods for chronic disease risk prevention (Kris-Etherton et al., 2001). Scientifically based dietary guidelines from the American Cancer Society (ACS) and the AICR reinforce these guidelines and further emphasize eating foods from plant sources (AICR, 2004). Dietary recommendations for women reiterated these health-promoting dietary guidelines (ADA & Dietitians of Canada, 2004). In addition, the Alternate Healthy Eating Index was developed to target food choices and nutrient intake associated with chronic disease risk (McCullough et al., 2002).

The dietary guidelines from these major health organizations agree in their basic message. The AICR stated, "Our research has shown that a diet that prevents cancer can also prevent other chronic diseases . . . the United States Department of Agriculture (USDA) and other major health organizations are now largely in agreement about specific dietary guidelines that protect overall health" (AHA, 2004).

The AHA, the ACS, the American Diabetes Association, the AICR, and the North American Association for the Study of Obesity concur with the new dietary recommendations (AHA, 2004). In July 2004 the ACS, the American Diabetes Association, and the AHA collaborated to work on health promotion and disease prevention (Eyre, Kahn, & Robertson, 2004). In their collaborative efforts these organizations are making unified health statements concerning the prevention of heart disease, cancer, diabetes, and related risk factors. Furthermore, these organizations agree on the following dietary patterns, which may help reduce the risk of chronic diseases (AHA, 2004; Eyre et al., 2004):

- Consume a diet that emphasizes whole grains and legumes, vegetables, and fruits.
- Decrease saturated fat and dietary cholesterol; limit red meat and full-fat dairy products.
- Limit intake of foods and beverages high in added sugars.

- Limit overall intake of calories and engage in regular physical activity to maintain a healthy body weight.

Despite the evidence of the importance of diet to health, vegetable and fruit consumption among adults continues to be below recommended amounts: Less than 25% of U.S. adults consume five servings a day (ACS, 2004). According to the USDA's 1994–1996 Continuing Survey of Food Intakes by Individuals and the Food Guide Pyramid, only 3% of individuals meet four of the five recommendations for the intake of grains, fruits, vegetables, dairy products, and meats (USDA, 1998).

The 2006 Dietary Guidelines for Americans was released in January 2005 by the USDHHS and the USDA. In the past a diet low in fat was recommended, but in 2000 this recommendation was changed to a diet "moderate" in total fat, and specifically low in saturated fat and cholesterol. The dietary guidelines have consistently encouraged the consumption of complex carbohydrates and fiber by eating more fruits, vegetables, and whole grains. In 2000 the guidelines separated the recommendations for eating fruits and vegetables and eating whole grains. The issue of safe foods was added. The two separate guidelines—"aiming for a healthy weight" and "increasing physical activity"—also were added in 2000.

In revising the Dietary Guidelines and the Food Guide Pyramid for 2006, the following revisions have been proposed (USDA, 2004):

- Balance calories from foods and beverages according to the amount of calories expended and using the food guide to determine appropriate caloric requirements based on age and physical activity levels.
- Select nutritional goals for food intake patterns.
- Propose food intake patterns for educating the American public about healthful eating patterns.
- Use "cups" and "ounces" instead of "servings" in educational materials.
- Select appropriate illustrations of food patterns for consumer materials.

In summary, diverse health organizations stress the similarities in the dietary recommendations for reducing disease risk. These recommendations are to eat less saturated fat and cholesterol (limit red meat and full-fat dairy products); increase consumption of fruits, vegetables, whole grains, and legumes; limit added sugar and sodium; drink alcohol in moderation; and increase physical activity. By using clear terms, public health nutrition and dietetic professionals can make the nutrition message easier for the public to understand, value, and implement.

Diet and Health: Nutrition Strategies and Risk Factors

Nutrition strategies are essential in the prevention and management of several chronic diseases and their risk factors.

● **Learning Point** When developing a public health program, risk factor assessment needs to be addressed. The following criteria can be assessed:

■ The risk factor must have a strong association with the development of a chronic disease (e.g., obesity and heart disease).
■ The risk factor must affect a significant number of people.
■ The risk factor must be modifiable, so it can be reduced or changed.
■ The risk factor must have a modification that, when changed or reduced, results in decreased mortality.

Because many risk factors can be modified by healthy life-style changes, early recognition of the risk factors for chronic disease prevention is critical.

Obesity

Obesity has reached epidemic proportions in the United States. In 1999–2000 nearly 65% of adults were overweight or obese (Eyre et al., 2004; USDHHS, 2004). Rates of excessive weight and obesity are steadily growing in our country. Nearly 55% of the U.S. adult population was overweight or obese in 1988–1994, compared with 46% in 1976–1980 (USDHHS, 2000b). The National Institutes of Health (NIH) Expert Panel uses BMI for defining excessive weight and obesity (National Heart, Lung, and Blood Institute [NHLBI], 1998). The cut-off point for *overweight* status is a BMI of 25 kg/m². *Obesity*, defined as having a BMI of 30 kg/m² or greater, has doubled among adults since 1980. Many diseases are associated with excessive weight and obesity, including CHD, stroke, high blood pressure, diabetes, arthritis-related disabilities, sleep apnea, gallbladder disease, and some cancers (USDHHS, 2000b).

The public health burden of excessive weight and obesity is overwhelming in terms of premature deaths and disability, lost productivity, and social stigmatization (USDHHS, 2001). In 2000 the total cost of obesity was estimated at $117 billion (USDHHS, 2004). Obesity rates are higher among certain population groups, such as Hispanic-Americans, African-Americans, Native Americans, and Pacific Islander-American women (USDHHS, 2000b). Research has reported, however, that overweight status has increased in *all* parts of the U.S. population (Mokdad et al., 2001; Flegal, Carroll, Ogden, & Johnson, 2002). The recent trend of overweight in the United States has become so severe that if it is not reversed in the next few years, poor diet and lack of physical exercise will likely become the leading preventable cause of mortality among adults (Mokdad et al., 2004).

Many factors contribute to excessive weight and obesity. For each individual, metabolic and genetic factors, as well as behaviors affecting dietary intake and physical activity, contribute to being overweight. Cultural, environmental, and socioeconomic influences also play a role. Most overweight and obese individuals eat more calories from food than they expend through physical activity. As body weight increases, so does the prevalence of health risks in an individual. For this reason, encouraging obese individuals to adopt new eating and physical activity habits is of vital importance.

Weight Management

The goals and outcomes of weight management programs should be guided by an assessment of an individual's weight (BMI) and health. The NHLBI guidelines recommend intervention for people who are overweight and have two or more risk factors associated with their weight (Kuczmarski & Flegal, 2000). Furthermore, according to the position paper of the ADA (2002) for weight management, assessment should incorporate the following areas:

■ *Anthropometrics:* The assessment of height, weight, BMI, and waist circumference (as waist measurement increases, so do health risks)
■ *Medical causes:* Identifying potential causes, age at onset, obesity-associated complications, and severity of obesity
■ *Psychological causes:* Eating disorders, possible psychological causes, and barriers to treatment
■ *Nutritional causes:* Weight history, diet history, current eating patterns, nutritional intake, environmental factors, meals eaten away from home, exercise history, and motivation to change

For an individual, the goal of a weight management program should focus on the prevention of weight gain as well as weight loss. This recommendation encourages indi-

Visit www.nhlbi.gov for more information about the NHLBI's recommendations.

viduals to adopt healthier life-styles, such as increasing physical activity and choosing less calorically dense foods. With this approach, weight loss will lead to reductions of health risks (Kassiger & Angell, 1998). A weight loss of as little as 10% can improve health risks associated with being overweight and obesity (NIH & NHLBI, 1998).

For effective weight management programs, a multidisciplinary team should be involved, including a physician, a dietitian, an exercise physiologist, and a behavioral therapist. Health care professionals should be especially dedicated and sensitive to the needs of overweight and obese individuals. It is appropriate to discuss realistic goals of weight loss and maintenance so that shared responsibility for weight management can develop between the provider and individual. Goals might include the following (ADA, 2002):

- Prevention or cessation of weight gain in an individual who is continuing to see an increase in his or her weight
- Progress in physical and emotional health
- Small realistic weight losses achieved through sensible eating and exercise
- Improvements in eating, exercise, and any behaviors apart from weight loss

Establishing both short- and long-term treatment goals and documenting measures before implementing the weight management plan and after the individual has started on the plan are important goals of care. Positive behavior changes, other than absolute weight, should be rewarded, because these can be very motivating.

Physical activity is highly recommended as an essential part of a weight management program. It is well established that to maintain weight loss, healthful dietary habits must be coupled with increased physical activity (USDHHS, 2000b). Physical activity contributes to weight loss not only by changing energy balance, but also by positively changing body composition by increasing lean body mass. Exercise decreases the risk of chronic disease and improves mood and quality of life. Many experts believe that physical inactivity is responsible for the increasing prevalence of excessive weight and obesity in the United States (USDHHS & NHLBI, 2001). Combining weight loss with regular physical activity reduces one's risk for chronic diseases such as heart disease and diabetes by reducing both blood cholesterol and blood glucose levels.

The biggest challenge in weight management is to maintain a healthy weight once it is achieved. It is essential to include physical activity in weight loss programs because regular physical activity is one of the best predictors of weight maintenance (Pavlou, Krey, & Stefee, 1989). Unfortunately, studies show that within 5 years, most people regain the weight they have lost (NIH Technology Assessment Conference Panel, 1993). The NIH recommends that both dietary and physical activity changes need to be continued indefinitely for weight loss to be maintained (NIH & NHLBI, 1998). A comprehensive lifestyle program that focuses on nutrition, exercise, cognitive behavioral changes, and medical monitoring has been shown to be most effective for longterm success (Jeffrey et al., 2000).

Because of the increased prevalence in overweight and obesity in the United States, weight management becomes crucial for primary prevention of many chronic diseases. It is the foundation of secondary and tertiary prevention of hypertension, high blood cholesterol, diabetes, arthritis, and some cancers. It is important for health care providers to lobby for public health policies that endorse the treatment and management of weight. Also, clients must be informed of the known healthy and positive outcomes achieved through weight management programs.

Cardiovascular Disease

Cardiovascular disease is the nation's leading cause of death, accounting for more than 38% of all deaths in the United States. In 2001 more than 930,000 Americans died of cardiovascular disease (AHA, 2004b). Three modifiable health behaviors—poor nutrition, lack of physical activity, and smoking—contribute greatly to the burden of heart disease.

Cardiovascular diseases include diseases of the heart and blood vessels: CHD, stroke, and peripheral vascular diseases. CHD is the most common form of cardiovascular disease and usually involves atherosclerosis and hypertension. Atherosclerosis is characterized by the buildup of plaques along the inner walls of the arteries, causing inadequate blood flow and leading to serious cardiovascular problems.

The consequences of cardiovascular disease are usually heart disease and stroke; these two diseases combined cause one death every 33 seconds (USDHHS, 2004). About 61 million Americans live with the effects of heart disease and stroke. The annual cost of cardiovascular disease and stroke is estimated at $194 billion (USDHHS, 2004). The death rate from cardiovascular disease fell by 17% in the last part of the 20th century; however, the number of deaths increased by 2.5% each year due to the growth and size of the population aged 65 years and older (CDC, 2004a). The decrease in the mortality rates due to cardiovascular disease is attributed to primary prevention (i.e., a decrease in dietary intake of saturated fat), secondary prevention (i.e., early detection and treatment of hypertension), and improved medical and surgical treatments (AHA, 2004b). In general, mortality and prevalence rates of cardiovascular disease could be improved by reducing the major risk factors: high blood pressure, high blood cholesterol, tobacco use, physical inactivity, and poor nutrition. Controlling one or more of these risk factors could have a major public health impact in our country.

Hypertension

High blood pressure, or hypertension, remains a "silent killer" in the United States, affecting about 50 million or 1 in 4 Americans (CDC, 2004a). High blood pressure is a major independent risk factor for cardiovascular disease. Hypertension increases the risk of heart attack, heart failure, stroke, and kidney disease (USDHHS, NIH, NHLBI, NHBPEP, & JCN 7 Express, 2003). This is significant because heart disease and stroke are, respectively, the first and third leading cause of death in the United States (USDHHS, 2004).

In the latest classification of blood pressure for adults, normal blood pressure is considered to be less than 120/80 mm Hg and prehypertension is designated as 120 to 139 systolic or 80 to 89 mm Hg diastolic pressure (USDHHS, NIH, NHLBI, NHBPEP, & JCN 7 Express, 2003). High blood pressure for adults is defined as a systolic pressure of 140 mm Hg or higher or a diastolic pressure of 90 mm Hg or higher. A recent finding has determined that systolic blood pressure is a more important predictor of CHD in older adults than diastolic blood pressure (Systolic Hypertension in the Elderly Program, 1991).

The number of people who were able to control their high blood pressure from life-style changes and the use of antihypertensive drugs rose from about 16% in 1971–1972 to about 65% in 1988–1994 (NHLBI, 1998). The age-adjusted death rate attributed to hypertension rose by about 36.4% over the past decade (data from 1991 to 2001), with the actual number of deaths increasing by 53% (Eyre et al., 2004). Twenty-five percent of people with hypertension are on medication but are inadequately controlled; only 34% are on medication and well controlled (NHLBI, 1998, USDHHS, NIH, NHLBI,

NHBPEP, & JCN 7 Express, 2003). Significant disparities exist among persons diagnosed with hypertension; for example, African-Americans have high blood pressure at an earlier age and in general have higher blood pressures (USDHHS, 2000c). Thirty percent of Americans are unaware they have hypertension (NHLBI, 2004).

The latest guidelines for the treatment of hypertension are found in The Seventh Report of the Joint National Committee on Prevention, Detection, Evaluation, and Treatment of High Blood Pressure (USDHHS, NIH, NHLBI, NHBPEP, & JCN 7 Express, 2003). This report advocates major life-style modifications shown to lower blood pressure, enhance antihypertensive drug efficacy, and decrease cardiovascular risk. General life-style modifications include weight reduction for overweight or obese individuals (the goal is for a BMI of 18.5 to 24.9) (Trials of Hypertension Prevention Collaborative Research Group, 1997; He, Whelton, Appel, Charleston, & Klag, 2000), the adoption of the Dietary Approaches to Stop Hypertension (DASH) eating plan (Sacks et al., 2001), reducing sodium intake (Chobanian & Hill, 2000), increasing physical activity (Whelton, Chin, Xin, & He, 2002), and moderating alcohol consumption (Xin et al., 2001). The DASH eating plan is a diet rich in calcium and potassium, consisting of fresh fruits, vegetables, and low-fat dairy products (Sacks et al., 2001; Vollmer et al., 2001). The DASH eating plan advocates a low sodium intake; intakes of 1,600 mg have been found to be as effective as single drug therapy in lowering blood pressure (Sacks et al., 2001). Other specific life-style modifications include reducing sodium to 2,400 mg a day, engaging in regular aerobic physical activity at least 30 minutes a day (most days of the week), and limiting alcohol consumption (two drinks a day for men and one drink a day for women) (USDHHS, NIH, NHLBI, NHBPEP, & JCN 7 Express, 2003). The report's guidelines recommend these life-style modifications for all individuals. For those people who have not achieved the goal blood pressure (<140/90 mm Hg), antihypertensive drugs, such as thiazide-type diuretics, may also be recommended (Psatsy et al., 1997).

● **Learning Point** A usual food intake in the United States, complete with convenience and fast foods, may provide 10,000 to 20,000 mg of sodium per day. Visit www.nhlbi.nih.gov/guidelines/hypertension/for more information about the Seventh Report of the Joint National Committee on Prevention, Detection, Evaluation, and Treatment of High Blood Pressure.

Cholesterol

High blood cholesterol is one of the major independent risk factors for heart disease and stroke (USDHHS, 2004). Modifying this risk factor is effective in reducing cardiovascular disease mortality. Animal, epidemiologic, and metabolic research show that having elevated blood cholesterol levels is associated with cardiovascular disease. In spite of recommended dietary guidelines and medications available, over 50% of Americans have total blood cholesterol levels of 200 mg/dL or greater and almost 46% have a low density lipoprotein (LDL) cholesterol of 130 mg/dL or higher (USDHHS, 2004).

Research from the 1980s showed that lowering high blood cholesterol significantly reduces the risk for heart attacks and reduces overall mortality rates. As a result, the National Cholesterol Education Program was launched in 1985 (Cleeman & Lenfant, 1998). Since its inception, the percentage of people who have had their cholesterol checked more than doubled, from 35% in 1983 to 75% in 1995 (NHLBI, 1995). Current guidelines recommend that all adults, aged 20 or older, have their blood cholesterol levels checked every 5 years as a preventive measure (USDHHS, 2000c). Nevertheless, over 80% of Americans who have high blood cholesterol do not have it under control.

In terms of dietary trends and blood cholesterol levels, as dietary consumption of total fat, saturated fat, and cholesterol declined in the 1980s and 1990s, average blood cholesterol levels in adults declined from 213 mg/dL in 1978 to 203 mg/dL in 1991 (Cleeman & Lenfant, 1998). Research shows that as little as a 10% decrease in total cholesterol levels can reduce the incidence of CHD by almost 30% (USDHHS, 2004).

In 2001 the National Cholesterol Education Program released updated clinical guidelines in its report of the Expert Panel on the Detection, Evaluation and Treatment of High Blood Cholesterol in Adults, referred to as the Adult Treatment Panel (ATP) III (USDHHS & NHLBI, 2001). This report updates the recommendations made in ATP II and I for people with high blood cholesterol levels and reinforces findings from studies that confirm elevated LDL cholesterol to be a major cause of CHD. The guidelines in ATP III focus on LDL lowering cholesterol strategies and on primary prevention in persons with multiple risk factors (USDHHS, NIH, NHLBI, NHBPEP, and JCN 7 Express, 2000). In 2004 an update was added to the National Cholesterol Education Program guidelines on cholesterol management that advised physicians to consider new more intensive medical treatments, such as statin drugs for people at high and moderately high risk for a heart attack (Grundy et al., 2004).

> ● **Learning Point** These lower blood cholesterol by inhibiting 5-hydroxy-3-methylglutaryl coenzyme A reductase, a liver enzyme that is responsible for producing cholesterol.

The ATP III report recommends a complete lipoprotein profile that includes total cholesterol, LDL cholesterol, high-density lipoprotein (HDL) cholesterol, and triglycerides as the preferred test rather than screening for total cholesterol and HDLs alone. For LDL-lowering therapy, a person's risk status needs to be assessed based on multiple risk factors, including cigarette smoking, hypertension, low HDL, family history of premature CHD, and age. Diabetes is considered as a CHD equivalent in assessing a person's risk. In addition, the current guidelines use the Framingham scoring projections of 10-year absolute CHD risk to identify people who need more intensive therapy and those with multiple metabolic risk factors. National Cholesterol Education Program defines high-risk patients as those who have CHD, or diabetes, or multiple (two or more) risk factors, such as hypertension or smoking, which gives them a greater than 20% chance of having a heart attack within 10 years (USDHHS & NHLBI, 2001). Very high-risk patients are those who have cardiovascular disease together with either multiple risk factors (especially diabetes), or badly controlled risk factors (e.g., smoking), or metabolic syndrome (a constellation of risk factors associated with obesity). For moderately high-risk and high-risk persons, the ATP III report and update recommend drug therapy in addition to therapeutic lifestyle changes, which include intensive use of nutrition, weight control, and physical activity (USDHHS & NHLBI, 2001; Grundy et al., 2004).

The specific parts of therapeutic life-style changes include the following: reducing intakes of saturated fat to less than 7% of total calories and decreasing cholesterol to less than 200 mg/day. Total fat from calories can be in the 25% to 35% range, as long as saturated and trans-fatty acids are kept low. Individuals are encouraged to use plant stanols and sterols in their diet (2 g/day). Small amounts of plant sterols, or phytosterols, occur naturally in pine trees and foods like soybeans, nuts, grains, and oils. Increasing soluble fiber to 10 to 25 g/day is also recommended with weight reduction and increased physical activity.

Because excessive weight and obesity are considered major underlying risk factors for CHD, weight reduction enhances LDL-lowering interventions.

In comparing the recommendations set forth in the ATP III report to the more recent updates, more intensive treatment options are delineated for very high-risk individuals. For high-risk patients, the goal in both reports remains an LDL level of less than 100 mg/dL; for very high-risk patients, a therapeutic option is to treat with statins to lower levels to less than 70 mg/dL. The update lowers the threshold for drug therapy to an LDL of 100 mg/dL or higher and recommends drug therapy for those high-risk people whose LDL is 100 to 129 mg/dL.

> ● **Learning Point** The decision to go on drug therapy for high LDL levels depends on a multitude of risk factors and is decided between the physician and the patient.

In ATP III, for moderately high-risk persons the LDL treatment goal is less than 130 mg/dL and drug therapy is recommended if LDL levels are 130 mg/dL or higher. In the update, there is a therapeutic option to set the treatment goal at LDL less than 100 mg/dL and to use statin drug therapy if LDL is 100 to 129 mg/dL to reach the goal. In the update, when LDL drug therapy is used it is advised that enough medication be used to achieve at least a 30% to 40% reduction in LDL levels. In both reports, anyone with LDL above the goal is a candidate for therapeutic life-style changes. In the update, any person at high or moderately high risk who has life-style-related risk factors should follow therapeutic life-style changes, regardless of LDL level (USDHHS & NHLBI, 2001; Grundy et al., 2004).

As individuals learn about their risk factors and begin therapeutic life-style changes, more registered dietitians and nutritionists will be asked to help people make necessary dietary changes. ATP III guidelines recommend that physicians refer individuals to dietitians for MNT (USDHHS & NHLBI, 2001). At all stages in the model of therapeutic life-style changes, the referral to a dietitian is recommended. This challenges public health providers to provide diet and exercise recommendations that will make a difference to those with elevated blood cholesterol levels.

> ● **Learning Point** Nutritionists also need to consider prevailing eating and ethnic habits when counseling people to lower blood cholesterol levels. In terms of adhering to the ATP III protocol guidelines (and the update), patients and health care providers are key players in realizing the benefits of cholesterol-lowering and in attaining the highest possible levels of CHD risk reduction.

Both screening for risk factors and compliance in adopting the lipid-lowering guidelines are essential. In reality, fewer than 50% of those persons eligible for meeting the criteria actually receive treatment (USDHHS & NHLBI, 2001).

Physical Activity

Research demonstrates that virtually all individuals benefit from regular physical activity. Yet, more than 60% of American adults are not regularly physically active (USDHHS, 1996). Twenty-five percent of all adults are not active at all. Inactivity increases with age and is more common among women than men. Also, those with lower incomes and less education exercise less than those with higher incomes or education (USDHHS, 1996). Thus, physical inactivity is a prevalent risk in the United States. People who are sedentary are almost twice as likely to develop CHD as people who engage in regular physical activity (USDHHS, 2000d). The risk imposed by physical inactivity is almost as high as other well-known CHD risk factors, such as high blood cholesterol, high blood pressure, or smoking (USDHHS, 1996, 2000d). Even moderate physical activity produces significant health benefits, such as a decreased risk of CHD (NIH Consensus Development Panel on Physical Activity and Cardiovascular Health, 1996). Research shows that moderate physical activity, such as walking 30 minutes a day five times a week, is more likely to be adopted and maintained than vigorous activity (Pate et al., 1995).

There are many health benefits to be gained from regular physical activity. It enhances cardiovascular function, reduces very low-density lipoprotein levels, raises HDL cholesterol, and can lower LDL cholesterol levels (USDHHS & NHLBI, 2001). Physical activity lowers blood pressure and reduces insulin resistance. Overall, physical activity improves muscle function, cardiovascular function, and physical performance and aids in weight management (USDHHS, 1996). Nutritionists should become aware of the different types of physical activity, especially moderate levels of activity, that can lower an individual's risk for cardiovascular disease.

Smoking

Cigarette smoking is responsible for more than 440,000 deaths each year and is the single largest preventable cause of death and disease among U.S. adults (USDHHS, 2004). Public health professionals, concerned about the risk factors for cardiovascular disease, need to discuss smoking with clients because it is a leading risk factor. Of the estimated 12 million deaths from smoking, almost half (5.5 million) are deaths from cardiovascular diseases (USDHHS, 2004). In 2003 an estimated 1.1 million Americans had a new or recurrent heart attack. Cigarette smoking was associated with sudden cardiac death in adult men and women (USDHHS, 2004). Smoking-related CHD may also contribute to congestive heart failure, causing 4.6 million to suffer from this disease (USDHHS, 2004). Smoking is also a major cause of stroke, which is the third leading cause of death in the United States. However, the risk of stroke decreases when an individual stops smoking.

Smoking cessation is also effective in preventing heart disease. In fact, after just 1 year of smoking abstinence, people who quit smoking have a 50% lower risk of death from CHD than those who continue to smoke (USDHHS, 1990). Studies have shown that secondhand smoke exposure causes heart disease among adults, with an estimated 35,000 deaths each year (Glanz & Parmely, 1995; USDHHS, 2004).

Smoking is a modifiable risk factor, and its modification is effective in preventing cardiovascular disease mortality. Smoking cessation is particularly important in people with other cardiovascular risk factors, such as high blood pressure and elevated blood cholesterol, because these risk factors work synergistically. Cigarette smoking is also a risk factor for other leading causes of death and disability, including several kinds of cancer and chronic lung diseases (USDHHS, 2004).

Trends

Progress has been made in decreasing mortality and risk factors for cardiovascular diseases. Between 1987 and 1996 the age-adjusted death rate for CHD declined by 22.2%, whereas deaths caused by stroke declined by 13.2% (CDC, 1999). However, the HP 2010 objectives on CHD and stroke were not reached. Hypertension rates climbed from 11% to 29%. The prevalence of high blood cholesterol, however, declined from 26% to 19% between 1988 and 1994. There was a slight decline in smoking between 1995 and 1999–2000, yet deaths from smoking, poor diet, and physical inactivity still accounted for almost one-third of all deaths in the United States (Mokdad et al., 2004).

Results from epidemiologic studies suggest that diets rich in fruits, vegetables, whole grains, and low-fat dairy foods are associated with a lower risk of mortality from many chronic diseases, including heart disease (McCullough et al., 2002). This nutritional pattern is supported by all the major health organizations. Nevertheless, a large gap remains between recommended dietary patterns and what U.S. adults actually eat. Only about one-fourth of U.S. adults eat the recommended five or more servings of fruits and vegetables each day (USDHHS, 2004). Recent research on frequency of fruit and vegetable consumption shows little change from 1994 to 2000 (Serdula et al., 2004). Caloric intake from total fat declined from 36% to 34% from 1976 to 1994 but fell short of the target goal of 30% set by HP 2010 (USDHHS, 2000c). According to data from the National Health and Nutrition Examination Surveys, decreases in calories from dietary fat and dietary cholesterol coincided with decreases in blood cholesterol levels (Ernst, Sempos, Briefel, & Clark, 1997).

From 1950 to 1996 age-adjusted death rates from cardiovascular diseases declined 60% (CDC, 1999). Although this is a positive trend, other health indicators have not improved significantly. Increasing prevalence rates in obesity and the continued high levels of blood pressure and stroke pose a continued public health challenge (CDC, 1999).

Cancer

Cancer is an umbrella term used to describe a large group of diseases characterized by uncontrolled growth and spread of abnormal cells (ACS, 2004). Cancer is the second leading cause of death in the United States, causing one in every four deaths. In 2004 an estimated 564,000 Americans died from this disease (USDHHS, 2004). According to the ACS (2004) about one-third of cancer deaths are preventable and are attributed to dietary factors, physical inactivity, being overweight, or obesity. For U.S. adults who do not smoke, dietary choices and physical activity are the most modifiable determinants of cancer risk. All cancers caused by cigarettes and the heavy use of alcohol could be prevented. The National Cancer Institute estimates that about 9.6 million Americans who had been diagnosed with cancer at some point in their lives were alive in 2000 (ACS, 2004). This estimate includes people living with cancer and those who were cancer free (Ries et al., 2003). The 5-year relative survival rate for all cancers is 63%, or about 4 in 10 persons, which represents people who are living 5 years after diagnosis of cancer (ACS, 2004).

Age-standardized death rates from all cancers decreased by 7.2% between 1991 and 2000 (Ries et al., 2003). Despite a decrease in the death rate from cancer, the total number of people who develop or die from cancer each year continues to increase because of our aging population (Stewart, King, Thompson, Friedman, & Wingo, 2004). The overall decrease in death rates from cancer is due to a decline in smoking and more effective detection and screening. The recent decrease in deaths from breast cancer in white women, for example, is due to a greater use of breast screening in regular medical care. Cancer death rates vary by gender, race, and ethnicity. For example, African-Americans are more likely to die from cancer than are whites (Key, Allen, Spencer, & Travis, 2002).

Although inherited genes play a significant role in cancer risk, they only explain part of all cancer incidences (ACS, 2004). Most of the variation in cancer incidence cannot be explained by inherited factors. The predominant causes of cancer are external factors such as cigarette smoking, diet or nutrition, weight, and physical inactivity (Key et al., 2002; ACS, 2004). These factors act to modify the risk of cancer at all stages. It is estimated that more than 50% of all cancers could be prevented through dietary improvements, such as reducing total fat and increasing fruit and vegetable consumption, and smoking cessation (Willett, 1996; USDHHS, 2004). Doll and Peto (1981) estimated that about 10% to 70% of deaths from cancer were attributable to diet. However, recent evidence showing actual causes of death in the United States found that 14% of cancer deaths occurring in 1990 could be attributed to diet (McGinnis & Forge, 1993). The science of nutrition and cancer is evolving but still is not as developed as that of diet and cardiovascular disease. Many large-scale studies are currently underway to further elucidate the relationship between various nutrients and cancer (McGinnis & Forge, 1993). Future research points to the areas of diet and gene interactions and biomarkers for cancer that will further our understanding in this area (Mandelson et al., 2000).

Current dietary recommendations are based on evidence from the ACS, the AICR/World Cancer Research Fund, and the Harvard Cancer Prevention Study (ACS, 2004; FANSA, 2004). In 2001 the ACS updated its guidelines on nutrition and physical activity after reviewing current scientific evidence (Byers et al., 2002). In general, the current dietary guidelines support the existing 2005 Dietary Guidelines for Americans and also encourage the consumption of plant-based diets, without relying on processed foods. The guidelines endorse eating a diet that promotes healthy weight control along with physical activity (ACS, 2004; FANSA, 2004). Specif-

ically, nutrition and food scientists agree on the following recommendations to lower cancer risk (ACS, 2004):

- Eat a plant-based diet that includes a wide variety of fruits, vegetables, whole grains, beans, and legumes. The recommendation is to choose whole grains over refined sources and eat three to five servings of vegetables and two to four servings of fruits per day.
- Eat less fat from all food sources.
- Limit excess calories and maintain a healthful weight throughout life. Eat a sound diet and incorporate moderate or vigorous physical activity 5 days a week or more to further reduce risks of cancer.
- Drink alcohol in moderation.

Nutrition supplements are not universally recommended for cancer prevention. Instead, the cancer prevention benefits of diet are considered among the best due to the interactions of many vitamins, minerals, and other plant-derived substances found naturally occurring in foods (ACS, 2004). However, the possible benefits of supplemental folate, calcium, and selenium are noted (Byers et al., 2002; ACS, 2004). By eating whole foods and following the cancer prevention dietary recommendations along with physical activity, the protection of the body's cells may take place during the initiation, promotion, and progression stages of cancer. These food substances may repair damage that has already occurred in cells. Some literature sources state that individuals do not need to be concerned about the pesticide residues on fruits and vegetables, because the benefits of eating fruits and vegetables far outweigh any potential risk (AICR, 2004). More long-term studies may help to state this definitively.

The study of diet and cancer prevention is relatively new. Dietitians and other public health care professionals need to stay abreast of these discoveries to give appropriate guidance to individuals at risk. The basis of MNT should include those recommendations set forth by the ACS and the World Cancer Research Fund/AICR (ACS, 2004; AICR, 2004).

Diabetes

Diabetes is a serious, costly, and increasingly common chronic disease that poses a significant public health challenge. In 2001 diabetes was the sixth leading cause of death in the United States (USDHHS, 2004). About 18 million Americans have diabetes, and over 5 million of these people are unaware they have the disease (USDHHS, 2004). Type 2 diabetes, once referred to as adult onset diabetes, may account for about 90% to 95% of all diagnosed cases of diabetes (NIH, 2004). By 2050 an estimated 29 million Americans are expected to have a diagnosis of diabetes. The increase in the number of cases has been particularly high within certain ethnic and racial groups in the United States (CDC, 2004).

Medical complications of type 2 diabetes include heart disease, kidney failure, leg and foot amputations, and blindness. Each year about 12,000 to 24,000 people become blind because of diabetic eye disease (USDHHS, 2004). Most deaths caused by diabetes are due to diabetes-associated cardiovascular disease. The presence of diabetes in adults is associated with a two- to fourfold increase in CHD compared with nondiabetic adults. Almost three-fourths of adults with diabetes have hypertension (USDHHS, 2004). Diabetes is the cause of 44% of end-stage renal disease cases. Severe forms of nervous system damage occur in 60% to 70% of diabetic adults. Approximately 60% of all nontraumatic amputations in the United States occur in people with diabetes (USDHHS, 2000d). Periodontal or gum disease is also more common among diabetics. As a result diabetes is a costly disease, with the total attributable costs (direct and indirect) estimated at $132 billion annually (USDHHS, 2000d).

Type 2 diabetes is associated with the following factors:

- *Age:* Diabetes is most common in people over 60 years of age (USDHHS, 2000d).
- *Ethnicity:* Deaths from diabetes are twice as high for African-Americans than for whites, Native Americans, and Hispanic-Americans; certain Pacific Islander-American and Asian-American populations also have higher rates.
- *Genetics and family history:* Genetic markers that indicate a greater risk for type 2 diabetes have been identified.
- *Obesity:* The increased prevalence of obesity among adults is positively associated with the increased rates of diabetes (Mokdad et al., 2000). Data from clinical trials strongly support the potential of moderate weight loss to reduce the risk of type 2 diabetes (Diabetes Prevention Program Research Group, 2003).
- *History of gestational diabetes in women:* Gestational diabetes is a form of glucose intoler-

ance that develops in some women during pregnancy. Obesity is associated with gestational diabetes. Women with a family history of gestational diabetes and Hispanic-American and African-American women are at an increased risk (Franz et al., 2004).

- *Impaired glucose metabolism:* People with prediabetes, or who at increased risk of developing diabetes, have impaired fasting blood glucose. Research studies suggest that weight loss and increased physical activity among people with prediabetes may return glucose levels to normal and prevent the onset of diabetes (CDC, 2004).
- *Physical inactivity:* If you are at higher risk and fairly inactive or exercise fewer than three times a week, you are more likely to develop type 2 diabetes.

In the United States recent life-style changes such as decreased physical activity and increased energy consumption, which contribute to the increased prevalence rates of obesity, are also strong risk factors for diabetes (Diabetes Prevention Program Research Group, 2003). On the other hand, positive life-style changes such as diet, weight loss of 5% to 7%, and moderate-intensity physical activity (e.g., walking 30 minutes a day) can delay the onset of diabetes.

> **● Learning Point** The Diabetes Prevention Program, a major large-scale study of over 3,000 people at high risk for developing diabetes, confirmed that positive lifestyle changes such as diet, weight-loss of 5–7 percent, and moderate-intensity physical activity (such as walking 30 min/day) can delay onset of diabetes and found a 58% reduction in the development of diabetes over a 3-year period. The findings from this study, sponsored by the NIH, showed that exercise, a healthy diet, and weight loss can reduce the risk of developing diabetes by as much as 71% in high-risk individuals (Diabetes Prevention Program Research Group, 2003).

MNT is an essential part of diabetes management for adults. Objectives for MNT include the following (Franz et al., 2004):

- Attaining and maintaining optimal metabolic outcomes, including normalizing blood glucose levels, maintaining a lipid profile that reduces vascular disease risk, and normalizing blood pressure levels
- Preventing, delaying, and treating the onset complications by modifying nutrient intake and life-style to prevent and treat obesity, cardiovascular disease, hypertension, and nephropathy

- Optimizing health through sensible food choices and physical activity
- Addressing personal and cultural preferences as well as life-style factors, including a person's willingness to change, when determining individual nutritional needs

In terms of specific nutrients and dietary recommendations for type 2 diabetes, studies in healthy subjects and those at risk for type 2 diabetes support the importance of including foods containing complex carbohydrates in the diet, particularly those from whole grains, fruits, vegetables, and low-fat milk (Franz et al., 2004). Reduced intake of total fat, especially saturated fat, may reduce the risk of diabetes.

In summary, life-style changes such as reduced energy intake, increased physical activity, and nutrition education (with the goal of promoting weight loss) represent essential aspects of type 2 diabetes management for adults. HP 2010 (USDHHS, 2000e) discusses the challenges of diabetes and the preventive interventions aimed at them: primary prevention, screening and early diagnosis, access, and quality of care. This includes secondary and tertiary prevention, such as glucose control and decreasing complications from diabetes (USDHHS, 2000e). As dietitians, public health professionals, and educators, many opportunities exist to contribute to the effective management of diabetes.

Osteoporosis

As one grows, bones develop and become larger, heavier, and denser. At approximately age 30 years, peak bone mass is achieved in both men and women. After this time period adults begin to lose bone mass, and this continues as they get older. Osteoporosis, or porous bone disease, develops when bone loss reaches the point of causing fractures under common everyday stresses. Because of increased bone fragility, there is a greater susceptibility to fractures of the hip, spine, and wrist. Both men and women suffer from osteoporosis.

Osteoporosis currently affects 44 million Americans, or 55% of people aged 50 and older, 68% of whom are women (NIH, 2003; National Osteoporosis Foundation, 2004). These rates correspond to one in two women and one in four men, aged 50 and older, who will experience an osteoporosis-related fracture in their lifetime (NIH, 2003). Osteoporosis causes significant disability with important economic consequences, costing about $14 billion each year in direct expenditures (hospitals and nursing homes) (NIH, 2001). Of the 1.5 million fractures occurring each year due to osteoporosis, over 300,000 are hip fractures, 700,000 are vertebral fractures, and 250,000 are wrist fractures. Of the 300,000 annual hip fractures, 24% result in death following complications from the fracture (National Osteoporosis Foundation, 2004).

Osteoporosis is often called the "silent disease" because it can occur without any overt symptoms. The technical standard for measuring bone mineral density is dual-energy x-ray absorptiometry. A low bone mass density is a strong predictor of fracture risk (National Osteoporosis Foundation, 2004). Bone density tests can detect osteoporosis before a fracture occurs and can serve as a predictor for future fracture risks.

The chances of developing osteoporosis are greatest in white women beyond menopause. Women have less bone tissue and lose bone more easily than men because of the hormonal changes involved in menopause. Those individuals who have a low dietary intake of calcium and vitamin D over a lifetime, who are physically inactive, who are cigarette smokers, who are excessive alcohol drinkers, who are thin and small-framed, and who have a family history of osteoporosis are at increased risk (NIH, 2003; National Osteoporosis Foundation, 2004). In addition, white and Asian-American women are at highest risk, whereas African-American and Hispanic-American women have lower risks (National Osteoporosis Foundation, 2004). Anorexia nervosa, the use of certain medications, and low testosterone levels in men are also risk factors for osteoporosis. The five factors that can be modified to prevent osteoporosis are (1) a diet rich in calcium and vitamin D, (2) weight-bearing exercise, (3) a healthy life-style that excludes smoking and excessive alcohol intake, (4) routine bone density measurements, and (5) the use of medication, when appropriate (National Osteoporosis Foundation, 2004).

Nutrition is an important modifiable risk factor in terms of both bone health and the prevention and treatment of osteoporosis. An adequate amount of calcium and vitamin D contributes significantly to bone health. Low calcium intakes are associated with low bone mass, rapid bone loss, and high fracture rates (Heany, 2002). Bone is a living growing tissue, and 99% of the body's calcium is found in bone. Throughout one's lifetime, bone formation and resorption occurs. This process, known as bone turnover, is responsive to dietary calcium regardless of age. Dietary calcium works to strengthen bone by suppressing bone resorption and parathyroid hormone (Heany, 2002).

According to the NIH (2001), calcium is the most important nutrient for the prevention of osteoporosis. In spite of this, actual calcium intakes for most of the U.S. population are considerably lower than the current Dietary Reference Intake (Institute of Medicine, 1999). Many studies have shown that adult skeletal health is improved by increasing dairy foods or calcium intake in the diet (Dairy Council, 2004). The DASH diet, used to treat hypertension, is a low-fat diet, rich in calcium and has been shown to reduce bone turnover and reduce the risk of osteoporosis (Sacks et al., 2001). Calcium requirements can be met with low-fat dairy products; however, low consumption of milk and other dairy products in the U.S. diet is mainly responsible for low calcium intakes among U.S. adults (Dairy Council, 2004). Other foods contain calcium, such as dark leafy greens, but these foods usually provide less calcium per serving than milk, and most Americans do not eat these vegetables often. For individuals who do not consume enough calcium in their diets, calcium supplements are recommended.

Vitamin D also plays an important role in calcium absorption and bone health. Vitamin D is a major determinant of intestinal calcium absorption. When skin is exposed to sunlight, the body synthesizes vitamin D. However, studies show decreased production of vitamin D in the elderly and individuals who are housebound, especially in the winter months (NIH, 2003). Because of inadequate intake of vitamin D in a high proportion of older adults, the most recent Dietary Reference Intake increased the vitamin D requirements for people 50 years and older (Institute of Medicine, 1999). Low-fat and non-fat milk, excellent sources of calcium, are fortified with 100 IU of vitamin D per serving.

> For those living in colder climates without much sunshine, vitamin D supplementation is suggested to accompany calcium intake.

In conclusion, osteoporosis is a serious public health disease and is largely preventable. Starting early in life both females and males should be advised on how to incorporate sources of calcium into their diets. The use of low-fat and non-fat dairy foods should be recommended, and if persons cannot consume dairy products, other food sources and calcium supplements are necessary. Adequate vitamin D intake needs to be addressed, as well. Public health nutritionists should encourage individuals to participate regularly in physical activity. Modifiable life-style factors should be discussed to promote bone health throughout life.

HIV/AIDS

In 1981 a new infectious disease, AIDS, was first identified in the United States. A few years later HIV was discovered, and this was identified as the viral agent that causes AIDS. HIV/AIDS has affected almost every ethnic, socioeconomic, and age group in the United States (CDC, 2001).

AIDS, a deadly disease, is the end stage of HIV infection. The infection progresses to overwhelm the immune system and leaves individuals defenseless against numerous other infections and diseases. HIV is spread through direct contact with contaminated body fluids, sexual intercourse, direct blood contact, or from mother to infant. In 1996, death rates from AIDS in the United States declined for the first time (CDC, 2001). Nevertheless, HIV/AIDS remains a significant cause of illness, disability, and death in the United States. According to the CDC, in 2001 the estimated number of diagnosed AIDS cases was about 890,000 (CDC, 2001). Death rates have dropped dramatically in the United States due to the introduction of antiretroviral therapies (CDC, 2001).

Health complications for people with HIV/AIDS are immune dysfunction and its associated complications, which include malnutrition and wasting. HIV targets the immune system, rendering an individual susceptible to infections and disease. The CDC defines the AIDS-related wasting syndrome as a 10% weight loss in a 6-month period accompanied by diarrhea or fever for more than 30 days (USDHHS, 2000f). Malnutrition and its complications can reduce one's tolerance to medications and other therapies. Malnutrition occurs in the form of tissue wasting, fat accumulation, increased lipid levels, and risk of other chronic disease. The ADA and the Dietitians of Canada (2000) strongly support nutrition evaluation and MNT as parts of the ongoing health care of HIV-infected individuals. In terms of MNT, this includes early assessment and treatment of nutrient deficiencies, the maintenance and restoration of lean body mass, and continued support for performing daily activities and maintaining quality of life. According to the ADA and the Dietitians of Canada (2000), nutrition education and guidance should incorporate the following aspects:

- Healthful eating principles
- Water and food safety issues
- Perinatal and breast-feeding issues
- Nutrition management for symptoms such as anorexia, swallowing problems, diarrhea, and so on

- Food–medicine interactions
- Psychosocial and economic issues
- Alternative feeding methods (supplementation, tube feeding, or parenteral nutrition)
- Additional therapies, including physical activity and disease management
- Guidelines for evaluating nutrition information, diet claims, and individual mineral and vitamin supplementation
- Strategies for treatment of altered fat metabolism

In addition, it is important for an HIV-infected individual to have adequate access to food, health care, and other support systems. The maintenance and restoration of nutrition stores are interrelated with recommended medical therapies; therefore it is essential that a public health nutritionist be an active participant in the healthcare team to provide optimal MNT.

Issues to Debate

1. What would you propose should be incorporated into public health programs that focus on nutrition as an important preventive factor in illness, disability, and death?
2. What advice would you give to the individual in the community with regard to preventing chronic disease risk factors such as obesity, physical inactivity, and smoking to reduce society's financial burden?
3. What proportion of public funds designated for nutrition services should be given for primary, secondary, and tertiary prevention versus acute medical care?
4. Programs such as for-profit weight loss centers are proliferating in this country. What are positive and negative aspects of this trend compared with public health weight-management programs?

Resource Websites

U.S. Dietary Guidelines www.health.gov/dietary guidelines/
Dietary Guidelines of the American Heart Association www.americanheart.org
American Cancer Society www.cancer.org
American Institute for Cancer Research www.aicr.org
America Dietetic Association www.eatright.org

Alternate Healthy Eating Index www.hsph. harvard.edu/nutritionsource/pyramids.html
American Diabetes Association www.diabetes.org
North American Association for the Study of Obesity www.naaso.org

References

American Cancer Society (ACS). (2004). *Cancer Prevention and Early Detection Facts and Figures 2004*. Atlanta, GA: ACS.

American Dietetic Association (ADA). (1996). Position paper: Nutrition education for the public. *Journal of the American Dietetic Association, 96*, 1183–1187.

American Dietetic Association (ADA). (1998). Position paper: The role of nutrition in health promotion and disease prevention programs. *Journal of the American Dietetic Association, 98*, 205–208.

American Dietetic Association (ADA). (2002). Position paper: Weight management. *Journal of the American Dietetic Association, 102*, 1145–1155.

American Dietetic Association (ADA) and Dietitians of Canada. (2000). Position paper: Nutrition intervention in the care of persons with human immunodeficiency virus infection. *Journal of the American Dietetic Association, 100*, 708–717.

American Dietetic Association (ADA) and the Dietitians of Canada. (2004). Position paper: Nutrition and women's health. *Journal of the American Dietetic Association, 104*, 984–1001.

American Dietetic Association (ADA), the Office of Disease Prevention and Health Promotion, Public Health Service, and the U.S. Department of Health and Human Services. (1993). *Worksite Nutrition: A Guide to Planning, Implementation, and Evaluation* (2nd ed.). Chicago: ADA.

American Heart Association (AHA). (2004a). AHA comment, May 31, 2004. Health agencies applaud HHS/USDA new dietary guidelines. Retrieved June 29, 2004 from www.americanheart.org.

American Heart Association (AHA). (2004b). *Heart Disease and Stroke Statistics: 2004 Update*. Dallas, TX: AHA.

American Institute of Cancer Research (AICR). (2001). The dietary guidelines: Surveillance issues and research needs. *Journal of Nutrition, 131*(Suppl.), 3154S–3155S.

American Institute of Cancer Research (AICR). (2004). Retrieved May 26, 2004 from www.aicr.org.

America on the Move. (2004). Retrieved May 26, 2004 from www.americaonthemove.org.

Brunner, E., White, I., Thorogood, M., Bristow, A., Curle, D., & Marmot, M. (1997). Can dietary interventions change diet and cardiovascular risk factors? A meta-analysis of randomized controlled trials. *American Journal of Public Health, 87*, 1415–1422.

Byers, T., Nestle, M., McTiernan, A., Doyle, C., Currie-Williams, A., Gansler, T., et al. (2002). American Cancer Society guidelines on nutrition and physical activity for cancer prevention: Reducing the risk of cancer with healthy food choices and physical activity. *Cancer Journal for Clinicians, 52*, 92–111.

Centers for Disease Control and Prevention (CDC). (1999). Decline in deaths from heart disease and stroke—United States, 1990–1999. *Morbidity and Mortality Weekly Report, 48*, 649–656.

Centers for Disease Control and Prevention (CDC). (2001). HIV/AIDS surveillance report. Addendum, 2002. Vol. 13(2). cdc.gov/hiv/topics/surveillance/resources/reports/2003 report.

Centers for Disease Control and Prevention (CDC). (2004). *Fact Sheet: High Blood Pressure*. Hyattsville, MD: CDC.

Centers for Disease Control and Prevention (CDC). (2004). *National Diabetes Fact Sheet: General Information and National Estimates on Diabetes in the U.S.* (2003. rev. ed.). Atlanta, GA: USDHHS, CDC.

Centers for Disease Control and Prevention (CDC), National Center for Chronic Disease Prevention and Health Promotion, and USDHHS. (2004). Preventing heart disease and stroke, addressing the nation's leading killers. *At a Glance* Summary Tables.

Centers for Disease Control and Prevention (CDC), National Center for Health Statistics. (1992). Effectiveness in disease and injury prevention; estimated national spending on prevention. U.S., 1988. *Morbidity and Mortality Weekly Report, 41*, 529–531.

Chobanian, A. V., & Hill, M. (2000). National Heart, Lung, and Blood Institute Workshop on Sodium and Blood Pressure: A critical review of current scientific evidence. *Hypertension, 35*, 858–863.

Cleeman, J. L., & Lenfant, C. (1998). The National Cholesterol Education Program: Progress and prospects. *Journal of the American Medical Association, 280*, 2099–2104.

Dairy Council. (2004). The benefits of dairy foods in health promotion. *Dairy Council Digest,* Vol. 75, No. 3.

Diabetes Prevention Program Research Group. (2003). Reduction in the incidence of type 2 diabetes with lifestyle intervention or metformin. *New England Journal of Medicine, 346*, 393–403.

Dietary Guidelines Advisory Committee. (2000). *Report of the Dietary Guidelines Advisory Committee on the Dietary Guidelines for Americans, 2000*. Washington, DC: USDA.

Dietary Guidelines Alliance. (1996). Do it yourself: Crafting consumer tips. In *Reaching Consumers With Meaningful Health Messages*. Washington, DC: Dietary Guidelines Alliance.

Doll, R., & Peto, R. (1981). The causes of cancer: Qualitative estimates of avoidable risks of cancer in the U.S. today. *Journal of the National Cancer Institute, 66*, 1191–1308.

Elo, S. L., & Caltrop, J. B. (2002). Health promotive action and preventive action model (HPA model) for the classification of healthcare services in public health nursing. *Scandinavian Journal of Public Health, 30*, 200–208.

Ernst, N. D., Sempos, S. T., Briefel, R. R., & Clark, M. B. (1997). Consistency between U.S. dietary fat intake and serum total cholesterol concentrations: The National Health and Nutrition Examination Surveys. *American Journal of Clinical Nutrition, 66*, 965S–972S.

Eyre, H., Kahn, R., & Robertson, R. M. (2004). Preventing cancer, cardiovascular disease, and diabetes. *Diabetes Care, 27*, 1812–1824.

FANSA. (2004). Statement on diet and cancer prevention in the U.S. Retrieved July 7, 2004 from www.eatright.org.

Flegal, K. M., Carroll, M. D., Ogden, C. L., & Johnson, C. L. (2002). Prevalence and trends of obesity among U.S. adults, 1999–2000. *Journal of the American Medical Association, 288*, 1723–1727.

Franz, M. J., Bantle, J. P., Beebe, C. A., Brunzell, J. D., Chiasson, J. L., Garg, A., et al. (2004). Nutrition principles and recommendations in diabetes. *Diabetes Care, 27*, S36.

Frazao, E. (1999). The high costs of poor eating patterns in the U.S. In E. Frazao (Ed.), *America's Eating Habits: Changes and Consequences.* Washington, DC: USDA, Economic Research Service, AIB-750.

Glanz, S. A., & Parmely, W. W. (1995). Passive smoking and heart disease: Mechanism and risk. *Journal of the American Medical Association, 272*, 1047–1053.

Goldberg, J. P. (1992). Nutrition and health communication: The message and the media over half a century. *Nutrition Review, 50*, 71–77.

Grundy, S. M., Cleeman, J. I., Merz, C. N., Brewer, Jr., H. B., Clark, L. T., Hunninghake, D.B., et al. (2004). For the coordinating committee of the National Cholesterol Education Program. Implications of recent clinical trials for the National Cholesterol Education Program Adult Treatment Panel III Guidelines. *Circulation, 110*, 227–239.

He, J., Whelton, P. K., Appel, L. J., Charleston, J., & Klag, M. J. (2000). Long-term effects of weight-loss and dietary sodium restriction on incidence of hypertension. *Hypertension, 35*, 544–549.

Heany, R. P. (2002). The importance of calcium intake for lifelong skeletal health. *Calcified Tissue International, 70*, 70–73.

Institute of Medicine. (1999). Standing Committee on the Scientific Evaluation of Dietary Reference Intakes. Food and Nutrition Board, Institutes of Medicine. *Dietary Reference Intakes for calcium, phosphorus, magnesium, vitamin D, and fluoride.* Washington, DC: National Academy Press.

Jeffrey, R. W., Drewsiowski, A., Epstein, L. H., Stunkard, A. J., Wilson, G. T., Wing, R. R., et al. (2000). Long-term maintenance of weight-loss: Current status. *Health Psychology, 1*(Suppl.), 5–16.

Kannel, W. B., Dawber, T. R., & McGee, D. L. (1980). Perspectives of systolic hypertension, the Framingham Study. *Circulation, 61*, 1179–1182.

Kassiger, J. P., & Angell, M. (1998). Losing weight—An ill-fated New Year's resolution. *New England Journal of Medicine, 1338*, 52–54.

Kaufman, M. (Ed.). (1990). *Nutrition in Public Health: A Handbook for Developing Programs and Services.* Rockville, MD: Aspen Publishers.

Key, T. J., Allen, N. E., Spencer, E. A., & Travis, R. C. (2002). The effect of diet on risk of cancer. *Lancet, 360,* 861–868.

Krauss, R. M., Eckel, R. H., Howard, B., Appel, L. J., Daniels, S. R., Deckelbaum, R. J., et al. (2000). AHA dietary guidelines: Revision 2000. A statement for healthcare professionals from the Nutrition Committee of the American Heart Association. *Circulation, 102,* 2284–2299.

Kris-Etherton, P., Daniels, S. R., Eckel, R. H., Engler, M., Howard, B. V., Krauss, R. M., et al. (2001). Summary of the scientific conference on dietary fatty acids and cardiovascular health. Conference summary from the Nutrition Committee of the American Heart Association. *Circulation, 103,* 1034–1039.

Koplan, J. P., & Dietz, W. H. (1999). Caloric imbalance and public health policy. *Journal of the American Medical Association, 282,* 1579–1581.

Kuczmarski, R. J., & Flegal, K. M. (2000). Criteria for definition of overweight in transition: Background and recommendations for the U.S. *American Journal of Clinical Nutrition, 72,* 1074–1081.

Mandelson, M. T., Oestreicher, N., Porter, P. L., White, D., Finder, C. A., Taplin, S. H., et al. (2000). Breast density as a predictor of mammographic detection: Comparison of interval- and screen-detected cancers. *Journal of the National Cancer Institute, 92,* 1081–1087.

McCullough, M. L., Feskanich, D., Stampfer, M. J., Giovannucci, E. L., Rimm, E. B., Hu, F. B., et al. (2002). Diet quality and major chronic disease in men and women: Moving toward improved dietary guidance. *American Journal of Clinical Nutrition, 76,* 1261–1271.

McGinnis, J. M., & Forge, W. H. (1993). Actual causes of death in the U.S. *Journal of the American Medical Association, 270,* 2207–2212.

Mokdad, A. H., Bowman, B. A., Ford, E. S., Vinicor, F., Macks, J. S., & Koplan, J. C. (2001). The continuing epidemics of obesity and diabetes in the U.S. *Journal of the American Medical Association, 286,* 1195–1200.

Mokdad, A. H., Ford, E. S., Bowman, B. A., Nelson, D. E., Engelgau, M. M., Vinicor, F., et al. (2000). Diabetes trends in the U.S.: 1990–1998. *Diabetes Care, 23,* 1278–1283.

Mokdad, A. H., Marks, J. S., Stroup, D. F., & Gerberding, J. L. (2004). Actual causes of death in the U.S., 2000. *Journal of the American Medical Association, 291,* 1238–1245.

Mokdad, A. H., Marks, J. S., Stroup, D. F., & Gerberding, J. L. (2005). Correction: Actual causes of death in the United States, 2000. *Journal of the American Medical Association, 293,* 293–294.

National Academy of Sciences, National Research Council, Food and Nutrition Board. (1989). *Diet and Health: Implications for Reducing Chronic Disease Risk.* Washington, DC: National Academy Press.

National Center for Chronic Disease Prevention and Health Promotion. (2004). *The Burden of Chronic Diseases and Their Risk Factors. Section 111: Risk Factors and Use of Preventive Services, United States.* Washington, DC: DHHS.

National Center for Health Statistics (NCHS). (1997). Report of the final mortality statistics, 1995. *Monthly Vital Statistics Report,* 5(Suppl. 2).

National Center for Health Statistics (NCHS). (2003). *Health.* Washington, DC: Government Printing Office.

National Heart, Lung, and Blood Institute (NHLBI). (1995). *Consumer Awareness Surveys.* Press conference. Bethesda, MD: NHLBI.

National Heart, Lung, and Blood Institute (NHLBI). (1998). *Morbidity and Mortality: 1998 Chartbook of Cardiovascular, Lung, and Blood Diseases.* Bethesda, MD: Public Health Service, NIH, NHLBI.

National Heart, Lung, and Blood Institute (NHLBI). (2004). National High Blood Pressure Education Program, program description. Retrieved May 19, 2004 from www.nhlbi.nih.gov.

National Institutes of Health (NIH). (2001). Consensus Development Panel on osteoporosis. *Journal of the American Medical Association, 285,* 785.

National Institutes of Health (NIH). (2003). Osteoporosis and related bone diseases, National Resource Center. Retrieved July 12, 2004, from www.osteo.org.

National Institutes of Health (NIH) Consensus Development Panel on Physical Activity and Cardiovascular Health. (1996). Physical activity and cardiovascular health. *Journal of the American Medical Association, 276,* 241–246.

National Institutes of Health (NIH), and National Heart, Lung, and Blood Institute (NHLBI). (1998). Clinical guidelines on the identification, evaluation, and treatment of overweight and obesity in adults—the evidence report. *Obesity Research, 6,* 1105.

National Institutes of Health (NIH), and National Institute of Diabetes and Digestive and Kidney Diseases (2004). Diabetes prevention program. Retrieved July 9, 2004, from www.preventdiabetes.com.

National Institutes of Health (NIH) Technology Assessment Conference Panel. (1993). Methods for voluntary weight loss and control. Consensus development conference. March 30–April 1, 1992. *Annals of Internal Medicine, 119,* 764–770.

National Osteoporosis Foundation. (2004). Osteoporosis, disease statistics. Retrieved July 12, 2004, from www.nof.org.

National Vital Statistics Report. (2003). Deaths: Preliminary data for 2001. March 14, 2003, p. 51.

Pate, R. R., Pratt, M., Blair, S. N., Haskell, W. L., Macera, C. A., Bouchard, C., et al. (1995). Physical activity and public health: A recommendation from the Centers for Disease Control and Prevention and the American College of Sports Medicine. *Journal of the American Medical Association, 273,* 402–407.

Pavlou, K. N., Krey, S., & Stefee, W. O. (1989). Exercise as an adjunct to weight-loss and maintenance in moderately obese subjects. *American Journal of Clinical Nutrition, 49,* 1115–1123.

Pender, N. J. (1996). *Health Promotion in Nursing Practice* (3rd ed.). Stamford, CT: Appelton-Lange.

Psatsy, B. M., Smith, N. L., Siscovick, D. S., Koepsell, T. D., Weiss, N. S., Heckbert, S. R., et al. (1997). Health outcomes associated with antihypertensive therapies used as first-line agents. A systematic review and meta-analysis. *Journal of the American Medical Association, 277,* 739–745.

Resnicow, K., Orlandi, M., Vaccaro, D., & Wynder, E. (1989). Implementation of a pilot school-site cholesterol reduction intervention. *Journal of School Health, 59,* 74–78.

Ries, L., Eisner, M., Kosary, C., Hankey, B. F., Miller, B. A., Clegg, L., et al. (2003). *SEER: Cancer Statistics Review, 1975–2000.* Bethesda, MD: National Cancer Institute.

Sacks, F. M., Syerkey, L. P., Vollmer, W. M., Appel, L. J., Bray, G. A., Harsha, D., et al. (2001). Effects on blood pressure of reduced dietary sodium and Dietary Approaches to Stop Hypertension (DASH) diet. DASH-Sodium Collaborative Research Group. *New England Journal of Medicine, 344,* 3–10.

Serdula, M. K., Gillespie, C., Kettel-Khan, L., Farris, R., Seymour, J., & Denny, C. (2004). Trends in fruit and vegetable consumption among adults in the U.S.: Behavioral Risk Factor Surveillance System, 1994–2000. *American Journal of Public Health, 94,* 1014–1018.

Shamansky, S. L., & Clausen, C. (1980). Levels of prevention: Examination of the concept. *Nursing Outlook, 28,* 104–108.

Sharlin, J., Posner, B. M., Gershoff, S., Zeitlin, M., & Berger, P. (1992). Nutrition and behavioral characteristics and determinants of cholesterol levels in men and women. *Journal of the American Dietetic Association, 92,* 434–440.

Stewart, S. L., King, J. B., Thompson, T. D., Friedman, C., & Wingo, P. (2004). Cancer mortality surveillance—U.S., 1990–2000. National Center for Chronic Disease Prevention and Health Promotion. *Morbidity and Mortality Weekly Report, 53*(S503), 1–108.

Systolic Hypertension in the Elderly Program (SHEP) Cooperative Research Group. (1991). Prevention of stroke by antihypertensive drug treatment in older persons with isolated systolic hypertension. Final results of the SHEP. *Journal of the American Medical Association, 265,* 3255–3264.

Trials of Hypertension Prevention Collaborative Research Group. (1997). Effects of weight-loss and sodium reduction intervention on blood pressure and hypertension incidence in overweight people with high-normal blood pressure. The Trials of Hypertension Prevention, Phase 11. *Archives of Internal Medicine, 157,* 657–667.

U.S. Department of Agriculture (USDA). (1998). *USDA Continuing Survey of Food Intakes by Individuals (CSFII), 1994–1996.* Washington, DC: USDA.

U.S. Department of Agriculture (USDA). (2004). News release: Scientific update of food guidance presented to the Dietary Guidelines Committee. Retrieved June 29, 2004 from www.usda.gov.

U.S. Department of Agriculture (USDA) and U.S. Department of Health and Human Services (USDHHS). (1992). *The Food Guide Pyramid.* Washington, DC: USDDA and USDHHS.

U.S. Department of Health and Human Services (USDHHS). (1990). *The Health Benefits of Smoking Cessation: A Report of the Surgeon General.* Atlanta, GA: USDHHS, CDC, Center for Chronic Disease Prevention and Health Promotion, Office on Smoking and Health.

U.S. Department of Health and Human Services (USDHHS). (1996). *Physical Activity and Health: A Report of the Surgeon General, 1996.* Atlanta, GA: CDC, National Center for Chronic Disease Prevention and Health Promotion.

U.S. Department of Health and Human Services (USDHHS). (1998). *The Surgeon General's Report on Nutrition and Health* (PHS Publication No. 88-50210). Washington, DC: USDHHS.

U.S. Department of Health and Human Services (USDHHS). (2000a). *Healthy People 2010: Understanding and Improving Health* (2nd ed.). Washington, DC: U.S. Government Printing Office.

U.S. Department of Health and Human Services (USDHHS). (2000b). Nutrition and overweight. In: *Healthy People 2010: Understanding and Improving Health* (2nd ed., pp. 19–49). Washington, DC: U.S. Government Printing Office.

U.S. Department of Health and Human Services (USDHHS). (2000c). Heart disease and stroke. In: *Healthy People 2010: Understanding and Improving Health* (2nd ed., pp. 12–23). Washington, DC: USDHHS.

U.S. Department of Health and Human Services (USDHHS). (2000d). Physical activity and fitness. In: *Healthy People 2010: Understanding and Improving Health* (2nd ed., pp. 22–26). Washington, DC: USDHHS.

U.S. Department of Health and Human Services (USDHHS). (2000e). Diabetes. In: *Healthy People 2010: Understanding and Improving Health* (2nd ed., pp. 5–34). Washington, DC: USDHHS.

U.S. Department of Health and Human Services (USDHHS). (2000f). HIV. In: *Healthy People 2010: Understanding and Improving Health* (2nd ed., pp. 13–27). Washington, DC: USDHHS.

U.S. Department of Health and Human Services (USDHHS). (2002). *Health, U.S., 2002* (DHHS Publication No. 1232). Rockville, MD: DHHS, CDC.

U.S. Department of Health and Human Services (USDHHS). (2004). *The Health Consequences of Smoking: A Report of the Surgeon General.* Atlanta, GA: CDC, National Center for Chronic Disease Prevention and Health Promotion, Office on Smoking and Health.

U.S. Department of Health and Human Services (USDHHS), Centers for Disease Control and Prevention (CDC), and National Center for Health Statistics (NCHS). (2003). National Health Interview Survey (NHIS). Retrieved May 26, 2004, from www.cdc.gov/nchs/.

U.S. Department of Health and Human Services (USDHHS), and National Heart, Lung, and Blood Institute (NHLBI). (2001). *National Cholesterol Education Program, third report of the Expert Panel on the Detection, Evaluation, and Treatment of High Blood Cholesterol in Adults (Adult Treatment Panel III)* (NIH Publication No. 01-367). Bethesda, MD: Author.

U.S. Department of Health and Human Services (USDHHS), and National Heart, Lung, and Blood Institute (NHLBI). (2004). National High Blood Pressure Education Program. Retrieved May 26, 2004 from www.nhlbi.nih.gov/about/nhbpep.

U.S. Department of Health and Human Services (USDHHS), National Institutes of Health (NIH), National Heart, Lung, and Blood Institute (NHLBI), NHBPEP, and JCN 7 Express. (2003). *The seventh report of the Joint National Committee on Prevention, Detection, Evaluation, and Treatment of High Blood Pressure* (NIH Publication No. 03-5233).

U.S. Department of Health and Human Services (USDHHS), Public Health Service, Office of the Surgeon General. (2001). *Surgeon General's Call to Action to Prevent and Decrease Overweight and Obesity.* Washington, DC: USDHHS.

U.S. Preventive Services Task Force. (2003). *Guide to Clinical Preventive Services* (3rd ed.). Washington, DC: USDHHS.

Vollmer, W. M., Sacks, F. M., Ard, J., Appel, L. J., Bray, G. A., Simons-Morton, D. G., et al. (2001). Effects of diet and sodium intake on blood pressure. Subgroup analysis of the DASH—sodium trial. *Annals of Internal Medicine, 135,* 1019–1028.

Whelton, S. P., Chin, A., Xin, X., & He, J. (2002). Effect of aerobic exercise on blood pressure: A meta-analysis of randomized, controlled trials. *Annals of Internal Medicine, 136,* 493–503.

Willett, W. (1996). Diet and nutrition. In D. Schottenfield & J. F. Frammeni, Jr. (Eds.), *Cancer Epidemiology and Prevention* (2nd ed., pp. 438–461). New York: Oxford University Press.

Wimbush, F. B., & Peters, R. M. (2000). Identification of cardiovascular risk: Use of a cardiovascular-specific genogram. *Public Health Nursing, 17,* 148–154.

Xin, X., He, J., Frontini, M. G., Ogden, L.G., Motsamai, O. I., & Whelton, P. K. (2001). Effects of alcohol reduction on blood pressure. A meta-analysis of randomized controlled trials. *Hypertension, 38,* 1112–1117.

CHAPTER 11

Special Topics in Adult Nutrition: Physical Activity and Weight Management

Stella Lucia Volpe, PhD, RD, LDN, FACSM

CHAPTER OUTLINE

Reader Objectives

After studying this chapter and reflecting on the contents, you should be able to

1. Describe the differences between overweight and obese and their implications for risk of disease.
2. Explain the components of energy balance and how they can impact weight management.
3. Describe the role of physical activity in maintaining a healthy body weight in adults based on scientific evidence.

Obesity has become a worldwide epidemic. Every country, despite its economic status, has shown some increase in body weight in its population. In the United States it has been estimated that more than 50% of adults and more than 30% of children are overweight and/or obese, and these numbers continue to rise. Many factors contribute to this rise in overweight status, and they include, but are not limited to, genetics, decrease in the thermic effect of food, environmental factors, and the effects of some medications. Nonetheless, though our genes have not changed over hundreds of years, people are consuming more energy than before and, subsequently, becoming more sedentary. This imbalance in total energy expenditure can explain the greatest reason for this obesity epidemic.

The purpose of this chapter is to present research in the areas of physical activity, exercise, and weight management. Before the discussion of physical activity and weight management, basic definitions of overweight and obesity are described as well as a basic description of the components of total energy expenditure.

Definitions of Obesity and Overweight

Overweight and obesity are both used as ranges of body weight that are above what is regarded as healthy for a given height (Centers for Disease Control and Prevention [CDC], 2006). Obesity and overweight also define ranges of body weight that increase the risk of chronic disease (CDC, 2006). There are a number of definitions of overweight and obesity. The universal definitions of overweight and **obesity** have been established using body mass index (BMI; kg of body weight / height [m²]). For adults a BMI between 25 and 29.9 kg/m² is considered overweight, whereas a BMI of 30 kg/m² or greater is defined as obese (CDC, 2006) (Table 11.1). BMI is a good tool to assess the rates of overweight status and obesity in a population, but it is not a good a tool to assess overweight status and obesity in individuals. Thus a person should be cautious when using BMI in a clinical setting. For most of the population, which is sedentary, BMI correlates well with percent body fat, but it is not a measure of percent body fat. Therefore, individuals who

Obesity: The universal definitions of overweight and obesity have been established using body mass index (BMI; kg of body weight/height [m²]). For adults, a BMI between 25 and 29.9 kg/m² is considered overweight, whereas a BMI of 30 kg/m² or greater is defined as obese. Note that this is not the best definition for individuals.

TABLE 11.1	Body Mass Index Categories
Category	Body Mass Index (kg/m²)
Underweight	<18.5
Normal weight	18.5–24.9
Overweight	25–29.9
Obese	≥30

Adapted from U.S. Department of Health and Human Services (USDHHS), National Institutes of Health, National Heart, Lung, and Blood Institute (2006). Retrieved November 29, 2006 from http://www.nhlbisupport.com/bmi/bmicalc.htm.

may be "overweight" but not "over fat," such as athletes, are not considered to be overweight or obese because they have more muscle mass (on average) (CDC, 2006).

Because of this discrepancy between BMI and percent body fat, other definitions of obesity and overweight are based on a percentage above ideal body weight or percent body fat. In general, it has been stated that a person is considered overweight if his or her body weight is 20% above ideal body weight. The ideal body weight of a person is typically assessed using the Hamwi equation. The Hamwi equation for ideal body weight in women is calculated as follows:

100 pounds for 5 feet, plus 5 pounds
for every inch over 5 feet, or minus 5 pounds
for every inch under 5 feet

The Hamwi equation for men is calculated as follow:

106 pounds for 5 feet, plus 6 pounds
for every inch above 5 feet, and minus 6 pounds
for every inch under 5 feet

For men and women, subtract or add 10%, respectively, if a person is considered small or large framed.

Percent body fat measured by under water (hydrostatic) weighing or by dual-energy x-ray absorptiometry is an ideal method of estimating a person's body fat and, hence, if they are overweight due to fatness or lean body mass. However, in most situations body fat assessment, even via skinfold measures or bioelectrical impedance measures, is impractical. Thus for the average population, BMI predicts overweight status and obesity fairly well. It does not predict overweight status and obesity well if someone is muscular and/or has dense bones. When a person who is obviously fit is said to have a high BMI, their exercise habits and body composition must be considered.

CRITICAL Thinking

What do you think is the major cause of obesity? Make a list of each cause (making sure that decreased energy expenditure, the topic of this chapter, is one of them), and find at least one recent (within the year) research article that pertains to each item on your list. If your list is short, find two to three research articles. From there, make a theoretical framework where you describe, based on the research, how these components are related and how they impact one another. Use thicker arrows for those components that have a greater impact on other components and thinner arrows for those that have less of an impact. If there is no relationship between one component or another, then no arrows are used.

Total Energy Expenditure

Energy expenditure: Kilocalories expended during the day. Total energy expenditure comprises basal metabolic rate, dietary induced thermogenesis, and the thermic effect of activity. A fourth component is nonexercise activity thermogenesis (NEAT).

Total **energy expenditure** comprises three main components: basal energy expenditure (or basal metabolic rate [BMR]), the thermic effect of food, and the thermic effect of activity. A fourth component, which has had a bit more attention paid to it in recent years, is nonexercise activity thermogenesis, which also is described. The measurement of total energy expenditure in humans is necessary to assess the metabolic needs of a person, in relation to the aforementioned components of total energy expenditure (Levine, 2005).

Basal Metabolic Rate

Basal energy expenditure and BMR are measured in kilocalories (kcal) per day, or kcal/kg body weight/day, or kcal/kg fat free mass/day. Basal energy expenditure or BMR is defined as the energy to maintain circulation, respiration, and so forth at rest. Sometimes basal energy expenditure is referred to as resting energy expenditure or resting metabolic rate (RMR). Although resting energy expenditure and RMR are interchangeable, BMR and RMR are actually not exactly the same, because RMR is typically about 5% greater than BMR. This is because with BMR, the individual being assessed via direct or indirect calorimetry does not have to travel to a site and therefore does not have an increased heart rate before the measurement. With RMR, however, the individual typically travels to a site to have his or her RMR assessed. More recent research (Levine,

2005), however, has shown that when given 10 to 15 minutes rest, RMR and BMR are virtually the same. Furthermore, Ventham and Reilly (1999) reported that the measurement of RMR is highly reproducible in children, 6 to 11 years of age, even when children were provided only 5 to 10 minutes of rest before indirect calorimetry measurements. Regardless, both RMR and BMR are measured when an individual has fasted for 8 to 12 hours.

RMR or BMR can be assessed via indirect calorimetry, direct calorimetry, or doubly labeled water. Although direct calorimetry and doubly labeled water provide more accurate evaluations of energy expenditure, indirect calorimetry is the most often used because of cost, but it too provides a high source of accuracy (Levine, 2005). Furthermore, doubly labeled water only allows the investigator to assess total energy expenditure, not just RMR or BMR. When resources are limited and/or high accuracy is not required, noncalorimetric methods and total collection systems may be used; however, the limitations of these systems must be noted (Levine, 2005). A more holistic and accurate approach to measure total energy expenditure is to combine any of the described methods with daily log entries of activity (Levine, 2005).

● Learning Point A rough method to assess BMR is to multiply a person's body weight by 10. Thus if someone weighs 150 pounds, then 150 × 10 = 1,500 kcal. Although this is a rough estimate of a person's BMR, it can provide an idea of his or her BMR.

Thermic Effect of Food

The thermic effect of food is another component of the total energy expenditure equation. The thermic effect of food, also known as dietary induced thermogenesis, is the amount of energy required for absorption and digestion of food. Using indirect calorimetry, the thermic effect of food is measured for a 4-hour period postprandially, with about 5 to 10 minutes given as a break to the individual at the end of each hour. The thermic effect of food comprises about 10% of total energy expenditure. It has been reported that obese individuals may have a slightly lower thermic effect of food than 10%.

Thermic Effect of Exercise

The thermic effect of exercise is perhaps the most variable component to the total energy expenditure equation. It can be as low as 10% in very sedentary individuals to as high as 100% in Olympic

TABLE 11.2	Activity Factors Used to Estimate Thermic Effect of Activity	
Activity	**Multiple of Basal Energy Expenditure**
Resting	= Basal energy expenditure
Very light (sitting, standing)	0.1
Light (leisure, housework)	0.25
Moderate (3.5–4.0 mph)	0.5
Heavy (fast walk +)	0.7

athletes or professional athletes, who work out from 6 to 10 hours per day. **Table 11.2** shows activity factors that are used to estimate thermic effect of food.

Nonexercise Activity Thermogenesis

Nonexercise activity thermogenesis (NEAT): The energy expenditure of all physical activities other than volitional sporting-like exercise. NEAT includes activities such as working, playing, and dancing.

Nonexercise activity thermogenesis (NEAT) is defined as "the energy expenditure of all physical activities other than volitional sporting-like exercise. NEAT includes all the activities that render us vibrant, unique, and independent beings such as working, playing, and dancing" (Levine, Vander Weg, Hill, & Klesges, 2006). This has been shown to account for up to 2,000 kcal/day, depending on the amount of NEAT a person accumulates throughout each day (Levine et al., 2006). It has been reported that lean individuals stand and move more than obese individuals, indicating that lean individuals have greater amount of NEAT than obese individuals (Levine et al., 2005). Even after lean and obese individuals gained weight, NEAT was still significantly greater in lean individuals, indicating central and humoral meditators that drive sedentary behaviors in obese individuals (Levine et al., 2005).

Obese individuals appear to have a natural predisposition to be seated for 2.5 hours a day more than their sedentary lean counterparts. If obese individuals could simply incorporate more NEAT into their daily routine and become more "NEAT-o-type" (Levine et al., 2006), they could expend about 350 more kcal per day, which could lead to a 15-kg weight loss over a year's period (Levine et al., 2005). Levine et al. (2006) stated that obesity reflects the surfacing of a "chair-enticing environment," where those who have a natural predisposition to sit have done so and, hence, have become obese. As a society, we need to assist individuals by promoting standing more often and becoming more active throughout the day. This can be done by reconfiguring work, school, and home environments to result in active life-styles (Levine et al., 2006).

Lower NEAT in obese individuals could be a result of a decreased production of neuromedin U (NMU), which has been associated with the control of energy intake and expenditure (Novak, Zhang, & Levine, 2006). NMU appears to affect the hypothalamic nuclei of the brain. Novak et al. (2006) applied varying doses of NMU directly into the paraventricular and arcuate hypothalamic nuclei of Sprague-Dawley rats. They reported increased physical activity and NEAT when NMU was applied to either nucleus; increased doses resulted in increased activity (Novak et al., 2006). Interestingly, they also reported that NMU decreased energy intake and body weight. Though the study of NMU is in its early stages, there could be promise of this peptide in combating obesity.

Despite the cause of a lower NEAT in obese individuals, a great deal of attention in the clinical and fitness industry has *not* been placed on NEAT. Nonetheless, focusing on NEAT would be a more realistic and simple approach to help obese individuals incorporate more activity into their daily lives, lose weight, and then begin to incorporate physical activity and exercise into their daily routines, after some initial weight has been lost, giving them more confidence to actually exercise.

Physical Activity and Obesity Prevention

Physical activity and exercise interventions, as well as a combination of physical activity/exercise and diet interventions, have been well researched in the area of obesity prevention. In 2005 the Dietary Guidelines for Americans listed physical activity and weight management as two of its nine key recommendations (U.S. Department of Health and Human Services [USDHHS] and U.S. Department of Agriculture, 2005). The main focus of this chapter is to present recent research in physical activity and a combination of physical activity and diet interventions and discuss the main outcomes of these trials. Though the most recent research is highlighted, some key older studies are also presented to lay the groundwork of where research in this area has been and where it will be moving toward.

Definitions of Physical Activity and Exercise

Before discussing research in the areas of physical activity and exercise and nutrition, it is important to de-

Physical activity: Body movement produced by the contraction of skeletal muscle and that substantially increases energy expenditure. Common categories of physical activity include occupational, household, leisure time, and transportation.

Exercise: Planned, structured, and repetitive bodily movement done to improve or maintain one or more components of physical fitness.

fine the differences between physical activity and exercise. **Physical activity** is defined as "bodily movement that is produced by the contraction of skeletal muscle and that substantially increases energy expenditure" (USDHHS, 1996). Common categories of physical activity include occupational, household, leisure time, and transportation (USDHHS, 1996). Occupational, household, and transportation physical activities are also known as "utilitarian" physical activities. In 2001 the Behavioral Risk Factor Surveillance System reported that in the United States from 28% to 55% of individuals performed leisure time physical activity (CDC, 2003). **Exercise** is defined as planned, structured, and repetitive bodily movement done to improve or maintain one or more components of physical fitness (USDHHS, 1996).

> **● Learning Point** The five components of physical fitness are cardiorespiratory endurance, muscular endurance, muscular strength, flexibility, and body composition (Ward, 1999). It has been reported that only about 20% of individuals in the United States exercise on a regular basis (three or more times per week, for at least 20 minutes per session).

Weight Loss Goals

Despite so few people participating in physical activity or exercise on a regular basis, individuals significantly ($p < 0.05$) overestimate their energy expenditure and underestimate their energy intake by approximately 500 kcal and 1,000 kcal, respectively (Lichtman et al., 1992). In addition, it has been reported that obese individuals have unrealistic weight loss goals. Before participating in a weight loss trial, individuals stated that a 38% reduction from their initial body weight (e.g., from an average of 218 pounds to an average of 135 pounds) would be their "dream weight" and that if they lost only 17% of their initial body weight (e.g., from 218 pounds to 180 pounds) they would be "disappointed" (Foster, Wadden, Vogt, & Brewer, 1997). In reality, individuals in most weight loss studies lose an average of about 15% of their initial body weight, which would be below their "disappointed" body weight loss.

Wadden et al. (2003) evaluated whether notifying obese participants that they would only lose a modest amount of body weight would then guide them to agree to more reasonable weight loss goals. At the baseline interview, Wadden and colleagues (2003) interviewed 53 obese women who stated that, on average, they expected to lose about 28% of their initial body weight after the first year of treatment with a weight loss medication. Before initiation of the trial, it was explained to the women, both in writing and verbally, that they should expect to lose about 5% to 15% of their initial body weight (Wadden et al., 2003). Regardless of this prior information, the women did not alter their weight loss expectations throughout the trial. These unrealistic expectations may be one of the many reasons for the high rate of recidivism after weight loss trials.

How Much Exercise or Physical Activity Is Enough?

In 1995 the Surgeon General, the CDC, and the American College of Sports Medicine established that individuals should accumulate *at least* 30 minutes or more of exercise per day for cardiovascular fitness. However, this amount of exercise, which on average represents about 150 minutes per week, may not be enough for weight loss. In 2005 the National Academy of Sciences of the Institute of Medicine established Dietary Reference Intakes for physical activity and exercise. In brief, the Dietary Reference Intake recommendation states that individuals should exercise at least 30 minutes per day at a high intensity or at least 60 minutes per day at a low intensity (Food and Nutrition Boards, Institute of Medicine, National Academy of Sciences, 2005).

In 2001 the American College of Sports Medicine published their position on effective weight loss methods (Jakicic et al., 2001). They stated, "the American College of Sports Medicine recommends that the combination of reductions in energy intake and increases in energy expenditure, through structured exercise and other forms of physical activity, be a component of weight loss intervention programs."

Physical Activity Interventions and Weight Loss

The research in the area of physical activity and weight loss has covered many types of study designs. In an effort to assess if multiple bouts of physical activity result in similar weight loss to one longer bout of physical activity, Jakicic and colleagues (1995) conducted a 20-week study in 56 overweight sedentary women, about 40 years of age, with a BMI of 34 kg/m². The long bout group was given instructions to walk 40 minutes per day in one session, whereas the short bout group was given instructions to walk for 40 minutes in two to four shorter sessions per day. Thus total exercise time remained the same between the two groups. The women wore accelerometers to assess energy expenditure. They were also told to maintain an energy intake of between 1,200 to 1,500 kcal/day, with about 20% of total energy intake derived from fat. Jakicic et al. (1995) reported significant ($p < 0.05$), and similar, weight loss for both groups of women and significant increases in cardiorespiratory fitness in both groups. It appears from this research that exercise in multiple bouts could be an encouraging method to increase physical activity in individuals; however, the study was only 20 weeks in duration, and therefore longer-term research is required to evaluate if the participants would continue with this exercise regimen.

Jakicic and coworkers (1999) conducted a longer-term study that somewhat paralleled the aforementioned research. They compared the effects of intermittent exercise with traditional long bout exercise on weight loss, but they also added another component: They examined the effects of intermittent exercise with that of using home exercise equipment. The participants were 148 sedentary overweight women (BMI = 32.8 ± 4.0 kg/m^2, 36.7 ± 5.6 years of age). The study was 18 months in duration, and the subjects were randomly assigned to one of three groups: long bout exercise, multiple short bout exercise, or multiple short bout exercise with home exercise equipment (SBEQ) using a treadmill. Their primary aims were to assess the differences among these three groups in body weight, body composition, cardiorespiratory fitness, and exercise adherence.

They reported that all three groups improved their cardiorespiratory fitness, with no difference among groups. Weight loss was significantly greater ($p < 0.05$) in participants in the SBEQ group compared with participants in the short bout group, with no differences in weight loss seen between the long bout group and either SBEQ or the short bout group (-7.4 ± 7.8 kg [SBEQ], -3.7 ± 6.6 kg [short bout group], -5.8 ± 7.1 kg [long bout group]).

Two interesting findings resulted from this study. First, the SBEQ group was able to sustain a significantly greater intensity of exercise than subjects in the short bout and long bout groups ($p < 0.05$). In addition, Jakicic et al. (1999) found a clear and significant ($p < 0.05$) dose–response relationship with the amount of exercise to the amount of weight loss. Thus participants who exercised more than 200 minutes per week for the 18-month intervention had a significantly greater weight loss than individuals who exercised from 150 to 200 minutes per week and compared with individuals who exercised less than 150 minutes per week (-13.1 ± 8.0 kg [200 min/wk], -8.5 ± 5.8 kg [150 to 200 min/wk], -3.5 ± 6.5 kg [<150 min/wk]). They concluded that access to home exercise equipment may assist in exercise adherence, resulting in weight loss in the long term. Furthermore, the dose–response relationship they reported, which would seem intuitive, clearly indicates that the greater energy expenditure, the more body weight the person will lose.

Physical Activity and Weight Loss in the Primary Care Setting

The primary care setting is becoming a more popular place to conduct research on weight loss, because the patients, for the most part, have developed a relationship with their primary care practitioners. Booth et al. (2006) evaluated the effect of primary care physicians writing prescriptions that recommended lifestyle changes to their patients. They called this the "active nutrition script," which included five nutrition messages and personalized exercise advice for the prevention of weight gain. This was a pilot study whereby family physicians were asked to write 10 active nutrition scripts over a 4-week period to 10 adult patients who had a BMI between 23 and 30 kg/m^2. The physicians recorded the patients' body weight, height, waist circumference, gender, date of birth, type and frequency of exercise prescribed, and nutrition messages on each script. Booth et al. (2006) reported that 19 family physicians (63% of them were women) provided approximately nine active nutrition scripts over a 4-week period. A total of 145 patients (57% were women) received the active nutrition scripts (54 ± 13.2 years of age, mean BMI = 31.7 ± 6.3 kg/m^2). Seventy-eight percent of the time the physicians wrote the active nutrition scripts for weight loss. Of the physicians interviewed by the researchers (17 of 19 physicians were interviewed), they all stated that the active nutrition scripts messages were clear and easy to deliver. Though the physicians found this script easy to deliver, they mainly prescribed it for weight loss instead of prevention of weight gain. This research needs to be taken to the next step, where body weight and BMI are actually measured over time in the patients who receive the active nutrition scripts. Although this was a pilot study, the primary care setting may be one of the best places for prevention of weight gain and for weight loss.

McQuigg et al. (2005) conducted a study in the United Kingdom in 80 primary care settings whose primary aim was to improve the management of obese adults in a primary care setting. The participants had a BMI $\geq$ 30 kg/m^2 or a BMI $\pm$ 28 kg/m^2 with at least one obesity-related comorbidity. This counterweight program consisted of four phases: audit and project development, practice training and support, nurse-led patient intervention, and evaluation. For the intervention portion, evidence-based pathways and incorporated approaches were used to empower the health care providers and patients in weight management. This program also had weight management advisers who were dietitians specializing in obesity.

McQuigg et al. (2005) reported a large number of intervention practices had been trained (almost 94%), and they recruited 1,549 patients. At 1 year after implementation, 33% of the patients achieved a weight loss of 5% or more, which is clinically significant, because only a small amount of weight loss has been shown to reduce the risk of chronic disease. It has been reported that for every kilogram of weight lost, there is a 16% reduction in the risk of type 2 diabetes mellitus (Hamman et al., 2006).

Although the aforementioned studies were successful, Morrato and colleagues asked the question, "Are health care professionals advising patients with diabetes or at risk for developing diabetes to exercise more?" Though the focus of this chapter is on physical activity and weight loss, one of the primary comorbidities developed as a result of obesity is type 2 diabetes mellitus. Morrato et al. (2006) accessed the Medical Expenditure Panel Survey, whereby more than 26,000 adults in the United States responded in 2002. They found that 73% of the adults with type 2 diabetes mellitus were told by a health care professional to exercise more, compared with 31% without diabetes mellitus. In addition, the number of people receiving exercise guidance increased as the amount of diabetes risk factors increased. These researchers reported that BMI and cardiovascular disease risk factors were the strongest predictors for practitioners to give exercise recommendations. They did report, however, that as the diabetes risk factors decreased, exercise advice to patients decreased, resulting in "missed opportunities for disease prevention" (Morrato et al., 2006). Despite the exercise advice, the patients did not always change behavior, which is still the most difficult part of the equation to change (Morrato et al., 2006).

How Can People Be Successful at Maintaining Weight Loss?

The maintenance of weight loss is probably the most difficult phase of any weight loss program. After a person feels successful losing weight, he or she often returns to eating the amount of foods consumed before weight loss and decreases physical activity. Though there may be many psychological, and even perhaps physiological, reasons behind this, there are practical ways people can incorporate physical activity into their day, which can help to increase energy expenditure and maintain weight loss and/or prevent weight gain.

Hill (2006) and colleagues (2006) stated that small changes can lead to big effects on the prevention of weight gain. They stated that if energy balance can be affected by a mere 100 kcal/day, this could lead to a large reduction in the obesity epidemic. People could achieve this small energy deficit by simply walking 15 minutes per day (and multiple bouts would be effective) and/or eat just a few less bites of food at each meal. These small changes are not daunting and may result in greater adherence to weight loss and maintenance.

Though the obesity epidemic is considered a gene–environment interaction (i.e., the human genotype is predisposed to ecologic influences that affect energy intake and expenditure), it is mostly a problem of energy balance (Hill, 2006). The most successful interventions are those that impact energy balance (increase expenditure and decrease intake) but that also take into consideration behavioral and environmental factors that play a big role in why

Cultural Diversity

It is important to respect and try to understand the different cultural practices of different ethnicities; however, it is equally important not to stereotype. For example, if one of your patients is Asian-American, you should not assume that he or she consumes traditional Chinese meals. You need to ask him or her first about dislikes, likes, and usual practices. Conversely, if one of your patients is white, you should not assume that he or she consumes typical "American" meals. Again, talk to the patient and find out likes, dislikes, usual practices, and ethnicity. As health care practitioners and researchers, we cannot make assumptions. We need to respect each person's individuality. However, there are cultural diversity issues in weight loss, obesity, and other chronic diseases; research has clearly shown differences. Just be certain you get to know your patient, client, or study participant as an individual.

Search for a recent research publication on ethnic/cultural diversity with respect to physical activity in obesity prevention and/or weight loss. Make a list of the major differences you find among different racial and ethnic groups as they pertain to weight loss and/or obesity with respect to physical activity.

individuals do not exercise or eat higher amounts of total energy (Hill, 2006). Hill (2006) stated the following:

> Our best strategy for reversing the obesity epidemic is to focus on preventing positive energy balance in the population through small changes in diet and physical activity that take advantage of our biological systems for regulating energy balance. Simultaneously we must address the environment to make it easier to make better food and physical activity choices. This is a very long-term strategy for first stopping and then reversing the escalating obesity rates, but one than can, over time, return obesity rates to pre-1980s levels.

Just as the primary care setting can be an ideal location to impact obesity, interventions that include the entire family could also lead to successful maintenance of weight loss. Rodearmel et al. (2006) focused on increasing steps walked per day and cereal consumption (for breakfast and snacks) as a weight reduction intervention for families. They included 105 families in their study who had at least one 8- to 12-year-old child who was at risk for becoming overweight or obese. This was a 13-week intervention, whereby 82 families were randomly assigned to the family-based intervention (increase steps to 2,000 per day and consume two servings of ready to eat cereal per day) and 23 families were randomly assigned to the control group. The intervention groups showed significant reductions in BMI and BMI-for-age in the adults and children, respectively, especially in mother–daughter pairs. Focusing on the family is a logical and practical way for individuals to maintain weight loss and/or prevent weight gain, because all individuals are making healthful changes together and provide a support system for one another.

Perhaps the most well-known registry of successful weight loss maintenance is the National Weight Control Registry. This is a registry of individuals who had an initial weight loss average of 33.1 kg and who were able to maintain a 13.6-kg weight loss for 5.8 years before enrolling in the Registry (Phelan, Wyatt, Hill, & Wing, 2006). Although many studies have been published on participants in the National Weight Control Registry, Phelan et al. (2006) evaluated whether dietary intake habits of registrants changed over the years, especially most recently, with the surge of low carbohydrate diets. They included 2,708 participants who were part of the National Weight Control Registry since 1995.

They reported that from 1995 to 2003 energy from fat intake increased from 23.8% to 29.4%, with an increase in saturated fat from 12.3 to 15.4 g/day. Subsequently, energy from carbohydrate declined from 56% to 49% ($p < 0.0001$), and those who consumed less than 90 g/day of carbohydrate increased from 5.9% to 17.1% ($p = 0.0001$). Except for 1995, where physical activity was calculated at 3,316 kcal/wk, the remaining years were stable at about 2,620 kcal/wk. Phelan et al. (2006) stated that weight regain over 1 year was primarily associated with greater energy intake, more fast food consumption, increased fat intake, and lower amounts of physical activity ($p < 0.03$). Table 11.3 lists practical ways people can incorporate more physical activity into their lives.

● **Learning Point** Though a small percentage of individuals in this registry reported consuming a low carbohydrate diet, the main factors that allowed these individuals to maintain weight loss over time remain the same: consumption of a low energy diet, moderate fat intake, limited consumption of fast food, and high amounts of physical activity or exercise (Phelan et al., 2006).

Summary

Obesity is a complex issue that requires a multifaceted approach to result in success. Although it is clearly a gene–environment interaction, the onus is still placed on greater energy expenditure combined with decreased energy intake. Increasing NEAT, mul-

TABLE 11.3 Practical Ways to Incorporate More Physical Activity into the Day

Take the stairs instead of the elevator.

Park farther away from the destination.

Sit on a balance ball while working at a desk.

Exercise during commercials while watching television (if made into a family event it will be even more fun and successful!).

Have a Thera-Band™ available by desks, couches, and so on so that strength training exercises can be performed.

Dance.

Stretch during the day.

Stand up during meetings.

Do chair exercises (leg lifts, work on core strength, etc.).

Move as much as possible throughout the day—be "inefficient."

tiple versus long bouts of exercise, and physical activity promotion in the primary care setting and family are all promising ways that the obesity epidemic can be reversed.

Issues to Debate

1. What are your views on bariatric surgery? Conduct a literature search to find at least one research article that showed a positive effect of bariatric surgery and one that does not. Find a recent (within a year) review article that describes each different type of bariatric surgery and when it needs to be performed. Debate both sides of this issue, providing background from your literature search. Include the pros and cons for prescribing physical activity to individuals who are morbidly obese and, hence, are candidates for bariatric surgery.

Case Study

Don is a 34-year-old African-American who is an attorney at a large practice in Chicago. He is fairly new to this firm and wants to make partner. His job is very stressful. He works about 100 hours per week and gets little time to eat well or exercise, but he would really like to start to exercise even a few days per week.

Body weight: 225 pounds
Height: 5 feet, 8 inches
Exercises once or twice a week "when I get time"

He says, in general, that he consumes his breakfast "on the run," usually in the car on his way to work. His wife is also an attorney at a large firm, and they are both often very busy. When he does eat breakfast, it is usually something quick, like a donut, or he may stop at a fast food restaurant drive-through to get an egg and cheese croissant sandwich. He drinks about five to six cups of coffee per day.

For lunch, it is either something from the vending machine or, the opposite, a large meal at an expensive restaurant with one of his clients. Thus his lunch energy intake varies drastically. For dinner he and his wife often eat takeout Chinese food, pizza, submarine sandwiches, or hamburgers and French fries. They do try to eat more "normally" on weekends, but both are often in the office at least one day on the weekend.

1. Calculate Don's BMI (kg/m^2).
2. Calculate Don's total energy expenditure.
3. Based on this crude "dietary recall," provide a rough estimate of his energy intake.
4. What ideas would you give Don to help him improve his eating? Be conscious of the fact that he has little time to prepare meals.
5. How might Don be able to incorporate any physical activity in his life? Be creative!

Website Resources

All websites were retrieved on December 8, 2006.

American College of Sports Medicine http://www.acsm.org//AM/Template.cfm?Section=Home_PageandWebsiteKey=3bb8c0a3-b699-44f5-99ca-4c9e64600c5e

American Dietetic Association http://www.eatright.org/cps/rde/xchg/ada/hs.xsl/index.html

American Obesity Association http://www.obesity.org/prevention/preventing.shtml

America on the Move http://aom.americaonthemove.org/site/c.krLXJ3PJKuG/b.1524889/k.BFFA/Home.htm

American Society for Bariatric Surgery http://www.asbs.org/

Centers for Disease Control and Prevention http://www.cdc.gov/nccdphp/dnpa/obesity/resources.htm

NAASO, The Obesity Society http://www.naaso.org/

National Institutes of Health Obesity Research http://obesityresearch.nih.gov/

References

Booth, A. O., Nowson, C. A., Huang, N., Lombard, C., & Singleton, K. L. (2006). Evaluation of a brief pilot nutrition and exercise intervention for the prevention of weight gain in general practice patients. *Public Health Nutrition, 9,* 1005–1061.

Centers for Disease Control and Prevention (CDC). (2003). Prevalence of physical activity, including lifestyle activities among adults—United States, 2000–2001. *Morbidity and Mortality Weekly Reports, 52,* 764–769.

Centers for Disease Control and Prevention (CDC). (2006). Obesity. Defining overweight and obesity. Retrieved November 29, 2006 from http://www.cdc.gov/nccdphp/dnpa/obesity/defining.htm

Food and Nutrition Board, Institute of Medicine, National Academy of Sciences. (2005). Dietary Reference Intakes for energy, carbohydrate, fiber, fat, fatty acids, cholesterol, protein, and amino acids (macronutrients). Washington, DC: The National Academy Press.

Foster, G. D., Wadden, T. A., Vogt, R. A., & Brewer, G. (1997). What is a reasonable weight loss? Patients' expectations and evaluations of obesity treatment outcomes. *Journal of Consulting and Clinical Psychology, 65,* 79–85.

Hamman, R. F., Wing, R. R., Edelstein, S. L., Lachin, J. M., Bray, G. A., Delahanty, L., et al. (2006). Effect of weight loss with lifestyle intervention on risk of diabetes. *Diabetes Care, 29,* 2102–2107.

Hill, J. O. (2006). Understanding and addressing the epidemic of obesity: An energy balance perspective. *Endocrine Reviews, 27*, 750–761.

Hill, J. O., Wyatt, H. R., Reed, G. W., & Peters, J. C. (2006). Obesity and the environment: Where do we go from here? *Science, 299*, 853–855.

Jakicic, J. M., Clark, K., Coleman, E., Donnelly, J. E., Foreyt, J., Melanson, E., et al. (2001). American College of Sports Medicine position stand. Appropriate intervention strategies for weight loss and prevention of weight regain for adults. *Medicine and Science in Sports and Exercise, 33*, 2145–2156.

Jakicic, J. M., Wing, R. R., Butler, B. A., & Robertson, R. J. (1995). Prescribing exercise in multiple short bouts versus one continuous bout: Effects on adherence, cardiorespiratory fitness, and weight loss in overweight women. *International Journal of Obesity and Related Metabolic Disorders, 19*, 893–901.

Jakicic, J. M., Winters, C., Lang, W., & Wing, R. R. (1999). Effect of intermittent exercise and use of home exercise equipment on adherence, weight loss, and fitness in overweight women: A randomized trial. *Journal of the American Medical Association, 282*, 1554–1560.

Levine, J. A. (2005). Measurement of energy expenditure. *Public Health Nutrition, 8*, 1123–1132.

Levine, J. A., Lanningham-Foster, L. M., McCrady, S. K., Krizan, A. C., Olson, L. R., Kane, P. H., et al. (2005). Interindividual variation in posture allocation: Possible role in human obesity. *Science, 307*, 584–586.

Levine J. A., Vander Weg, M .W., Hill, J. O., & Klesges, R. C. (2006). Non-exercise activity thermogenesis: The crouching tiger hidden dragon of societal weight gain. *Arteriosclerosis, Thrombosis, and Vascular Biology, 26*, 729–736.

Lichtman, S. W., Pisarska, K., Berman, E. R., Pestone, M., Dowling, H., Offenbacher, E., et al. (1992). Discrepancy between self-reported and actual caloric intake and exercise in obese subjects. *New England Journal of Medicine, 327*, 1893–1898.

McQuigg, M., Brown, J., Broom, J., Laws, R. A., Reckless, J. P., Noble, P. A., et al. (2005). Empowering primary care to tackle the obesity epidemic: The Counterweight Programme. *European Journal of Clinical Nutrition, 59* (Suppl. 1), S93–S100.

Morrato, E. H., Hill, J. O., Wyatt, H. R., Ghushchyan, V., & Sullivan, P. W. (2006). Are health care professionals advising patients with diabetes or at risk for developing diabetes to exercise more? *Diabetes Care, 29*, 543–548.

Novak, C. M., Zhang, M., & Levine, J. A. (2006). Neuromedin U in the paraventricular and arcuate hypothalamic nuclei increases non-exercise activity thermogenesis. *Journal of Neuroendocrinology, 18*, 594–601.

Phelan, S., Wyatt, H. R., Hill, J. O., & Wing, R. R. (2006). Are the eating and exercise habits of successful weight losers changing? *Obesity, 14*, 710–716.

Rodearmel, S. J., Wyatt, H. R., Barry, M. J., Dong, F., Pan, D., Israel, R. G., et al. (2006). A family-based approach to preventing excessive weight gain. *Obesity, 14*, 1392–1401.

U.S. Department of Health and Human Services (USDHHS). (1996). Physical activity and health: A report of the Surgeon General. Atlanta, GA: USDHHS, and CDC, National Center for Chronic Disease Prevention and Health Promotion.

U.S. Department of Health and Human Services (USDHHS) and U.S. Department of Agriculture. (2005). *Dietary Guidelines for Americans*.

Ventham, J. C., & Reilly, J. J. (1999). Reproducibility of resting metabolic rate measurement in children. *British Journal of Nutrition, 81*, 435–437.

Wadden, T. A., Womble, L. G., Sarwer, D. B., Berkowitz, R. I., Clark, V. L., & Foster, G. D. (2003). Great expectations: "I'm losing 25% of my weight no matter what you say." *Journal of Consulting and Clinical Psychology, 71*, 1084–1089.

Ward, A. (1999). Exercise and exercise intervention in the prevention of coronary artery disease. In J .M. Rippe (Ed.), *Lifestyle Medicine* (pp. 90–97). Malden, MA: Blackwell Science.

Special Topics in Nutrition and the Older Adult: Diet, Life-Style, Disease, and Pharmacologic Considerations

Roschelle Heuberger, PhD, RD

CHAPTER OUTLINE

After studying this chapter and reflecting on the contents, you should be able to

1. Identify controversies surrounding the definition of an "older adult."

2. Categorize the emerging elderly population by demographics and specifically by socioeconomics.

3. Define cellular senescence and successful aging.

4. Itemize the direct and indirect determinants of aging and cellular senescence.

5. Delineate differences between biochemical/physiologic and life-style/environmental contributions toward inflammation, oxidative stress, apoptosis, and free-radical-induced damage with aging processes.

6. Discuss the processes and their determinants for disease states that accompany aging.

7. Identify issues in the hospitalized/institutionalized older adult. Relate those issues to morbidity and mortality through nutriture.

8. Describe the pharmacologic considerations in the treatment of diseases in older persons, inclusive of the issues of polypharmacy.

9. Define strategies for the treatment of obesity in an older adult, with attention to future directions for pharmacotherapeutic agents.

Older adults are a diverse and extremely heterogeneous population group. Differentiation between chronologic age and **senescence** must be taken into account. Some 70-year-old persons are more fit and less "aged" from a cellular and functional standpoint than some 40-year-olds, due to a variety of genetic and life-style characteristics. However, functional declines naturally occur with aging and the oldest old (>85 years) generally exhibit changes associated with senescence (Singer & Manton, 1998). An overview of the older adult population and issues surrounding senescence, determinants of health and nutritional status, and consequences of aging and disease is given.

Senescence: The process of aging taking into account cellular death and dysregulation leading to functional decline.

Older adults comprise the most rapidly growing demographic in the United States as well as in other industrialized countries. Life expectancies have increased as a result of a number of factors:

- Declines in mortality from infectious diseases
- Increases in technologic ability to detect disease at an early juncture
- Advent of new pharmacotherapies for a variety of acute and chronic disease states
- Increases in awareness of antecedents for disease among the general population
- Overall better access to health care
- Overall better nutriture and sanitation
- Overall technologic enhancements or preventative measures that may determine better health status over the life span (i.e., better automotive safety or stricter seat belt regulations)

As a result of the population living longer and the aging of the "baby boomers," there is a current critical need for education regarding the requirements of older adults. Because of interrelationships of nutritional status with socioeconomics, life-style characteristics, environmental considerations, comorbid conditions and genetics, all must be evaluated concurrently with dietary intake in this population.

Older Adults

Definitions of *elderly, older adult, geriatric, frail, senior,* and/or *aged* vary widely. This is problematic for the purposes of identifying or classifying individuals to determine policy or procedure. For the purposes of the government, such as with food assistance programs, taxation, and retirement, the person over age 65 is considered to be an older adult or senior. This is not the case when talking with persons trained in gerontology. In the social sciences, the definition of "aged" is related to functional status and not chronologic age. Functional ability is most often related to psychological status, ability to perform tasks of daily living (i.e., bathing, cooking), medical status, and socioeconomics.

For the subspecialty of geriatrics, which is more focused within the health professions, the terms "geriatric patient" or "frail elderly" are tied to medical status and cellular or mechanistic processes as opposed to holistic definitions (Woods et al., 2005). The term "frailty" is misrepresented in the literature, because it was most often in the past associated with being underweight with or without frank vitamin and mineral malnutrition (Sullivan, Lui, Roberson, Bopp, & Rees, 2004). There has been a recent shift to include normal or overweight persons in the category of frail, if they have **sarcopenia**, several diagnoses, poor nutritional status, and a decreased ability to function (Weinrebe, Guneysu, & Welz-Barth, 2002). This trend is a consequence of the obesity epidemic across all age groups, including elderly persons.

Sarcopenia: Decrements in muscle mass that result in declining functional ability.

There is an increasing need to develop a uniform classification system for older adults, just as we have for the differing developmental stages of infants, children, and adolescents. Currently, the information regarding subgroups within the older adult population is lacking, and gross generalizations often result from research in this area. Each older adult must therefore be considered individually for preventative measures, nutritional recommendations, and treatment options based on the totality of the information available (Keller & Ostbye, 2003).

Epidemiology

The "graying" of America currently taking place with the aging of the baby boomers is considered to be a health care crisis, with insufficient practitioners, facilities, or accommodations for the changing demographics.

● **Learning Point** If current trends hold, by the year 2050 one in four persons in the United States will be over the age of 65. The "oldest old" are the most rapidly increasing segment of this population. Women (minority women in particular) will soon be the dominant demographic in this oldest old category (National Institute on Aging, 2005; U.S. Bureau of the Census, 2005).

There will be fewer working adults and an enormous drain on the economy with large numbers of poor elderly persons requiring extended care. Efforts to promote a healthy aging agenda for the population are beginning to get underway, despite the fact that this national campaign should have commenced three decades ago to maximize effects in late life.

Characteristics of the U.S. population that are over the age of 65 include a number of regional differences, and warmer climate states usually have an over-representation of certain segments of the elderly population. Florida has the highest percentage of older adults at nearly 20% of the population. Mississippi, Alabama, Louisiana, and Puerto Rico have 15% to 20% of their older adults living under the poverty level. Older adults are among the poorest of the poor, especially older women who were homemakers and do not receive added benefits from having worked. Women also live longer than men, and when they reach the oldest old category they have depleted any resources they may have had and require more medication, health care, and assistance, which results in the need for greater fiscal resources. Minority women make up the poorest of the poor among this demographic.

The number of elderly that live alone is estimated at 10%, and households containing an elderly person are above 23%. Asian and Hispanic descent is correlated with increased numbers of elderly as part of households, whereas African-American and white descent correlates with increased numbers of elderly living alone. Details of the national averages are shown in **Table 12.1**.

Epidemiologic data on older adults are available from a number of federal, state, local, nonprofit, and private sector sources. The federal government National Health and Nutrition Examination Survey, which has been ongoing, collected data on an over-sampling of the elderly population in the United States. A variety of statistics is available regarding socioeconomics, blood values, and dietary data. Medical and behavioral measures were also obtained for the older population in the National Health and Nutrition Examination Survey series. Behavioral Risk Factor Surveillance Studies have also included older adults. Conducted at the state level, these assessments are available for specific samples of elderly in most of the 48 contiguous states. Variables regarding demographics, health risk factors, and some dietary information are available.

The National Institute on Aging, a branch of the National Institutes of Health, promotes epidemiologic inquiry on older Americans, and organizations such as the American Association for Retired Persons and the Association on Aging also routinely collect information on the over-65 population. In addition, a number of gerontologically focused educational institutions across the nation have centers on aging and conduct aging research.

Health maintenance organizations and corporations that deal with the elderly also have available data sets. Corporate data from assisted living facilities or long-term care are extremely useful as an index of the utilization of different providers and resources for the aged population and, more important, provide critical data for the oldest old, who are routinely under-represented in governmental monitoring because of those initiatives being targeted at the noninstitutionalized (free-living) population in the United States.

Information on the oldest old has been sparse in the past, but due to the increasing numbers of this demographic, new directives have been issued to try to capture as much information as possible on this age group to enhance care and better understand issues of concern for healthcare providers, family, and the oldest old themselves.

Assessment Methodology

A number of methods for assessing the older adult on a large scale, such as with national nutritional

TABLE 12.1	Demographic Characteristics (United States)[a]		
Unadjusted Percentages for the U.S. Population		Male	Female
Percentage over the age of 65 years in the U.S. (2000)		5%	7%
Percentage of persons over the age of 85 in the U.S. (2000)		0.5%	1.0%
Percentage of persons over the age of 85 within the elderly population in the U.S. (2000)		30%	70%
Projected increases in the over-85-year age range among the elderly population in the U.S. by 2010		+1.5%	+3.5%
Rates for persons over the age of 65 in the U.S.		2000	2002
Percentage of older adults with a disability		35%	36%
Percentage of older adults widowed, single		31%	32%
Percentage of older adults with caretaking responsibilities		42%	n/a[b]

[a]U.S. Census. Retrieved December 20, 2005 from www.census.gov
[b]Not yet available from www.census.gov

monitoring systems or in community studies, have been used over the years. Quick screening tools such as the DETERMINE (Disease, Eating poorly, Tooth loss /mouth pain, Economic hardship, Reduced social contact, Multiple medications, Involuntary weight loss or gain, Needs assistance in self care, Elder years > 80) checklist and the Mini Nutritional Assessment have been shown to be useful in large-scale surveillance and in small-scale clinical settings (see http://www.aafp.org and http://www.mna-elderly.com/index.htm to access these screening tools). Both instruments have been shown to be effective for flagging older adults with issues related to nutritional status and health. The Mini Nutritional Assessment in particular has been the subject of recent research as it has been tested in a variety of populations and languages (Gazzotti, Albert, Pepinster, & Petermans, 2000; Beck, Ovensen, & Schroll, 2001).

National Health Objectives

The National Institute on Aging has reported that levels of disability among the older adult population in the United States have been falling since 1982 because of a variety of factors, such as better technology and increased access to health care. However, the National Institute on Aging proposed the following initiatives with regard to national efforts toward bettering the older segment of United States society:

- Sustain decreases in disability, maintaining health and function in older adults.
- Improve strategies for promoting healthy behaviors among the older population, including:
  - Diet
  - Smoking
  - Alcohol abuse
  - Safety
  - Exercise
  - Evaluation of hormone replacement therapy
  - Evaluation of dietary supplements
  - Improved interaction with the healthcare system
  - Reduction in caregiver and family stress
  - Improvement in individual coping with chronic disease

Each area was identified as being critical to maintaining the current decline in morbidity and mortality, despite the increasing numbers of older adults within the population. (http:///www.nia.gov/

initiatives.html). These recommendations to researchers and healthcare professionals were borne out of the epidemiologic evidence collected over the past few decades. In addition, public health campaigns, such as *Healthy People 2010*, have provided general objectives for improvement that target the lay person over the age of 65. Other groups have also targeted the lay older adult, including the American Diabetes Association and the American Cancer Institute, with media campaigns specifically targeting elderly diabetics and cancer survivors.

Aging

Aging Theories

Theories regarding aging include population-based, organ-system-based, and cellular-based theories. Population-based theories involve type I or "rate of living" and type II or the collagen theories of aging. Rate of living theories assume that the time it takes for development and maturity determines how long one lives. Collagen theories state that collagen cross-linking over time results in decreased longevity (Morley, Glick, & Rubenstein, 1995).

Organ system theories involve endocrine, immune, and "pacemaker" errors increasing over time and thus decreasing life span. In endocrine theories, hormonal changes or decrements result in decreased viability of organs and systems. In immune theories, failure of immunocompetence results in aging and death, and the pacemaker of aging theory involves predetermined organ system failure as a result of the body's own life clock ticking down (Morley et al., 1995).

Cellular aging theories have the most experimental evidence to back them. "Wear and tear" theories, as they are sometimes called, state that continuous use coupled with decreases in the division and maturation of new cells causes aging and ultimately death. **Apoptosis** eventually results in decreased numbers of viable cells. Somatic mutation, error catastrophe, free radical, glycation, and alteration of genetic code theories are encompassed in this category. The somatic mutation theory involves mutations that are present in cells that, over time, cause malfunction on a system-wide level, leading to death. Error catastrophe theory states that over time the number of cellular errors increase until a threshold is reached that results in catastrophe and death. The free radical

Apoptosis: Preprogrammed cell death.

theory of aging involves cumulative damage as a result of natural free radical oxidative changes, which over time result in increased antigenicity, protein changes, and oxidative DNA damage.

The sum of these processes results in cellular senescence and organ system failure, ending in death. Glycation theory assumes that posttranslational protein modification by the linking of glucose to lysine residues results in diminished protein functionality, which in turn decreases organ system viability and ends in death. The "alterations in genetic coding theory" proposes that aging is the result of changes in protein synthesis and messenger RNA processing. Chemical alterations in DNA over time, coupled with translational aberrations, are the cause of aging and death (Morley et al., 1995; Rimkus, Melinchok, McEvoy, & Yeager, 2005).

Caloric restriction, with adequate vitamin and mineral nutriture, has been associated with longevity. This is thought to be the result of decreases in oxidative stress, less metabolic free radical generation, and decrements in the abnormal compounds generated as a result of redox damage. The underlying mechanisms have yet to be fully established, but fewer glycation products, less lipid peroxidation, and fewer genetic anomalies with improved genetic expression over time seem to be causal in delayed cellular senescence (Warner, Fernandes, & Wang, 1995; Roth, Ingram, & Lane, 1999).

Determinants

Determinants of successful aging with little disease or disability involve many factors. Dietary considerations across the life span, such as increased intake of fiber, antioxidants, and minerals or caloric restriction, have been correlated with increased longevity and decreases in morbidity. Patterns of intake have also shown relationships to successful aging. Characteristics such as small frequent meals, sitting down with family, having a glass of wine with dinner, and eating until 80% full seem to have beneficial effects over the long term.

Life-style characteristics such as maintenance of a normal body weight, decreased exposure to known carcinogens such as tobacco or heavy metals or better coping mechanisms for stress seem to promote healthy aging. Adequate exercise and sleep are also important. Drug and alcohol use along with life course levels of stress have been shown to have significant impact on cellular senescence.

There are other indirect determinants of successful aging with decreased cellular senescence. Some of these include mental status, mental activity, pet ownership, and social interaction. Sociodemographic characteristics also play a role, such as marital status, level of education, income, race, and ethnicity. Quality of life and perceptions of the quality of life along with spirituality, civic engagement, and coping abilities are moderating influences on the mechanisms involved in healthy longevity. Ultimately, genetic makeup and the propensity toward maintaining cellular protection against environmental influences determine the course of the individual's life span (De Groot, Verheijden, de Henauw, Schroll, & van Staveren, 2004; Bamia, 2005).

Diet

Dietary determinants of successful aging include issues with both macro- and micronutrient intake. Caloric content across the life span, adequate (but not excessive) protein intake with moderate to high bioavailability, and high complex carbohydrate consumption are all associated with decreases in morbidity and mortality (Millward, 2004; Jungjohann, Luhrmann, Bender, Blettner, & Neuhäuser-Berthold, 2005). Decreased total fat intake, with greater proportions of monounsaturates, long chain mega-3 fatty acids, and low trans/saturated fats, are associated with decrements in vascular anomalies and chronic disease with mortality (Hjerkinn et al., 2005). Micronutrient content of the diet across the life span is directly related to disease and indirectly, but ultimately, related to mortality.

Healthy aging has been associated with increased intake of antioxidants, including phytochemicals; selenium (part of glutathione peroxidase); vitamins C, E, and A; the carotenoids; and zinc (as part of metallothionein) (Gonzalez et al., 2004; Chernoff, 2005; Faure, Ducros, Couzy, Favier, & Ferry, 2005) (Figure 12.1). In addition, bone health is improved with increased calcium, vitamin D, vitamin K, adequate magnesium, and lower intakes of phosphorus during the course of the life span (Bischoff-Ferrari et al., 2004; Ryan-Harshman & Aldoori, 2004). Increased dietary potassium and lower levels of sodium are important for blood pressure and vascular health, and the B vitamins are critical for decrements in homocysteine levels (Hamilton & Hamilton, 1997; Demingné, Sabboh, Rémésy, & Meneton, 2004; Gori et al., 2005).

Macronutrients

In older adults, adequate protein intake is essential for the prevention of muscle mass losses, pressure ulcers, and decreased immunocompetence. Sarcopenia in the

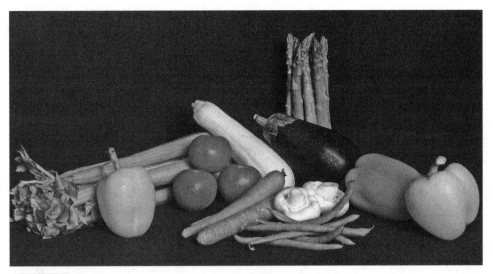

Figure 12.1 Vegtables are an excellent source of fiber, minerals, vitamins, phytochemicals, and organic constituents, all known to be beneficial for health due to a variety of effects, including their antioxidant capabilities. Increased vegetable consumption over the life span is associated with decreased cellular senescence, morbidity, and mortality.

elderly is associated with poor outcome, frailty, and falls. Investigations into the roles of essential amino acids in prevention of the above have shown that adequate protein intake is important to replacement of aging muscle tissue as well as in the maintenance of bone health. In conjunction with weight-bearing exercise, essential amino acids can increase the concentrations of insulin-like growth factor I, which has a permissive effect on bone and muscle cellular repair and, to some extent, replication. It should be noted that protein consumption is related to calcium intake, which mediates the relationships seen between protein intake and bone health (Devine, Dick, Islam, Dhaliwal, & Prince, 2005; Gori et al., 2005).

Another set of variables related to protein adequacy are socioeconomics and institutionalization. Poor and institutionalized elderly have reduced high-quality protein intakes and often have other factors that impact muscle mass, bone health, and wound healing, which cloud direct relationships in the research, such as decreased access to health care, altered mental status, or long-standing chronic disease. The provision of protein supplements to these populations has been shown to be beneficial in decreasing morbidity (Ginty, 2003; Collins, Kershaw, & Brockington, 2005; Milne, Potter, & Avenell, 2005).

Fiber intake in older persons is important for decreasing constipation, which results from enteromuscular changes consistent with aging. Both soluble and insoluble fiber sources are needed to slough abnormal cells from the gut, increase stool quality and frequency, and trap bilious cholesterol, drug metabolites, and car-

cinogens. In addition, fiber sources reduce calories and improve blood glucose level stability (Marlett, McBurney, & Slavin, 2002).

Fiber from whole foods is also rich in micronutrients, but this form of intake is often reduced in older persons, especially in those with poor dentition. Edentulous older persons often cannot chew high-fiber whole foods and avoid them. Poorer older persons may not be able to afford fresh, high-fiber, whole foods, such as produce, which is more expensive. Older persons who have not had dietary patterns consistent with high-fiber foods are reluctant to introduce them in late life and often exclude fruits, vegetables, legumes, and whole grains. Older adults may also have issues with fresh high-fiber foods because of their gas-forming potential. The addition of soluble and insoluble fiber sources to the diet of the older adult should be gradual. The use of bulking agents or fiber supplements may provide an acceptable option, and the untoward effects may be reduced by the addition of a supplemental form of normal gut flora, such as Bifidobacterium or other probiotics (Zunft et al., 2004).

Blood glucose control is important for decreasing glycation products, which according to theory is a contributing factor to senescence. Antioxidants from high-fiber fruits and vegetables are important for controlling free radical damage. Another theory regarding cellular senescence and the decrease in caloric content seen in high-fiber diets is associated with the maintenance of normal body weight, another factor in healthy aging and longevity. In addition, the sloughing of abnormal cells Figure 12.2 with high-fiber intake reduces carcinogenesis and disease and trapping cholesterol by fiber reduces atherosclerotic tendencies, which again is associated with healthier aging.

Cholesterol, trans fats, saturated fats, and total fat intake over the life span have been shown to impact morbidity and mortality in the aged (Anderson, Suchindran, Kritchevsky, & Barrett-Connor, 2004). In terms of overall macronutrient intake, these compounds have been shown to interact with genetic

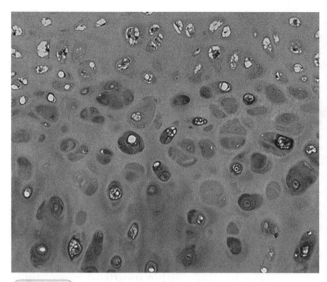

Figure 12.2 Abnormal Cell. Cellular abnormalities increase with age. The etiology of these changes is complex and multifactorial. Several mechanisms are thought to be integral to the disruption of cellular processing and homeostatic capability.

© Phototake/Alamy Image

predisposition to increase vascular adverse events and morbidity more than any other dietary constituent. Inflammatory processes that mediate the effects involve a multitude of eicosanoids, **cytokines**, blood constituents such as platelets, hormones, and other cellular signals. In addition, body weight, energy expenditure, and environmental exposure serve to moderate the progression of disease in the face of increased intake (Okuyama, Ichikawa, Fujii, Ito, & Yamada, 2005). Cellular senescence as a result of increased fat and cholesterol intake may be related to free radical and nitric oxide generation and decrements in cellular repair with continued inflammatory response. Inflammatory markers such as C-reactive protein, sP-selectin, and sICAM-1 decrease with low fat intake over time.

Cytokines: A class of cellular chemical messengers often involved in cascade reactions such as with inflammatory response.

Micronutrients
In terms of micronutrient status, several vitamins and minerals have been linked to healthy aging. The associations between maintenance of normal cellular function and vitamin or mineral status is also moderated by cumulative oxidative stress and inflammatory response. It is common knowledge that antioxidants from fruits, vegetables, and whole grains prevent oxidative damage. Because oxidative stress is related to disease state from atherosclerosis to bone and joint health, investigations into the use of foods versus vitamin and mineral supplementation have been performed (Ganesan, Tekle-

haimanot, Tran, Asuncion, & Norris, 2005; Lichtenstein & Russell, 2005).

Whole fresh foods are preferable to increasing antioxidant capabilities because so many additional compounds are contained within the food in forms that make them potentiate the action of select micronutrients. The ancillary compounds in foods include organic acids, sulfur and nitrogenous compounds that aid in uptake, and activation and utilization of vitamins and minerals, in addition to having their own direct benefits (Boudville & Bruce, 2005).

> **● Learning Point** Nutritional supplementation should be used when intake cannot provide fresh whole foods high in nutrient density (Dawson-Hughes, 2004). For certain fat-soluble vitamins like D and E or minerals such as calcium, there may be benefits of supplementation over whole foods, when dairy or fatty foods are not advisable due to the macronutrient content of the product (Deplas, Debiais, Alcalay, Bontoux, & Thomas, 2004; Nieves, 2005).

The relationships of the B vitamins to indices of cellular senescence have been the focus of recent research. Because homocysteine has been related to oxidative damage and diseases ranging from cardiovascular disease to neurodegenerative diseases of aging, such as Alzheimer's disease, vitamin B12, vitamin B6, and folate have been studied for their impact on disease over the life span (Bottiglieri & Diaz-Arrastia, 2005). Although **neurodegenerative disease** is thought to have a genetic component that makes the individual more susceptible with the appropriate environmental and dietary stimuli, dietary components have been shown to turn on select genes in a wide variety of models (Lewis et al., 2005).

Neurodegenerative disease: Diseases that involve malfunction of the central and peripheral nervous tissue. These are often diseases that progress slowly but insidiously and result in progressive loss of function and eventual mortality. Examples include Alzheimer's and Parkinson disease.

Neurodegenerative diseases, which involve atherosclerotic changes such as vascular dementia, are also linked through the cycle involving methionine conversion, with methylmalonate, homocysteine, and S-adenosyl-methionine intermediates, each playing a role in cellular dysregulation and changes to DNA blueprinting (Quadri et al., 2004). The B vitamins, in their active and unconverted forms, and the pathways involved in the conversion process of methionine, along with the intermediates, are shown in Figure 12.3 through Figure 12.9 .

Homocysteine is also thought to be a modifiable risk factor for neurodegenerative diseases because of its direct neurotoxicity at high levels. Alterations

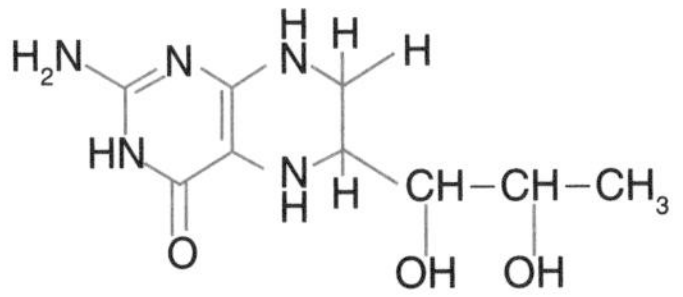

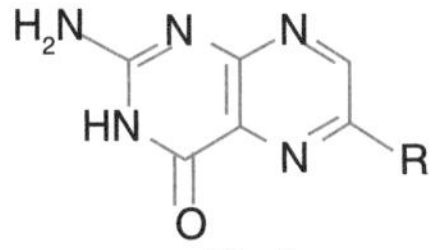

Figure 12.3 Tetrahydrobiopterin and pterin. These compounds are the intermediates in the synthesis of stable, oxidized, and activated tetrahydromethylfolate AKA pteroyl glutamate. What we know as folic acid is actually pterin + p-aminobenzoic acid + three to seven glutamic acids + one or more methyl groups.

Methylation reactions: The process of attaching a methyl group to an existing compound through 1 C transfer by several vitamin/mineral cofactors.

in the **methylation reactions** essential for normal neurotransmitter synthesis are impaired at high levels of homocysteine and its metabolites (Tucker, Qiao, Scott, Rosenberg, & Spiro, 2005). High homocysteine levels are a result of low folate levels, and low folate levels are thought to be endemic in the elderly population in areas where mandatory folate fortification is not practiced (Wolters, Hermann, & Hahn, 2005). Decreased B12 absorption is also common in elderly persons who have atrophic gastritis or some other risk for the reduction of intrinsic factor production from the parietal cells lining the stomach. Older adults are also more vulnerable to B vitamin insufficiency due to dietary choices and medication usage, which potentially interferes with bioavailability (Ravaglia et al., 2005). Cellular uptake and conversion of folates and cyanocobalamin may also be diminished as a function of aging. Receptor function and transporter capabilities naturally decline with aging. **Transcobalamin** synthesis and IF-complex reception decline, and conversion enzymes for methyl-tetrahydrofolate are diminished.

Transcobalamin: Transport protein classes for cyanocobalamin in blood and tissues.

Supplementation with B vitamins or the addition of B vitamins to foods as with fortification may be an option for elderly persons (Dhonukshe-Rutten et al., 2005). In the absence of severe decrements in transport and absorption, oral supplementation can raise levels of serum B vitamins in an older adult, thus decreasing **hyperhomocystinemia**. Additional benefits of increasing the vitamin B12, folate, and pyridoxine vita-

Hyperhomocystinemia: Elevated blood levels of homocysteine, the sulfur-containing amino acid metabolite.

min content of foods include decreasing other diseases for which the elderly are more susceptible, such as pernicious anemia, decrements in immune function, and depressive disorders. These B vitamins are essential to cellular division and successful replication (Pfeiffer, Caudill, Gunter, Osterloh, & Sampson, 2005). Rapidly dividing cells, such as the red and white blood cells, are impacted by the insufficiency, hence the benefit from additional oral intake (Woodman, Ferrucci, & Guralnik, 2005).

In regard to depressive symptoms, the B vitamins (folate in particular) are related to the ability to synthesize de novo methionine and S-adenosylmethionine (SAM-e). SAM-e is a universal methyl donor. Methylation reactions are essential for the synthesis of neurotransmitters such as serotonin in the brain and throughout the body. Serotonin receptors are not exclusive to the brain, and there are colonies of serotonin receptors throughout every organ system in the body. Serotonin is a chemical mediator for many homeostatic processes, including but not limited to mood. SAM-e has been shown to have potential as an antidepressant. Folate is necessary for SAM-e participation in methylation reactions, and elevated SAM-e production can be achieved through supplementation of folate in older adults (Ramos, Allen, Haan, Green, & Miller, 2004).

Dietary intake and functional B vitamin status is thus linked to cellular senescence through a number of pathways. The impact of hyperhomocystinemia on increasing oxidative stressors, with concomitant inflammatory response, is a modifiable risk factor for aging and cellular pathology. B vitamins are essential to the regulation of homocysteine. Therefore B vitamin status is thought to be of importance to healthy aging.

Dietary Patterns

Dietary patterns are important to aging processes and cellular senescence, albeit indirectly. Differences have been investigated in the relationship between consumption patterns and inflammatory response in older persons, and the indirect relationships seem to have an effect on the progression of cellular dysregulation and ultimately disease. This can be seen in the advent of type 2 diabetes, where patterns of intake high in refined sugars and processed foods have been tied to inflammatory markers. Intake of high levels of sugared soft drinks, refined grains, diet drinks, lunch meat, and processed foods with low intake of vegetables is thought to increase CRP (C-Reactive

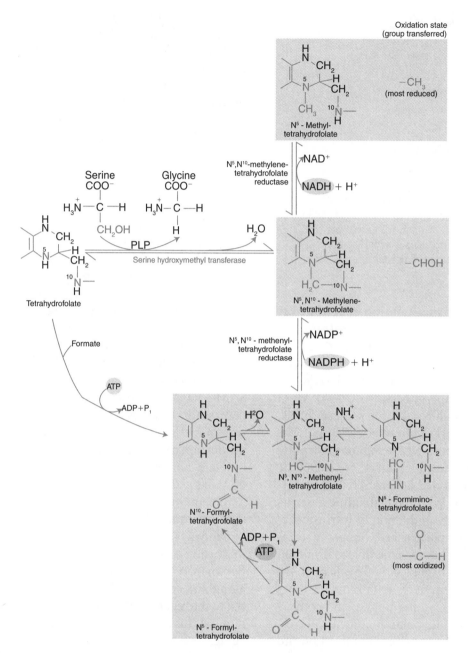

Figure 12.4 Activated folic acid. The attaching of methyl groups onto the pteroylglutamate at various positions. All methylated intermediates are considered "folate." "Folate" is actually a group of many different compounds with varied physiologic abilities and functions.

Tumor necrosis factor-alpha: An indicator of inflammatory response and a mediator of several cascade mechanisms involved in immune function and homeostasis.

Protein), interleukin-6, and **tumor necrosis factor-alpha** (Schulze et al., 2005).

A Westernized dietary pattern of highly processed, high-fat foods has also been linked to morbidity through inflammatory processes and oxidative stress. Acculturation and the transition of other peoples to this consumption pattern has resulted in an increase of cellular changes and chronic diseases of aging as they move away from traditional dietary patterns of fresh whole foods (Iso, Date, Noda, Yoshimura, & Tamakoshi, 2005). Increases in patterns of consumption with fish as the dietary protein staple or of omega-3 oils from other sources have been shown to modify inflammation through the eicosanoids and their mediating influences on the inflammatory cascade (Payet et al., 2004). This decrement in inflammation over time with omega-3 fatty acid intake is directly related to cellular senescence through prolonged accumulation of oxidative stressors.

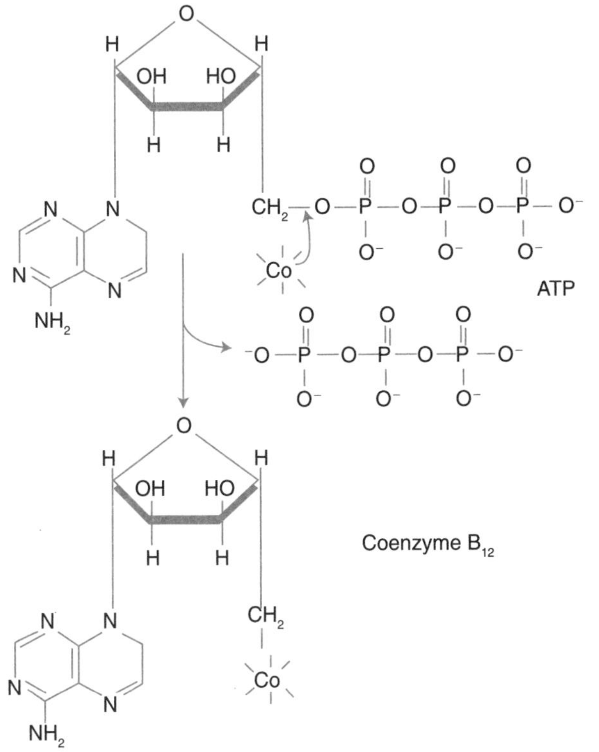

Figure 12.5 Vitamin B$_{12}$. Cyanocobalamin, or vitamin B$_{12}$, is the only vitamin cofactor with a cobalt in the center. The vitamin shown here is stable after insertion and breaking of the high-energy phosphate bonds.

Increased low-fat dairy consumption has also been shown to be a healthful dietary pattern. Increased levels of several regulatory nutrients, not just calcium and vitamin D, may be obtained from dairy foods (McCabe et al., 2004). Encouraging older adults to consume low-fat dairy products as part of an overall dietary pattern is important. A caveat is that lactose intolerance increases with age, and arrangements must be made for use of lactose-free products, many of which are unfamiliar to older adults and may be rejected because of novelty or taste differences.

Immune function declines also occur in old age and are mediated by nutritional status. Increased infection results in increased oxidative stress. Cellular damage occurs with decrements in the immune system's ability to ward off pathologic changes such as in cancer or autoimmune disease.

● **Learning Point**

Chemokines: A class of chemical messengers that constitute cellular signals which respond to very specific levels of a particular compound in a defined area of tissue.

Immunity and host defense are directly related to the ability to produce white blood cells, **chemokines,** and other cellular components; which ultimately depend on minerals such as iron and zinc and vitamins such as folate, in addition to other micro- and macronutrients.

Iron deficiency anemia in older adults may be due to other factors, such as the anemia of chronic disease, blood loss, or impaired absorption due to **achlorhydria.** However, regardless of the etiology, more iron is needed for red blood cell synthesis and tissue oxygenation, and poor iron status due to increased needs ultimately results in impaired immunity. Iron deficiency results in decreases in cell-mediated immune function, with decrements in T-cell proliferation and T-lymphocyte function (Ahluwalia, Sun, Krause, Mastro, & Handte, 2004).

Achlorhydria: Absence or decrement in the level of hydrochloric acid due to decreased production of the parietal cells in the fundus of the stomach.

Phagocytosis and **bacteriostatic** capabilities are diminished. Inflammatory response cytokines increase with poor iron status. It should also be noted that iron in and of itself is a potent **pro-oxidant** and must be bonded to a carrier or incorporated into a compound such as hemoglobin, because it cannot travel freely without inducing free radical damage. Therefore carrier proteins and compounds such as myoglobin and hemoglobin must be synthesized correctly and in adequate amounts. Protein must be adequate to synthesize these components, and all cofactors for cellular differentiation and maturation must also be available in addition to the iron.

Phagocytosis: The ability to engulf foreign bodies by white blood cells.

Bacteriostatic: The ability of immune cells to incapacitate bacterial invaders through engulfing, dissolution, or direct toxicity.

Pro-oxidant: A compound that normally has the potential to act as a free radical in its present oxidative state.

Similarly for zinc, older adults are more susceptible to poorer zinc status. Zinc-containing foods are more expensive and may be prohibitive for older adults in lower socioeconomic strata. Zinc needs may be elevated in older adults suffering from comorbid conditions. Zinc malabsorption may take place because of gastrointestinal changes associated with aging, or deficiencies may result from dietary choices that are low in zinc. Metallothionein, the transporter for zinc, must be synthesized at optimal levels, which requires adequate protein, kilocalories, and other micronutrients. Because zinc is so tightly controlled in human serum through negative feedback homeostasis, it is often difficult to determine if older adults are deficient. Tests for zinc lack sensitivity and **specificity.** Zinc is inherently involved in the genetic up-regulation of immune component synthesis. Because zinc is so closely tied to immune function, there are rapid changes in cellular components such as lymphocytes and inflammatory factors such as interleukin-2 and

Specificity: The ability to actually measure the component which is of interest.

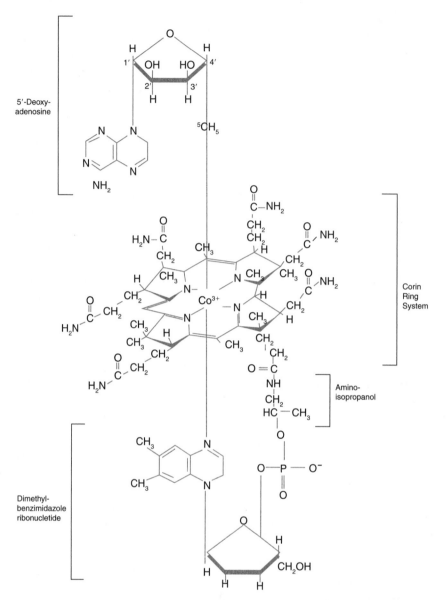

Coenzyme B12

Figure 12.6 Vitamin B_{12} in coenzyme form. Coenzyme B_{12} participates in numerous functions on a cellular level. Decreased levels due to impaired absorption or long-term vegan vegetarianism result in pernicious anemia, which may go undetected until peripheral neuropathy is seen in the older adult.

interleukin-6 (Andree et al., 2004). Representations of red and white cell types are shown in Figure 12.10 through Figure 12.14.

Dietary intake of vitamins such as folate and vitamin C and adequacy of macronutrient intake are also essential to normal immune function. Because immunity is tied to cellular senescence through inflammatory responses, oxidative stressors, and glycation products, protein, total kilocalories, carbohydrates, and vitamins such as folate and C are essential to healthy **normative** aging. Provision of adequate micro- and macronutrients to older adults has been shown to increase immune response, regardless of form. Dietary intake of nutrient-dense whole foods is always preferable, but supplementation with enriched products also produces desirable increases in immune function (Wouters-Wesseling et al., 2005).

Normative: Based on a normal distribution of a population, representing the "average" or normal individual within a given set of parameters.

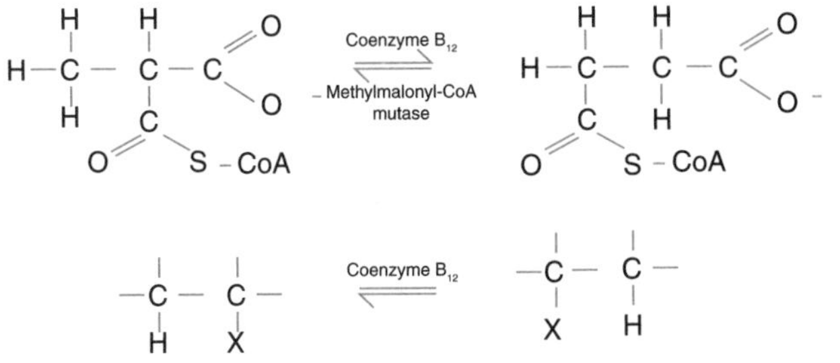

Figure 12.7 B$_{12}$ involvement in methylmalonic acid conversion. Cyanocobalamin plays a major role in the conversion of methylmalonic acid (MMA). MMA is an intermediary in the reactions involving methione, SAM-e, and homocysteine, a potent oxidant and a risk factor for cardiovascular disease and general inflammation.

Nutritional status impacts morbidity and mortality in older adults. Mediating factors for cellular senescence and overall homeostasis include dietary pattern, macro- and micronutrient intake and impact on cumulative oxidative stressors, increases in glycation, and damage induced by free radical production over time. Successful aging with improved long-term outcome is inherently attributable to macro- and micronutrient availability (Donini et al., 2004).

Life-Style

Life-style characteristics of an individual can have a marked impact on cellular senescence, when interacting with genetic predisposition. Many life-style attributes have been investigated in this regard:

- Physical activity
- **Body habitus**
- Environmental contaminant exposure
- Alcohol use
- Methylxanthine use
- Cigarette smoking
- Oral health
- Pet ownership
- Reproductive hormone levels
- Marital status
- Mental status
- Mental activity
- Socioeconomics
- Education
- Social support

Body habitus: The size and shape of the body; may also include perceptions of the size and shape of the body.

This noncomprehensive listing of variables all mediate and/or moderate successful aging. The interactions that occur are extremely complex, and it is

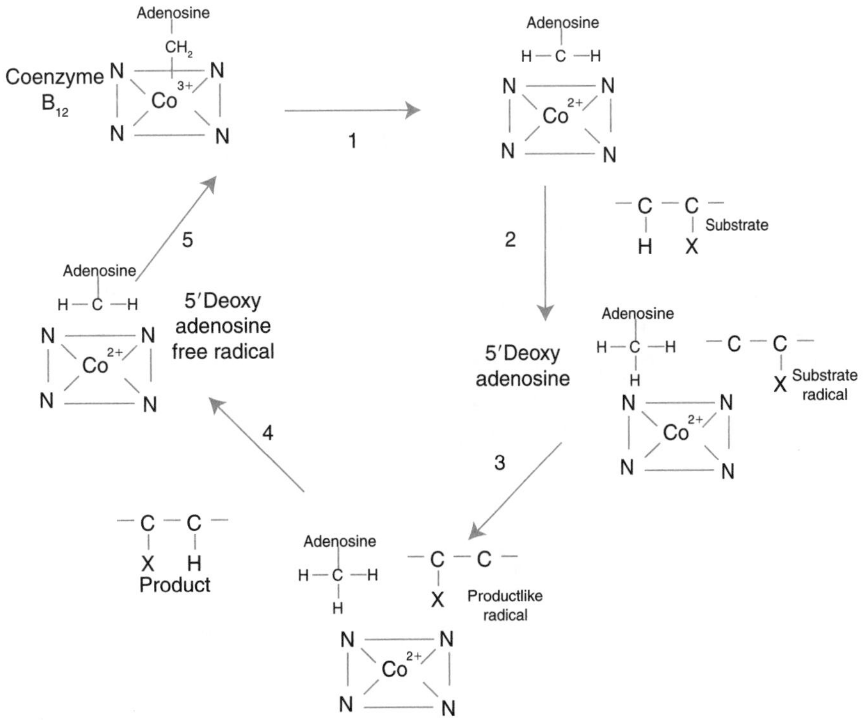

Figure 12.8 Cyanocobalamin coenzyme cycle. The coenzyme cycle for Vitamin B$_{12}$ produces intermediates that act as free radicals and produce oxidative stress when in contact with strong reducing agents. Cyanocobalamin is a nutrient primarily obtained from animal products or bacteria, yeast, or other organisms, which is stored in large quantities over long periods of time in liver tissue.

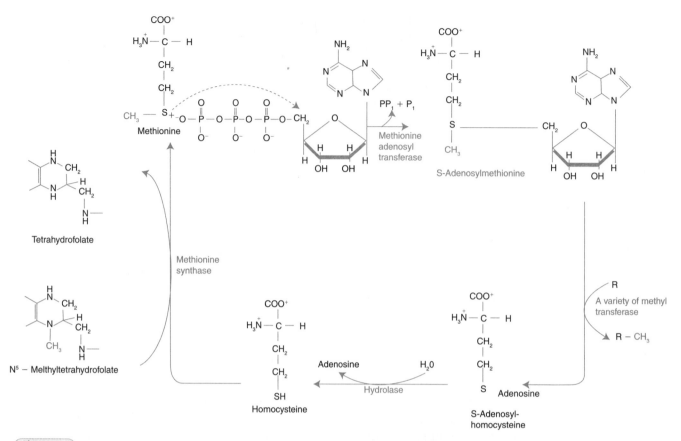

Figure 12.9 Methionine SAM-e cycle. The interconversion of methionine and S-adenosylmethionine with homocysteine is outlined. Activated coenzyme B_{12} is essential in this process. Note the involvement of N-methyl-tetrahydrofolate in the process as well.

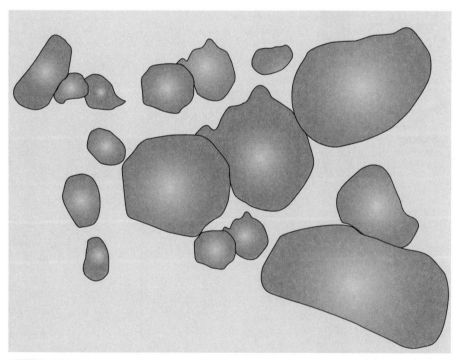

Figure 12.10 Megaloblastic cell. Immature red blood cells are often associated with nutritional deficiency and anemia. This is especially deleterious for an older person, who may be experiencing age-related declines in absorption and utilization of micronutrients.

extremely difficult to assess the level of impact for any one of these factors alone. Therefore research efforts have opted to use these variables as a means of broadly classifying risk for morbidity and mortality (Brach, Simonsick, Kritchevsky, Yaffe, & Newman, 2004). The more risk factors per individual, the greater the cumulative effects in terms of cellular damage through oxidative stress, glycation, and free radical production.

Physical Activity

Physical activity over the life span is important to healthy aging, preventing functional decline. Improvements in balance, decrements in the sarcopenia of old age, and better mood and sleep are all important to overall health in the aged. It should be

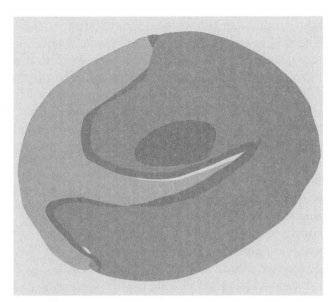

Figure 12.11 Red blood cells. Normal red blood cells are enucleated and have a life span of approximately 3 to 4 months. Their normal development requires several macronutrients, including vitamins A, K, and E; all the B vitamins; and iron, copper, and zinc. Anemia is common in older adults because of a variety of factors, including decreased micronutrient intake, absorption, distribution, and utilization.

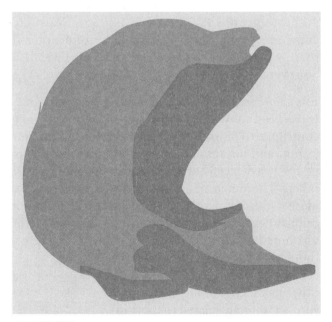

Figure 12.12 Abnormal red blood cells. Abnormal red blood cell production, activation, and destruction are important contributors as well as indices of disease. There are several diseases or circumstances in which abnormalities in erythropoiesis are present, besides nutritional deficiency. Some of these include autoimmune disease, environmental contaminant exposure with lead or mercury, or marrow failure as in cancer or prolonged sepsis.

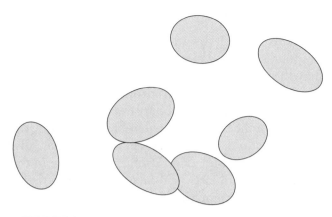

Figure 12.13 Normocytic cell. Normal cell size and shape as well as full maturation of the cell with normal functional capabilities are important tools in the evaluation of an older adult. Nutritional anemias (as well as a variety of other factors) influence cell size, shape, and activity.

noted that increased physical activity is associated with increased oxidative stress, normally a result of oxygen utilization in aerobic metabolism. However, physical activity is also associated with improved ability to combat the increases in free radical production, and sustained lifelong activity improves counterregulation of oxidative cellular damage. Physical activity should be encouraged throughout the life span, thus improving appetite, enhancing weight control, decreasing visceral adiposity, and improving immune responsivity and glycemic control (Nied & Franklin, 2002; Lee et al., 2004).

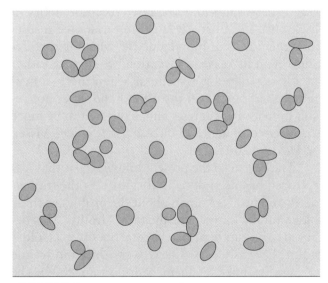

Figure 12.14 Cell size. Microcytic cells can be a result of nutritional anemias in the older adult but must be differentiated from other causes for interrupted maturation of blood cells, such as from medications, carcinogenesis, or heavy metal exposure.

Body Habitus

Visceral adiposity is an extremely strong risk factor for disease, and metabolic syndrome associations have been well studied (Wannamethee, Shaper, Morris, & Whincup, 2005). Android (apple shape) versus gynoid (pear shape) obesity has been investigated in terms of the cellular contributions this adipose tissue makes to disease over time. *Body habitus*, displaying an "apple" deposition, plays a role in the dysregulation of fatty acid flux from adipocytes located in and around the visceral organs that are fed by portal circulation. Increased free fatty acid flux, with resultant increases in lipoprotein transport, increased synthesis of cholesterol, and increased redistribution of triglycerides in portal circulation, is thought to increase inflammatory response (Farin, Addasi, & Reaven, 2006). This has been shown through increased levels of mitochondrial leakage of superoxides and higher levels of serum isoprostanes, indicative of increased oxidative stress. Oxidation products and the deposition of oxidized low-density lipoprotein cholesterol into vessel endothelia dysregulate many of the ancillary feedback mechanisms for homeostatic control. One of these includes insulin responsivity (Weinbrenner et al., 2006).

Insulin resistance increases over time due to the increased levels of macronutrients in blood and alterations of the fluidity of membranes on cells that hold the receptors for insulin, among others (Jaques, Moeller, & Hankinson, 2003). Insertion of saturated fats into the membrane lipid bilayer results in stiffness and decreased receptor ability to lock onto its substrate. Insulin resistance results in higher levels of blood glucose, which in turn results in an increase in glycation products, another factor associated with cellular senescence. Gluteal femoral adiposity, on the other hand, does not result in the same changes and is thought to be more "protective" in terms of disease risks (Snijder, Visser, & Dekker, 2005).

The caveat to the present knowledge is that less research has been done in this area on the frail elderly and little is known about the profiles of these older adults. In the past, the term "frailty" was believed to be antithetical to visceral obesity in an older adult, because frail elderly were thin and fragile (Kennedy, Chokkalingham, & Srinivasan, 2004). The terminology is slowly changing to include older persons who may be obese but are still fragile (Gause-Nilsson & Dey, 2005).

A factor that determines healthy aging is body habitus. Efforts to reduce visceral obesity in older adults, both men and women, should be undertaken. The risk for increased visceral adipose accumulation increases postmenopause for women, such that it mirrors the risk for men at the same age (Chen et al., 2005). Estrogen production in women serves to increase gluteal femoral deposition over android deposition, thus protecting women to some extent from swift development of metabolic syndrome (syndrome X) in the absence of other risk. It should be noted that BMI does not account for body habitus, and **skin fold thickness measures** have not been shown to be effective for assessing visceral adiposity (Snijder, Visser, & Dekker, 2002). These measures are very widely used despite these known issues, because they are easy, inexpensive, and historical.

Skinfold thickness measures: Measurements done with the use of calipers; historically used and standardized for the measurement of subcutaneous adiposity from a variety of target points, such as the triceps area, the scapula, and the waist.

There are population standards for these measures, so practitioners can evaluate their patients against known cut-off points. Pathologic processes stemming from visceral deposition result in increased cellular senescence, morbidity, and ultimately mortality. Therefore assessment of abdominal stores should be routine for older persons. Waist circumference data are now being standardized for a variety of age, sex, and race groups (Snijder et al., 2005). Waist circumference may be a better predictor of health risk than waist-to-hip ratio in older persons (Welch & Somwers, 2000).

Environmental Contaminant Exposure

It has been shown that environmental contaminants contribute to morbidity through carcinogenesis, mutation, and inflammation. Known risks include asbestos, heavy metals, and ambient air pollution, among others. The mutagenesis, metabolic dysregulation, oxidative stress, and inflammation lead to alterations in cellular development, function, and homeostasis. Environmental contaminant exposure is therefore thought to be a **permissive effect** of cellular senescence. Coupled with other risk factors, long-term exposure is indirectly related to morbidity, aging, and cellular senescence (Pope et al., 2004).

Permissive effect: Factors that aid in the pathologic effect of another factor or set of antecedents.

Alcohol Use

Alcohol intake is highly controversial with respect to morbidity, mortality, and aging in general. Differences in drinking patterns and the type of alcohol consumption have varied risks associated with them. Those risks are significantly different between races, gender, and age and interact with life-style issues across the board. An example is a person who drinks one glass of red wine with dinner several nights per week for many years versus a person who engages in **binge drinking** of distilled spirits late in life as a result of depression or loss. The former is considered a healthy behavior; the latter is unhealthy and associated with morbidity. The interactions between alcohol intakes at a variety of levels with diet, exercise, and other issues are extremely complex. Because older adults are at risk for falls, take many different medications, and already suffer from a variety of conditions, it is best to recommend that alcohol intake be avoided in advanced age.

> **Binge drinking:** The consumption of five or more standardized ethanol equivalents in one sitting. A standardized ethanol equivalent is 12 ounces of beer, 4 ounces of wine, or 1.5 ounces of distilled spirits.

Ethanol is broken down in a healthy liver to a variety of metabolites all with known oxidative properties. Liver function declines in advanced age, and the metabolites such as acetaldehyde are thought to take more time for disposal. The use of the dehydrogenases, catalase, and the MEOSAQ2 systems for ethanol catabolism detract from these enzymes' abilities to deal with other reactions essential for drug disposition, nutrient activation, and toxin removal. Increased levels of circulating ethanol, acetaldehyde, and other intermediates (Figure 12.15) are known to induce oxidative stress (Lieber, 1992).

Methylxanthine Use

Methylxanthines such as theobromine, theophylline, and caffeine are consumed in increased amounts over the life span. These compounds are found in coffee, tea, chocolate, and cocoa as well as in over-the-counter preparations such as pain relievers and cold remedies. Methylxanthines alter neurotransmission and, ultimately, vascular response. They are inhibitors of adenosine reception and permissive for sympathetic nervous system firing. They require catabolism, and the intermediates are pro-oxidants (Shils, 2005). These compounds profoundly affect hydration and water homeostasis. They are diuretics and increase urinary calcium losses, ultimately affecting bone density in older women in particular (Shils, 2005). Methylxanthines also interact with a variety of medications used by older adults. There have been concerns regarding interactions with prescribed diuretics for blood pressure control, **sympathomimetic** drugs used to treat neurodegenerative conditions, and drugs that influence calcium uptake and disposition (Watson, 2001).

> **Sympathomimetic:** Having the effect of upping sympathetic response, mimicking sympathetic response or acting synergistically with sympathetic response.

Cigarette Smoking

Cigarettes, chewing tobacco, and even pipe smoking are all considered deleterious to health over the long term. Known carcinogens are present in these preparations and interact with a variety of other factors to influence cellular senescence, morbidity, and mortality. Increased pro-oxidant status plus effects of contaminants contained in tobacco (such as cadmium) of smokers requires the diversion of available antioxidant mechanisms toward interruption of the pathologic changes induced by tobacco products (Chen, Pu, & Lin, 2001). Even with adequate antioxidant capabilities, the number of oxidative events eventually surpasses response, and carcinogenic and inflammatory processes cause cellular alteration with continued tobacco use. Over time, an increase in a variety of disease states can be seen in tobacco users. Cancer, cardiovascular disease, stroke, and osteoporosis are significantly correlated with tobacco product usage; extent, duration, and type of usage should always be assessed in the older adult (Kato, Toniolo, Zeleniuch-Jacquotte, Shore, & Koenig, 2000). Other variables impact these tobacco effects in a **synergistic** manner; thus poor diet quality, lack of exercise, body habitus, and heavy drinking elevate risk for morbidity. These variables are often seen clustered in an individual, creating a profile that is very strongly correlated with risk. Those with less education, lower economic status, and high stress often exhibit this variable profile (Burke et al., 2001).

> **Synergistic:** The outcome of two influential factors is greater than the sum of each alone (such as $1 + 1 = 3\times$ the effect).

Oral Health

Oral health is important for being able to consume foods and provide adequate nutriture. Nutritionally

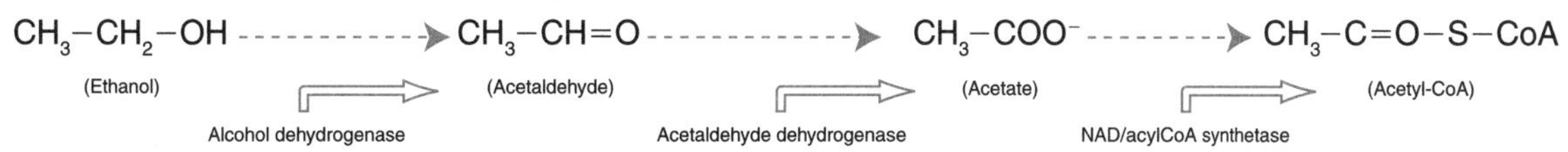

$$CH_3-CH_2-OH \dashrightarrow CH_3-CH=O \dashrightarrow CH_3-COO^- \dashrightarrow CH_3-C=O-S-CoA$$

| (Ethanol) | (Acetaldehyde) | (Acetate) | (Acetyl-CoA) |

Alcohol dehydrogenase   Acetaldehyde dehydrogenase   NAD/acylCoA synthetase

Figure 12.15 Induced oxidative stress.

dense foods such as fruits and vegetables are not consumed in adequate amounts by persons with dentition problems or periodontal disease. Decreased salivation, ill-fitting dentures, and mouth sores or pain are just some of the factors involved in poor nutritional status due to decrements in oral intake. In addition to the lack of antioxidants, vitamins, minerals, and proteins are not adequately consumed; these include the relationship between oral health and systemic inflammatory response (Avcu et al., 2005). The oral cavity is home to many different species of bacteria.

> **● Learning Point** During aging, the bacteriostatic potential of saliva is decreased, the amount of saliva produced declines, and the ability to perform oral hygiene tasks declines (Mojon, Budtz-Jorgensen, & Henri, 1999). Increased ingestion of bacteria, aspiration of foreign antigens, and oral infections that can spread systemically are increased over the life span.

Increases in the chemokine response are associated with increased oxidative effects and inflammatory cascades. All cause mortality rises with poor oral health, although much research has focused on heightened vascular infiltration and plaque formation with cardiovascular disease (Nakashini, Fukada, Takatorige, & Tatara, 2005).

Pet Ownership

Evidence of the positive effects of pet ownership on health have been documented with respect to lowering of blood pressure, decreased risk of cardiovascular disease, decreased depression and loneliness, and overall desensitization to antigens with decreases in immune and inflammatory response. Community-dwelling older adults may also see a significant impact of pets, especially dog ownership, in terms of heightened social interaction, increased physical activity, and indirectly toward better nutritional status Figure 12.16 (McNicholas et al., 2005). Alternatively, studies on cohorts of persons in specific geographic areas have found anecdotal support for these findings but no statistically significant evidence (Parslow, Jorm, Christensen, Rodgers, & Jacomb, 2005). Three potential relationships exist to explain the benefits of pet ownership on health in older people:

1. Pet ownership is associated with specific personality traits, age, and economic status, and it is these associated traits that mediate the positive effects of pet ownership on human health.
2. Pet ownership enhances social interactions and leads to decreased social isolation, thus providing an indirect mechanism for increased health.

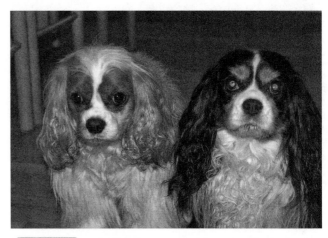

Figure 12.16 Benefits of pet ownership. Pet ownership, especially dog ownership, may have mediating effects on disease and cellular senescence. Walking a dog increases social interaction and physical activity among older peopole, which is shown to benefit overall health.

Courtesy of Judith Sharlin

3. Pet ownership itself reduces stress, increases physical activity, and changes levels of hormones involved in the inflammatory process Figure 12.17. These direct effects may also interact with the indirect effects previously outlined.

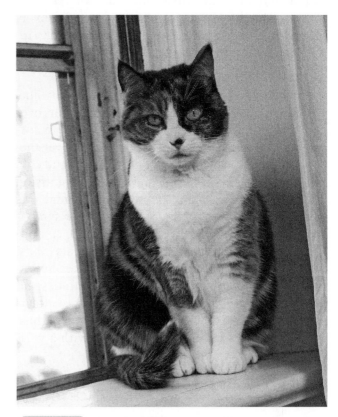

Figure 12.17 Pet Ownership. Pet ownership may offer more than companionship to an elderly person living alone. Pets may alleviate depression, decrease inflammatory processes, and elevate nutritional intake.

Pet ownership and its effects on overall health may require additional research to statistically obviate findings, but it should not be overlooked as a contributing factor to healthy aging.

Reproductive Hormone Levels

Declines in circulating sex steroids are known to alter inflammatory mediators such as cytokines and acute phase proteins. Several inflammatory mediators, including tumor necrosis factor-alpha, interleukin-6, and interleukin-8, are modulated by sex steroids. Aging and its declines in sex steroid production may indirectly influence cellular senescence via increased oxidative stress. In addition, the protective effects of sex steroid hormones have long been documented in terms of bone health for women, with postmenopausal women showing increased bone density losses. It has also been shown that the sex steroids in premenopausal women are protective for coronary artery disease, which can be seen in numerous surveys that have corrected for other variables known to influence risk (Krabbe, Pederson, & Brüünsgaard, 2004).

Hormone replacement therapy has become increasingly widespread among postmenopausal women, and it is also thought that gluteal femoral adiposity is favored in these women and visceral adiposity is not. This may be a mediating relationship in the hypothesis that estrogen and other female sex steroids reduce oxidative risk in older women.

Age-related inflammatory cytokine increases may have multiple etiologies and may interact with a number of other compounds through a variety of mechanisms. The upshot is that inflammation increases morbidity and mortality in older adults through partial mediation by declines in the sex steroid hormones (Brüünsgaard & Pedersen, 2003).

Marital Status

Marital status is thought to have a moderating influence on healthy aging, especially in older men. Some of the reasons may involve decreased social isolation; spousal aid in procuring foods, cooking, and serving meals; or increased caregiving in general (Schone & Weinick, 1998). Widowhood is associated with increased morbidity and mortality in both older men and women and is associated with greater disability (Hokby, Reimers, & Laflamme, 2003; Iwashyna & Christakis, 2003). Nutritional status among older men is also associated with marital status, with unmarried or widowed men having poorer intakes and living alone without caregiver support being associated with poorer dietary intake in both genders (Larrieu et al., 2004).

Mental Status

Depression, declines in cognitive function, and neurodegenerative disease have profound effects on the nutritional status of the older adult (Salerno-Kennedy & Cashmanl, 2005). These conditions also impact morbidity, mortality, and cellular senescence, although the exact mechanisms are not fully understood (Robertson & Montagnini, 2004). There are probably a number of factors that are moderators of this effect, including decreased physical activity, increased stress hormone production, and alterations in neurotransmission leading to metabolic dysregulation, among others (Yaffe et al., 1999; Loucks, Berkamn, Gruenewald, & Seeman, 2005). Loneliness, social isolation, and depression can result in poor dietary intake, frank anorexia, self-neglect, and debilitation in an older person (Abrams, Lachs, McAvay, Keohane, & Bruce, 2002; Ferry, Sidobre, Lambertin, & Barberger-Gateau, 2005).

Mental Activity

Mental activity is thought to delay the progression of age-related cognitive declines and improve mood. The benefits of "psychological well-being" on morbidity and mortality have been documented in the elderly, but the exact mechanisms are not yet fully understood (Depp & Jeste, 2006). The role of mental activity in delaying cellular senescence is thought to involve the effects of nonspecific immune and inflammatory factors, which decline with improved mood, increased physical activity, more social integration, and better nutritional and life-style characteristics (Fortes et al., 2003). Having multiple roles, motivation, "personal projects," and varied activities and having one's basic needs met have been shown to impact aging, disability, disease, and mortality (Adelman, 1994; Herzog, Regula, Markus, & Holmberg, 1998; Powell, Moss, & Winter, 2002; Blazer & Sachs-Ericsson, 2005).

Socioeconomics

Socioeconomics impacts nutritional status and overall health, especially in the aged. Lack of access to health care, less money available to purchase foods, and fewer resources to procure, prepare, and consume nutritious foods are all consequences. The elderly make up some of the poorest poor, with increasing costs for medications and fixed incomes dedicated to paying for housing and other basic needs (U.S. Department of Health and Human Services, 2003). Declines in nutrient-dense food intake among the elderly result in deficiencies in calcium, iron, zinc, vitamin B12, and vitamin E. Foods high in these particular micronutrients are also more expensive and are often protein sources as well (Drewnowski & Schultz, 2001). Socioeconomic hardship is associated with poorer outcome in terms of nutritional status, morbidity, and mortality.

Education

Education may be a surrogate for socioeconomic standing or may in and of itself be related to general health and nutritional status. Increased education is associated with more successful aging, perhaps through more informed dietary choices and life-style characteristics, better access to health care, or increased mental activity. Less-educated minority persons have been shown to have increased risks for nutritional deficiency as well as poorer overall health. Increased educational attainment is also associated with increased social and psychological resources, which may also mediate the relationships (Ross & Mirowsky, 1999).

Social Support

Social support and networks of friends, relatives, community resources, and religious organizations are associated with improved health and decreased disability, morbidity, and mortality among the elderly. This may be related to the provision of care by others, increased mental activity, healthier lifestyle, more physical activity, and less social isolation. Improved nutritional status with an extended network is also probable, with more resources for the procurement and provision of nutritious foods. In addition, place within a social hierarchy may also provide benefit, just by virtue of increased resources available (Lavis, McLeod, Mustard, & Stoddard, 2003). In older adults there are benefits to increased social networks and support on mental status, nutritional status, functional status, and overall successful aging (Koukouli, Vlachonikolis, & Philalithis, 2002; Yeh & Liu, 2003; Kirby, Coleman, & Daley, 2004).

Disease

Older adults with multiple conditions often require continuous care. Whether acute or chronic, comorbidity in the aged presents challenges in terms of health care costs and availability of facilities and staffing. The processes involved in cellular senescence along with overt disease often result in the need for hospitalization, institutionalization, or prolonged rehabilitation, because the older person does not have the recuperative capacity of a younger adult.

Malnutrition is correlated with institutionalization, hospitalization, and rehabilitative care. Poor nutritional status is a major risk factor for complications and delayed recovery. Unintentional weight loss, disease-related malnutrition, and depression-related anorexia rates are estimated to be up to 45% for older adults in the acute or subacute care setting (Brantervik, Jacobsson, Grimby, Wallén, & Bosaeus, 2005). Falls and functional decline with hospitalization often result in further complications, including sarcopenia, and constitute the sixth leading cause of death in persons over 65 years of age. This is due in part to malnutrition, reduced physical activity, reduction in sex hormone levels, and impairment in growth and insulin-like growth hormones (Borst, 2004).

Hospitalized elderly have increased rates of **nosocomial** infections with malnutrition and decrements in immune function consistent with aging. Inflammation results in hypermetabolic state, which increases needs while intakes remain marginal. Length of hospitalization worsens these effects, and the outcomes are generally poorer with longer duration of stay (Kyle, Genton, & Pichard, 2005). Generally, the type of institution also plays a role in the declines experienced by the ailing older adult. Larger institutions and/or institutions with more resources tend to offer more comprehensive care and have improved or cutting-edge practices that decrease the level of the malnutrition and improve the outcome of elderly patients.

Nosocomial: Hospital-acquired infection, usually with an antibiotic-resistant strain of organism.

Skilled nursing facilities also differ in the amount of resources and staff provided to ill elderly residents. Recent advances in low-cost formulations that are high in protein, supplemented with vitamins and minerals, and easily digested have made it easier and more feasible to deal with nutritional support in this population; however, these advances do not address the fundamental problem of poor oral feeding and the quality of life issues regarding eating of pleasurable foods (Levinson, Dwolatzky, Epstein, Adler, & Epstein, 2005). Holistic treatment of the issues regarding hospitalized or institutionalized frail older adults is essential, and clinical outcome in terms of morbidity and mortality should not be the only endpoints. Quality of life should be considered and is comprises health and physical functioning and social and emotional functioning, both measured and perceived (Keller, 2004).

Hospitalization or institutionalization of the frail older person results in decrements in nutritional status just by virtue of changes to the eating environment. Institutional surroundings, lack of attention to the appearance, or preparation of foods impacts intake and dietary choices (Gibbons & Henry, 2005). Several key macro- and micronutrients are affected, such as vitamin D, zinc, calcium, and protein (Meydani, 2001; Pepersack et al., 2001). In the case of vitamin D, less exposure to sunlight with no time spent outdoors complicates vitamin D and calcium nutriture in the geriatric patient (Lyman, 2005). Smaller macro- and micronutrient enriched meals, properly prepared and nicely presented, may aid in improving nutritional status and preventing further debilitation among the institutionalized elderly (Kannus, Uusi-Rasi, Palvanen, & Parkkari, 2005; Lorefält, Wissing, & Unosson, 2005).

Common problems in comorbid hospitalized or institutionalized elderly include aspiration, infection due to aspiration or nosocomial acquisition, and pressure ulcers (Kikawada, Iwamoto, & Takasaki, 2005). All are inherently tied to nutriture and to increases in inflammatory response and cellular senescence. It is extremely difficult to treat these conditions, and they often result in further debilitation and ultimately in increased mortality (Mathus-Vliegen, 2004; Loeb & High, 2005). Several strategies have been used to augment treatment in the compromised older adult in these environments, including nutritional support with added select amino acids, such as glutamine or arginine; use of appetite enhancers such as megestrol; and single supplement augmentation of oral intake with zinc, chromium, copper, manganese, or antioxidant vitamins such as A and C (Rabinovitz et al., 2004; Reuben, Hirsch, Zhou, & Greendale, 2005; Stechmiller, Langkamp-Kenken, & Childress, 2005).

Benefits of these artificial feeding and hydration strategies have met with mixed results, and the use of nutrition support or supplementation must be weighed against quality of life issues, such as pleasurable eating in the end of life. Implementation of best practice for nutrition in the frail older adult must be considered, taking into account personal preferences, involvement of a multidisciplinary health care team approach to oral intake, permissivity of the diet order, and incorporation of social interaction into mealtimes (Booth, Leadbetter, Francis, & Tolson, 2005). Continuous improvement of the approach to provision of nutrition to the insti-

tutionalized or hospitalized geriatric patient is essential (Pepersack, 2005). It is also important to accept that mortality is inevitable, and provision of nutrition and fluids at the end of life may not be in the best interest of the patient.

Indicators of whether or not to provide additional support to the geriatric patient may be evaluated using a number of tools, including laboratory indices, the Mini Nutritional Assessment, the minimum data set, anthropometry, and assessment of unintentional weight loss or gain (Salva, Corman, Andrieu, Salas, & Vellas, 2004; Zulkowski & Coon, 2004; Ranhoff, Gjoen, & Mowé, 2005). Regardless of physical state, the older adult should be granted autonomy in health care decisions; if the older adult is unable to make decisions due to mental status issues, a legally appointed guardian should be allowed to direct continuance of care. The wishes of the older adult should always be in the forefront when making decisions regarding medical procedures and feeding and hydration at the end of life (Stuck et al., 2005).

Artificial feeding and provision of fluids not by oral means is a burden in terms of health care costs, inefficient use of medical resources, and increased patient suffering in an elderly person at the end of life. Artificial provision of food and fluids in this stage is thought to cause continued pain and discomfort. Complications resulting from nasogastric tubes, total parenteral nutrition, or tube feeding include increases in infection, aspiration, and inflammation. Patients often have to be restrained so they do not dislodge tubes, and restraint in and of itself increases distress even in a patient with severely altered mental state (Slomka, 2003).

Dying from dehydration is a pain-free, natural, and peaceful process. Dry mouth is the only symptom associated with this course of action and is easily treated with lip balm and ice chips. Death through dehydration reduces nausea, diarrhea, and urinary output with concomitant urinary tract infection or bedsores from catheterization, wet bed sheets, and use of bedpans. Pulmonary secretions decrease, resulting in less discomfort from shortness of breath, choking, coughing, and congestion. Measures of physical pain show that in persons who are dying there is significantly less pain and in most cases mild euphoria with dehydration (Hoefler, 2000). It is unfortunate that societal norms are such that death is viewed as something that must be staved off at all costs, and the medical community has done little to inform itself and the public of the burden of keeping a dying older adult alive through artificial measures, even in situations where the individuals' own wishes are overturned.

Pharmacologic Considerations

Polypharmacy is common among older persons. In addition to prescribed medications, older adults report more frequent use of over-the-counter preparations and herbal supplements (Figure 12.18). Nonvitamin nonmineral supplement use complicates the interactions between over-the-counter, prescribed medications, and nutrients derived from oral intake or vitamin and mineral preparations (Figure 12.19).

The use of herbals, botanicals, and amino acid supplements is significantly under-reported by older adults and is thought to interact with a variety of other preparations, especially the vitamin K antagonist anticoagulants, such as warfarin, Coumadin, and dicoumarol (Figure 12.20) (Archer, 2005). Compounds from herbals such as garlic, ginkgo biloba, Co-Q10, and others mediate the clotting cascade by the same mechanisms as the vitamin K antagonists (Figure 12.21). In addition, several botanicals have known interactions with the inflammatory cascade with potent lymphocytic activation (Figure 12.22).

Aging is associated with increases in chronic and acute disease, for which multiple medications are prescribed (Soini, Routasalo, & Lagstrom, 2005). Nutritional status is often impaired as a result of the use of a variety of medications and other preparations (Eriksson, Dey, Hessler, Steen, & Steen, 2005). Polypharmacy is defined as "the use of excessive drugs or compounds with drug-like effects" or "the prescription of multiple medications given at one

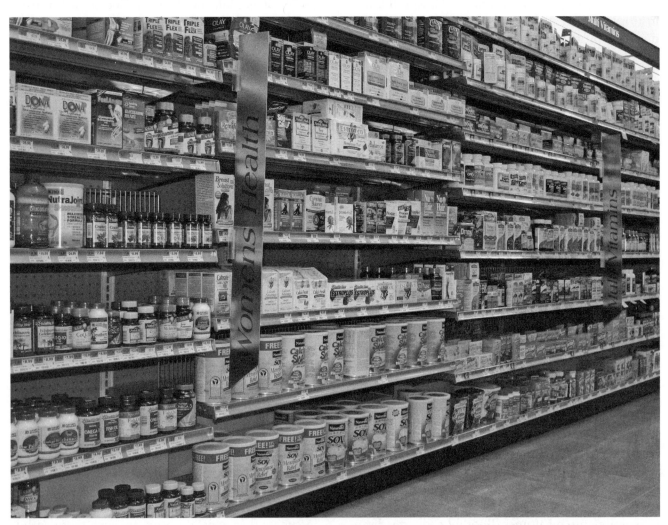

Figure 12.18 Supplements. Many supplements are marketed specifically to older adults. Several formulations exist for many herbal and other supplements with minimal standardization of dose or active ingredient. These products are largely uncontrolled by governmental agencies, and it is the burden of manufacturers to prove purity, efficacy, and legitimacy of any health claims.

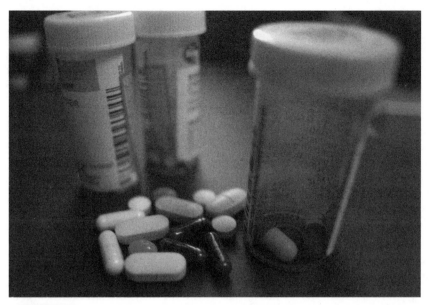

Figure 12.19 Drugs. Many older persons take a variety of medications every day. Average estimates of numbers of drugs taken by elderly persons, both prescribed and over-the-counter, are greater than eight per day in 70+-year-olds in the United States.

time" (Pugh, 2000). Current trends include the movement away from the use of nutritionally dense foods as a means of preventing or treating age-related concerns to the use of drugs, supplements, or herbal products in their stead (Solomons, 2005). Over 250 different medications alter food intake due to sensory side effects, and hundreds more have direct effects on the absorption, disposition, and utilization of nutrients.

> **● Learning Point** The number of prescribed medications taken by community-dwelling elderly is estimated at three or more per day, with almost half taking additional over-the-counter and supplemental products. The number of medications taken by institutionalized elderly persons is estimated at six or more per day (Bales, Ritchie, & Russell, 2004).

Polypharmacy involves a complex set of problems in that foods alter drug disposition, drugs alter other drug disposition, and drugs alter nutrient disposition through a variety of mechanisms. The addition of cellular senescence, organ system deterioration, and alterations in catabolic potential for compounds, such as medications or herbal supplements, result in reductions in total homeostatic control in an older person (Bauer, 2001). Several classes of compounds are known for their interactions and nutritional effects:

- Anticholinergic medications: impair sensory perception, leading to declines in intake and increased gastrointestinal distress
- Glycosides: alter nutrient absorption, increase gastrointestinal distress and anorexia, and promote electrolyte disturbances

- Diuretics: affect mineral excretion, hydration, and electrolyte balance
- Beta-adrenergic antagonists: alter gastrointestinal function, cause gastrointestinal distress, and impair glycogen metabolism
- Vasodilators: interact with B vitamins such as pyridoxine, cause gastrointestinal distress, and depress food intake
- Antiarrhythmic agents: cause gastrointestinal distress, anorexia, dysgeusia, dysosmia, and dry mouth
- Anticoagulants: cause gastrointestinal distress and interact with vitamins K and E and calcium
- Hypolipidemics: may alter the absorption of fat-soluble vitamins and cause gastrointestinal distress and severe constipation
- Central nervous system or psychotherapeutic agents: interact with a wide range of amino acids, vitamins, and minerals in addition to altering sensory perception, depressing or increasing appetite (depends on the drug), causing gastrointestinal disturbance, and altering the disposition of many metabolic intermediates (Mallarkey, 1999; Bauer, 2001).

Older adults use more than 30% of all medications prescribed, and one in three older persons have been prescribed an unnecessary, ineffective, or potentially dangerous medication. Among Medicare patients there has been documentation of more than 1,500 adverse events in a single year. Most adverse events are the result of interactions, and the estimated incidence of interaction increases from 6% in persons taking two or more drugs to 50% in persons taking five medications per day (Wootan & Galavis, 2005). Polypharmacy has also been linked to falls, worsening cognitive status, and poorer overall outcomes in both free-living and institutionalized older adults (Perr et al., 2005; Ziere et al., 2006). Because of the plethora of medications, each with its own set of drug–drug and drug–nutrient interactions, it is impossible to cover the entire spectrum of available information. There are several guides available for interactions between nutrients and drugs, herbals and drugs, and drugs and other drugs.

As a result of the increasing obesity problem in the United States, there has been an effort to assess

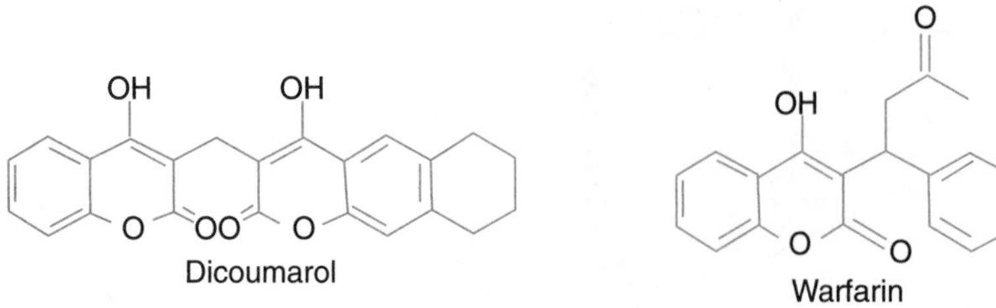

Figure 12.20 Warfarin. Coumadin, dicoumarol, and warfarin are potent inhibitors of the vitamin K-aided clotting cycles with gamma glutamic acids.

excessive weight and obesity in the elderly population, with or without frailty. The prevalence of obesity is thought to increase to about 40% in 2010 in the oldest age groups, bringing with it an increase in cellular senescence, morbidity, and mortality along with increasing health care costs and fiscal burden in the United States (Arterburn, Crane, & Sullivan, 2004; Boyle & Holben, 2006). Drug treatment of obesity is due to come into the forefront for older adults, who will be prescribed drugs to decrease the effects of visceral adiposity, delaying metabolic syndrome complications and improving obesity related disease (Hoekstra, Geleijnse, Schouten, Kok, & Kluft, 2005).

Pharmacotherapeutic Intervention in Obesity

In light of the changing demographics in the United States, the issues of weight and weight control in older persons will become increasingly important, and little is known about the treatment efficacy of anorexigenic drugs in this population or the likelihood of interactions between these drugs and other medications, nutrients, or herbal products. More is known about appetite stimulation in this population (Lee et al., 2005). Intuitively, this population would be better served by using diet, exercise, and nutrient density as a first response to weight change (Keller, Hadley, Hadley, Wong, & Vanderkooy, 2005). Unfortunately, societal propensity to medicate and health professionals' response to prescribe may result in an overuse of anorexigenics in older persons in the near future.

Several drugs have been used to treat obesity with limited success. The "phen/fen" regimen came under scrutiny when mitral valve abnormalities and primary pulmonary hypertension were identified as adverse events with prolonged use. Subsequently, fenfluramine was removed from the market. Phentermine (Ionamin), an amphetamine-like compound, which reduces appetite through hypothalamic mediation, is still available. Phentermine is an older drug, available since the late 1970s, and is infrequently prescribed because of inconsequential long-term weight loss and ineffective weight maintenance with increased interactions with other drugs (Heuberger, 1998).

Xenical or Orlistat, a lipase inhibitor, has recently been approved for sale over the counter, causes malabsorption of fat-soluble nutrients, without stellar weight loss. Because of the action of Orlistat on the gastrointestinal tract, there is considerable potential for steatorrhea, anal leakage, flatulence, bloating, nausea, and vomiting. Because of age-related declines in gut function, the impact of lipid malabsorption on vitamins E, D, and K are extreme. In addition, there may be loss of several minerals, through entrapment in the undigested materials in the gut, with subsequent elimination. In older persons, the prescription of a drug that causes malabsorption of key nutrients with gastrointestinal distress is not recommended (Kasper et al., 2005).

Serotonin reuptake inhibitors have also been used. Fluoxetine (Prozac) and sertra-

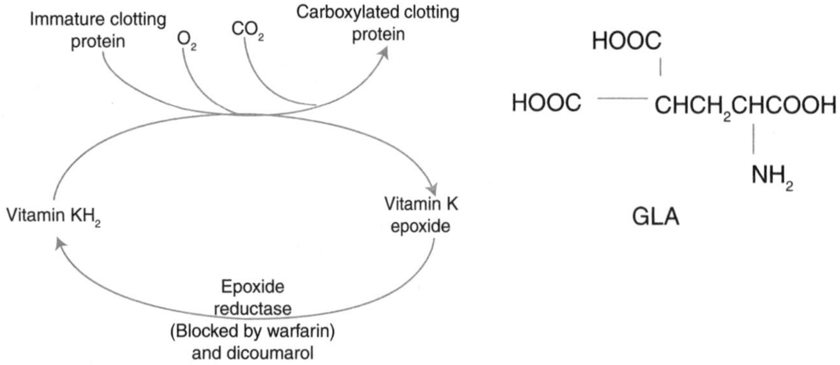

Figure 12.21 Vitamin K cycle. The vitamin K-dependent cycle for the activation of the proteins involved in the blood-clotting cascade. Several clotting factors are affected, including factors IX, X, and VII.

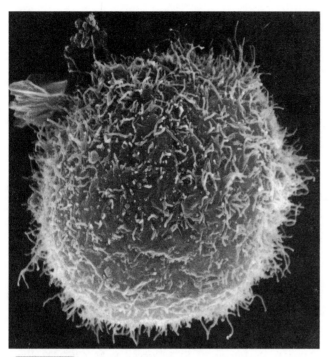

Figure 12.22 Lymphocyte, white blood cell. Inflammation and the resultant chemokine response are intertwined with the immune system and its components. Lymphocytic activity correlates well with increases in response that increase risk for cellular senescence.

Courtesy of Dr. Timothy Triche/National Cancer Institute

line (Zoloft) are just two examples. The weight change can go up or down, and decrements are not substantial or sustained when weight declines. Sibutramine, which affects norepinephrine, dopamine, and serotonin, has also been shown to have undesirable side effects and minimal efficacy for substantial loss and maintenance of weight loss over time. Sibutramine works through central reuptake inhibition of these neurotransmitters, which in turn affects heart rate and blood pressure and is unsuitable for use in older patients. Newer generations of endogenous hypothalamic 5- hydroxytryptophan medications are being developed to specifically target receptors for satiety (Fairburn & Brownell, 2002; Halford, Lawton, & Blundell, 2005; Kasper et al., 2005).

Several targets have been identified as having an influence on weight and appetite. New drugs that either reduce food intake or increase oxygen consumption and energy expenditure are being tested. Beta-3 agonists that increase energy expenditure and uncoupling proteins to convert white to brown fat and result in elevated thermogenesis have been undergoing evaluation. Both result in increased oxidative stress and elevations in blood pressure, resting heart rate, and other side effects, making future use

in elderly unlikely. Alternatively, drugs that act hypothalamically to induce satiety and reduce cravings are also of interest (Sidahaye & Cheskin, 2006).

There are a variety of these drugs under investigation, which include compounds that affect the endocannabinoid receptor systems in the brain and are thought to decrease appetite and cravings for specific macronutrients along with decreasing the desire for nicotine and smoking. The endocannabinoids are endogenous lipids that bind to specific receptors in the hypothalamic portions of the brain, including CBAQ2, CB-1AQ2, CB-2AQ2, and others. These receptors are also present in the gastrointestinal tract and peripherally in both soft tissue and adipocytes. Blocking these receptors decreases the inherent rewards of eating (Kirkham, 2005; Pagotto, Vincenati, & Pasqual, 2005).

Recent evidence also points to the influence of stimulation of these CBAQ2 receptors on fatty acid synthesis through synthetase expression. Blockage would result in decreased hepatic lipogenesis and that in turn modulates metabolic homeostasis for weight and feeding, as well as oxidative stress (Osei-Hyiaman et al., 2005; Di Marzo & Matias, 2005). These compounds are still in clinical trial but show promise in terms of the reduction of body weight and long-term weight-loss maintenance among subjects, with few adverse effects. Rimonabant™ is one such CB-1AQ2 receptor antagonist (Boyd & Fremming, 2005).

Investigations into receptor agonists for NPYAQ2, a protein inherently tied to body weight stability and satiety, have been done with rodent models with mixed results (Boggiano et al., 2005). Lipoprotein lipase activation is also under consideration in animal models. NO-1886AQ2 increases the expression of uncoupling protein, thermogenin, with concomitant decreases in fat pads in obese animals (Kusunoki, Tsutsumi, & Iwata, 2005). Research is being conducted on drugs that will induce apoptosis in white adipose tissue, including extracts from green tea and fenugreek seeds (Handa, Yamaguchi, Sono, & Yazawa, 2005; Nelson-Dooley, Della-Fera, Hamrick, & Baile, 2005). It is unknown what the adverse potential of these novel compounds will be or whether they will ever come to clinical trial in humans.

Obesity in older adults presents unique challenges, but the treatment of obesity warrants even greater concern. Most pharmacotherapeutic interventions for obesity in the older adult are contraindicated, with the elderly having multiple conditions and polydrug use. It remains to be seen if drug treatment can play a significant role in the upcoming obesity epidemic among older persons in the United States

Summary

The concept of "successful" or "healthy" aging involves many factors. Some of these include complex interactions between nutritional status, genetics, life-style, and environmental considerations. Nutritional adequacy with caloric restriction over the life span is thought to be critical to the expression of genetic tendencies toward apoptosis or cellular senescence. Mediation of oxidative stresses and apoptotic events is thought to include exposure to environmental contaminants as well as alcohol, drug, and tobacco use. Other moderating factors that may directly or indirectly influence senescence include mental status, mental activity, pet ownership, marital status, economics, education, and parity, among others. Health conditions and acute or chronic disease requiring medication each impact the aging process. Body habitus and obesity with their concomitant influences on disease and cellular senescence are inherently tied to overall morbidity and mortality. In summary, healthy aging involves multiple factors, each with its own set of complex interactions. Older adults must be evaluated holistically, accounting for the multitude of factors that influence overall quality of life and longevity.

Issues for Debate

1. Discuss examples of health factors that have affected older people you have known.
2. How could some of these health factors have been improved?
3. What will be the impact of health factors on the aging baby boomer population?

References

Abrams, R. C., Lachs, M., McAvay, G., Keohane, D. J., & Bruce, M. L. (2002). Predictors of self neglect in community dwelling elders. *American Journal of Psychiatry, 159,* 1724–1730.

Adelman, P. K. (1994). Multiple roles and psychological well being in a national sample of older adults. *Journal of Gerontology, 49,* 277S–285S.

Ahluwalia, N., Sun, J., Krause, D., Mastro, D., & Handte, G. (2004). Immune function is impaired in iron-deficient, homebound, older women. *American Journal of Clinical Nutrition, 79,* 516–521.

Anderson, J. J., Suchindran, C. M., Kritchevsky, S. B., & Barrett-Connor, E. (2004). Macronutrient intakes of elderly in the Lipid Research Clinics Program Prevalence Study. *Journal of Nutrition, Health, and Aging, 8,* 395–399.

Andree, K. B., Kim, J., Kirschke, C. P., Gregg, J. P., Paik, H., Joung, H., et al. (2004). Investigation of lymphocyte gene expression for use as biomarkers for zinc status in humans. *Journal of Nutrition, 134,* 1716–1723.

Archer, S. L. (2005). Nonvitamin and nonmineral supplement use among elderly people. *Journal of the American Dietetic Association, 105,* 63–64.

Arterburn, D. E., Crane, P. K., & Sullivan, S. D. (2004). The coming epidemic of obesity in elderly Americans. *Journal of the American Geriatric Society, 52,* 1907–1912.

Avcu, N., Ozbek, M., Kurtoglu, D., Kurtoglu, E., Kansu, O., & Kansu, H. (2005). Oral findings and health status among hospitalized patients with physical disabilities, aged 60 or above. *Archives of Gerontology and Geriatrics, 41,* 69–79.

Bales, C. W., Ritchie, C. S., & Russell, R. M. (2004). *Handbook of Clinical Nutrition and Aging* (pp. 214–271). Totowa, NJ: Humana Press.

Bamia, C. (2005). Dietary patterns among older Europeans: The EPIC-Elderly study. *British Journal of Nutrition, 94,* 100–113.

Bauer, L. A. (2001). *Applied Clinical Pharmacokinetics* (pp. 226–229). New York: McGraw-Hill.

Beck, A. M., Ovesen, L., & Schroll, M. (2001). A six month prospective follow up of 65 and older patients from general practice classified according to nutritional risk by the MNA. *European Journal of Clinical Nutrition, 55,* 1028–1033.

Bischoff-Ferrari, H. A., Dietrich, T., Orav, E. J., Hu, F. B., Zhang, Y., Karlson, E.W., et al. (2004). Higher 25-hydroxyvitamin D concentrations are associated with better lower-extremity function in both active and inactive persons aged > 60 y. *American Journal of Clinical Nutrition, 80,* 752–758.

Blazer, D. G., & Sachs-Ericsson, N. H. (2005). Perception of unmet needs as a predictor of mortality among community dwelling older adults. *American Journal of Public Health, 95,* 299–304.

Boggiano, M. M., Chandler, P. C., Oswald, K. D., Rodgers, R. J., Blundell, J. E., Ishii, Y., et al. (2005). PYY3-36 as an anti-obesity drug target. *Obesity Review, 6,* 307–322.

Booth, J., Leadbetter, A., Francis, M., & Tolson, D. (2005). Implementing a best practice statement in nutrition for frail older people: Part 2. *Nursing Older People, 17,* 22–24.

Borst, S. E. (2004). Interventions for sarcopenia and muscle weakness in older people. *Age and Ageing, 33,* 548–555.

Bottiglieri, T., & Diaz-Arrastia, R. (2005). Hyperhomocystinemia and cognitive function: More than just a casual link? *American Journal of Clinical Nutrition, 82,* 493–494.

Boudville, A., & Bruce, D. G. (2005). Lack of meal intake compensation following nutritional supplements in hospitalised elderly women. *British Journal of Nutrition, 93*, 879–884.

Boyd, S. T., & Fremming, B. A. (2005). Rimonobant—A selective CB-1 antagonist. *Annals of Pharmacotherapy, 30*, 684–690.

Boyle, M. A., & Holben, D. H. (2006). *Community Nutrition in Action: An Entrepreneurial Approach* (4th ed., pp. 135–140). Belmont, CA: Thomson Wadsworth.

Brach, J. S., Simonsick, E. M., Kritchevsky, S., Yaffe, K., & Newman, A. B. (2004). The association between physical function and life-style activity and exercise in the health, aging and body composition study. *Journal of the American Geriatrics Society, 52*, 502–509.

Brantervik, A. M., Jacobsson, I. E., Grimby, A., Wallén, T. C., & Bosaeus, I. G. (2005). Older hospitalized patients at risk of malnutrition: Correlation with quality of life, aid from the social welfare system and length of stay? *Age Aging, 34*, 444–449.

Brüünsgaard, H., & Pedersen, B. K. (2003). Age-related inflammatory cytokines and disease. *Immunology and Allergy Clinics of North America, 23*, 15–39.

Burke, G. L., Arnold, A. M., Bild, D. E., Cushman, M., Fried, L. P., Newman, A., et al. (2001). Factors associated with healthy aging: The cardiovascular health study. *Journal of the American Geriatrics Society, 49*, 254–262.

Chen, Y. C., Pu, Y. S., & Lin, R. S. (2001). Blood and urine levels of cadmium in relation to demographic and life style in middle age and elderly men. *Bulletin on Environment Contamination Toxicology, 66*, 287–294.

Chen, Z., Bassford, T., Green, S. B., Cauley, J. A., Jackson, R. D., LaCroix, A. Z., et al. (2005). Postmenopausal hormone therapy and body composition—a substudy of the estrogen plus progestin trial of the Women's Health Initiative. *American Journal of Clinical Nutrition, 82*, 651–656.

Chernoff, R. (1999). *Geriatric Nutrition: Health Professional's Handbook* (2nd ed., pp. 356–368). Gaithersburg, MD: Aspen Publishers.

Chernoff, R. (2005). Micronutrient requirements in older women. *American Journal of Clinical Nutrition, 81*, 1240S–1245S.

Collins, C. E., Kershaw, J., & Brockington, S. (2005). Effect of nutritional supplements on wound healing in home-nursed elderly: A randomized trial. *Nutrition, 21*, 147–155.

Dasgupta, M., Sharkey, J. R., & Wu, G. (2005). Inadequate intakes of indispensable amino acids among homebound older adults. *Journal of Nutrition for the Elderly, 24*, 85–99.

Dawson-Hughes, B. (2004). Racial/ethnic considerations in making recommendations for vitamin D for adult and elderly men and women. *American Journal of Clinical Nutrition, 80*, 1763S–1766S.

De Groot, L. C., Verheijden, M. W., de Henauw, S., Schroll, M., & van Staveren, W. A. (2004). Life-style, nutritional status, health, and mortality in elderly people across Europe: Our view of the longitudinal results of the SENECA study. *Journals of Gerontology. Series A, Biological Sciences and Medical Sciences, 59*, 1277–1284.

Demingné, C., Sabboh, H., Rémésy, C., & Meneton, P. (2004). Protective effects of high dietary potassium: Nutritional and metabolic aspects. *Journal of Nutrition, 134*, 2903–2906.

Deplas, A., Debiais, F., Alcalay, M., Bontoux, D., & Thomas, P. (2004). Bone density, parathyroid hormone, calcium and vitamin D nutritional status of institutionalized elderly subjects. *Journal of Nutrition, Health & Aging, 8*, 400–404.

Depp, C. A., & Jeste, D. V. (2006). Definitions and predictors of successful aging: A comprehensive review of larger quantitative studies. *American Journal of Geriatric Psychiatry, 14*, 6–20.

Devine, A., Dick, I. M., Islam, A. F., Dhaliwal, S. S., & Prince, R. L. (2005). Protein consumption is an important predictor of lower limb bone mass in elderly women. *American Journal of Clinical Nutrition, 81*, 1423–1428.

Dhonukshe-Rutten, R. A., van Zutphen, M., de Groot, L. C., Eussen, S. J., Blom, H. J., & van Staveren, W. A. (2005). Effect of supplementation with cobalamin carried either by a milk product or a capsule in mildly cobalamin-deficient elderly Dutch persons. *American Journal of Clinical Nutrition, 82*, 568–574.

Di Marzo, V., & Matias, I. (2005). Endocannibinoid control of food intake and energy balance. *Nature Neuroscience, 8*, 585–589.

Donini, L. M., De Bernardini, L., De Felice, M. R., Savina, C., Coletti, C., & Cannella, C. (2004). Effect of nutritional status on clinical outcome in a population of geriatric rehabilitation patients. *Aging Clinical and Experimental Research, 16*, 132–138.

Drewnowski, A., & Schultz, J. M. (2001). Impact of aging on eating behaviors, food choices, nutrition and health status. *Journal of Nutrition, Health, and Aging, 5*, 75–79.

Eriksson, B. G., Dey, D. K., Hessler, R. M., Steen, G., & Steen, B. (2005). Relationship between MNA and SF-36 in a free-living elderly population aged 70 to 75. *Journal of Nutrition, Health, and Aging, 9*, 212–220.

Fairburn, C. G., & Brownell, K. D. (2002). *Eating Disorders and Obesity: A Comprehensive Handbook* (2nd ed., pp. 555–559). New York: The Guilford Press.

Farin, H. M., Abbasi, F., & Reaven, G. M. (2006). Body mass index and waist circumference both contribute to differences in insulin mediated glucose disposal in non-diabetic adults. *American Journal of Clinical Nutrition, 83*, 47–51.

Faure, P., Ducros, V., Couzy, F., Favier, A., & Ferry, M. (2005). Rapidly exchangeable pool study of zinc in free-living or institutionalized elderly women. *Nutrition, 21*, 831–837.

Ferry, M., Sidobre, B., Lambertin, A., & Barberger-Gateau, P. (2005). The SOLINUT study: Analysis of the interaction between nutrition and loneliness in persons aged over 70 years. *Journal of Nutrition, Health, and Aging, 9*, 261–268.

Fortes, C., Farchi, S., Forestiere, F., Agabiti, N., Pacifici, R., & Zuccaro, P. (2003). Depressive symptoms lead to impaired cellular immune response. *Psychotherapy and Psychosomatics, 72,* 253–260.

Ganesan, K., Teklehaimanot, S., Tran, T. H., Asuncion, M., & Norris, K. (2005). Relationship of C-reactive protein and bone mineral density in community-dwelling elderly females. *Journal of the National Medical Association, 97,* 329–333.

Gause-Nilsson, I., & Dey, D. K. (2005). Percent body fat estimation from skinfold thickness in the elderly. Development of a population-based prediction equation and comparison with published equations in 75-year-olds. *Journal of Nutrition, Health, and Aging, 9,* 19–24.

Gazzotti, C., Albert, A., Pepinster, A., & Petermans, J. (2000). Clinical usefulness of the mini-nutritional assessment (MNA) scale in geriatric patients. *Journal of Nutrition, Health, and Aging, 4,* 176–181.

Gibbons, M. D., & Henry, C. J. (2005). Does eating environment have an effect on food intake in the elderly? *Journal of Nutrition, Health, and Aging, 9,* 25–29.

Ginty, F. (2003). Dietary protein and bone health. *Proceedings of the Nutrition Society, 62,* 867–876.

Gonzalez, S., Huerta, J. M., Alvarez-Uria, J., Fernandez, S., Patterson, A. M., & Lasheras, C. (2004). Serum selenium is associated with plasma homocysteine concentrations in elderly humans. *Journal of Nutrition, 134,* 1736–1740.

Gori, A. M., Corsi, A. M., Fedi, S., Gazzini, A., Sofi, F., Bartali, B., et al. (2005). A proinflammatory state is associated with hyperhomocystinemia in the elderly. *American Journal of Clinical Nutrition, 82,* 335–341.

Halford, J. C., Harrold, J. A., Lawton, C. L., & Blundell, J. E. (2005). Serotonin drugs: Effects on appetite expression and the use for the treatment of obesity. *Current Drug Targets, 6,* 201–213.

Hamilton, B. P., & Hamilton, J. H. (1997). Hypertension in elderly persons. *Endocrine Practice, 3,* 29–41.

Handa, T., Yamaguchi, K., Sono, Y., & Yazawa, K. (2005). Effects of fenugreek seed extract in obese mice fed a high fat diet. *Bioscience, Biotechnology, and Biochemistry, 69,* 1186–1188.

Herzog, A., Regula, F., Markus, H., & Holmberg, D. (1998). Activities and well being in older age: Effects of self concept and educational attainment. *Psychological Aging, 13,* 179–185.

Heuberger, R. A. (1998). *Combination Drug Treatment of Obesity.* Ann Arbor, MI: UMI Publications.

Hjerkinn, E. M., Seljeflot, I., Ellingsen, I., Berstad, P., Hjermann, I., Sandvik, L., et al. (2005). Influence of long-term intervention with dietary counseling, long chain n-3 fatty acid supplements, or both on circulating markers of endothelial activation in men with long-standing hyperlipidemia. *American Journal of Clinical Nutrition, 81,* 583–589.

Hoefler, J. M. (2000). Making decisions about tube feeding for severely demented patients at the end of life: Clinical, legal and ethical considerations. *Death Studies, 24,* 233–254.

Hoekstra, T., Geleijnse, J. M., Schouten, E. G., Kok, F. J., & Kluft, C. (2005). Relationship of C-reactive protein with components of the metabolic syndrome in normal-weight and overweight elderly. *Nutrition, Metabolism, and Cardiovascular Disease, 15,* 270–278.

Hokby, A., Reimers, A., & Laflamme, I. (2003). Hip fractures among older people: Do marital status and type of residence matter? *Public Health, 117,* 196–201.

Iso, H., Date, C., Noda, H., Yoshimura, T., & Tamakoshi, A. (2005). Frequency of food intake and estimated nutrient intake among men and women: The JACC Study. *American Journal of Epidemiology, 15*(Suppl. 1), S24–S42.

Iwashyna, T. J., & Christakis, N. A. (2003). Marriage, widowhood and health care use. *Social Science and Medicine, 57,* 2137–2147.

Jaques, P. F., Moeller, S. M., & Hankinson, S. E. (2003). Weight status, abdominal adiposity, diabetes and early age related lens opacities. *American Journal of Clinical Nutrition, 78,* 400–405.

Jungjohann, S. M., Luhrmann, P. M., Bender, R., Blettner, M., & Neuhäuser-Berthold, M. (2005). Eight-year trends in food, energy and macronutrient intake in a sample of elderly German subjects. *British Journal of Nutrition, 93,* 361–378.

Kannus, P., Uusi-Rasi, K., Palvanen, M., & Parkkari, J. (2005). Non-pharmacological means to prevent fractures among older adults. *Annals of Medicine, 37,* 303–310.

Kasper, D. L., Fauci, A. S., Longo, D. L., Braunwald, E., Hauser, S. L., & Jameson, J. L. (2005). *Harrison's Principles of Internal Medicine* (16th ed., pp. 428–429). New York: McGraw-Hill.

Kato, I., Toniolo, P., Zeleniuch-Jacquotte, A., Shore, R. E., & Koenig, K. L. (2000). Diet, smoking and anthropometric indices and postmenopausal bone fractures: A prospective study. *International Journal of Epidemiology, 29,* 85–92.

Keller, H. H. (2004). Nutrition and health-related quality of life in frail older adults. *Journal of Nutrition, Health & Aging, 8,* 245–252.

Keller, H. H., & Ostbye, T. (2003). Nutritional risk and time to death: Predictive validity of SCREEN. *Journal of Nutrition, Health, and Aging, 7,* 274–279.

Keller, H. H., Hadley, M., Hadley, T., Wong, S., & Vanderkooy, P. (2005). Food workshops, nutrition education, and older adults: A process evaluation. *Journal of Nutrition for the Elderly, 24,* 5–23.

Kennedy, R. L., Chokkalingham, K., & Srinivasan, R. (2004). Obesity in the elderly: Who should we be treating, and why, and how? *Current Opinion in Clinical Nutrition and Metabolic Care, 7,* 3–9.

Kikawada, M., Iwamoto, T., & Takasaki, M. (2005). Aspiration and infection in the elderly: Epidemiology, diagnosis and management. *Drugs & Aging, 22,* 115–130.

Kirby, S. E., Coleman, P. G., & Daley, D. (2004). Spirituality and well being in frail and non-frail older adults. *Journal of Gerontology, 59,* 123–129.

Kirkham, T. C. (2005). Endocannibinoids in the regulation of appetite and body weight. *Behavioral Pharmacology, 16*, 297–313.

Koukouli, S., Vlachonikolis, I. G., & Philalithis, A. (2002). Sociodemographic factors and self reported functional status—The significance of social support. *BMC Health Service Research, 2*, 20.

Krabbe, K. S., Pedersen, M., & Brüünsgaard, H. (2004). Inflammatory mediators in the elderly. *Experimental Gerontology, 39*, 687–699.

Kusunoki, M., Tsutsumi, K., & Iwata, K. (2005). NO-1886 (Ibrolipim), an LPL activator, increases expression of UCP-3 in skeletal muscle and suppresses fat accumulation in high fat diet induced obesity in rats. *Metabolism: Clinical and Experimental, 54*, 1587–1592.

Kyle, U.G., Genton, L., & Pichard, C. (2005). Hospital length of stay and nutritional status. *Current Opinion in Clinical Nutrition and Metabolic Care, 8*, 397–402.

Larrieu, S., Letenneur, L., Berr, C., Dartigues, J. F., Ritchies, K., & Alperovitch, A. (2004). Sociodemographic differences in dietary habits in a population based sample of elderly subjects: The 3C study. *Journal of Nutrition, Health, and Aging, 8*, 497–502.

Lavis, J. N., McLeod, C. B., Mustard, C. A., & Stoddard, G. I. (2003). Is there a gradient in lifespan by position in the social hierarchy? *American Journal of Public Health, 93*, 771–773.

Lee, J. S., Kritchevsky, S. B., Harris, T. B., Tylavsky, F., Rubin, S. M., & Newman, A. B. (2005). Short-term weight changes in community-dwelling older adults: The Health, Aging, and Body Composition Weight Change Substudy. *American Journal of Clinical Nutrition, 82*, 644–650.

Lee, J. S., Kritchevsky, S. B., Tylavsky, F. A., Harris, T., Everhart, J., Simonsick, E. M., et al. (2004). Weight-loss intention in the well-functioning, community-dwelling elderly: Associations with diet quality, physical activity, and weight change. *American Journal of Clinical Nutrition, 80*, 466–474.

Levinson, Y., Dwolatzky, T., Epstein, A., Adler, B., & Epstein, L. (2005). Is it possible to increase weight and maintain the protein status of debilitated elderly residents of nursing homes? *Journals of Gerontology, Series A, Biological Science, 60*, 878–881.

Lewis, M. S., Miller, L. S., Johnson, M. A., Dolce, E. B., Allen, R. H., & Stabler, S. P. (2005). Elevated methylmalonic acid is related to cognitive impairment in older adults enrolled in an elderly nutrition program. *Journal of Nutrition for the Elderly, 24*, 47–65.

Lichtenstein, A. H., & Russell, R. M. (2005). Essential nutrients: Food or supplements? Where should the emphasis be? *Journal of the American Medical Association, 294*, 351–358.

Lieber, C. (1992). *Medical and Nutritional Complications of Alcoholism.* New York: Plenum Publishing.

Loeb, M., & High, K. (2005). The effect of malnutrition on risk and outcome of community-acquired pneumonia. *Respiratory Care Clinics of North America, 11*, 99–108.

Lorefält, B., Wissing, U., & Unosson, M. (2005). Smaller but energy- and protein-enriched meals improve energy and nutrient intakes in elderly patients. *Journal of Nutrition, Health, and Aging, 9*, 243–247.

Loucks, E. B., Berkamn, L. F., Gruenewald, T. L., & Seeman, T. E. (2005). Social integration is associated with fibrinogen concentration in elderly men. *Psychosomatic Medicine, 67*, 353–358.

Lyman, D. (2005). Undiagnosed vitamin D deficiency in the hospitalized patient. *American Family Physician, 71*, 299–304.

Mallarkey, G. (1999). *Drug Treatment Considerations in the Elderly* (pp. 61–64). Hong Kong: Adis International.

Marlett, J. A., McBurney, M. I., & Slavin, J. L. (2002). Position of the American Dietetics Association: Health implications of dietary fiber. *Journal of the American Dietetics Association, 102*, 993–1000.

Marshall, J. A., Lopez, T. K., Shetterly, S. M., Morganstern, N. E., Baer, K., Swenson, C., et al. (1999). Indicators of nutritional risk in a rural elderly Hispanic and non-Hispanic white population: San Luis Valley Health and Aging Study. *Journal of the American Dietetic Association, 99*, 315–322.

Mathus-Vliegen, E. M. H. (2004). Old age, malnutrition, and pressure sores: An ill-fated alliance. *Journals of Gerontology Series A: Biological Sciences and Medical Sciences, 59*, M355–M360.

McCabe, L. D., Martin, B. R., McCabe, G. P., Johnston, C. C., Weaver, C. M., & Peacock, M. (2004). Dairy intakes affect bone density in the elderly. *American Journal of Clinical Nutrition, 80*, 1066–1074.

McNicholas, J., Gilbey, A., Rennie, A., Ahmedzai, S., Dono, J., & Ormerod, E. (2005). Pet ownership and human health: A brief review of evidence and issues. *British Medical Journal, 331*, 1252–1254.

Meydani, M. (2001). Nutrition interventions in aging and age-associated disease. *Annals of the New York Academy of Sciences, 928*, 226–235.

Millward, D. J. (2004). Macronutrient intakes as determinants of dietary protein and amino acid adequacy. *American Society for Nutritional Sciences, 134*, 1588S–1596S.

Milne, A. C., Potter, J., & Avenell, A. (2005). Protein and energy supplementation in elderly people at risk from malnutrition. *Cochrane Database System Review,* CD003288.

Mojon, P., Budtz-Jorgensen, E. R., & Henri, C. (1999). Relationship between oral health and nutrition in very old people. *Age and Aging, 28*, 463–468.

Morley, J. E., Glick, Z., & Rubenstein, L. Z. (1995). *Geriatric Nutrition: A Comprehensive Review* (2nd ed.). New York: Raven Press.

Nakashini, N., Fukada, H., Takatorige, T., & Tatara, K. (2005). Relationship between self assessed masticatory ability and 9 year mortality in a cohort of community residing elderly people. *Journal of the American Geriatrics Society, 53*, 54–58.

National Institute on Aging. (2005). Strategic plan research goals. Retrieved December 22, 2005, from www.nia.nih.gov.

Nelson-Dooley, C., Della-Fera, M. A., Hamrick, M., & Baile, C. A. (2005). Novel treatments for obesity and osteoporosis: Targeting apoptotic pathways in adipocytes. *Current Medicinal Chemistry, 12*, 2215–2225.

Nied, R. J., & Franklin, B. (2002). Promoting and prescribing exercise for the elderly. *American Family Physician, 65*, 419–426.

Nieves, J. W. (2005). Osteoporosis: The role of micronutrients. *American Journal of Clinical Nutrition, 81*, 1232S–1239S.

Okuyama, H., Ichikawa, Y., Fujii, Y., Ito, M., & Yamada, K. (2005). Changes in dietary fatty acids and life style as major factors for rapidly increasing inflammatory diseases and elderly-onset diseases. *World Review of Nutrition and Dietetics, 95*, 52–61.

Osei-Hyiaman, D., DePetrillo, M., Pacher, P., Lui, J., Radaeva, S., & Batkai, S. (2005). Endocannabinoid activation at hepatic CB1 receptors stimulates fatty acid synthesis and contributes to diet-induced obesity. *Journal of Clinical Investigation, 115*, 1298–1305.

Pagotto, U., Vincenati, V., & Pasquali, R. (2005). The endocannabinoid system and the treatment of obesity. *Annals of Medicine, 37*, 270–275.

Parslow, R. A., Jorm, A. F., Christensen, H., Rodgers, B., & Jacomb, P. (2005). Pet ownership and health in older adults. *Gerontology, 51*, 40–47.

Payet, M., Esmail, M. H., Polichetti, E., Le Brun, G., Adjemout, L., Donnarel, G., et al. (2004). Docosahexaenoic acid-enriched egg consumption induces accretion of arachidonic acid in erythrocytes of elderly patients. *British Journal of Nutrition, 91*, 789–796.

Pepersack, T. (2005). Outcomes of continuous process improvement of nutritional care program among geriatric units. *Journals of Gerontology, Series A: Biological Sciences and Medical Sciences, 60*, 787–792.

Pepersack, T., Rotsaert, P., Benoit, F., Willems, D., Fuss, M., Bourdoux, P., et al. (2001). Prevalence of zinc deficiency and its clinical relevance among hospitalized elderly. *Archives of Gerontology and Geriatrics, 33*, 243–253.

Perr, M., Menon, A. M., Deshpande, A. D., Shinde, S. B., Jiang, R., Cooper, J. W., et al. (2005). Adverse outcomes associated with inappropriate drug use in nursing homes. *Annals of Pharmacotherapy, 39*, 405–411.

Pfeiffer, C. M., Caudill, S. P., Gunter, E. W., Osterloh, J., & Sampson, E. J. (2005). Biochemical indicators of B vitamin status in the US population after folic acid fortification: Results from the National Health and Nutrition Examination Survey. *American Journal of Clinical Nutrition, 82*, 442–450.

Pope, A. C., Hansen, M. L., Long, R. W., Meilsen, K. R., Eatogh, N. L., & Wilson, W. E. (2004). Ambient air pollution, heart rate variability and blood markers of inflammation in a panel of elderly subjects. *Environmental Health Perspective, 112*, 339–345.

Powell, L. M., Moss, M. S., & Winter, L. H. (2002). Motivation in later life: Personal projects and well being. *Psychological Aging, 17*, 539–547.

Pugh, M. B. (2000). *Stedman's Medical Dictionary* (27th ed.). Philadelphia: Lippincott Williams & Wilkins.

Quadri, P., Fragiacomo, C., Pezzati, R., Zanda, E., Forloni, G., Tettamanti, M., et al. (2004). Homocysteine, folate, and vitamin B-12 in mild cognitive impairment, Alzheimer's disease, and vascular dementia. *American Journal of Clinical Nutrition, 80*, 114–122.

Rabinovitz, H., Friedensohn, A., Leibovitz, A., Gabay, G., Rocas, C., & Habot, B. (2004). Effect of chromium supplementation in elderly patients. *International Journal for Vitamin and Nutrition Research, 74*, 178–182.

Ramos, M. I., Allen, L. H., Haan, M. N., Green, R., & Miller, J. W. (2004). Plasma folate concentrations are associated with depressive symptoms in elderly Latina women despite folic acid fortification. *American Journal of Clinical Nutrition, 80*, 1024–1028.

Ranhoff, A. H., Gjoen, A. U., & Mowé, M. (2005). Screening for malnutrition in elderly acute medical patients: The usefulness of MNA-SF. *Journal of Nutrition, Health, and Aging, 9*, 221–225.

Ravaglia, G., Forti, P., Maioli, F., Martelli, M., Servadei, L., Brunetti, N., et al. (2005). Homocysteine and folate as risk factors for dementia and Alzheimer disease. *American Journal of Clinical Nutrition, 82*, 636–643.

Reuben, D. B., Hirsch, S. H., Zhou, K., & Greendale, G. A. (2005). The effects of megestrol acetate suspension for elderly patients with reduced appetite after hospitalization: A phase II randomized clinical trial. *Journal of the American Geriatrics Society, 53*, 970–975.

Rimkus, A., Melinchok, M. D., McEvoy, K., & Yeager, A. K. (2005). *Thesaurus of Aging Terminology* (8th ed.). Washington, DC: AARP.

Robertson, R. G., & Montagnini, M. (2004). Geriatric failure to thrive. *American Family Physician, 70*, 343–350.

Ross, C. E., & Mirowsky, J. (1999). Refining the association between education and health. The effects of quantity, credential and selectivity. *Demography, 36*, 445–460.

Roth, G. S., Ingram, D. K., & Lane, M. A. (1999). Calorie restriction in primates: Will it work and how will we know? *Journal of the American Geriatric Society, 47*, 896–903.

Ryan-Harshman, M., & Aldoori, W. (2004). Bone health. New role for Vitamin K? *Canadian Family Physician, 50*, 993–997.

Salerno-Kennedy, R., & Cashmanl, K. D. (2005). Relationship between dementia and nutrition-related factors and disorders: An overview. *International Journal for Vitamin and Nutrition Research, 75*, 83–95.

Salva, A., Corman, B., Andrieu, S., Salas, J., & Vellas, B. (2004). Minimum data set for nutritional intervention studies in elderly people. *Journals of Gerontology, Series A: Biological Sciences and Medical Sciences, 59*, M724–M729.

Schone, B. S., & Weinick, R. M. (1998). Health related behaviors and the benefits of marriage for elderly persons. *Gerontologist, 38*, 618–627.

Schulze, M. B., Hoffmann, K., Manson, J. E., Willett, W. C., Meigs, J. B., Weikert, C., et al. (2005). Dietary pattern, inflammation, and incidence of type 2 diabetes in women. *American Journal of Clinical Nutrition, 82*, 675–684.

Shils, M. E. (2005). *Modern Nutrition in Health and Disease* (10th ed.). Philadelphia: Lippincott Williams & Wilkins.

Sidahaye, A., & Cheskin, L. J. (2006). Pharmacologic treatment of obesity. *Advances Psychosomatic Medicine, 27*, 42–52.

Singer, B. H., & Manton, K. G. (1998). The effects of health changes on projections of health service needs for the elderly population of the United States. *Proceedings of the National Academies of Sciences of the United States, 95*, 15618–15622.

Slomka, J. (2003). Withholding nutrition at the end of life: Clinical and ethical issues. *Cleveland Clinic Journal of Medicine, 70*, 548–552.

Snijder, M. B., Visser, M., & Dekker, J. M. (2002). The prediction of visceral fat by dual x-ray absorptiometry in the elderly: A comparison with computed tomography and anthropometry. *International Journal of Obesity and Related Metabolism Disorders, 26*, 984–993.

Snijder, M. B., Visser, M., & Dekker, J. M. (2005). Low subcutaneous thigh fat is a risk factor for unfavorable glucose and lipid levels independent of high abdominal fat. The Health ABC study. *Diabetologia, 48*, 301–308.

Soini, H., Routasalo, P., & Lagstrom, H. (2005). Nutritional status in cognitively intact older people receiving home care services—A pilot study. *Journal of Nutrition, Health, and Aging, 9*, 249–253.

Solomons, N. W. (2005). Nutritional dilemmas of long term health: Implications of evolution and ageing for policies and food industry practices affecting chronic diseases. *Asia Pacific Journal of Clinical Nutrition, 14*(Suppl.), S1–S9.

Stechmiller, J. K., Langkamp-Henken, B., & Childress B. (2005). Arginine supplementation does not enhance serum nitric oxide levels in elderly nursing home residents with pressure ulcers. *Biology Research in Nursing, 6*, 289–299.

Stuck, A., Amstad, H., Baumann-Hölzle, R., Fankhauser, A., Kesselring, A., Leuba, A., et al. (2005). Treatment and care of elderly persons who are in need of care: Medical-ethical guidelines and recommendations. *Journal of Nutrition, Health, and Aging, 9*, 288–295.

Sullivan, D. H., Liu, L., Roberson, P. K., Bopp, M. M., & Rees, J. C. (2004). Body weight change and mortality in a cohort of elderly patients recently discharged from the hospital. *Journal of the American Geriatric Society, 52*, 1696–1701.

Tucker, K. L., Qiao, N., Scott, T., Rosenberg, I., & Spiro III, A. (2005). High homocysteine and low B vitamins predict cognitive decline in aging men: The Veterans Affairs normative aging study. *American Journal of Clinical Nutrition, 82*, 627–635.

U.S. Bureau of the Census. (2005). Retrieved December 22, 2005, from www.census.gov.

U.S. Department of Health and Human Services. (2003). Health, United States, 2003: Special excerpt: Trend tables on 65 and older population. Hyattsville, MD: Centers for Disease Control and Prevention.

Wannamethee, S. G., Shaper, A. G., Morris, R. W., & Whincup, P. H. (2005). Measures of adiposity in the identification of metabolic abnormalities in elderly men. *American Journal of Clinical Nutrition, 81*, 1313–1321.

Warner, H. R., Fernandes, G., & Wang, E. (1995). A unifying hypothesis to explain the retardation of aging and tumorigenesis by caloric restriction. *Journals of Gerontology, Series A, Biological Sciences and Medical Sciences, 50*, B107–B109.

Watson, R. R. (2001). *Alcohol and Coffee Use in the Aging*. Boca Raton, FL: CRC Press.

Weinbrenner, T., Schroder, H., Escurriol, V., Fito, M., Elosua, R., Vila, J., et al. (2006). Circulating oxidized LDL is associated with increased waist circumference independent of BMI in men and women. *American Journal of Clinical Nutrition, 83*, 30–36.

Weinrebe, W., Guneysu, S., & Welz-Barth, A. (2002). Low muscle mass of the thigh is significantly correlated with delirium and worse functional outcome in older medical patients. *Journal of the American Geriatric Society, 50*, 1310–1311.

Welch, G. W., & Somwers, M. R. (2000). The interrelationship between body topology and body composition varies with age among women. *Journal of Nutrition, 130*, 2371–2377.

Wolters, M., Hermann, S., & Hahn, A. (2005). Effect of multivitamin supplementation on the homocysteine and methylmalonic acid blood concentrations in women over the age of 60 years. *European Journal of Nutrition, 44*, 183–192.

Woodman, R., Ferrucci, L., & Guralnik, J. (2005). Anemia in older adults. *Current Opinion in Hematology, 12*, 123–128.

Woods, N. F., LaCroix, A. Z., Gray, S. L., Aragaki, A., Cochrane, B. B., Brunner, R. L., et al. (2005). Frailty: Emergence and consequences in women aged 65 and older in the Women's Health Initiative Observational Study. *Journal of the American Geriatric Society, 53*, 1321–1330.

Wootan, J., & Galavis, J. (2005). Polypharmacy: Keeping the elderly safe. *RN, 68*, 44–51.

Wouters-Wesseling, W., Vos, A. P., Van Hal, M., De Groot, L. C., Van Staveren, W. A., & Bindels, J. G. (2005). The effect of supplementation with an enriched drink on indices of immune function in frail elderly. *Journal of Nutrition, Health, and Aging, 9*, 281–286.

Yaffe, K., Blackwell, T., Gore, R., Sands, L., Reus, V., & Browner, W. S. (1999). Depressive symptoms and cognitive decline in non-demented elderly women. *Archives of General Psychiatry, 56*, 425–430.

Yeh, S. C., & Liu, Y. Y. (2003). Influence of social support on cognitive function in the elderly. *BMC Health Service Research, 3*, 9.

Ziere, G., Dieleman, J. P., Hofman, A., Pols, H. A., vander Cammen, T. J., & Stricker, B. H. (2006). Polypharmacy and falls in the middle age and elderly population. *British Journal of Clinical Pharmacology, 61*, 218–223.

Zulkowski, K., & Coon, P. J. (2004). Comparison of nutritional risk between urban and rural elderly. *Ostomy/ Wound Management, 50*, 46–58.

Zunft, H. J., Hanisch, C., Mueller, S., Koebnick, C., Blaut, M., & Dore, J. (2004). Symbiotic containing *Bifidobacterium animalis* and insulin increases stool frequency in elderly healthy people. *Asia Pacific Journal of Clinical Nutrition, 13*(Suppl.), S112.

Special Topics in Age-Related Risks: Unique Nutrition Issues in the Older Adult

Karen M. Funderburg, MS, RD, LD, and Migy K. Mathews, MD

CHAPTER OUTLINE

Reader Objectives

After studying this chapter and reflecting on the contents, you should be able to

1. List the unique physiologic changes that occur with aging that affect nutrient intake and nutritional status.

2. List key psychosocial changes associated with aging that can affect the desire or ability to consume an adequate diet.

3. Discuss the impact that age-related changes have on nutritional status and quality of life.

4. Understand the consequences of age-related malnutrition and nutrient deficiencies on overall health status and quality of life.

5. Identify nutrition interventions that can improve nutritional status and enhance quality of life.

The older adult is faced with physiologic and social changes that are unique to aging. These changes lead to a wide array of conditions that impair appetite, the ability to eat, and the utilization of nutrients, resulting in an increased risk for malnutrition and nutrition-related health problems and decreased

Quality of life: Personal sense of physical and mental health and the ability to react to physical and social environments.

quality of life. This chapter focuses on the unique and complex nutrition issues facing the older population. Malnutrition, key nutrient deficiencies, impaired appetite, eating ability, osteoporosis, and other nutrition-related health problems are discussed. The roles of nutrition interventions that improve nutritional status and enhance quality of life are presented.

CRITICAL **Thinking**

How Are Appetite and Hunger Similar and Different?

Appetite is defined as "any of the instinctive desires necessary to keep up organic life; especially the desire to eat. *Hunger* is defined as "a craving or urgent need for food or a specific nutrient; an uneasy sensation occasioned by the lack of food."

Compare loneliness to social isolation. Relate these conditions to health and nutritional status in the older adult. *Loneliness* is sadness from being alone or separation from a loved one. *Social isolation* is characterized by the lack of pleasant companionship. A state of being alone is thought of as being imposed by others and seen as negative.

Age-Related Risks for Malnutrition

The demographic challenge of the growing population of older adults calls for solutions to reduce chronic diseases and compress morbidity. Diet presents itself as a key part of the solution. Age-related changes in physiology and metabolism affect all organ systems, with the response of the older adult often differing from that of a younger counterpart (Kinney, 2004). In addition, this age group faces socioeconomic changes that can impact availability of food and desire to eat. Nutritional status surveys of the older population have shown a relatively low prevalence of frank nutrient deficiencies but a marked increase in risk of malnutrition and evidence of subclinical deficiencies with a direct impact on function (Blumberg, 1997). In this section we discuss key changes that increase the risk of malnutrition in the older individual; in the next section we suggest nutritional interventions and strategies to reduce the chances that an inadequate diet will be consumed.

Impaired Appetite

At all ages in the life cycle appetite is associated with physiologic well-being. The intake of food not only

provides necessary nutrients but is an important part of special occasions such as holidays, birthdays, weddings, and anniversaries. The intake of food is a daily contributor to social, cultural, and psychological quality of life. Changes in the gastrointestinal tract, decreased taste and smell acuity, medication side effects, diet modifications, depression, or altered mental status are just a few conditions that can take away the desire to eat. Table 13.1 provides a comprehensive list of factors than may affect appetite. A diminishing appetite can lead to smaller meals, skipping meals, and poor food choices. A decline in intake of total calories and essential nutrients leads to increased risk of illness and infections. Infections may lead to a higher metabolic rate and increased nutritional needs, affecting weight and nutritional status. Ultimately, an impaired appetite may lead to significant risks to overall health and well-being (American Dietetic Association [ADA], 2005b). Early detection and creative strategies are needed to combat appetite loss and prevent serious health complications.

Appetite Assessment

Declining food intake and **anorexia** are predictors for undernutrition in older adults in community and institutional settings (ADA, 2005b). Early detection is necessary to prevent compromised nutritional status and decreased quality of life. Nutrition screening

Anorexia: Diminished appetite.

TABLE 13.1	Conditions That May Affect Appetite

Decreased or altered taste
Decreased smell
Decreased thirst acuity
Hypochlorhydria
Early satiety
Dyspepsia
Decreased caloric needs
Lack of hunger
Eating impairment
Diet modifications
Dining environment
Limited food choices
Lack of control over food choices
Medication side effects
Dementia
Depression
Loneliness
Social isolation

tools designed for the older population exist and screen for a variety of nutrition risk factors. The Determine Your Nutritional Health Checklist screens for number of meals eaten per day, diet modifications, prescription drug use, and social interaction at mealtime (Nutrition Screening Initiative, 1991). The Mini Nutritional Assessment looks at declining food intake, psychological stress, neuropsychological problems, medication use, and number of full meals consumed per day (Nestle Clinical Research, 1998). The main objective of both screening tools is to determine nutritional risk. Because a decline in appetite may indicate or lead to serious health problems, tools designed specifically to assess appetite are important. When a problem is identified, early detection and treatment may prevent weight loss and improve health outcomes (Wilson et al., 2005).

An appetite self-assessment tool was used in seven countries during the Survey in Europe on Nutrition and the Elderly, a Concerted Action (SENECA) study (Mathey, de Jong, de Groot, de Graaf, & Van Staveren, 2001). The SENECA study was a three-part study with the last phase occurring in 1999, when the protocol used the Appetite, Hunger, Sensory Perception (AHSP) questionnaire (de Jong, Mulder, de Graaf, & Van Staveren, 1999). (The questionnaire consists of 29 items that estimate energy intake, appetite and hunger sensations, and taste and smell perceptions in the elderly. Before the European study, the tool had been validated as reliable in providing accurate descriptive data on elderly self-assessment of appetite.) In the SENECA study the researchers used the AHSP in three population groups. They wanted to determine if the tool could distinguish differences in sensations of appetite, hunger, and sensory perception between healthy elderly people living independently, frail elderly living independently, and nursing home residents (Mathey et al., 2001). As a subset of the SENECA study, data from the Dutch population were analyzed. Results of the Dutch study revealed that appetite is related to the health status of the elderly. In healthy subjects appetite was a good indicator of body weight. In the frail subjects disease state rather than appetite affected body weight (Mathey et al., 2001).

The Council for Nutritional Strategies in Long-Term Care developed another appetite assessment tool. The Council was formed in 1998 and is an interdisciplinary panel comprising of experts from academia and the medical community, including geriatricians, dietitians, pharmacists, and nurse practitioners. The Council's charge is to examine issues related to diagnosis, prevention, and treatment of undernutrition in older adults and to identify evidence-based recommendations for the treatment of undernutrition in long-term care (Wilson et al., 2005). They developed the Council of Nutrition Appetite Questionnaire (CNAQ), which scores eight questions to determine a person's risk for anorexia. The questionnaire addresses appetite, hunger, early satiety, taste perception and changes, gastrointestinal tolerance of food intake, mood, and frequency of meals. The total points scored on the questionnaire identify a person's risk for impaired appetite.

Researchers at St. Louis University conducted a study to determine the reliability and validity of the CNAQ. Study subjects were residents in nine long-term care facilities and community-dwelling elderly. Subjects were asked to complete the simple short CNAQ and the longer questionnaire used in the European study, the AHSP tool. Because the AHSP had been validated, the researchers used it to facilitate validation of the CNAQ. During data analysis, the reliability analysis indicated that questions 3, 5, 7, and 8 were reliability reducers. Therefore questions 1, 2, 4, and 6 were separated out to form the Simplified Nutritional Appetite Questionnaire (SNAQ). In this study the CNAQ and SNAQ were validated for use in older adults to identify persons at risk for significant weight loss. Use of the CNAQ and the SNAQ as clinical tools can promptly identify problems and facilitate early intervention. Because the researchers found SNAQ to have comparable reliability to the CNAQ, its four-question length may be preferred in a clinical setting (Wilson et al., 2005).

Diet Modification

In December 2005 the ADA released an updated position paper that stated, "Food is an essential component of quality of life; an unacceptable or unpalatable diet can lead to poor food and fluid intake, resulting in weight loss and undernutrition and a spiral of negative health effects" (ADA, 2005a, p. 1955).

> ● **Learning Point** Special diets that alter texture or consistency because of poor dentition or disease are often unpalatable. Restriction of certain nutrients, such as sodium or fat, can also create an unacceptable diet. The insult of a restrictive diet may lead to poor intake, depression, and malnutrition.

A previously prescribed dietary restriction may no longer be necessary based on the person's current health, age, and dietary intake. The need for diet modifications should be carefully evaluated. In the face of declining appetite, the decision to restrict choices may do more harm than good. Diet prescriptions should be as liberal as possible for optimum intake and quality of life. According to the ADA position paper, "Overall health goals may not warrant the use of a therapeutic diet because of the possible negative effect on quality of life. Often, a more liberalized nutrition intervention allowing a resident to participate in his or her diet-related decisions can provide for nutrient needs and allow alterations contingent on medical conditions while simultaneously increasing the desire to eat and enjoyment of food" (ADA, 2005a, p. 1956). Diet modifications along with other conditions that affect appetite may result in limited food enjoyment and compromised food intake, potentially leading to unintentional weight loss and malnutrition (ADA, 2003b).

Physiologic Changes

Food intake decreases even in healthy older adults as physical activity and metabolic rate decline. This decrease is often called anorexia of aging (ADA, 2005a). Physiologic changes can reduce hunger and lead to early satiety. Body composition changes result in decreases in muscle mass, bone density, total body water, and metabolic rate. Older adults are generally less active than in their younger years, causing a further reduction in energy requirements. These changes reduce caloric need without reducing nutritional needs, making food selection more challenging than for the younger adult.

Changes in the gastrointestinal tract are common with aging and may include problems with **dentition**, oral health, swallowing, diarrhea, constipation, and decreased hydrochloric acid in the stomach. The decrease in acid may diminish hunger and decrease vitamin B_{12} absorption. Medications that reduce stomach acid may have the same effect. Other gastrointestinal changes may cause alteration in food selections as the patient attempts to compensate for losses in gastrointestinal function or chewing and swallowing abilities.

Dentition: The natural teeth, as considered collectively.

Sensory loss is common in the aging process (ADA, 2005a). Appetite is stimulated by the sight and aroma of food. Taste and smell are intertwined and significant contributors to recognizing flavors and the enjoyment of food and beverages. Aging, chronic health problems, and medications can alter olfactory and taste perceptions (Morley, 2001). Smell sensation that declines with aging is called **presbyosmia**. According to the National Institutes of Health, Senior Health Website (see Website Resources, below), problems with the sense of smell occur in about 30% of Americans between the ages of 70 and 80. The problem increases to two of three persons over the age of 80 (National Institute on Deafness and Other Communication Disorders, 2006). Smell plays a key role in food enjoyment. A smell disorder can decrease the appreciation of food flavors and the desire to cook and consume a variety of foods. Food taste, temperature, texture, and aroma combine to create the perceived flavor of food. Like smell, the loss of taste sensitivity can cause a loss of appetite.

presbyosmia: Loss of the sense of smell.

The older adult is at greater risk for food-borne illness due to the physiologic changes of aging. Risk factors for food-borne illness are decreased taste and smell, diminished immune function, **hypochlorhydria**, and altered mental status (ADA, 2003a). Food safety education targeted for seniors is available from the Food Safety Inspection Service of the U.S. Department of Agriculture and other government agencies such as the U.S. Food and Drug Administration and the National Institutes of Health.

Hypochlorhydria: Presence of an abnormally small amount of hydrochloric acid in the stomach.

Additional physiologic changes come in the form of disabilities and diseases. Accumulating disease and disability may rob a patient of their independence. The loss of the ability to shop, cook, and even eat may decrease the desire to eat. For many people disability leads to a more sedentary life-style often accompanied by social isolation (ADA, 2005b).

Cognitive Changes

Impaired mental health can have an impact on food intake and appetite. Persons may forget to eat, may have no desire to eat, or may have difficulty swallowing due to stroke, Alzheimer's disease, or other diseases such as Parkinson disease or cancer. Impaired cognition may decrease the ability to self-feed, alter appetite, impair movement, and affect memory. The loss of family members and friends can lead to loneliness, isolation, and depression. Persons who eat most of their meals alone are at increased risk for malnutrition. Depression, anxiety, and bereavement may result in a loss of interest in food and may trigger substance abuse.

One form of **dementia** is Alzheimer's disease. The Alzheimer's Association provides tips to improve intake on their Website (see Website Resources, below). Decreasing distraction at mealtime, providing easy-to-use dishes and utensils, serving finger foods,

Dementia: The loss, usually progressive, of cognitive and intellectual function.

and limiting food choices to one or two items at a time are some helpful tips (Alzheimer's Association, 2006).

The Mini Mental State Examination is widely used to assess the cognitive impairment of the older adult. Eleven items measure orientation, registration, attention and calculation, recall, and language. It is an effective screening tool for older adults in all settings (Kurlowitz & Wallace, 1999).

Psychosocial Changes

Nutritional risk is associated with economic hardship and loneliness. Objectives of the Elderly Nutrition Program include combating these two barriers to nutritional health. The Administration on Aging of the U.S. Department of Health and Human Services is responsible for providing funding for congregate and home-delivered meals through state-run elderly nutrition programs. The funds are authorized under Title III and Title IV of the Older Americans Act. Programs are provided through local Area Agency on Aging or Tribal Senior Services. Participants can build an informal support system and develop friendships and receive a well-balanced lunch meal, educational programs, and health screenings. Persons that qualify for homebound status can have a lunch meal delivered 5 days per week. The program participants are primarily at high nutritional risk. The success of the Elderly Nutrition Program is well documented (U.S. Administration on Aging, n.d.-a).

A study was done by Gollub and Weddle (2004) to determine if the addition of breakfast as a second home-delivered meal could improve the well-being of at-risk older adults. Most study participants lived alone, were low income, and had trouble shopping or preparing food. A demonstration project, The Morning Meals on Wheels Program, delivered breakfast 5 days per week to subjects who also received home-delivered lunch meals for at least 6 months. A comparison group only received the five home-delivered lunch meals each week. Both groups received the same lunch items, which provided one-third of the Dietary Reference Intake. The breakfast meals also provided one-third of the Dietary Reference Intake. Several surveys were used to assess participants' perceived global quality of life, health, loneliness, food security, enjoyment of food, and depression. The study found that breakfast participants had greater energy and nutrient intakes, less food insecurity, and less depressive days than the other group. The addition of the breakfast meal reduced malnutrition risk and improved appetite, perceived health, and outlook on life (Gollub & Weddle, 2004).

Medication Use

Increased disease leads to increased medication use. Many medications have side effects such as dry mouth, altered taste sensation, sedation, diarrhea, constipation, and decreased appetite. Medications that sedate patients may decrease waking active hours and affect mealtimes and intake.

Medications that stimulate appetite and produce weight gain continue to be explored. Current medications are megestrol, dronabinol, oxandrolone, testosterone, metoclopramide, and cyproheptadine. More research is needed to verify the benefits of these drug therapies.

Interventions for Impaired Appetite

Treating impaired appetite requires an individual approach. The first step is to determine the root causes or factors contributing to a decreased desire to eat. Using tools that aid in assessing appetite and mental status can assist in discovering the most significant problems. Providing choices in food selection, decreasing meals eaten alone, providing assistance with meals, maintaining independence, and using flavor enhancers are first-line strategies. Exploring medication options to decrease negative side effects should also be a part of the action plan. Table 13.2 provides a list of strategies to increase food and nutrient intake.

Multiple factors and conditions result in decreased food intake in the older adult. Often these go hand-in-hand with impaired appetite and are just

TABLE 13.2	Strategies to Increase Food and Nutrient Intake
Liberalized diet	
Freedom in food selection	
Eating with others	
Congregate meals or home-delivered meals	
Providing assistance	
Providing specialized utensils	
Finger foods	
Flavor enhancers	
Adding nutrients to food	
Adding nutrient-dense snacks	
Adding commercial supplements	
Pleasant eating environment with minimal distractions	
Providing praise and encouragement	
Appetite stimulants	

as complex. Impaired eating ability can have significant negative effects on nutritional status and quality of life. **Table 13.3** lists the common problems associated with decreased eating ability that include poor oral health and dentition, swallowing problems, and altered physical ability due to decreased motor skills, mental status, visual impairment, and range of motion.

Oral Health Problems

Oral health problems can lead to pain, tooth loss, and alterations in the diet and have a significant impact on quality of life (Ritchie, 2002). National Health and Nutrition Examination Survey (NHANES) data from 1999 to 2002 confirm that oral health is an increasing problem with age and is compounded by poor income status and lower education level (National Center for Chronic Disease Prevention and Health Promotion, 2005). Information on tooth decay revealed that only 9% of adults aged 20 to 39 years had decay on the roots of their teeth compared with 32% in adults 60 years or older. Forty-one percent of low-income adults (100% federal poverty level) had untreated tooth decay as compared with 16% in the higher income group (.200% federal poverty level). Edentulousness was also affected by income. The prevalence was 15% in adults below 100% of the federal poverty level compared with only 5% in the higher income group (.200% federal poverty level).

Education level also was shown to have a significant impact on oral health. Forty-one percent of adults who had less than a high school education had tooth decay compared with 14% of adults who had a higher than high school education. Fourteen percent of adults who had not completed high

school were **edentulous** compared with 9% with a high school education and 4% with a post–high school education.

Other interesting oral health data from NHANES showed that smoking increases tooth decay. The data showed that 13% of current smokers were edentulous, compared with 8% of former smokers and 5% of people who had never smoked. The greatest disparities in the prevalence of root caries were seen for current smokers. Twice as many current smokers (28%) as nonsmokers (14%) had root caries (National Center for Chronic Disease Prevention and Health Promotion, 2005).

Edentulous: Toothless; having lost the natural teeth.

> **Cultural Diversity:** Non-Hispanic whites had a great prevalence of tooth decay (93%) compared with African-Americans (85%) and Mexican-Americans (84%). However, the percentage of untreated decay was the lowest in non-Hispanic whites at 18%, followed by 36% in Mexican-Americans and 41% in African-Americans. Edentulousness was highest in African-Americans at 10% and lowest in non-Hispanic whites at 6% (National Center for Chronic Disease Prevention and Health Promotion, 2005).

Persons who wear dentures may avoid certain foods because they are hard to chew. Dietary quality and nutrient intake can be compromised, particularly in persons who perceive that their dentures are ill-fitting (Sahyoun & Krall, 2003). An analysis of dietary quality and selection was conducted by Sahyoun and Knall (2003) using data from 4,466 NHANES III participants. Dietary intake, dietary quality, and serum nutrient values were analyzed for denture wearers and compared with participants with natural teeth. A denture wearer is someone who wears at least a full denture on the upper or lower jaw. As part of NHANES III data collection, denture wearers completed a four-item questionnaire to assess their perception of denture use and fit. The results showed that denture wearers had significantly lower serum levels of vitamins C and E, beta-carotene, lycopene, and lutein zeaxanthin than the dentate group. Participants who believed they had ill-fitting dentures consumed fewer fruits and vegetables and had less variety in their diet than the participants who perceived they had good-fitting dentures or participants who had at least 18 natural teeth.

Data from 181 rural residents of Pennsylvania enrolled in a managed-risk Medicare program were surveyed regarding mouth pain and chewing and swallowing problems. Participants were surveyed twice with a year between surveys. Twenty-two participants reported persistent oral health problems. Results of analysis revealed that these participants had significantly greater medical problems than the

TABLE 13.3	Problems That Affect Eating Ability

Tooth loss
Edentulousness
Dentures
Mouth pain
Xerostomia
Dysphagia
Visual impairment
Impaired motor skills
Arthritis
Altered mental status

participants who reported no oral health problems. They were also more likely to have lower intakes of fiber and vitamins C, A, and B$_6$. There was no significant difference in carbohydrate, protein, and fat between the groups (Bailey, Ledikwe, Smiciklas-Wright, Mitchell, & Jensen, 2004).

Oral hygiene after each meal can reduce oral health problems. Brushing, flossing, and using antimicrobial mouthwashes can help maintain oral health and prevent tooth decay, periodontal disease, and halitosis. Residents in long-term care facilities have multiple barriers to daily oral care. They frequently have functional decline due to chronic diseases or disabilities that make routine brushing and flossing difficult or not possible (Ship, 2002). Medication side effects such as dry mouth (**xerostomia**) can also impact oral health. Residents may have ill-fitting dentures due to weight loss or bone loss. Every resident of long term care should have access to routine dental examinations and treatment.

Xerostomia: A dryness of the mouth.

Decreases in tooth extraction due to dental caries or periodontal disease are addressed in *Healthy People 2010* in Focus Area 21, Oral Health (Office of Disease Prevention and Health Promotion, n.d.). Two objectives specifically target the older adult. Objective 21-4 is to reduce the proportion of adults aged 65 to 74 who have had all their natural teeth extracted. The baseline data from 1997 showed that 26% of adults in this age group had full mouth extractions. The 2010 objective calls to reduce the number to 20%. Objective 21-11 aims to increase the proportion of long-term care residents who use the oral health care systems each year. The target is 25% verses 19% from the 1997 baseline data. Federal regulations require long-term care facilities that receive Medicare and/or Medicaid funds to ensure that each resident attains and maintains the highest practicable physical, psychosocial, and mental well-being (National Center for Chronic Disease Prevention and Health Promotion, 2005).

Ironically, Medicare does not cover dental services, regardless of cause or complexity, unless the procedure itself requires inpatient hospitalization or is necessary for another medical treatment. Coverage is not based on the value or the necessity of dental care but rather on the service required. Oral care that involves treatment, removal, or replacement of teeth or structures supporting teeth, removal of diseased teeth in an infected jaw, or preparing the mouth for dentures is not covered (Centers for Medicare and Medicaid Services, n.d.). If a person has a nondental medical condition, such as a tumor, that requires teeth to be extracted, Medicare does not cover the cost of dental appliances or dentures, even though the covered medical service resulted in the need for the teeth to be repaired or replaced. The exclusion from the Social Security Act can be found on the Center for Medicare Services Website (see Website Resources, below). The dental exclusion was included as part of the initial Medicare Program. Congress did not limit the exclusion to routine dental services but included a blanket exclusion of dental services.

The expense of dental services and artificial teeth can be prohibitive for many people in their older years. Like other income barriers, a lack of dental care can profoundly affect a person's ability to eat and thus their nutritional status. Prevention and treatment programs for older adults are needed and should be incorporate as an interdisciplinary team approach. Further research is needed to determine the consequences of poor oral health on overall health and nutritional status.

Swallowing Problems

Swallowing problems can result from a variety of etiologies. Dementia, stroke, neurologic disease such as Parkinson disease, muscle disease such as multiple sclerosis, head and neck surgery, and weakened muscles due to aging are among the conditions that may require precautionary measures to prevent choking and **aspiration**. Impaired swallowing may lead to decreased food intake, malnutrition, dehydration, and decreased quality of life.

Aspiration: Inhalation into the airways of fluid or foreign body; when food or liquid actually enters the lungs.

The assessment and diagnosis of a swallowing problem is usually triggered by signs and symptoms in the person experiencing difficulty. These include coughing before, during, or after swallowing; frequent throat clearing; hoarse breathy voice; drooling; pocketing of food; and attempting to swallow multiple times with each bite (Deering, Russell, & Womack, 2001). Silent aspiration can occur in which no warning signs are present.

If **dysphagia** is suspected, then a swallowing evaluation by a swallowing therapist, such as a speech pathologist, should be obtained. A videofluoroscopic study or barium swallow can identify specific swallowing problems (Deering et al., 2001). The results of testing are used to determine what diet modifi-

Dysphagia: Difficulty in swallowing.

cations are the most beneficial in protecting the person from aspiration.

Modifying food and beverage consistency and positioning during swallowing are the most common interventions. Before the introduction of the National Dysphagia Diet (NDD) in 2002, there was no standardized language regarding diet consistency and thickened liquids. NDD provides a multilevel approach to diet consistency and liquid viscosity (National Institute of Dental and Craniofacial Research, 2005). Dysphagia pureed (NDD1), dysphagia mechanically altered (NDD2), and dysphagia advanced (NDD3) identify three levels of food textures that range from pudding-like to nearly normal texture solids. The four liquid viscosities are "thin," "nectar-like," "honey-like," and "spoon thick." It is vital that foods and liquids have the appropriate texture and consistency for the swallowing ability of the impaired person or aspiration can occur. Unfortunately, texture, consistency, and viscosity modifications make food less appealing and lead to decreased intake. Persons who require thickened liquids may not consume adequate liquids. Dysphagia increases the risk for dehydration and malnutrition.

Dry Mouth

Saliva plays an important role in chewing and swallowing. It also protects teeth from decay and fights mouth infections (National Institute of Dental and Craniofacial Research, 2005). Although xerostomia is not a normal part of aging, it is often the result of certain medication side effects. Common medications used for urinary incontinence, allergies, high blood pressure, and depression can alter the function of the salivary glands. Over 400 prescription and over-the-counter medications can produce this side effect. Dry mouth can also be the result of a medical condition such as diabetes, Parkinson disease, **Sjögren syndrome,** or head and neck radiation therapy or chemotherapy (National Institute of Dental and Craniofacial Research, 2005).

Sjögren syndrome: Dryness of mucous membranes.

The first step in treating dry mouth is to identify the cause. Once the cause is known, a course of treatment can be implemented. Eating moist foods and drinking water or sugarless beverages with meals are front-line solutions. Sucking on sugarless candy can stimulate the salivary glands, and keeping a water bottle close by can help moisten the mouth between meals (National Institute of Dental and Craniofacial Research, 2005).

Malnutrition and Nutrient Deficits

In the United States it is estimated that 40% of nursing home residents and 50% of hospitalized elderly patients are malnourished (Chen, Schilling, & Lyder, 2001). In the literature there are two clinical approaches to define malnutrition in the older adult. The first definition characterizes malnutrition as any insufficient dietary intake among essential nutrients. The second approach refers to malnutrition as protein–energy undernutrition. Protein–energy undernutrition is the progressive loss of both lean body muscle mass (**sarcopenia**) and adipose tissue resulting from insufficient consumption of protein and energy, although one or the other may play the dominant role in the elderly (Chen et al., 2001).

Sarcopenia: Progress reduction in muscle mass with aging.

From the literature, three measurement systems have been used in identifying malnutrition in the older population, including dietary intake, biochemical indices, and **anthropometrics.** Most nutritional assessment instruments also use all three aspects of measurement plus some clinical assessment such as anorexia or comorbid conditions. The Mini Nutritional Assessment is an example of this mixing of measurement systems. It should be noted that, to date, no single measurement has emerged as optimal in defining malnutrition in the older person (Chen et al., 2001).

Anthropometrics: Measurements of the human body.

● Learning Point Malnutrition in the older individual affects muscle mass even more than in younger individuals with the same degree of weight loss; also, correcting malnutrition in the older person is more difficult than in the younger person with a similar degree of weight loss. The importance of prevention should therefore be stressed (Kinney, 2004).

Weight Loss

The older adult must be evaluated periodically for unintended weight loss. Weight and height should be obtained at each visit using the same scale and without shoes. Body mass index is a ratio of body weight in kilograms divided by the height in square meters. The body mass index can guide the health care provider in determining the overall weight status of the patient. A body mass index of less than 18.5 kg/m^2 is considered underweight, 18.5 to 24.9 kg/m^2 is normal, 25 to 29.9 kg/m^2 is overweight, and higher than 30.0 kg/m^2 is considered obese (Amin, Kuhle, & Fitzpatrick, 2003).

Weight loss exceeding 5% in 1 month or 10% in 6 months deserves a complete evaluation, including a detailed physical examination, review of age-indicated preventive measures, pertinent screening tools, psychosocial assessment, review of medications, medical history, and laboratory and radiologic testing when indicated. Risk factors for poor nutritional status and subsequent weight loss are listed in **Table 13.4**.

Energy and Caloric Intake

Numerous studies have shown energy intake declines with age, making a nutritionally adequate diet more difficult to achieve. A reduction in **basal metabolic rate** is partly responsible for this decline in energy and caloric intake, but a reduction in lean body mass and decreased physical activity appear to be the major causes (Wahlqvist & Savige, 2000).

> **Basal metabolic rate:** The minimal amount of energy required to sustain life in the waking state.

Protein-Energy Malnutrition

Protein plays an important role in the maintenance of the elderly person's health. Illness or inadequate intake may result in protein–energy malnutrition, a condition more common among elderly patients, especially those in institutionalized care (Wahlqvist & Savige, 2000). Chronic deficiency of protein in the elderly person's diet may result in poor wound healing, **decubitus ulcer** development, depressed immune function, osteoporosis, and loss of muscle strength (Chrnoff, 1996). Protein

> **Decubitus ulcer:** Focal ischemic necrosis of skin and underlying tissue at sites of constant pressure or recurring friction in patients immobilized by illness or disability.

TABLE 13.4	Risk Factors for Weight Loss

Alcohol or substance abuse
Cognitive dysfunction
Depression
Functional limitations
Inadequate financial resources
Limited education
Limited mobility
Transportation issues
Chronic medical illness
Poor dentition
Restricted diet
Poor eating habits
Social isolation

foods are rich in other essential nutrients as well; their inclusion in the elderly individual's diet should be encouraged.

Vitamin D

Vitamin D deficiency has special implications for the elderly, especially those who are institutionalized or homebound. Although dietary consumption of vitamin D through fortified dairy products, sardines, and egg yolks can provide part of the daily allowance, natural sunlight is another important source. Aging skin, deteriorating renal function, and physical inactivity (with the possible consequence of less sunlight exposure) are factors that contribute to a greater likelihood of vitamin D deficiency in older adults, thus making them more susceptible to osteoporosis (Wahlqvist & Savige, 2000). The Dietary Reference Intake for vitamin D is 15 mg, three times higher than the younger adult (National Academy Press, n.d.).

Thiamin

Thiamin intakes vary considerably between different elderly populations. Thiamin deficiency is usually associated with poor intakes rather than an increased need, although some studies have shown that the biochemical status of older adults can indicate the presence of thiamin deficiency despite seemingly adequate intakes (Wahlqvist & Savige, 2000). Thiamin deficiency is often responsible for symptoms of peripheral neuropathy.

Vitamin B_6

A number of studies have suggested that age-related changes occur in both the absorption and metabolism of this vitamin, and as a consequence, aged adults may have a higher requirement. Vitamin B_6 is commonly found in meat and leafy greens, and deficiency of this vitamin often lead to impaired immune function and impaired cognitive function.

Vitamin B_{12}

Vitamin B_{12} deficiency is more common among older adults because of the prevalence of pernicious anemia and atrophic gastritis, which appear to increase with age. Also, the prevalence of *Helicobacter pylori* increases with age and has been shown to be associated with vitamin B_{12} malabsorption, possibly because it contributes to gastric atrophy. Deficiency of vitamin B_{12} increases the risk of irreversible neurologic damage and can likely contribute to homocysteine concentrations that are associated with vascular disease (Wahlqvist & Savige, 2000).

Fluid

Aging adults are more susceptible to the risk of dehydration due to alterations in thirst responses, decreasing renal function, and certain medical conditions. Moreover, a reduction in total body water with age also increases the susceptibility of elderly people to dehydration (Wahlqvist & Savige, 2000).

Nutrition-Related Health Problems

Although nutrition-related health problems can occur at any age, the older adult is at risk for accumulation of health problems due to years of life. In this section, vascular conditions, incontinence, visual function, and osteoporosis are discussed.

Cardiovascular Disease

Cardiovascular disease is the most common cause of death and disability in the developed world. Dietary habits may contribute to or provide protection against the risk factors associated with cardiovascular disease (Wahlqvist & Savige, 2000). Diet influences the pathogenesis of coronary artery disease in a variety of ways. The principal mechanism by which fat and cholesterol ingestion translate into increased cardiovascular risk is the induced elevation of serum lipoproteins, especially low-density lipoprotein. The initial development of fatty streaks in coronary arteries is mediated by serum lipid levels and free radical oxidation, both of which are modified by nutrients (Katz, 2000).

An inverse relationship was found between fish consumption and coronary heart disease mortality. Also, excess alcohol consumption is associated with hypertension, a risk factor for cardiovascular disease, yet moderate consumption may be protective against cardiovascular disease through its favorable effect on high-density lipoprotein cholesterol. Elevated homocysteine levels have been identified as an independent risk factor for cardiovascular disease,

and it was found that elderly adults with better folate status had lower homocysteine levels. Foods that have high amounts of folate include breakfast cereal, fruit, orange juice, and leafy green vegetables.

Dietary counseling is an essential component in the primary prevention of heart disease. It is also an essential component in the clinical management of all patients with established coronary heart disease and in those with risk factors (Katz, 2000).

Peripheral Vascular and Cerebrovascular Disease

The dietary recommendations for the prevention and modification of cardiovascular risk generally are pertinent for peripheral vascular disease and cerebrovascular disease. Peripheral vascular disease is associated with elevated plasma homocysteine levels and, therefore, may be amenable to treatment with B vitamin and folate supplementation in certain patients. Also, elevated postprandial insulin levels appear to be an independent risk factor, suggesting that dietary intervention to improve glycemic control may play a role in the prevention and control of peripheral vascular disease (Katz, 2000).

The predominant risk factor for stoke is hypertension, which can be prevented and modified by dietary interventions. Dietary sodium restriction and generous intake of potassium, magnesium, and calcium may lower blood pressure (Katz, 2000).

Incontinence

Urinary and fecal **incontinence** are common and often debilitating conditions in older people. Urinary incontinence is reported to afflict approximately half the elderly living in institutions and 15% to 30% of community-based elderly (Wahlqvist & Savige, 2000). Dietary interventions that encourage an adequate intake of fluid and a variety of plant foods that are a good source of dietary fiber may assist in alleviating some of the problems that can cause incontinence (Wahlqvist & Savige, 2000).

Incontinence: Inability to control the discharge of urine or feces.

Visual Function

Cataracts and age-related **macular degeneration** are common causes of visual impairment in older adults. Nutrients may play a very important role in vision; for example, the antioxidants alpha-tocopherol, beta-carotene, and ascorbic acid may help to prevent cataract formation and macular degeneration (Wahlqvist & Savige, 2000). Therefore a diet rich in fruits and green leafy

Cataract: Complete or partial opacity of the ocular lens.

Macular degeneration: An eye disease that affects the macula, a part of the retina.

vegetables should be recommended as primary prevention of age-related eye disease. In those over the age of 50 or with less than judicious diets, supplementation with vitamin C 500 mg, vitamin E 400 to 800 IU, and zinc may be helpful in the prevention of age-related eye disease (Katz, 2000).

Osteoporosis

According to the 2004 Surgeon General's report on bone health and osteoporosis, the cost of caring for bone fractures from osteoporosis is $18 billion each year (U.S. Department of Health and Human Services, 2004). According to the National Institute of Arthritis and Musculoskeletal and Skin Diseases

Osteoporosis: Reduction in the quantity of bone.

(2006), **osteoporosis** affects more than 10 million adults in the United States, and millions more are at risk for the disease. Risk factors for osteoporosis are numerous and include gender, ethnicity, and life-style. **Table 13.5** provides a comprehensive list.

Dietary management is fundamental to the primary and secondary prevention of osteoporosis. The origins of osteoporosis are in childhood and adolescence, during which time adequate physical activity and dietary calcium are particularly important. Peak bone density is reached by around the end of the third decade (Katz, 2000). Many dietary factors have implications for bone health.

> **● Learning Point** Sodium, caffeine, and alcohol have been negatively associated with bone status. Specific nutrients that may play an important role in maintaining bone health include protein, vitamin D, calcium, vitamin K, and boron (Wahlqvist & Savige, 2000).

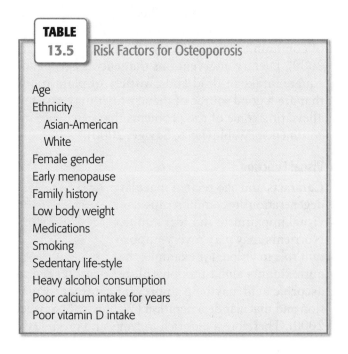

TABLE 13.5 Risk Factors for Osteoporosis

Age
Ethnicity
   Asian-American
   White
Female gender
Early menopause
Family history
Low body weight
Medications
Smoking
Sedentary life-style
Heavy alcohol consumption
Poor calcium intake for years
Poor vitamin D intake

Dietary recommendations should focus on diversity in the diet, consumption of low-fat dairy products, calcium and vitamin D fortified foods, avoiding or quitting smoking, limiting alcohol intake, and engaging in consistent weight-bearing physical activity, at least some of which should be outdoors in sunlight. In older adults at risk, vitamin D supplementation with 400 to 600 IU and calcium intake of about 1,500 mg/day is advisable (Katz, 2000).

Special Considerations for the Older Woman

Women face unique challenges with aging, partially due to their long life expectancy. According to the Centers for Disease Control and Prevention, a female born in 2003 has a life expectancy of 80.1 years compared with 74.8 years for a male born in the same year. White women have a longer life expectancy than African-American women, reported at 80.5 years compared with 76.1 years, respectively (National Center for Health Statistics, n.d.). Disease and disability increase with advanced aging. Women live longer but have more chronic health conditions than men. These conditions include osteoporosis, depression, Sjögren syndrome, rheumatoid arthritis, and other autoimmune diseases (U.S. Department of Health and Human Services, n.d.-a). Older women are also more likely than older men to live in poverty, live in long-term care, or live alone (ADA, 2005b).

One of the conditions unique to women is menopause. Like adolescence, it is a natural process in a woman's life span. A woman is in menopause when she has not had a menstrual cycle for 12 consecutive months. Although normally this occurs in the late forties or early fifties, a woman who has had her ovaries surgically removed will experience the physiologic condition.

For many women menopause brings unpleasant side effects such as hot flashes, mood swings, sleep disturbances, night sweats, depression, and weight gain. Menopause can also bring serious health concerns because it increases the risk for bone loss and heart disease. Eighty percent of adults with osteoporosis are women (National Institute of Arthritis and Musculoskeletal and Skin Diseases, 2006). Historically, hormone replacement therapy has been used to prevent bone loss and to treat the symptoms of menopause. This practice has known benefits for bone health but has been linked to breast, uterine, and ovarian cancer and heart disease. Prescribing hormone replacement therapy is no longer routine, and recommendations are based on the woman's family history and degree of symptoms. Soy isoflavones, exercise, vitamin supplements, and stress reduction techniques are some alternatives for women who choose to forgo hormone replacement therapy due to the risks.

Summary

Aging brings unique challenges that encompass physical, mental, social, and financial changes. Special attention to food selection is important to meet the demands of the aging process and accompanying health issues. The ultimate goal of maintaining the highest quality of life possible through the life span is as important in the older adult as with any other age. Independence, dignity, well-being, and social interaction are desired by all human beings. Regular nutrition screening with early interventions, when problems are identified, can enhance the quality of life of the older adult.

Issue to Debate

Hormone Replacement Therapy: Benefits and Risks

Perimenopause and the transition to menopause are marked by a time in a woman's life when progesterone and estrogen levels are changing in response to an aging body. These changes are companied by symptoms ranging from mild to severe that can disrupt a woman's daily life. Unfortunately, other "silent" but significant changes are occurring. Bone mineral density can be lost during this time, placing the woman at risk for fractures, tooth loss from declining jawbone, pain, and disability.

The National Heart, Lung, and Blood Institute and the National Cancer Institute, parts of the National Institutes of Health, sponsored the Women's Health Initiative Hormone Program that examined the effects of hormone replacement therapy on women's health. Researchers conducted two studies using hormone therapy. One study involved estrogen alone and the other tested estrogen plus progestin. The estrogen plus progestin study was stopped in 2002 when researchers determined that the risks of heart disease, stroke, blood clots, and breast cancer outweighed the benefits. The estrogen alone study was stopped in 2004 due to increased risk of stroke and blood clots. Researchers found no significant effect on the risk of breast or colorectal cancer in the estrogen only group (National Institute on Aging, 2005).

Hormone replacement therapy can assist in preserving bone loss, reduce the risk of colorectal cancer, and assist in managing unpleasant symptoms of menopause.

1. Considering the known risks and benefits of hormone replacement therapy, how should a woman choose which course to take?

Case Study

A 79-year-old woman was evaluated in an outpatient clinic. She lives with her 81-year-old husband, who is her primary caregiver. He reports that approximately 2 years ago his wife began to lose interest in the things she enjoyed, like shopping, cooking, and sewing. Gradually, she become less interested in food and has lost 18 pounds in the past year. He has tried commercial nutritional supplements but has not been successful in getting her to consume them. He stated he is not much of a cook but has been trying his best. He is frustrated and concerned about his wife's weight loss and lack of appetite. He believes he is constantly trying to get her to eat. He does not have any family support because he and his wife never had children. Her medical evaluation revealed cognitive impairment using the Mini Mental State Examination. She does not appear to have any chewing or swallowing problems but has not seen a dentist in over 3 years. She takes one prescription medication for her arthritis.

1. What questions would you like to ask her husband?
2. What strategies might be appropriate for her treatment plan?
3. Do you have concerns about her husband and his ability to care for her?

Case Study

Mrs. Walker is a 74-year-old non-Hispanic white woman. She is 62 inches tall and weighs 112 pounds. She has lost 2 inches in height in the past 20 years. She smokes half a pack of cigarettes a day and has been a smoker for 54 years. About 18 months ago she began to experience mouth pain. A dental examination revealed several loose teeth due to severe gum disease. She has had significant dental work in the past year, which has resulted in five extracts. A partial plate with false teeth was attempted but due to continued mouth pain was not worn regularly. Mrs. Walker has altered her diet due to her poor dentition. She no longer eats fresh fruits, salad, steak, nuts, or other hard-to-chew foods. She rarely eats out anymore. It takes her twice as long to eat as a few years ago. She plans to have a full upper jaw extraction and be fitted for a full denture when she has the money. Since her dental problems began, she has lost 11 pounds. She is depressed and frustrated by the changes she has had to make in her diet. Eating has become a chore and has lost the pleasure it once had.

1. What risk factors does Mrs. Walker have for developing malnutrition?
2. What concerns you the most about this case?
3. What suggestions to do have for Mrs. Walker?

Website Resources

Alzheimer's Association www.alz.org

Administration on Aging www.aoa.gov

Food Safety Information for Seniors www. foodsafety.gov

Nestle Nutrition; Mini Nutritional Assessment www.nma-elderly.com

NIH Senior Health www.nihseniorhealth.gov

Centers for Disease Control and Prevention www.cdc.gov

Center for Medicare Services www.cms.hhs.gov

National Osteoporosis Foundation www.nof.org

Women's Health Information www.womenshealth. gov

National Institute on Deafness and Other Communication Disorders www.nidcd.nih.gov

References

Amin, S. H., Kuhle, C. L., & Fitzpatrick, L. A. (2003). Comprehensive evaluation of the older woman. *Mayo Clinic Proceedings, 78*, 1157–1185.

Alzheimer's Association. (2006). Fact sheet: Eating. Retrieved May 12, 2006, from http://www.alz.org.

American Dietetic Association (ADA). (2002). The National Dysphagia Diet Task Force. *The National Dysphagia Diet: Standardization for Optimal Care.* Chicago: American Dietetic Association.

American Dietetic Association (ADA). (2003a). Position of the American Dietetic Association: Food and water safety. *Journal of the American Dietetic Association, 103*, 1203–1217.

American Dietetic Association (ADA). (2003b). Position of the American Dietetic Association: Oral health and nutrition. *Journal of the American Dietetic Association, 103*, 615–623.

American Dietetic Association (ADA). (2005a). Position of the American Dietetic Association: Liberalization of the diet prescription improves quality of life for older adults in long-term care. *Journal of the American Dietetic Association, 105*, 1955–1965.

American Dietetic Association (ADA). (2005b). Position of the American Dietetic Association: Nutrition across the spectrum of aging. *Journal of the American Dietetic Association, 105*, 616–633.

Bailey, R. L., Ledikwe, J. H., Smiciklas-Wright, H., Mitchell, D. C., & Jensen, G. L. (2004). Persistent oral health problems associated with comorbidity and impaired diet quality in older adults. *Journal of the American Dietetic Association, 104*, 1273–1276.

Blumberg, J. B. (1997). Nutritional needs of seniors. *Journal of the American College of Nutrition, 16*, 517–523.

Centers for Medicare and Medicaid Services. (n.d.). Dental coverage. Retrieved March 18, 2006, from http://www.cms.hhs.gov/MedicareDentalCoverage.

Chen, C. C., Schilling, L. S., & Lyder, C. H. (2001). A concept analysis of malnutrition in the elderly. *Journal of Advanced Nursing, 36*, 131–142.

Chrnoff, R. (1996). Nutrition. In D. Jahnigen & R. Schrier (Eds.), *Geriatric Medicine* (2nd ed.). Cambridge, MA: Blackwell Science.

Council for Nutritional Strategies in Long-Term Care. Council on Nutrition Appetite Questionnaire. Retrieved March 18, 2006 from http://medschool.slu.edu/agingsuccessfully/pdfsurveys/appetitequestionnaire.pdf.

de Jong, N., Mulder, I., de Graaf, C., & Van Staveren, W. A. (1999). Impaired sensory functioning in elders: The relationship with its potential determinants and nutritional intake. *The Journals of Gerontology. Series A, Biological Sciences and Medical Sciences, 54*, B324–B331.

Deering, C., Russell, C., & Womack, P. (2001). *Perspectives on Dysphagia: A Continuing Education Self-Study Guide for Dietetics Professionals.* Chicago: American Dietetic Association.

Gollub, E. A., & Weddle, D. O. (2004). Improvement in nutritional intake and quality of life among frail homebound older adults receiving home-delivered breakfast and lunch. *Journal of the American Dietetic Association, 104*, 1227–1235.

Katz, D. L. (2000). *Nutrition in Clinical Practice* (1st ed.). Philadelphia: Lippincott Williams and Wilkins.

Kinney, J. M. (2004). Nutritional frailty, sarcopenia and falls in the elderly. *Current Opinion in Clinical Nutrition and Metabolic Care, 7*, 15–20.

Kurlowitz, L., & Wallace, M. (1999). *The Mini Mental State Examination (MMSE). Best Practices in Nursing Care to Older Adults.* New York: Hartford Institute for Geriatric Nursing.

Mathey, N., de Jong, C. P. G. M., de Groot, C., de Graaf, W. A., & Van Steveren (2001). Assessing appetite in Dutch elderly with the Appetite, Hunger, Sensory Perception (AHSP) questionnaire. *Journal of Nutrition, Health, and Aging, 5*, 22–28.

Morley, J. E. (2001). Decreased food intake with aging. *The Journals of Gerontology. Series A, Biological Sciences and Medical Sciences, 56*, 81–88.

National Academy Press. (n.d.). National Academy of Science. Dietary Reference Intake tables. Retrieved May 12, 2006, from www.nap.edu.

National Center for Chronic Disease Prevention and Health Promotion. (2005). Fact sheet: Key findings from NHANES 1999–2002. Retrieved March 18, 2006, from http://www.cdc.gov/oralhealth/factsheets/nhanes_findings.htm.

National Center for Health Statistics. (n.d.). Life expectancy at birth, at 65 years of age, and at 75 years of age according to race and sex, United States selected years, 1900–2003. Retrieved June 30, 2006, from http://www.cdc.gov/nchs/data/hus/hus05.pdf#027.

National Eye Institute. (2005). Age-related macular degeneration. Retrieved on May 14, 2006 from http://nihseniorhealth.gov/agerelatedmaculardegeneration.

National Institute on Aging. (2005). Hormones after menopause. Retrieved on May 14, 2006, from http://www.niapublications.org/agepages/hormonafter.asp.

National Institute of Arthritis and Musculoskeletal and Skin Diseases. (2006). Osteoporosis. Retrieved on May 12, 2006, from www.nihseniorhealth.org.

National Institute of Dental and Craniofacial Research. (2005). Dry mouth. Retrieved on May 14, 2006, from http://www.nihseniorhealth.org/drymouth.

Nestle Clinical Research. (1998). Mini Nutritional Assessment. Retrieved on May 14, 2006, from http://mna-elderly.com.

Nutrition Screening Initiative. (1991). Determine Your Nutritional Health Checklist. Retrieved on February 25, 2006, from http://www.aafp.org/x17367.xml.

Office of Disease Prevention and Health Promotion, U.S. Department of Health and Human Services. (n.d.). *Healthy People 2010.* Retrieved on March 18, 2006, from www.healthypeople.gov.

Ritchie, C. S. (2002). Oral health, taste, and olfaction. *Clinics in Geriatric Medicine, 18,* 709–717.

Sahyoun, N. R., & Krall, E. (2003). Low dietary quality among older adults with self-perceived ill-fitting dentures. *Journal of the American Dietetic Association, 103,* 1494–1499.

Ship, J. A. (2002). Improving oral health in older people. *Journal of the American Geriatrics Society, 50,* 1454–1455.

U.S. Administration on Aging. (n.d.-a). The Elderly Nutrition Program. Retrieved June 30, 2006, from http://www.aoa.gov/press/fact/alpha/fact_elderly_nutrition.asp.

U.S. Administration on Aging. (n.d.-b). Addressing diversity. Retrieved May 14, 2006, from http://www.aoa.gov/prof/adddiv/adddiv.asp.

U.S. Department of Health and Human Services. (n.d.-a). Sex differences in autoimmune disease. Retrieved on May 14, 2006, from http://www.womenshealth.gov.

U.S. Department of Health and Human Services. (n.d.-b). Sex differences in musculoskeletal health. Retrieved on May 14, 2006, from http://www.womenshealth.gov.

U.S. Department of Health and Human Services. (2004). The 2004 Surgeon General's report on bone health and osteoporosis: What it means to you. Retrieved on May 14, 2006, from http://www.surgeongeneral.gov.

Wahlqvist, M. L., & Savige, G. S. (2000). Intervention aimed at dietary and lifestyle changes to promote healthy aging. *European Journal of Clinical Nutrition, 54,* S148–S156.

Wilson, M. M., Thomas, D. R., Rubenstein, L. Z., Chibnall, J. T., Anderson, S., Baxi, A., et al. (2005). Appetite assessment, simple appetite questionnaire predicts weight loss in community-dwelling adults and nursing home residents. *American Journal of Clinical Nutrition, 82,* 1074–1081.

Special Topics Related to the Registered Dietitian and Older Adults: Roles and Responsibilities of the Registered Dietitian in Long-Term Care

Victoria Hammer Castellanos, PhD, RD, and Angela Sader, RD, LD, MBA

CHAPTER OUTLINE

After studying this chapter and reflecting on the contents, you should be able to

1. Discuss the fundamental differences between nutrition care delivery in the long-term care setting compared with other care settings, including prioritization of resident quality of life and a regulatory environment that drives patient care.

2. Describe the clinical and management responsibilities that regularly fall to the dietitian within the long-term care setting.

3. Identify the management opportunities for long-term care dietitians within the areas of clinical care, food service management, survey management, and **risk management.**

Risk management: Identification of areas where harm may occur to an individual, such as in the case of a fall with injury. Taking precautions to limit the number of times this situation may occur is the responsibility of facility management.

Unique Characteristics of Long-Term Care

Approximately 1.5 million older adults currently reside in long-term care (LTC) facilities. Having its own unique culture and challenges, a number of factors set apart the delivery of nutrition care in nursing homes compared with other care settings (Castellanos, 2004). The nursing home environment has the following characteristics:

- The facility is considered to be the resident's home. Although some residents stay in the facility only for a few weeks or months, many residents live out the remainder of their life in this setting.
- A large segment of the population is both very old and quite frail. However, a growing number of residents are somewhat younger adults who are suffering from an acute illness or injury and who expect to return home after a period of recovery or rehabilitation.
- Usually, both long-term and short-term stay residents suffer from a host of chronic and acute disease conditions.
- The resident's physical ability to eat enough food is often greatly reduced because of aging and/or disease processes.
- Nutrition care is, at the same time, both driven and hindered by the regulatory environment. The characteristics of skilled nursing facilities and the residents themselves make nutritional well-being difficult to achieve in this setting but present a rare opportunity for the nutrition professional to significantly impact both the health outcomes and quality of life of a significant number of people.

Types of LTC Centers

LTC is a designation given to any facility-based operation that has accepted the responsibility of caring for patients deemed to require some form of 24-hour-a-day supervision to meet their care-related needs. The types of LTC centers are described in Table 14.1. The goals of all LTC facilities are similar; each is expected to help the patients under their care reach the highest level of living and activity possible through the administration of nonskilled and/or skilled services.

Whether or not a person is qualified to reside in an LTC facility primarily depends on a certified physician recommending that individual for LTC ser-

TABLE 14.1 Types of LTC Centers	
Facility Type	**Function**
Skilled nursing facilities (SNFs, pronounced "sniffs")	Facilities approved to accept Medicaid and Medicare for payment when the resident qualifies. The resident population of most SNFs represents a variety of payer sources, i.e., Medicaid, Medicare, insurance, hospice, and self-pay.
Hospital-based facilities	LTC facilities under the umbrella of a hospital organization. These are usually SNFs but may be private placement or government sponsored. Because the billing mechanism is quite different in an acute care hospital from that of an LTC facility, the RD employed in this environment will be required to keep careful track of hours spent in each unit.
Private placement facilities, also called private pay facilities	Facilities in which the resident assumes all responsibility for payment of stay, either through insurance or self-pay.
Government-sponsored facilities	Medicaid certified but not Medicare certified

vices. There are state and **federal regulations** that provide guidance to the physicians regarding placement decisions. The acuity level of LTC residents varies from residents who have a relatively small need for services to residents who require extensive observation, care, and oversight to ensure quality care.

Federal regulations: Documents published by the Centers for Medicare and Medicaid Services for use in the survey process for long-term care facilities.

Significant cost is associated with LTC. There are programs designed to reduce the personal financial burden, including Medicare (federally funded), Medicaid (state indigent care funds), Medicare Part B (federally funded), Veterans Administration (federally funded), insurance, and hospice (federally funded). All these payer sources are designed to help individuals requiring LTC services to receive those benefits even if personal funds are not available.

LTC facilities range in size from a few to over 200 residents. Depending on their business classification, facilities may be designated as "for profit" or "not for profit," "private ownership," or "publicly traded." Expectations for resident care are similar across business classifications, but internal rules and policies may vary depending on acuity of residents, number of residents involved, and reimbursement from external sources.

The exact cost of care in an LTC facility varies depending on many factors. Pricing is affected by the number of associates the individual requires to assist them with care (i.e., does it require one or two persons to move them?), room size, age of facility, services offered, the level of care, acuity of the resident, and many other factors. It is common practice for a daily rate sheet to be provided to a potential resident that lists the services covered for a flat daily fee. This varies from facility to facility. Additional services must be reimbursed by the resident's personal funds. For example, the daily rate may not cover the cost of services provided by the beautician, cable television, and so on. Although residents receive similar care regardless of payer source, out of consideration for the resident, it is important that registered dietitians (RDs) are aware of services that may cause a financial burden to the resident. For example, if a resident is not covered under Medicare or if he or she does not have private insurance, the resident is responsible for the cost of goods and services such as adaptive eating devices and laboratory blood work. Where possible, the RD should strive to achieve positive results with care approaches that are not a financial burden to the resident or family (e.g., only recommend that additional blood work be completed when the results of the laboratory analysis are clearly necessary to determine whether or not the current plan of care should be modified).

Nursing Home Regulation Drives Nutrition Care

The regulatory environment has a tremendous impact on nutrition care in the LTC setting. Nursing homes are heavily regulated at both the federal and state levels. This is in contrast to community-based care and other types of LTC that are regulated only by the states; regulations for community-based care are generally sparse. The **Centers for Medicare and Medicaid Services** enforces many specific regulations related to food and nutrition care delivery in nursing homes (American Health Care Association, 2005). The Centers for Medicare and Medicaid Services normally contracts with state health depart-

Centers for Medicare and Medicaid Services: The federal agency responsible for nursing home regulations and their enforcement. The Centers for Medicare and Medicaid Services is part of the U.S. Department of Health and Human Services.

ments to complete the surveys according to federal regulations (i.e., "state survey"). Each state has additional regulations that must also be followed and are enforced by the state surveyors.

One cannot underemphasize the extent to which the state and federal regulations drive nutrition care delivery in the nursing home setting. Success as an LTC practitioner requires one to become intimately familiar with these regulations. To help drive this point home, we have referred to some of the relevant federal nursing home regulations throughout this chapter. A summary of the **Federal Nursing Home Regulation for Nutrition Services** can be found at the American Health Care Association Website at www.ahcancal.org.

Federal Nursing Home Regulation for Nutrition Services: Documents published by the Centers for Medicare and Medicaid Services for use in the survey process for long-term care facilities that focus on the nutritional oversight and delivery to the residents in the facility.

Structure of the Nutritional Services Department

The nutritional services department is composed of the RD, the dietary service manager (DSM), dietetic technician, and all staff involved in food production and service. It is the standard division of responsibilities in most nursing homes that the nutritional services department is responsible for getting the appropriate food and drinks to the resident's dining area, whereas it is the responsibility of the nursing staff to feed the resident. Licensed nurses are responsible for supervising the provision of food and fluid to residents by certified nursing assistants. During their training, certified nursing assistants are taught techniques to assist and/or feed residents with various kinds of health problems, including dysphagia (swallowing disorders). Federal regulation also allows for paid feeding assistants to help feed residents at low risk for choking, although not all states allow paid feeding assistants.

The basis for nutritional services staffing in the LTC facility begins with regulations F361 and 362, which state that the facility must have adequate personnel to provide dietary services and that a qualified dietitian is utilized in planning, managing, and implementing dietary service activities. The RD staff is then expanded to meet the requirements of the residing state and the needs of the facility residents.

State staffing requirements are highly variable. A particular state may go so far as to define the components of a nutritional assessment and identify the professionals appropriate to complete the task as a whole or parts of the task. A state may also specify the minimum number of hours an RD must be present in a facility to provide services or dictate the number of RD hours based on facility census or the number of nursing stations. Some states have requirements related to the dietary manager that affect both DSM and RD staffing. For example, if a state requires that the DSM complete an approved course by the Dietary Managers Association to become a "certified dietary manager," completion of the course requires oversight and training of the DSM by the RD. The assignment of responsibilities within the nutritional services department varies depending on facility characteristics and state regulations.

> **● Learning Point**   The RD is responsible for reviewing the menu (for nutritional adequacy, appropriate therapeutic combinations, serving sizes, etc.), providing staff education, and providing residents with medical nutrition therapy (MNT) through assessment and appropriate intervention.

Facilities frequently use a DSM to manage department staffing, meal production, procurement, food service sanitation, and the budget. As per regulation the DSM must be under the oversight of an RD. In a smaller facility, and if state regulation allows, it is not uncommon for the DSM to be the staff member responsible for the collection of subjective and objective resident information to be used by the RD in his or her resident assessment. In this scenario, it is the responsibility of the RD to review the DSM's completion of the aforementioned activities. If a facility is larger or if a state requires that a licensed/registered health care practitioner complete documentation in the medical record, the facility may hire a dietetic technician to assist with clinical documentation. Various other staffing scenarios are also possible.

After meeting the regulatory requirements, RD staffing in a facility is largely determined by the facility census, the level of care provided, and the average number of admissions per week. Individual facilities usually have a predetermined number of beds set aside for Medicare (i.e., short term) versus long-term residents. Residents who are admitted under Medicare after discharge from an acute care facility are usually more medically complex than long-term stay residents. These residents are more likely to be on dialysis, have pressure ulcers, require enteral therapy, or require other types of MNT. Further, Medicare beds turn over more frequently, and with each new admission it is necessary for the RD to spend a significant amount of time on the initial nutritional as-

sessment and development of comprehensive **care plans.**

For example, it is a common mistake to assume nutritional services staffing should be the same for equivalently sized facilities (e.g., 120 beds) in the same state. However, the facility with 25 Medicare beds (resulting in an average of seven new admissions per week) and 10 residents receiving enteral feeding requires more RD time for admission assessments, MNT documentation, and enteral therapy follow-up than a facility with only 4 Medicare beds and 2 residents receiving enteral feeding.

> **Care plans:** As per the Centers for Medicare and Medicaid Services regulation, a facility must use an interdisciplinary approach to develop a comprehensive care plan for each resident that includes measurable objectives and timetables to meet a resident's medical, nursing, mental, and psychosocial needs. These care plans must be revised as the resident's status changes.

Roles of the Dietitian Within the Nutritional Services Department

Whether the services of an RD are provided by a consultant dietitian or regular employee of the company, the role of the RD in the LTC setting is central to the health and well-being of the residents and goes far beyond the responsibility of patient assessment. The RD's time in the facility is not only spent on MNT but in review of the nutritional services department and all the processes related to providing nutrition care to the residents. In the LTC setting the RD must be prepared to use skills in staff and patient education, quality management, menu planning, food production, food safety, product selection and purchasing, emergency planning, and budget management, including labor utilization.

One of the most critical functions of the dietitian in the nursing home setting is to make sure that the facility is meeting both federal and state regulations relevant to nutrition services. The nutrition professional in the nursing home setting will use a wide variety of skills and training to assist a facility in maintaining compliance with regulations and provide appropriate care to residents.

Clinical Care Delivery in the LTC Setting

Regulations require nursing facilities to meet the nutritional needs of residents (F325-327 and F360-367) while maintaining their dignity and quality of life (F240 and F241). This is also the ethical responsibility of providers. After all, the LTC facility is "home" for this population of older adults.

Residence in a nursing home is unlike a brief admission to a hospital, where limited choice and reduced quality of life are justified by short-term clinical goals. But, like a hospital, decisions regarding the menu and the exact nature of meal and snack service are made on a facility-wide basis. The implications for LTC residents are that each food, dining environment, and staffing decision made at the facility level will serve to either limit or expand the nutrition and eating pleasure available to that individual for a significant portion of his or her life.

Although such decisions bring with them significant responsibility, they also afford tremendous opportunity for the care provider. That is to say that the nursing home has both the infrastructure and consistency of client contact that make it possible to move beyond a *reactive* medical model and to adopt a *proactive,* prevention-focused, home-like approach to nutrition care. For example, weight loss and pressure ulcer prevention committees are often created in facilities. These committees meet frequently to review individual residents who have risk factors for weight loss or pressure ulcers and to initiate interventions designed to prevent weight loss or wounds from developing.

The nutritional needs of nursing home residents are likely to be affected by both illness and advanced age. Most nursing home residents are medically frail, with at least five chronic health conditions, and suffer intermittent bouts of acute illnesses, such as infection and diarrhea. These disease states tend to increase nutrient needs. Further, some aspects of institutional living may affect nutritional needs; for example, little or no exposure to sunlight makes residents highly dependent on dietary and supplemental sources of vitamin D (Institute of Medicine, 1997).

Most nutrition-related problems in nursing homes are a consequence of undernutrition. These may include unintended weight loss, protein–energy malnutrition, pressure ulcers, and dehydration (American Dietetic Association [ADA], 2005). A host of additional nutrient deficiencies are likely to occur as an accompaniment to inadequate food intake, including vitamin and mineral deficiencies. For most nursing home residents, the risk of morbidity and mortality related to undernutrition exceeds the potential for adverse outcomes of chronic disease (ADA, 2005). Having said this, there are few data on which to base standards of nutrition care for the frail oldest adults.

There are few published data regarding the food and fluid intake patterns of LTC residents. Some reports suggest that LTC residents consume a greater proportion of their breakfast meal than they do of other meals, especially dinner (Chapman, Samman, & Liburne, 1993; Endres, Welch, Ashraf, Banz, & Gower, 2000; Simmons & Reuben, 2000; Young, Binns, & Greenwood, 2001; Castellanos, Surloff, & Giordan, 2003c); however, there is typically a smaller quantity of food served at breakfast than at lunch and dinner. A study by Young et al. (2001) found that older adults with dementia tend to eat less food as the day progresses. Also, a study looking at snack interventions found that residents consumed significantly less during the evening snack period than during the morning or afternoon snack (Simmons & Schnelle, 2004).

Inadequate hydration is a significant issue in the LTC setting (Chidester & Spangler, 1997; Kayser-Jones, Schell, Porter, Barbaccia, & Shaw, 1999). Older adults in nursing facilities are likely to be unwell, have limited access to palatable fluids, and are at greater risk for suboptimal hydration than other older people (Chidester & Spangler, 1997). Inadequate water intake can contribute to acute confusion, urinary tract infections, pressure ulcers, constipation, and adverse drug responses (American Medical Directors Association, 2002). These problems can lead to increased morbidity and mortality and can escalate health care costs (Chidester & Spangler, 1997; American Medical Directors Association, 2002).

Older people do not always feel thirsty, even when they are dehydrated (Rolls & Phillips, 1990). It may be difficult or impossible for older people with neurologic or musculoskeletal disabilities to obtain or consume liquids independently. In addition, it is not uncommon for nursing home residents to have medical conditions (diarrhea, vomiting, and dysphagia) or to be prescribed treatments (diuretic medications) that put them at increased risk for dehydration. Fortunately, systems put in place to ensure adequate resident assistance with eating are likely to have the added benefit of supporting adequate intake of fluids. For example, one study found that verbal prompting increased fluid intake in 71% of residents, with the range of increase of 5 to 20 oz/day (Simmons, Alessi, & Schnelle, 2001a). Also, hydration programs can be implemented to ensure that fluids offered between meals or with medications are of significant volume, frequency, and palatability to appreciably increase overall fluid intake.

LTC facilities are also filled with people suffering from acute and medically complex illnesses that were once found only in hospitals. For example, knee and hip replacement therapy is now occurring in the LTC facility instead of the hospital. At one time hospitalized people stayed in the hospital until they were well enough to be discharged home. In the current health care system these "patients" are becoming "residents" of skilled nursing facilities. Thus the LTC facility must also have the clinical staff and infrastructure to provide adequate care to severely ill people who often do not eat or drink enough to meet their nutritional needs.

Nutrition Care Process and Timeline

It is important to identify current nutrition problems and the risk of future nutrition problems in a timely fashion. This requires a logical and preplanned sequence of screening, assessments, and reviews. Many of the timeframes are dictated by federal standards, but an individual facility may choose to monitor its residents more closely than required. The policy and procedure manual in the facility should outline the timeframe for all phases of nutrition care.

Within 24 hours of admission to the facility, a member of the nutritional services department should conduct an initial interview to greet the resident, confirm the diet prescription, identify meal preferences and food dislikes, screen the resident for nutrition risk, and introduce the resident to the food service system. The DSM, dietetic technician, or RD may conduct this interview. A brief chart note should be written, and the note should state that the diet order has been confirmed and the resident has been interviewed and screened. Many times, this type of note will conclude by stating that a complete **nutrition assessment** will follow.

A **nutrition screening** is a quick review to determine if the resident meets any known factors for nutrition risk. Each facility should outline a screening process to identify which residents need immediate assessment and which residents should be given a chance to settle in to the facility before the assessment takes place. Typically, a nutrition screening ascertains weight history, albumin level, diagnosis, the presence of feeding tubes, and skin condition. The nutrition screening or interview process should be sensitive enough to identify new residents with feeding tubes, intravenous lines, a diagnosis of malnutrition or dehydration, and other significant nutrition problems. An immediate assessment is warranted with certain diagnoses or the presence of a feeding tube.

Nutrition assessment: A thorough evaluation of the resident's food and eating preferences, medical and nutritional status, estimation of nutritional needs, and identification of medical conditions/treatments and other factors that might make the resident at risk of developing malnutrition in the future. This information is used to develop the individualized plan of nutrition care for the resident.

Nutrition screening: A quick review to determine if the resident meets any known factors for nutrition risk that would require an immediate assessment by a registered dietitian.

Per regulations (F272 and F276), a complete nutrition assessment should be conducted within the first 14 days of admission. Many facilities improve on this standard and make it a policy to complete the assessment by the 7th day of admission. It is often advisable to wait until the resident has been in the facility for several days before completing an assessment. This short delay allows time for the resident to become accustomed to the new surroundings and for body weight and baseline laboratory data to be obtained, dining location secured, and hospital records copied for the nursing home chart. There are a number of resources available to assist the RD in completing the complete assessment. The ADA described in detail the components of the nutritional assessment, which is an essential part of the nutrition care process (Lacey & Pritchett, 2003). In addition, the ADA practice group, Consultant Dietitians in Health Care Facilities, developed written resources that are specifically designed to support the assessment process in the LTC setting (http://www.cdhcf.org).

A **reassessment** of each resident must be performed a minimum of every 3 months (i.e., quarterly). A quarterly review is not as in-depth as a full initial assessment but should determine if the current nutritional regimen is adequate to meet the resident's nutritional needs. If the resident has had a change in medical condition or suffers a significant weight loss, a reassessment must be done even if it is not scheduled. A full assessment, equivalent to the initial assessment, must be completed at the end of each year of residency.

Reassessment: A resident assessment that takes place after a significant change in the resident's status or after 4 months, whichever comes first. The purpose is to determine if the current nutritional regimen is adequate to meet the resident's nutritional needs.

One unique component of the medical record in nursing homes is the **minimum data set (MDS)**. The MDS is an electronic summary of the medical status of each resident. The MDS Section K, Oral/Nutritional Status, is usually completed after the initial nutrition assessment is complete. It is helpful to complete the MDS as soon after the assessment as possible while the information is easily accessible and memorable. It is recommended that the same person who completes the nutrition assessment also completes the MDS. Often, facilities will use an MDS coordinator to complete the entire MDS, but it is preferable that the nutrition care professional be responsible for completing the nutrition section. In some cases the MDS Section K

Minimum data set (MDS): An electronic summary of the medical status of each resident mandated by the Centers for Medicare and Medicaid Services.

may be completed by the DSM because it is just the gathering of objective data from the chart. In this case the MDS coordinator, either a registered nurse or RD, reviews and signs off that Section K was completed accurately.

Dietitians within the facility use the MDS as one way to identify residents who may be experiencing a nutritional problem or who are at risk for a nutritional problem. The use of the MDS in identifying individuals at nutrition risk was validated by Blaum et al. (1997). Once a resident has been identified as being at nutritional risk, the clinician must follow up using **resident assessment protocols**. The resident assessment protocol for malnutrition is "triggered" if any of the following are indicated on the MDS: resident has a weight loss or gain of 5% or more in last 30 days or 10% or more in last 180 days; complains about the taste of many foods; leaves 25% or more food uneaten at most meals; receives a parenteral/intravenous feeding; receives a mechanically altered, syringe (oral feeding), or therapeutic diet; or has a pressure ulcer for which the highest stage is 2, 3, or 4. Once a resident assessment protocol for malnutrition is triggered, the problem must be evaluated and the response documented. This evaluation must be completed by a licensed professional, because it requires clinical judgment as to whether a problem actually exists that would need to be addressed through a care plan. Sometimes, after the assessment a determination is made that a care plan is not necessary. For example, a resident assessment protocol may be triggered because the MDS indicates a resident requires a texture-modified diet. However, subsequent assessment by the RD reveals that the resident has no difficulties eating the texture-modified food that is being provided, her dentures are in good repair, her intake is adequate to meet her needs, and her weight is stable. Because the resident is not experiencing a nutritional problem, there is no need for a care plan.

The process of completing the MDS requires care plans must be complete by the 21st day of admission. The care planning process is an interdisciplinary process, and the nutrition team member should initiate those who relate directly to nutrition and contribute to nursing care plans. The nutritional department usually writes care plans that involve weight loss, dehydration, tube feedings, and nutritional deficiencies, with other disciplines adding their approaches on as necessary. Nutrition interventions should be found on all care plans that involve any diet-related approaches. For example, nutrition plays a role in many care plans seen as nursing issues, such as hypertension, pressure ulcers, congestive heart failure, and risk of aspiration. Care plans should be updated whenever there is a new intervention or, otherwise, at least quarterly.

Resident assessment protocols: Protocols developed by the Centers for Medicare and Medicaid Services to be used for guiding resident assessment after a "trigger" on the minimum data set. These protocols have been developed for a number of nutrition-related issues.

Clinical RD Accountability in the LTC Setting

What is expected of the clinical dietitian, including what is written in the medical record, is significantly different in a nursing home compared with an acute care facility. The paradigm is fundamentally different due to the length of time the person spends in the facility, the regulatory environment of an LTC facility, and the central role the resident and the resident's family play in determining what care will be provided.

The average length of stay in an acute care facility is days to weeks, which compares with an average length of stay of about 2.5 years in an LTC facility (ElderWeb, n.d.). This extended stay provides significantly more opportunity for the RD to have an impact on the resident's health but brings with it a proportional increase in the RD's accountability for resident care and outcomes. In the LTC setting there is sufficient opportunity to identify the full extent of the resident's nutritional issues, as well as other factors that contribute to a resident's nutritional risk, and there is a higher expectation that each nutritional issue and risk factor will be addressed. At the same time invasive assessment and treatment methods that are used in the acute setting, such as frequent laboratory blood analysis, may be limited unless the outcome of the procedure is expected to result in a change in care that will improve the resident's quality of life.

The LTC regulations also go much further in specifying the details of clinical care. The interpretive guidelines, which have been developed to assist surveyors in evaluation and providers to comply with the intent of the federal regulations, are often quite specific regarding how care for various conditions should be provided: "Unless contraindicated, nutritional goals for a resident with nutritional compromise who has a pressure ulcer or is at risk of developing pressure ulcers should include protein intake of approximately 1.2–1.5 gm/kg body weight daily (higher end of the range for those with larger, more extensive, or multiple wounds)" (American Health Care Association, 2005). This is very different from the approach used by the Joint Commission on Accreditation of Healthcare Organizations, the accrediting body for hospitals, which does not identify such specific standards of care for various conditions. Thus it is incumbent upon the LTC RD to have a detailed knowledge of the interpretive guidelines and other regulatory language and to conduct assessments and to provide care in a manner that is consistent with them.

There is also an expectation that the dietitian will be proactive and intervene *before* a problem becomes significant. For example, an RD should recognize when a resident has a nutrition risk factor and bring the issue to the care team so it can be addressed before nutritional status is compromised.

Another aspect of LTC that is different from acute care is the care plan process. In LTC, the care plans for an individual resident should be as much the resident's and family's plan of care as it is the provider's (i.e., it should be individualized to meet the needs and desires of the resident and be interdisciplinary in nature). If a resident or a responsible family member refuses some aspect of care, relevant conversations with family members must be documented, including documentation that the risks and benefits have been explained. It is also the case that the members of the care plan team (nurses, therapists, dietitians, social workers, etc.) have significantly more authority in the LTC setting than they would in the acute care setting. The care planning team can, and often does, make recommendations to the physician based on their assessments.

Discharge Education

Discharge education occurs in the LTC facility less often than in an acute care setting but is needed for individuals who will discharge to a setting that provides a lower level of care, either after rehabilitation or strengthening. The dietitian needs to make sure that educational materials are available and that training is provided to both nursing staff and the DSM so that, in the dietitian's absence, discharge education may be provided to the resident, family, or other caregivers. Materials often are taken from the diet manual of the facility or are available through other resources, such as the ADA, the American Heart Association, or the National Dairy Council.

Modified Diet Menu Writing and Approval and Modified Diet Prescriptions

The nutrition care for the resident begins with a menu made up of standardized recipes in an accepted regional pattern to meet the nutritional needs of the general elderly population. Federal regulation requires that the meals meet the needs of residents in accordance with the Recommended Dietary Allowances and that planned menus are followed (F363). A complete understanding of menu and recipe mechanics and the systems related to them are key to the RD's ability to help a facility succeed in meeting its clinical and operational goals. A menu must be nutritionally sound to have a chance of meeting clinical goals, and the financial impact of a poorly planned menu is enormous. Before altering or building a menu for a facility, an RD should become familiar with the procurement process, products available through the process, nutritional content of the foods available, the budget around labor and food cost, staff skill set, equipment available, the diet manual adopted, the ADA's position on therapeutic diets, and the facility's goals regarding customer satisfaction.

If the RD is serving in the capacity of a consultant, his or her involvement in menu creation will vary based on the operational support provided by the facility, for example, whether menus are available from a corporate office, if menus are purchased from a vendor, if diets are software available, and whether purchasing programs are set up with a vendor. The assistance needed by the facility may include all or part of the following:

- Writing the entire menu, including finding recipes for texture modifications and therapeutics such as dialysis diets
- Writing the occasional combination diet for which there is no menu extension, such as a puree diet that is also a consistent carbohydrate diet
- Approving menu changes in response to facility/resident preferences or a food availability issue
- Reviewing disaster menus and plans or creating disaster menus and plans for multiple scenarios, such as no electricity, partial electricity, or evacuation to a local school or church

Many resources are available regarding disaster planning, including information in diet manuals and from consultant companies.

As discussed previously, the LTC facility is viewed as the resident's home, and the approaches should be the same as they would be at home: to maintain health and to have the highest quality of life possible. One area where this philosophy dramatically affects care is in the area of therapeutic diet prescriptions. Although there may be an occasion where a therapeutic restriction is necessary, the position of the ADA (2005) is, "the quality of life and nutritional status of older residents in the LTC facility may be enhanced by liberalization of the diet prescription." Food consumption is frequently compromised because of a combination of acute and chronic disease conditions, such that any additional restrictions that would reduce food acceptability and intake would be counterproductive to achieving the care goals.

In addition to making diet recommendations intended to maintain each resident's health and quality of life, the RD in the LTC setting also has the responsibility to evaluate the success of those recommendations over time. Because the facility provides care to most residents over a period of weeks to months, the RD must regularly reassess the resident and determine whether the current diet prescription is resulting in significant clinical progress or is otherwise meeting the resident's care goals.

Increasing and Maintaining Resident Food Intake

Dining is much more than just the consumption of food; it is the smells, sounds, conversations, and anticipation and recall of memories that inspires us to eat (Beverly Healthcare, 1999).

● **Learning Point** One of the most important contributions of the RD is to make sure the dining environment is one that optimizes resident food intake.

A multifacility study conducted by the UCLA Borun Center examined the relationships between 16 nutrition care processes and prevalence of weight loss in nursing facilities (Simmons et al., 2003a). There were no identifiable differences in the RD medical record documentation between the low-weight-loss and the high-weight-loss facilities. Instead, the major difference between the high- and low-weight-loss facilities was the dining environment. The staff at the low-weight-loss nursing homes consistently provided verbal prompting and social interaction during meals to a greater proportion of the residents, including those most at risk for weight loss. These data suggest that it is in the area of meal service and dining that the expertise of the RD may not be fully utilized in the many LTC facilities.

The provision of feeding assistance at meals (social interaction throughout the mealtime period, graduated verbal prompting that enhances self-feeding

capabilities, and physical assistance to the degree required) has been found to have a dramatic effect on food intake. One study found that 50% of residents previously identified as having low food intake responded to feeding assistance by increasing their food intake more than 10%. A subset of the residents (39%) in this study were identified as "highly responsive" to the intervention and increased their meal intake over 2 days from 48% to an average of 74% consumed (Simmons, Lam, Rao, & Schnelle, 2001b). Across studies, Simmons and coworkers (2001a,b, 2004) consistently found that 40% to 50% of residents who had one-on-one feeding assistance significantly increased their oral food and fluid intake during mealtime.

Similarly, some residents have responded to additional feeding assistance with snacks, and enhancing between-meal snack programs is one alternative for increasing dietary intake (Rahman & Simmons, 2005). A study by Simmons and Schnelle (2004) found that 70% of the residents who were not responsive to increased feeding assistance at meals did significantly increase their between-meal intake when targeted for additional attention and assistance during snacks. With the snacking intervention, calories consumed between meals (supplement + snacks) increased to 380 kcal/day from 96 kcal/day under usual care (Simmons & Schnelle, 2004). The second and third most preferred nutrition interventions among family members of residents were improved feeding assistance and the provision of multiple small meals and snacks, respectively (Simmons et al., 2003b).

Family members of nursing home residents most prefer an intervention that includes the provision of more nutritious food (Simmons et al., 2003b). This is often referred to by dietitians as a "food first" approach, and many facilities have a policy for such an offering. There is some evidence that the energy and nutrient intakes of nursing home residents can be significantly increased by increasing the energy/nutrient density of several foods across two or more meals each day (Olin et al., 1996, 2003; Barton, Beigg, Macdonald, & Allison, 2000; Castellanos et al., 2003c), where the energy density of a food is defined as the energy content per weight or volume of food served (Kral & Rolls, 2004). Increasing the nutrient density of the foods residents are already choosing to eat, instead of providing substitute foods or supplements, also allows residents both choice and control over their environment (Castellanos et al., 2003b; Simmons et al., 2003b). Further, research has shown that food preferences and acceptability are important determinants of amounts consumed (de Jong, Chin-A-Paw, de Graff, de Groot, & van Staveren, 2001), particularly for residents who are cognitively intact (Simmons et al., 2001a). Often, the enhanced items are varied or rotated to limit the chance of taste fatigue for the resident.

Provision of liquid nutrition supplements is one of the nutrition interventions least preferred by residents' family members (Simmons et al., 2003b). Although the data are limited, studies suggest that some residents are willing to consume supplements and do benefit from them (Johnson, Dooley, & Gleick, 1993). However, as many as 40% of residents do not consume the liquid supplements they are provided (Johnson et al., 1993; Ross, 1999). Dietitians, however, perceived supplemental products to be second only to tube feedings in terms of effectiveness for increasing intake (Cluskey & Kim, 1997). It should be noted that there is some evidence that supplements consumed with meals cause early satiation (reduce intake of other foods provided in the meal) (Wilson, Purushothaman, & Morley, 2002); thus the greatest benefit to residents is likely to occur when liquid supplements are provided between meals. For residents with poor appetite, replacing restrictive diets with a wider range of food choices may also improve intake and quality of life (ADA, 2005).

> **● Learning Point** Providing residents with a choice of preferred foods and drinks has been found to significantly increase food and fluid intake, particularly in residents who are cognitively intact (Simmons et al., 2001a).

Medications thought to stimulate appetite are sometimes used to improve food intake and weight status, but their use is controversial. It is a common belief that some older people eat better when they are provided with "small portions." Here a note of caution is warranted. Although the impact of portion size on food intake in older people has not been thoroughly studied, the few studies that do speak to this issue have found that some LTC residents eat *less,* whereas others are unaffected when portion sizes are reduced (Cluskey & Dunton, 1999; Young et al., 2001; Castellanos, Georgian, & Wellman, 2003a). That is to say, there is no evidence that smaller portions enhance food intake in this population. This is consistent with a large number of studies in younger people showing that food intake decreases when smaller portions are served (Kral & Rolls, 2004).

Qualified dietitians should be responsible for managing facility-wide dining and snack programs and should optimize menus to meet the unique needs of this population. It is both a necessity and an opportunity for the nutrition professional to take responsibility for all the processes and systems in the facility that support adequate food and fluid intake of residents.

Cultural Diversity in LTC Facilities

LTC facilities are distinctly different from both acute care and community settings in that they are both residential and institutional. That is to say that the facility is "home" to the client for at least a few weeks, and many residents live out the remaining months or years of their life in this care setting. At the same time the provider, not the individual resident, is in the position to make decisions regarding the nature of the food that is available, the manner of food service, and the timing of resident access to food. It is not difficult to imagine that these factors can have a tremendous impact, both negatively and positively, on the quality of life of the residents.

For example, the availability of culturally acceptable foods can impact a resident's food and nutrient consumption, affecting both health and quality of life. Staple foods are very culture specific, and people from a given culture prefer to eat their particular staple food (e.g. tortillas, bread, rice, beans, or pasta) many times a week, if not several times a day. If a resident is not able to regularly obtain the foods that are staples of his or her culture and instead receives the staples of another culture (e.g., an Asian immigrant who receives bread at most meals instead of rice), the menu is unlikely to be acceptable to that individual. Further, the standard of a well-planned menu is determined by the cultural perspective of the evaluator. For example, a menu writer of Northern European descent may not think twice that bread is served at every evening meal but would never develop a menu where rice and beans are served at every evening meal. However, this same menu writer may be responsible for a facility with a large number of Hispanic residents. Some Hispanics, depending on their country of origin, would expect to eat rice and beans at almost every noon and evening meal and perceive different beans and legumes (e.g., black, white, red, garbanzo, etc.) as entirely different foods and consider beans served on rice as entirely different from beans cooked with rice. In short, planning a single menu for a group of residents from varying cultures can be a challenging task.

To make food provision in the LTC setting more complicated, people reside in facilities because they suffer from a number of acute and chronic diseases such that they cannot be cared for at home. Federal regulations require that food be served in a form and nutrient content to meet individual needs and to support treatment and plan of care. Further, this population is known to be at high risk for deficiencies in energy, protein, fiber, and water, as evidenced by the high prevalence of unintended weight loss, compromised protein status, constipation, and dehydration. Unfortunately, any resident provided a culturally unacceptable menu is unlikely to eat well, which is likely to result in weight loss and undernutrition and a spiral of negative health effects.

Federal regulation specifies the facility's responsibilities toward creating and maintaining an environment that humanizes and individualizes each resident, including how each resident is treated at mealtime. This is consistent with the position of the ADA that nutrition care in LTC facilities must promote quality of life. Because of this, it is the standard of practice for LTC facilities to provide menus that are consistent with regional and cultural norms (e.g., rice and beans may be on the menu frequently in Miami but will be rarely if ever served in Kansas City). Facilities are also adopting new attitudes toward providing care, as described by the ADA (2005). A "resident-centered" or "person-centered" care approach involves residents in decisions about schedules, menus, and dining locations. This approach is one way to honor the relationship between food and culture in the LTC setting while at the same time meeting the intent of the federal statutes.

Food Preparation

Food preparation and service are critical functions in the LTC facility, yet they often receive insufficient attention from the RD. Tags F362 to F365, F368, and F369 address various aspects of the proper preparation and service of food, and the dietitian is responsible for ensuring that the facility is in compliance. However, the health and well-being of the residents and the financial viability of the company are both equally important reasons for dietitians to give adequate time and attention to the food service operation.

From both the financial and the resident outcomes point of view, the most expensive meal to a facility is the one that is not consumed. Food and dining are important quality of life issues for residents, and food of poor nutritional quality or food that is not consumed in adequate amounts result in a decline in the health and nutritional status of residents. Further, food service operations are resource intensive, and if the food service in an LTC facility is poorly managed, scarce resources available for resident care will be wasted. However timely and thorough a dietitian may be in completing clinical assessments and care plans, if the food leaving the kitchen is not nutritionally adequate or if it is not consumed by residents (because is unpalatable, not served at an acceptable temperature, not in the proper form, or served at an acceptable time), then the documentation in the medical record is of little use.

The RD has tremendous opportunities to assist the facility in improving resident care through their expertise in staff management, food preparation, food service systems, training skills, and financial management. For example, to verify the use of standardized recipes and instructions and compliance with the menu, the dietitian can periodically observe food preparation. Staff can be reminded or educated in regard to cooking methods that preserve nutritional quality and texture, such as limiting water when heating vegetables and batch cooking. The tray line can also be observed periodically to verify that the menu is being followed for therapeutic diets and that alternates are available. Further, the RD can minimize food waste by making sure that items on the tray line are portioned correctly according to the recipes (e.g., correct pan size and the number of cuts per pan) and the menu (e.g., use of a no. 8 scoop for ½-cup servings). Food safety and palatability are always of paramount importance, and the RD can spot check to verify that tray line temperatures meet both **Hazard Analysis Critical Control Point (HACCP)** process and palatability requirements. Although the DSM and/or the cook should observe a dining room at every meal to determine resident acceptance, the RD should also routinely observe dining to identify any issues with the service of the meal, the dining environment, the provision of feeding assistance, and meal acceptance.

> **Hazard Analysis Critical Control Point (HACCP):** A process used in cooking to identify steps and points in food preparation that are deemed as critical in preventing food-borne illness.

Food Safety and Sanitation

The most common deficiency in LTC surveys is F371: Store, prepare, distribute, and serve food under sanitary conditions. Over 40% of LTC facilities are cited for deficient practice under this tag. Per the federal guidelines, the intent of this regulation is "to prevent the spread of food-borne illness and reduce those practices, which may result in food contamination and compromise food safety in nursing homes. Food-borne illness is often fatal to nursing home residents and can and must be avoided" (American Health Care Association, 2005).

The federal guidelines suggest the use of the U.S. Food and Drug Administration **Food Code** as a resource, but the regulation does not mandate its use. Since the advent of this guideline, several states have adopted the Food Code, and several counties are mandating its use, especially in reference to HACCP. HACCP is a process used in cooking to identify steps and points in food preparation deemed critical in preventing food-borne illness. Although all chapters of the Food Code are relevant, chapters 1 through 4 tend to be the most applicable to LTC settings. The Food Code is one of the most heavily used reference books in the LTC industry, and a copy should be placed in every nutritional services department and should be the foundation for all sanitation training. It should be noted that the Food Code is updated approximately every 2 years, and it is common for a state to adopt a specific version of the Food Code and not recognize newer versions (e.g., a state may use the 2002 Food Code instead of the 2005 version). Thus it is important for a facility RD to be aware of and follow the version of the Food Code that his or her state uses.

Because F371 is such a problem in LTC settings, most facility administrators and nursing home com-

> **Food Code:** Published by the U.S. Food and Drug Administration, this is a model that assists food control jurisdictions at all levels of government by providing them with a scientifically sound technical and legal basis for regulating the retail and food service segment of the industry.

panies focus efforts on avoiding this citation. These stakeholders look to the RD to assist them in making sure the facility practices help them achieve that goal. A study by the RD Council for Quality Nursing Home Care identified the three most common surveyor observations associated with F371 in 95 surveys across nine different LTC companies (Nevins, Gluch, Castellanos, & RD Council for Quality Nursing Home Care, 2003):

- In 45.3% of F371 citations, surveyors observed problems with soiled equipment.
- In 41.1% of F371 citations, surveyors observed problems with food storage. This included a range of problems from food not labeled and dated to improper thawing and cooling of food.
- In 35.8% of F371 citations, surveyors observed problems with the cleanliness and condition of the physical structure of the kitchen. This covers dirty walls and surfaces, broken floor tiles, and holes in screens or gaps in windows.

A dietitian can significantly improve a facility's ability to achieve compliance with F371. On a routine basis the RD should review cooling and thawing practices, educate staff on proper procedures, and conduct spot checks in the kitchen. The RD should regularly inspect equipment sanitation, assist the facility in the use of cleaning schedules, and provide training on the proper use and cleaning of equipment. The RD should also make sure there is an effective system for the fulfillment of maintenance requests and completion of the routine types of cleaning normally performed by facility maintenance (e.g., refrigerator fans). Finally, the RD can review facility policies to make sure they are consistent with the Food Code currently being used by that state.

Critical Thinking on Nutrition Issues in LTC Facilities

Nursing home regulations are intended to ensure the provision of quality care to all residents. Unfortunately, few of the nutrition regulations or the interpretive guidelines used to assist providers and surveyors are based on clinical studies, as there are very few in this population or this care setting. Thus the standard of practice in LTC is often based on consensus opinion rather than on evidence. Further, when research findings do become available, federal regulations are slow to change and accommodate these advances. When a standard of care is not clearly defined, surveyors are instructed to verify that the facility has developed its own policy and procedures, optimally based on the literature. The survey process then assesses whether the facility is following its own care standards. Although state surveyors assert that they do not mandate *how* care is delivered, providers often perceive the federal regulations, inter-

pretive guidelines, and survey process as barriers to making changes in nutrition care delivery. In other words, practitioners often believe they are at increased risk of receiving a citation if they provide care in a manner that varies from what the surveyor is familiar with or expects and that belief inhibits them from making changes, even improvements, to facility policies and procedures.

An example of a common practice that remains in place simply because it is perceived by providers to be required for compliance with regulations is the recording of meal intake estimates. It is the standard of practice in most nursing homes for nursing assistants to record estimates of meal consumption for every resident at every meal during the entire length of their stay. Maintaining this practice takes a significant amount of time and effort by nursing staff and generates a tremendous amount of paperwork for the facility. It is the mistaken belief of many nurses, dietitians, and others that federal regulation requires estimates of meal intake at every meal. In point of fact, to be in compliance with the regulation the facility must record each resident's intake for several days before the MDS is completed, which is within the 14 days following admission, after a significant change of status, and annually.

Beyond the few days of meal intake estimates required to complete the MDS, the primary reason given for estimating resident food intake is to identify those individuals who are eating poorly. However, there are many reasons to justify the abandonment of daily estimates of meal intake in favor of a more accurate and objective assessment of intake adequacy:

1. Meal intake estimates are inherently inaccurate (Castellanos & Andrews, 2002).
2. Meal intake estimates do not reflect whether meal intake is sufficient to meet the individual resident's nutritional needs.
3. Meal intake estimates divert limited resources away from activities proven to be associated with quality care.
4. Meal intake estimates constitute a barrier to more home-like meal service options because they make intake estimates more difficult or impossible.
5. Meal intake estimates offer the illusion that there is a valid and reliable system in place to identify those residents who are eating poorly.
6. Meal intake estimates provide fodder for lawyers in civil litigation if the record is incomplete or obviously erroneous, which is often.

It has been suggested that practitioners should rely on body weight measures to assess whether food intake is adequate to meet resident energy needs (Castellanos & Andrews, 2002). Body weight change is known to be a valid and reliable way to assess whether individual people are getting adequate nutrition, particularly energy (Gibson, 2005). Amount, rate, and timing of weight loss have also been found to be associated with physiologic impairment and clinical outcomes in hospitalized patients (Gibson, 2005). Further, accurate weighing and documentation are important for defining needs and monitoring MNT success (Splett, Roth-Yousey, & Vogelzang, 2003), and weight loss has been shown to be a valid indicator of quality nutrition care in the LTC setting (Simmons et al., 2003a). Although body weight change is not a valid measure of energy adequacy in all individuals (i.e., those with edema), if done correctly it would be valid and reliable for the vast majority of residents. Nursing home regulation does require weekly weights on short-term stay residents covered under Medicare and monthly weights on all others, but most nursing homes do not go beyond these minimums to take full advantage of body weight change as an assessment tool.

In summary, there are instances when the nature of the care provided to nursing home residents is as much about avoiding citations as it is about utilizing the best care process. The practice of recording meal intake estimates is an example of how regulations, perceptions of regulations, or the survey process can become a barrier to improvements in nursing home care. For most residents weekly body weights during the entire length of their stay would be a valid, reliable, inexpensive, and noninvasive way to identify those who are eating poorly. The availability of frequent weights over time enables both the identification of inadequate food intake and the evaluation of various interventions on weight outcomes. From a purely scientific point of view, utilization of weekly weights as an assessment tool would justify the abandonment of daily meal intake estimates, which are known to be both invalid and unreliable. Yet because daily meal estimates are expected by surveyors and many RDs and registered nurses are of the mistaken belief that they are required and because federal regulations do not require weekly body weights on long term stay residents, most facilities are reticent to alter their current practice.

Survey Management

Numerous times in this chapter we have referenced the regulations the LTC facility must follow when caring for their residents. An annual survey to determine the facility's compliance with the regulations occurs a minimum of once every 18 months. Other surveys do occasionally take place, such as a "complaint survey" for review of a complaint made to the state about the facility. A **state survey** team can enter the facility at any time, including the middle of the night or on weekends. Occasionally, a federal survey team, whose job it is to review the state team's results for accuracy, follows them a few days later. At times the federal survey team will actually accompany the state survey team. Thus there may be anywhere from three to nine surveyors in a facility at one time. The survey teams usually include nurses, sanitarians, and social workers and may occasionally include an RD.

State survey: The process of the state department of health entering a facility to determine if the Centers for Medicare and Medicaid Services and state requirements are being met.

The survey experience can be unsettling to both residents and staff. The best way to make this experience a positive one is to plan for the survey in conjunction with the DSM and be prepared to manage the survey. Some steps in planning for and managing a survey are listed in Table 14.2. Knowledge is power and confidence. These planning steps, and many others, can be taken to give staff the tools and confidence they need to succeed under pressure. Taking steps to manage the survey helps to keep everyone calm and focused during the actual survey.

Quality Management

In most businesses quality assessment and assurance is optional and is used for business improvement. In LTC settings quality management is required by the federal government (F520 and 521). Dietitians in the LTC setting play a critical role in ensuring that the facility meets quality care standards in both clinical care and meal production. Well-designed systems must be in place to ensure appropriate and timely nutrition assessment of residents, execution of the nutrition care plan, minimal weight loss and pressure ulcers, proper sanitation, food preparation, and de-

TABLE 14.2	Planning for and Managing the LTC Survey
Planning	**Managing**
Educating staff about the federal and state regulations, interpretive guidelines, and investigative protocols.	Identifying the contact person in the nutritional services department to communicate with the surveyor.
Educating staff regarding the procedures used by surveyors. This clarifies the expectations of the survey process and how staff should respond in anticipation of the next step in the process.	Determining who will stay with the surveyor assigned to nutritional services throughout the survey process so that resources, documentation, justifications/ explanations, and so on can be provided as needed.
Ensuring systems are in place so that proper meal production and service can be practiced every day.	Responding to potential deficiency areas discovered during the survey using a predetermined approach, e.g., fix any problematic issues immediately.
Attending resident council meetings periodically and probing for issues or complaints that residents may bring to surveyors so that they can be addressed beforehand.	Holding staff meetings at the beginning and the end of the day to review issues such as surveyor comments, ingredient availability, and staffing.
Participating in the facility plan for the surveyor visit, such as determining where the surveyors will be given space to work so as to minimize interference with resident activities and planning what food and beverages will be provided to them so that those items can be on hand.	Determine a plan for management to follow-up on potential issues mentioned by surveyors.

livery of the meals. Quality assurance activities are necessary to ensure the delivery of high quality nutritional services.

The essential elements of traditional **quality assurance** are to (1) identify potential problems that may exist that can be measured through review of data and outcomes, (2) set a performance standard, (3) screen to ensure compliance to the performance standard, (4) gather individual feedback and identify deficiencies, (5) review systems and processes to determine where breakdown is occurring, (6) institute corrective action to achieve performance standard, and (7) emphasize health care structure, process, and outcome.

Quality assurance: A system for ensuring that quality care is being delivered and that the activities required to maintain quality are being performed at an acceptable level.

Step 5 of the quality assurance process is critical for ensuring that quality care is being delivered and that the activities required to maintain quality are being performed at an acceptable level. The efficacy of the quality assurance committee depends on their ability to evaluate the systems and processes in a facility. Although quality assurance may not be a responsibility of the dietitian in other care settings, the nature of the LTC setting demands that dietitians use a wide range of management skills to ensure that residents receive quality care during the entire length of their stay. Although the dietitian may not be in attendance for all quality assurance meetings (e.g., if the facility RD is a consultant), the RD should review the minutes of quality assurance meetings and assist the DSM in the system analysis.

The Centers for Medicare and Medicaid Services also has a focus on quality management. State and federal regulators use facility data from the MDS to monitor various **quality indicators**; the MDS Quality Indicator Report for Nutrition/Eating includes "prevalence of weight loss," "prevalence of tube feeding," and "prevalence of dehydration."

Quality indicators: A quality indicator report is generated from a facility-wide minimum data set to be used by surveyors during the survey process. The quality indicator report is used to help surveyors identify potential quality problems in the facility. The quality indicator report for nutrition/eating includes "prevalence of weight loss," "prevalence of tube feeding," and "prevalence of dehydration."

The Centers for Medicare and Medicaid Services has also made certain data available to the public so that they, the consumers, can use it to compare nursing homes. Selected MDS data from each facility are available nationally at the Nursing Home Compare Website (www.medicare. gov/NHCompare/). These data, called **quality measures**, are intended to represent the quality of care provided at nursing facilities so that consumers can make an informed decision. Of particular relevance to nutrition services is the "weight loss quality measure." The quality measure reports the percentage of residents with a significant weight loss, excluding residents receiving hospice care; that is, residents who have experienced a weight loss of more than 5% of their body weight in 1 month or 10% of their body weight in 6 months.

Quality measures: Selected minimum data set made available to the public by the Centers for Medicare and Medicaid Services at the Nursing Home Compare website (www.medicare. gov/NHCompare/). These data are intended to represent the quality of care provided at nursing facilities so that consumers can make an informed decision. Prevalence of weight loss is one of the quality measures from each nursing home that the Centers for Medicare and Medicaid Services shares with the public.

It is appropriate that the facility RD take the lead in efforts to improve the facility's weight loss quality measure. The etiology of unintentional weight loss and undernutrition is multifactorial and is likely related to both psychological factors and physiologic changes (Morley, 2003). Studies have suggested that behavioral and environmental factors may be the most important determinants of food intake in the nursing home setting (Simmons et al., 2001a, 2002). It is critical that nutrition care processes focus on underlying causes and emphasize prevention of weight loss (Beck & Ovesen, 1998).

Unique Role of the Consultant Dietitian in LTC

Consultant, as defined by Webster, is a person who is called on for professional or technical advice or opinions. RD consultants are in a unique position because they not only have the clinical training necessary to provide MNT, they are also highly valued for their knowledge in the areas of food preparation, sanitation, and food service systems. If the facility RD is a consultant and not a full-time employee of the facility or company, it is important to remember that the resident is not the only customer. The clients of the consultant RD also include the facility administrator, the director of nursing services, and the DSM.

Consultants are in an LTC facility a limited number of hours per week. If the activities of a consultant are limited only to charting and pointing out sanitation or production errors, then the facility is not able to take full advantage of the expertise of the consultant in helping them to develop in-house staff and improve their performance over time. On the other hand, if the consultant takes the time to identify and understand the current issues or concerns of the facility, he or she may be able to provide relevant staff education and/or offer several possible solutions to ongoing problems. This approach allows the facility team the opportunity to develop their own competency in the area of concern and affords staff the opportunity to choose and take ownership of the solution. Staff development and buy-in are essential for long-term correction of any problem.

An example consultant report is as follows: Cross-contamination between clean and dirty dishes in the dish room observed. An alternative consultant report that provides more information and solutions follows: At entrance conference facility expressed concern regarding sanitation. Sanitation tour completed, see attached. Provided in-service to staff on dish machine procedures. Recommend two options for change: (1) Move the hand sink closer to the dish area as discussed and/or (2) Restructure staffing to allow for one associate on each end of the dish machine, thus eliminating need to crossover from clean to dirty side.

Summary

In summary, the role for the RD in LTC settings is much more complex than it is in many other care settings. In LTC it is the expectation that the dietitian will not only be proficient in MNT but will have expertise in the regulatory environment, food preparation, sanitation, dining, and survey and quality management. The provision of nutrition care in this setting also requires a proactive and system-oriented approach, where residents' quality of life is a primary consideration in every decision, and care should be provided in the most home-like manner possible. The potential for the RD to make a significant difference in the quality of life of residents and to be valued by the facility are limited only by the aspirations of the individual practitioner.

Issues to Debate

1. Discuss the effects of being unregulated on the residents of an LTC facility.
2. Discuss the effects of making a dietitian's consultation optional to the residents of an LTC facility.
3. Discuss the potential differences between a private and public LTC facility.

Website Resources

American Dietetic Association www.eatright.org

American Dietetic Association Evidence Analysis Library www.adaevidencelibrary.org

American Health Care Association http://www.ahca.org/

American Society for Parenteral and Enteral Nutrition http://www.nutritioncare.org/

Centers for Medicare and Medicaid Services http://www.cms.hhs.gov/default.asp?fromhcfadotgov=true and http://www.cms.hhs.gov/CertificationandComplianc/

Consultant Dietitians in Health Care Facilities www.cdhcf.org

Dietary Managers Association http://www.dmaonline.org/index.html

Drug Bank http://redpoll.pharmacy.ualberta.ca/drugbank/

2005 Food Code http://vm.cfsan.fda.gov/~dms/foodcode.html

International Food Information Council www.ific.org

National Academy of Sciences www.nas.edu/health/

Nursing Home Compare http://www.medicare.gov/NHCompare/

National Quality Measures Clearinghouse http://www.qualitymeasures.ahrq.gov/

Nursing Home Quality Initiatives http://www.cms.hhs.gov/NursingHomeQualityInits/

The Clinician's Ultimate Guide to Drug Therapy http://www.globalrph.com/

UCLA Borun Center for Gerontological Research http://borun.medsch.ucla.edu/

U.S. Department of Agriculture, MyPyramid www.mypyramid.gov

USDA Nutrient Data Laboratory http://www.nal.usda.gov/fnic/foodcomp

PubMed http://www.pubmed.gov

National Resource Center on Nutrition, Physical Activity and Aging, Long Term Care Institute http://nutritionandaging.fiu.edu/about_long_term.asp

References

American Dietetic Association (ADA). (2005). Position of the American Dietetic Association: Liberalization of the diet prescription improves quality of life for older adults in long term care. *Journal of the American Dietetic Association, 105,* 1955–1965.

American Health Care Association. (2005). *The Long Term Care Survey.* Washington, DC: Author.

American Medical Directors Association. (2002). *Clinical Practice Guidelines: Dehydration and Fluid Maintenance.* Columbia, MD: Author.

Barton, A. D., Beigg, C. L., Macdonald, I. A., & Allison, S. P. (2000). A recipe for improving food intakes in elderly hospitalized patients. *Clinical Nutrition, 19,* 451–454.

Beck, A. M., & Ovesen, L. (1998). At which body mass index and degree of weight loss should hospitalized elderly patients be considered at nutritional risk? *Clinical Nutrition, 17,* 195–198.

Beverly Healthcare. (1999). *Enhanced Dining Resources.* Little Rock, AR: Author.

Blaum, C. S., O'Neill, E. F., Clements, K. M., Fries, B. E., & Fiatarone, M. A. (1997) Validity of the minimum data set for assessing nutritional status in nursing home residents. *American Journal of Clinical Nutrition, 66,* 787–794.

Castellanos, V. H. (2004). Food and nutrition in nursing homes. *Generations, 28,* 65–71.

Castellanos, V. H., & Andrews, Y. N. (2002). Inherent flaws in a method commonly used to report food intake in long term care facilities. *Journal of the American Dietetic Association, 102,* 826–830.

Castellanos, V. H., Georgian, M. E., & Wellman, N. S. (2003a). Fluid intake increased when larger portions were offered to nursing home residents with medications. *FASEB Journal, 17,* A285.

Castellanos, V. H., Silver, H. J., Gallagher-Allred, C., & Smith, T. (2003b). Nutrition issues in home, community, and long-term care setting. *Nutrition Clinical Practice, 18,* 21–36.

Castellanos, V. H., Surloff, S. C., & Giordan, W. L. (2003c). Systematic enhancement of food over short term increased calorie intake by residents with dementia. *Journal of the American Dietetic Association, 103,* A40.

Chapman, K., Samman, S., & Liburne, A. M. (1993). Are the guidelines for nutritional care and food service in nursing homes being implemented? *Australian Journal of Nutrition and Diet, 50,* 39–45.

Chidester, C., & Spangler, A. A. (1997). Fluid intake in the institutionalized elderly. *Journal of the American Dietetic Association, 97,* 23–28.

Cluskey, M., & Dunton, N. (1999). Serving meals of reduced portion size did not improve appetite among elderly in a personal-care section of a long-term-care community. *Journal of the American Dietetic Association, 99,* 33–35.

Cluskey, M., & Kim, Y. (1997). Use and perceived effectiveness of strategies for enhancing food and nutrient intakes among elderly persons in long-term care. *Journal of the American Dietetic Association, 101,* 111–114.

de Jong, N., Chin-A-Paw, M. J., de Graff, C., de Groot, L., & van Staveren, W. A. (2001). Appraisal of 4 months' consumption of nutrient-dense foods within the daily feeding pattern of frail elderly. *Journal of Aging and Health, 13,* 200–216.

ElderWeb. (n.d.). Average length of nursing home stay. Retrieved May 1, 2006, from http://www.elderweb.com/home/node/2770.

Endres, J., Welch, P., Ashraf, H., Banz, W., & Gower, E. (2000). Acceptance of soy foods by the elderly in a long-term care facility. *Journal of Nutrition in the Elderly, 19,* 1–17.

Gibson, R. S. (2005). *Principles of Nutritional Assessment* (2nd ed.). New York: Oxford University Press.

Institute of Medicine. (1997). *Dietary Reference Intakes for Calcium, Phosphorus, Magnesium, Vitamin D, and Fluoride.* Washington, DC: National Academy Press.

Johnson, L. E., Dooley, P. A., & Gleick, J. G. (1993). Oral nutritional supplement use in elderly nursing home patients. *Journal of the American Geriatrics Society, 41,* 947–952.

Kayser-Jones, J., Schell, E. S., Porter, C., Barbaccia, J. C., & Shaw, H. (1999). Factors contributing to dehydration in nursing homes: Inadequate staffing and lack of professional supervision. *Journal of the American Geriatrics Society, 47,* 1187–1193.

Kral, T. V., & Rolls, B. J. (2004). Energy density and portion size: Their independent and combined effects on energy intake. *Physiology & Behavior, 82,* 131–138.

Lacey, K., & Pritchett, E. (2003). Nutrition care process and model: ADA adopts road map to quality care and outcomes management. *Journal of the American Dietetic Association, 103,* 1061–1072.

Morley, J. E. (2003). Anorexia and weight loss in older persons. *Journal of Gerontology, 58A,* 131–137.

Nevins, D. A., Gluch, L. A., Castellanos, V. H., & RD Council for Quality Nursing Home Care. (2003). Most common causative factors for F371 deficiencies in long-term care state surveys. *Journal of the American Dietetic Association, 103,* A42.

Olin, A. O., Armyr, I., Soop, M., Jerstrom, S., Classon, I., Cederholm, T., et al. (2003). Energy-dense meals improve energy intake in elderly residents in a nursing home. *Clinical Nutrition, 22,* 125–131.

Olin, A. O., Osterberg, P., Hadell, K., Armyr, I., Jerstrom, S., & Ljungqvist, O. (1996). Energy-enriched hospital food to improve energy intake in elderly patients. *Journal of Parenteral and Enteral Nutrition, 20,* 93–97.

Rahman, A. N., & Simmons, S. F. (2005). Individualizing nutritional care with between-meal snacks for nursing home residents. *Journal of the American Medical Directors Association, 6,* 215–218.

Rolls, B. J., & Phillips, P. A. (1990). Aging and disturbances of thirst and fluid balance. *Nutrition Reviews, 48,* 137–143.

Ross, F. (1999). An audit of nutritional supplement distribution and consumption on a care of the elderly ward. *Journal of the Human Nutritional Diet, 12,* 445–452.

Shatenstein, B., & Ferland, G. (2000). Absence of nutritional or clinical consequences of decentralized bulk food portioning in elderly nursing home residents with dementia in Montreal. *Journal of the American Dietetic Association, 100*, 1354–1360.

Simmons, S. F., Alessi, C., & Schnelle, J. F. (2001a). An intervention to increase fluid intake in nursing home residents: Prompting and preference compliance. *Journal of the American Geriatrics Society, 49*, 926–934.

Simmons, S. F., Osterweil, D., & Schnelle, J. F. (2001b). Improving food intake in nursing home residents with feeding assistance. A staffing analysis. *Journal of Gerontology. Series A, Biological Sciences and Medical Sciences, 56*, M790–M794.

Simmons, S. F., Babinou, S., Garcia, E., & Schnelle, J. F. (2002). Quality assessment in nursing homes by systematic direct observations: Feeding assistance. *Journal of Gerontology. Series A, Biological Sciences and Medical Sciences, 57*, M665–M671.

Simmons, S. F., Garcia, E. T., Cadogan, M. P., Al-Samarrai, N. R., Levy-Storms, L. F., Osterweil, D., et al. (2003a). The minimum data set weight-loss quality indicator: Does it reflect differences in care processes related to weight loss? *Journal of the American Geriatrics Society, 51*, 1410–1418.

Simmons, S. F., Lam, H. Y., Rao, G., & Schnelle, J. F. (2003b). Family members' preferences for nutrition interventions to improve nursing home residents' oral food and fluid intake. *Journal of the American Geriatrics Society, 51*, 69–74.

Simmons, S. F., & Reuben, D. (2000). Nutritional intake monitoring for nursing home residents: A comparison of staff documentation, direct observation, and photography methods. *Journal of the American Geriatrics Society, 48*, 209–213.

Simmons, S. F., & Schnelle, J. F. (2004). Individualized feeding assistance care for nursing home residents: Staffing requirements to implement two interventions. *Journal of Gerontology. Series A, Biological Sciences and Medical Sciences, 59A*, 966–973.

Splett, P. L., Roth-Yousey, L. L., & Vogelzang, J. L. (2003). Medical nutrition therapy for the prevention and treatment of unintentional weight loss in residential healthcare facilities. *Journal of the American Dietetic Association, 103*, 352–362.

Wilson, M.-M. G., Purushothaman, R., & Morley, J. E. (2002). Effect of liquid dietary supplements on energy intake in the elderly. *American Journal of Clinical Nutrition, 75*, 944–947.

Young, K. W., Binns, M. A., & Greenwood, C. E. (2001). Meal delivery practices do not meet needs of Alzheimer patients with increased cognitive and behavioral difficulties in a long-term care facility. *Journal of Gerontology. Series A, Biological Sciences and Medical Sciences, 56*, M656–M661.

Judith Sharlin, PhD, RD, and I. David Todres, MD

CHAPTER OUTLINE

Reader Objectives

After studying this chapter and reflecting on the contents, you should be able to

1. Address the appropriate uses and methods for artificial nutrition and hydration and the role of the registered dietitian at the end of life.

2. Describe the benefits, risks, and burdens associated with artificial nutrition and hydration.

3. Apply an ethical framework for decision-making regarding the appropriateness of artificial nutrition and hydration.

4. Learn the legal application of ethical principles and understand two seminal cases regarding tube-feeding termination.

5. Understand the use of advanced directives and how they affect decision-making in long-term tube feeding care.

Artificial Nutrition and Hydration: Definition, Indications, and Prevalence

Nutrition and hydration and the end of life are considered by health care professionals to be medical interventions (American Dietetic Association, 2002). It is the patient's articulated desires for extent of medical care that should be the driving force for determining the level of nutrition intervention (American Dietetic Association, 2002). Before any medical, nutritional, or ethical decisions can be made about a patient's care, however, it is important to understand the definitions of artificial nutrition and hydration. Artificial nutrition and hydration (ANH) is defined as "any nutrition and/or hydration support of an invasive nature requiring placement of a tube into the alimentary tract or parenterally via intravenous or subcutaneous means" (Burge et al., 1995). Tube feeding is used for patients with a functioning gastrointestinal tract who cannot eat or who are unable to swallow (McMahon, Hurley, Kamath, & Mueller, 2005). Tube feeding can include nasoenteric, gastrostomy, and jejunostomy tubes. Since medical advancements in the 1980s, percutaneous endoscopic gastrostomy (PEG) tubes have become the method of choice for long-term tube feeding (Ponsky & Gauderer, 1981).

The benefits to the use of the PEG tube in patients with certain diseases include that these tubes may prolong life and may help alleviate the discomfort of symptoms and enhance quality of life (Ganzini, 2006). PEG feeding tubes extend life by improving nutrition, lessening dehydration, reducing aspiration, and helping to heal pressure sores. Health care professionals, patients, and families also perceive tube feeding to be less invasive than parenteral nutrition. In addition, tube feeding has fewer complications and is less costly than parenteral nutrition (McMahon, 2004; Hurley & McMahon, 2005).

There has been a dramatic increase in the placement of PEG tubes in patients—from 61,000 in 1988 to 121,000 in 1995. About 30% of those patients receiving PEG tubes had dementia (Rabeneck, Wray, & Petersen, 1996). Studies of PEG tubes and patients with dementia have shown 30-day post-PEG mortality to be as high as 25% to 30% (Cox, 2006). The use of PEG tubes and its negative outcomes in older adults with advanced dementia has been documented. In reviewing studies from 1966 through 1999 on tube-feeding patients with advanced dementia, none of them showed any of the (previously mentioned) benefits to the patient: prolonged life, reduced risk of pressure sores or infections, preventing aspiration pneumonia, or palliative care (Finucane, Christmas, & Travis, 1999). There is also no evidence showing survival benefits with the PEG tube in patients suffering terminal diseases, including Alzheimer's disease, amyotrophic lateral sclerosis, and terminal stages of cancer (Rabeneck et al., 1996). More education is needed among health care professionals and families to alleviate conflicts around feeding problems in patients with dementia.

In many states there are financial incentives in nursing facilities for tube feeding, even though many experts believe it is more ethical and effective to spoon feed these patients (Ganzini, 2006). Many nursing home settings are, unfortunately, driven by profit and state regulations. Although it is more labor intensive to feed patients by hand (Mitchell, Buchanan, Littlehale, & Hamel, 2003), it is more nurturing for patients. Hand feeding may provide patients with appropriate social and sensory stimulation that enhances quality of life.

The major complication associated with tube feeding is aspiration. Aspiration occurs between 25% and 40% of patients who are receiving tube feeding (McClave & Chang, 2003). Major risk factors include a history of previous aspiration, depressed level of consciousness, neuromuscular disease, vomiting, and prolonged supine position (McClave et al., 2002).

Dehydration

There is a current debate whether or not terminally ill patients facing imminent death benefit from dehydration. Deprivation of water causes a decrease in secretions, urinary output, edema, and ascites and increases an endogenous dynorphin that acts as a very potent opiate, which calms the patient (Printz, 1992). Dehydration also causes confusion and lethargy in dying patients secondary to hyponatremia (Sullivan, 1993). However, other researchers have shown dehydration to be isotonic in the dying patient and have discounted the hyper- and hyponatremic effects (Cox, 2006). Studies of cancer patients have shown that more than two-thirds complain of thirst or dry mouth at the end of life (Huang & Ahronheim, 2000). Contrary to healthy individuals, however, thirst in advanced cancer patients appears to be unrelated to dehydration and serum sodium and is not relieved by fluids. In fact, some terminally ill patients have experienced uncomfortable and painful effects from the administration of fluids, including increased urinary output, diarrhea, nausea, and respiratory problems (Viola, Wells, & Peterson, 1997).

Fluid overload from artificial hydration increases pulmonary and gastrointestinal secretions, urinary output, and pharyngeal secretions that could lead to the choking and gurgling sounds known as the "death rattle" (Gallagher, 1989). A study showed increased peripheral edema, ascites, and pleural effusions with modest hydration and no difference in bronchial secretion or delirium (Morita et al., 2005). Research has shown oral disease to be strongly associated with the cause of thirst in terminally ill patients (Byock, 1995). Most healthcare professionals in palliative care promote the use of good mouth care and sips of water and ice chips, when desired (Ersek, 2003). At the end of life, a decrease in food and fluid intake seems to be part of the natural physiology of dying (Burge et al., 1995). Data from hospice health workers suggest that not eating and drinking at the end of life causes little suffering.

Meaning of Food and Drink

In patient care both food and drink have psychological and physical functions as well as many social meanings. Giving food and drink encompasses strong cultural and emotional values that are often equated with nurturing and caring. Providing nutrition and hydration is, however, not synonymous with eating or with feeding someone. Normally, people eat through the mouth with utensils. A medical intervention such as ANH is not considered socially normative (Slomka, 2003). In fact, until recently the term "tube feeding" was called "forced feeding."

In the position paper of the American Dietetic Association (2002) concerning ethical and legal issues in nutrition, hydration, and feeding, the following guidelines were proposed for oral intake (nutrition and hydration):

1. Oral feeding should be advocated whenever possible.
2. The patient's physical and emotional enjoyment of food should be the primary consideration. Staff and family members should be encouraged to assist in feeding the patient.
3. Nutrition supplements should be used to encourage oral intake and alleviate painful symptoms associated with hunger, thirst, or malnutrition.

4. Diet restrictions should be reevaluated.
5. The patient has the right to determine whether he or she wants to consume foods outside of the "diet prescription."
6. Suboptimal oral feedings may be more appropriate than tube or parenteral feeding.

Finally, it seems appropriate for the health care professional to ask the following questions: Is withholding or withdrawing ANH the same as denying food and drink? Is there a "moral imperative" required by human decency to provide nutrition and hydration (Slomka, 2003)?

Roles of the Registered Dietitian

Registered dietitians are in a unique position, because of their education and background, to work collaboratively with the health care team to make nutrition, hydration, and feeding recommendations. Registered dietitians are trained to assess patients' nutritional needs, offer nutritional counseling, and provide meals that reduce side effects of medicine and treatment. Dietitians can also encourage patients and families to suggest or supply their own favorite meals, if appropriate, and to assist in hand feeding patients. Often, a registered dietitian's familiarity with practical aspects of food and fluid at the end of life are helpful to answer families' concerns and questions about chewing, swallowing, and the cessation of thirst and hunger.

A registered dietitian may be able to best express "knowing what is wanted" by the patient because they are the main conversation partners about feeding issues with the patient and family (American Dietetic Association, 2002). They are in a position to contribute the most accurate information on nutritional value judgments. The registered dietitian is trained in medical nutrition therapy and teaching so that he or she can assume the responsibility of keeping the patient's understanding of the options and outcomes about feeding in the center of the deliberation. The registered dietitian has the responsibility to make sure all options about feeding are deliberated, rather than assuming that one strategy is obligatory. For example, a situation might occur with a patient where tube feeding seems to be the only option when, in fact, careful hand feeding may be a better alternative for adequate nutrition. Finally, the dietitian's role, along with the rest of the health care team, is to promote a compassionate and positive experience for the patient, family, and loved ones at the end of life.

Ethical Principles as a Framework for Decision-Making

The practice of long-term tube feeding has escalated over the past two decades as a result of an aging population and new technology. Ensuring that the patient is given food and water is an important symbolic nurturing act that is deeply rooted in cultural and religious traditions. However, in special circumstances it may be morally correct to consider it inappropriate to provide ANH to the patient. This consideration raises strong emotional reactions and leads to anguished decision-making for patients, families, and health care workers. Appreciating the ethical principles underlying these decisions is helpful in ensuring that the patient's care rests on a strong moral foundation (Mueller, Hook, & Fleming, 2004; Casarett, Kapo, & Caplan, 2005; McMahon et al., 2005).

The Terri Schiavo Case

To understand the ethical issues raised in the appropriateness of long-term tube feeding, it is helpful to review the recent case of Terri Schiavo (Gostin, 1997). This case highlighted the complexities of medicine, ethics, law, and family dynamics in deciding on the appropriateness of ANH for Terri Schiavo. The patient had suffered a cardiac arrest in 1990 as a result of an electrolyte imbalance precipitated by an eating disorder. The patient had been sustained by ANH through a feeding tube for 15 years. A struggle that was fought out in the courts and the public resulted from a wish by the patient's husband to discontinue ANH and the patient's parents and siblings insisting on ANH being continued.

The facts of the case clearly demonstrated that Ms. Schiavo was in a permanent vegetative state (PVS), a state in which there is no higher cortical functioning and therefore no cognition. Initially, PVS is considered a persistent state, and after a period of 1 year this state becomes permanent. This was attested to by multiple neurologic examinations and is an important point because the facts have to be clear and consistent for a successful ethical discussion. Because there was no conscious awareness, there would be no suffering on her part. Ms. Schiavo was not in a position to state her own wishes—the principle of autonomy rooted in the precept of respect for the person—but her wishes would have been known had she left an advance directive regarding her future care. Because no advance directive was left, the principle of **substituted judgment** was applied through statements by her closest family. Legally, the designated decision-maker was Terri Schiavo's husband, who requested withdrawal of the tube feeding.

> **Substituted judgment:** A legal term used to describe what a person would decide if he or she were able to decide; used when the individual is not competent to provide an autonomous decision.

When the patient's wishes cannot be ascertained (e.g., an infant or one who has always been incompetent to rationally choose), then treatment decisions are based on the patient's best interests, that is, what a reasonable person would most likely want in the same circumstances (Annas, 2004). Ms. Schiavo's family (parents and siblings) did not accept the diagnosis of PVS and believed the condition would improve with further rehabilitative care. The parents strongly believed that withdrawal of the feeding tube would violate their daughter's Catholic belief and be tantamount to euthanasia. This belief, that the withdrawal of feeding would be morally wrong, had the support of a recent allocution by the late Pope John Paul II, who stated that for patients in PVS, "the administration of water and food even when provided by artificial means of preserving life, [is] not a medical act . . . and as such is morally obligatory" (Pope John Paul II, 2004). According to Paris (2005), this interpretation of the Catholic position on the sanctity of life is not consistent with traditional church teaching, and Paris cites the 2001 directive of the U.S. Catholic bishops that states, "A person may forgo means that in the patient's judgment do not offer a reasonable hope or benefit and entail an excessive burden . . ." (Paris, 2005).

There were multiple court hearings and repeated episodes of tube withdrawal and replacement. The case was also politicized, until finally it involved the President of the United States. However, in the end the judicial court ruling of withdrawal of the tube was carried out (Quill, 2005). Ms. Schiavo died a few days after the withdrawal of tube feeding.

Surveys of the attitudes of the American public regarding the Terri Schiavo case were carried out (Blendon, Benson, & Herrmann, 2005). Twelve national opinion surveys showed that most Americans opposed efforts by elected politicians to intervene in the Schiavo case. However, the public was more divided on the question of whether Schiavo's feeding tube should be removed. A substantial minority, 24%

to 42%, opposed it. Of interest too is that one-third of respondents believed she could experience pain and discomfort when the feeding tube was withdrawn.

The Nancy Cruzan Case

The 1990 Nancy Cruzan case also illustrates the legal and ethical approach to withdrawal of tube feeding (*Cruzan v. Director*, 1990). Ms. Cruzan was a patient who had been diagnosed as in a PVS. Her parents brought the issue of withdrawal of tube feeding to the courts. The family was united in this. The Missouri Supreme Court noted that tube feeding could be discontinued on the basis of Nancy's right of self-determination. However, because she was in a PVS she was unable to make that decision, and the court stated that tube feeding could be stopped only if those speaking for her could produce "clear and convincing" evidence that she would refuse the tube feeding if she could speak for herself. Eventually, evidence was brought forward to this effect and the tube feeding was discontinued.

Advance Directives

The Nancy Cruzan case stimulated the public to ensure that individuals could convey personal wishes regarding their care through advance directives or assignments of durable power of attorney. The advance directive would take the form of a "living will" or designation of a health care proxy (Hanson & Rodgman, 1996; Hofmann et al., 1997; Tulsky, Fischer, Rose, & Arnold, 1998; Gillick, 2004). By 2000 every state had passed some form of living will or healthcare proxy law.

The optimal way in which an advance directive should be implemented is to designate one or more persons to act on our behalf to make the treatment decisions when we are unable to make them ourselves (Annas, 2004). This is done in writing using a health care proxy form. It is also important to inform the person or persons designated (often family) how one wants to be treated in specific situations, for example, "do not wish to be tube fed." Doing this verbally is acceptable, but it is preferred to have the instructions in a written letter or living will.

A living will also has its shortcomings. Interventions will be employed by the medical team that the patient may not want to have. This is often difficult to predict. However, with a trusted health care agent who is made aware of your goals of care and your values, the right decision will be made that is in your best interests. The healthcare proxy assumes responsibility when the patient becomes incompetent. Despite the ethical advantages of an **advanced directive,** however, only one-fifth of the public have one in place (Morrison, Zayas, Mulvihill, Baskin, & Meier, 1998).

> **Advanced directive:** Information in written or oral form provided by the patient that outlines the competent adult's wishes regarding medical treatment should he or she become incompetent in the future.

The Anthony Bland Case

This seminal case in Britain involved a young man, Anthony Bland, who was in a PVS for 3 years and in which the courts were asked to adjudicate the withdrawal of food and water administered by a tube. The case eventually reached the highest court in Britain, the law lords in the High Court. The overall decision was to support the withdrawal of ANH. However, of ethical interest are the different approaches by which the justices came to this decision. Some stated it would be an assault to continue to treat without his consent. Others stated that continued treatment would be futile; still others stated it could not be in his best interests to continue to provide treatment that had no prospect of improving his condition. They made the distinction that because he required assisted feeding via a tube, he was unable to feed himself. Therefore it was held that ANH was a medical treatment, which could be withdrawn on the grounds of futility (McClean & Mason, 2003).

Special Condition of Dementia

The wisdom of providing tube feeding in patients with severe dementia has come under question (Finucane et al., 1999; Mitchell, Tetroe, & O'Connor, 2001; Post, 2001; Meier, Ahronheim, Morris, Baskin-Lyons, & Morrison, 2002). Tube feeding seldom achieves its intended medical aims in this condition and rather than prevent suffering can cause it; thus it should not be recommended to patients with advanced dementia (Gillick, 2000). These patients often pull out their tubes and therefore have to be restrained, leading to further agitation and distress, with the need for pharmacologic sedation. Also, the feeding tube fails to prevent pulmonary aspiration, because this usually occurs as a result of gastric reflux and aspiration of saliva. Survival rates in patients with tube feeding are not extended (Sanders et al., 2000). Overall, there is little benefit for gastrostomy tubes and much potential for harm.

Withdrawing or Withholding Treatment

Many believe it is more acceptable to withhold a treatment than to withdraw it. This distinction is not supported by currently accepted ethical and legal reasoning (Beauchamp & Childress, 2001; Meisel & Cerminara, 2004).

Some have argued that there is an analogy between tube feeding and mechanical ventilation: Both are seen as medical treatments, and withdrawal of one has the same ethical and legal foundation as the other. Others have argued, however, that mechanical ventilation replaces the capacity to breathe, whereas a tube does not replace the capacity to digest but merely delivers food to the stomach (Keown, 2002).

With regard to withholding or withdrawing ANH from terminally ill or permanently unconscious patients, the courts have decreed that administration of ANH is like any other medical treatment and may be withdrawn if the patient refuses the treatment or, in the case of the incapacitated patient, the appropriate standard is met (Meisel, Snyder, Quill, & the American College of Physicians–American Society of Internal Medicine End-of-Life Care Consensus Panel, 2000). This followed the U.S. Supreme Court's 1990 Cruzan decision giving qualified approval to this practice. In this situation the death of the patient results from the patient's underlying condition so there is no legal liability for the patient's death.

Quality of Life

Quality of life at the end of life is receiving increasing attention. In considering the patient at the end of life, the whole person's physical, psychological, social, and spiritual parts need to be considered because they significantly affect the person's experience of illness (Singer, Martin, & Kelner, 1999). It is estimated that almost 85% of Americans who continue to die in hospitals and nursing homes are denied the benefits of palliative care at this time (Rummans, Bostwick, & Clark, 2000). Modern sophisticated technologies are often accompanied by increased suffering, pain, and emotional distress. It is important for health care workers to recognize that their own biases and misconceptions can greatly influence patients' emotional, social, and spiritual distress.

Moral Distinction Between Killing and Letting Die

Of concern in the act of withdrawing tube feeding is the moral distinction between killing and letting die. It is legally and ethically acceptable to allow a patient to die when the burdens and risks of life-prolonging treatment clearly outweigh their benefits. Legally, an act of killing is murder if it was intended and is prohibited in our culture. When ANH is with-

drawn the foreseen death occurs from natural causes. There can be ambiguity around the cause of death when the feeding tube is withdrawn. Some argue that withdrawal of the tube is the cause of death. However, death is caused by the underlying failure of an organ system; the fundamental cause of death is the patient's condition, not the withdrawal of treatment. The life support has on a temporary basis postponed the death. If there is no reasonable hope of recovery, further life-sustaining treatment cannot benefit the patient, and therefore it is not in the patient's interests to continue it. When it is removed, the body's own causality results in the death (Randall & Downie, 1999).

Communication

Effective communication often helps to prevent ethical dilemmas. In communicating with the patient we need to learn the patient's values, goals, and beliefs. It is also very important that the prognosis and facts associated with the patient's condition are clearly spelled out and mutually understood. The process of informed consent should be carefully carried out, not rushed, and with a mutual understanding of the patient's goals of care (Brett & Rosenberg, 2001). Deep-rooted cultural and religious beliefs affect the patient's approach to the consideration of the appropriateness of long-term tube feeding (Orr, Marshall, & Osborn, 1995; Helman, 2000). Some patients and especially families consider removal of tube feeding as unethical because it is a state of "starvation" (Helman, 2000; Pope John Paul II, 2004).

Patients' families at times believe that lack of ANH causes suffering and will demand that "everything be done" to avoid this, including placement of PEG and long-term tube feeding. However, clinicians are not obligated to provide futile treatment (Snyder, Leffler, & the Ethics and Human Rights Committee, American College of Physicians, 2005). It is necessary to clearly define what is meant by futile. This judgment must take into account the goals of care, the proposed treatment, and the outcome so that we are virtually certain the goal cannot be achieved.

How the issue of ANH is presented to the patient and family requires compassion and appropriate choice of words that are clearly communicated. An example of this was provided by clinicians caring for amyotrophic lateral sclerosis patients based on their clinical experience. They explained that PEG had risks, such as infection at the site of the tube, disfigurement of body shape, and diarrhea or constipation that may not always be transient. They also explained that tube feeding was cumbersome and with loss of hand movement required an assistant at every meal. The clinicians told patients that to decide against tube feeding was okay and they wouldn't starve because their bodies would adjust and not feel hunger. However, many patients have stated that they wished they'd chosen it sooner (Mitsumoto & Rabkin, 2007).

Many health care workers, unfamiliar with the ethical arguments, the law in the state in which they practice, and the fact that the Supreme Court justices decreed ANH to be a form of medical treatment and could be terminated, align themselves with family concerns that their loved one would "starve to death." In a study of physicians regarding ANH appropriateness, 34% of medical attending physicians and 45% of surgical attending physicians that responded believed that even if life support in the form of mechanical ventilation of dialysis was stopped, nutrition and hydration should always be continued (Solomon et al., 1993).

Summary

The increasing use of tube feeding has led to a consideration of the appropriateness based on the benefits and burdens associated with the procedure. Studies have been carried out to assess the patients' and families' preferences and the experience of tube feeding being withheld.

When a decision is considered that enteral tube feeding is indicated, the patient is informed of the risks and benefits of the intervention and alternatives, including doing nothing. This is the basis of informed consent, and the patient demonstrates a clear understanding of the issues and appropriate decision-making capacity. Respecting the patient's choice is the principle of **autonomy** and in our culture has come to override the other principle of **beneficence,** that is, doing good (or nonmalfeasance, that is, not doing harm). The need for advanced directives is stressed as a means to ensure the patient's wishes are respected at all times. Optimal care of the patient involves a multidisciplinary approach in which the registered dietitian should play an active role in all decisions made by the health care team.

Autonomy: The paramount ethical principle that states the competent adult has the right to make choices about treatment options.

Beneficence: The ethical principle of doing good; for example, proposing a therapy that is worthwhile for the patient (patient centered). This agrees with the ethical principle of nonmalfeasance, which is "not doing any harm."

Case Study and Issues to Debate

The patient is an 82-year-old with severe Alzheimer's dementia. He has had repeated episodes of aspiration pneumonia. He lacks decision-making capacity and had not left an advance directive as to his care wishes. Identifying the ethically relevant facts is considered under the following in this case (Jonsen et al., 2002):

1. Medical indication for long-term tube feeding: The principles of beneficence and nonmalfeasance (do no harm) are applied. Will the patient benefit from the procedures and will the procedure hurt more than help?
2. Patient preferences: Respect for autonomy is the primary principle. Does the patient have decision-making capacity? Lacking this capacity, is there an appropriate surrogate?
3. Quality of life: The principles of beneficence, nonmalfeasance, and autonomy are considered. In this case the evidence appears to indicate no worthwhile benefits to tube feeding, whereas the procedure has significant risks.
4. Contextual features: Cultural and religious traditions need to be taken into account. If there is a conflict of interest with regard to the clinician's or institution's standards, consideration should be given to transfer to another clinician or institution.

References

American Academy of Hospice and Palliative Medicine. (December 8, 2006). Statement on the use of nutrition and hydration. Retrieved July 24, 2007 from http://www.aahpm.org/positions/nutrition.html.

American Dietetic Association. (2002). Ethical and legal issues in nutrition, hydration and feeding. *Journal of the American Dietetic Association, 102,* 716–726.

American Nurses Association. (April 2, 1992). Position statement on foregoing nutrition and fluid. ANA Nursing World. Retrieved July 24, 2007 from http://www.nursingworld.org/readroom/position/ethics/etnutr.htm.

Annas, G. J. (2004). *The Rights of Patients* (3rd ed.). New York: New York University Press.

Annas, G. J. (2005). "Culture of life" politics at the bedside: the case of Terri Schiavo. *New England Journal of Medicine, 352,* 1710–1715.

Beauchamp, T. L., & Childress, J. F. (2001). *Principles of Biomedical Ethics* (6th ed.). New York: Oxford University Press.

Blendon, R. J., Benson, J. M., & Herrmann, M. J. (2005). The American public and the Terri Schiavo case. *Archives of Internal Medicine, 65,* 2580–2584.

Brett, A. S., & Rosenberg, J. C. (2001). The adequacy of informed consent for placement of gastrostomy tubes. *Archives of Internal Medicine, 161,* 745–748.

Burge, F., Byock, I., Daniels, D., Mueller, F., Schmale, J., & William, C. (1995). Artificial hydration and nutrition in the terminally ill: A review. *Academy of Hospice Physicians.*

Byock, I. (1995). Patient refusal of nutrition and hydration: Walking an ever-finer line. *American Journal of Hospice Palliative Care, 12*, 8–13.

Casarett, D., Kapo, J., & Caplan, A. (2005). Appropriate use of artificial nutrition and hydration: Fundamental principles and recommendations. *New England Journal of Medicine, 353*, 2607–2612.

Cox, A. (2006). End-of-life nutrition and hydration: Issues and ethics. *Today's Dietitian, 7*, 35–40.

Cruzan v. Director, Missouri Department of Health, 110 S.Ct. 2841 (1990).

Ersek, M. (2003). Artificial nutrition and hydration: Clinical issues. *Journal of Hospice Palliative Care Nursing, 5*, 221–230.

Finucane, T. E., Christmas, C., & Travis, K. (1999). Tube feeding in patients with advanced dementia: A review of the evidence. *Journal of the American Medical Association, 282*, 1365–1370.

Gallagher, A. C. R. (1989). *Nutritional Care of the Terminally Ill*. Rockville, MD: Aspen Publishers.

Ganzini, L. (2006). Artificial nutrition and hydration at the end of life: Ethics and evidence. *Palliative and Supportive Care, 4*, 135–143.

Ganzini, L., Goy, E. R., Miller, L. L., Harvath, T. A., Jackson, A., and Delorit, M. A. (2003). Nurses' experiences with hospice patients who refuse food and fluids to hasten death. *New England Journal of Medicine, 349*, 359–365.

Gillick, M. R. (2000). Rethinking the role of tube feeding in patients with advanced dementia. *New England Journal of Medicine, 342*, 206–210.

Gillick, M. R. (2004). Advance care planning. *New England Journal of Medicine, 350*, 7–8.

Gostin, L. O. (1997). Deciding life and death in the courtroom: From Quinlan to Cruzan, Glucksberg, and Vacco: A brief history and analysis of constitutional protection of the "right to die." *Journal of the American Medical Association, 278*, 1523–1528.

Hanson, L. C., & Rodgman, E. (1996). The use of living wills at the end of life: A national study. *Archives of Internal Medicine, 156*, 1018–1022.

Helman, C. (2000). *Culture, Health, and Illness* (4th ed.). Oxford, England: Butterworth–Heinemann.

Hofmann, J. C., Wenger, N. S., Davis, R. B., Teno, J., Connors, A. F. Jr., Desbiens, N., et al. (1997). Patient preferences for communication with physicians about end of life decisions. *Annals of Internal Medicine, 127*, 1–12.

Huang, Z. B., & Ahronheim, J. C. (2000). Nutrition and hydration in terminally ill patients: An update. *Clinics in Geriatric Medicine, 16*, 313–325.

Hurley, D. L., & McMahon, M. M. (2005). Diabetes mellitus. In R. H. Rolandelli, R. Bankhead, J. I. Boulatta, & C. W. Compher (Eds.), *Clinical Nutrition: Enteral and Tube Feeding* (4th ed., pp. 498–505).

Jonsen, A. R., Siegler, M., & Winslade, W. J. (2002). *Clinical Ethics: A Practical Approach to Ethical Decisions in Clinical Medicine* (5th ed.). New York: McGraw-Hill.

Keown, J. (2002). *Euthanasia, Ethics and Public Policy*. Cambridge, England: Cambridge University Press.

McClave, S. A., & Chang, W. K. (2003). Complications of enteral access. *Gastrointestinal Endoscopy, 58*, 739–751.

McClave, S. A., DeMeo, M. T., DeLegge, M. H., DiSario, J. A., Heyland, D. K., Maloney, J. P., et al. (2002). North American Summit on Aspiration in the Critically Ill Patient: Consensus statement. *JPEN. Journal of Parenteral and Enteral Nutrition, 26*(6 Suppl.), 580–585.

McClean, S., & Mason, G. K. (2003). *Legal and Ethical Aspects of Health Care* (p. 165). London: Greenwich Medical Media.

McMahon, M. M. (2004). Parenteral nutrition. In L. Goldman & D. Aussiello (Eds.), *Cecil's Textbook of Medicine* (vol. 2, 22nd ed., pp. 1322–1326). Philadelphia: WB Saunders and Co.

McMahon, M. M., Hurley, D. L., Kamath, P. S., & Mueller, P. S. (2005). Medical and ethical aspects of long-term enteral tube feeding. *Mayo Clinic Proceedings, 80*, 1461–1476.

Meier, D. E., Ahronheim, J. C., Morris, J., Baskin-Lyons, S., & Morrison, R. S. (2002). High short-term mortality in hospitalized patients with advanced dementia: Lack of benefit of tube feeding. *Archives of Internal Medicine, 161*, 594–599.

Meisel, A., & Cerminara, K. L. (2004). *The Right to Die: The Law of End-of-Life Decision Making* (3rd ed.). New York: Aspen.

Meisel, A., Snyder, L., Quill, T., & the American College of Physicians–American Society of Internal Medicine End-of-Life Care Consensus Panel. (2000). Seven legal barriers to end-of-life care: Myths, realities, and grains of truth. *Journal of the American Medical Association, 284*, 2495–2501.

Mitchell, S. L., Buchanan, J. L., Littlehale, S., & Hamel, M. B. (2003). Tube feeding versus hand feeding nursing home residents in advanced dementia. *Journal of the American Geriatrics Society, 51*, 129–131.

Mitchell, S. L., Tetroe, J., & O'Connor, A. M. (2001). A decision aid for long-term tube feeding in cognitively impaired older persons. *Journal of the American Geriatrics Society, 49*, 313–316.

Mitsumoto, H., & Rabkin, J. G. (2007). Palliative care for patients with amyotrophic lateral sclerosis. *Journal of the American Medical Association, 298*, 207–216.

Morita, T., Hyodo, I., Yoshimi, T., Ikenaga, M., Tamura, Y., Yoshizawa, A., et al. (2005). Association between hydration volume and symptoms in terminally ill cancer patients with abdominal malignancies. *Annals of Oncology, 16*, 640–647.

Morrison, R. S., Zayas, L. H., Mulvihill, M., Baskin, S. A., & Meier, D. E. (1998). Barriers to completion of health care proxies: An examination of ethnic differences. *Archives of Internal Medicine, 158*, 2493–2497.

Mueller, P. S., Hook, C. C., & Fleming, K. C. (2004). Ethical issues in geriatrics: A guide for clinicians. *Mayo Clinic Proceedings, 79*, 554–562.

Orr, R. D., Marshall, P. A., & Osborn, J. (1995). Cross-cultural considerations in clinical ethics consultations. *Archives of Family Medicine, 4*, 159–164.

Paris, J. J. (2005). To feed or not to feed: Terri Schiavo and the use of artificial nutrition and fluids. *Southern Medical Journal, 98*, 757–758.

Ponsky, J. L., & Gauderer, M. W. L. (1981). Percutaneous endoscopic gastrostomy, a non-operative technique for feeding gastrostomy. *Gastrointestinal Endoscopy, 27*, 9–11.

Pope John Paul II. (2004). Address to the participants in the International Congress on Life Sustaining Treatments and Vegetative States: Scientific advances and ethical dilemmas. *Origins, 33*, 738–740.

Post, S. G. (2001). Tube feeding and advanced progressive dementia. *Hastings Center Report, 31*, 36–42.

Printz, L. A. (1992). Terminal dehydration, a compassionate treatment. *Archives of Internal Medicine, 152*, 697–700.

Quill, T. E. (2005). Terri Schiavo: A tragedy compounded. *New England Journal of Medicine, 352*, 1630–1633.

Rabeneck, L., Wray, N. P., & Petersen, N. J. (1996). Long-term outcomes of patients receiving percutaneous endoscopic gastrostomy tubes. *Journal of General and Internal Medicine, 11*, 287–293.

Randall, F., & Downie, R. S. (1999). *Palliative Care Ethics* (2nd ed., p. 271). Oxford, England: Oxford University Press.

Rummans, T. A., Bostwick, T. M., & Clark, M. M. (2000). For the Mayo Clinic cancer center quality of life working group. *Mayo Clinic Proceedings, 75*, 1305–1310.

Sanders, D. S., Carter, M. J., D'Silva, J., James, G., Bolton, R. P., & Bardhan, K. D. (2000). Survival analysis in percutaneous endoscopic gastrostomy feeding: A worse outcome in patients with dementia. *American Journal of Gastroenterology, 95*, 1472–1475.

Singer, P. A., Martin, D. K., & Kelner, M. (1999). Quality end-of-life care: Patients' perspectives. *Journal of the American Medical Association, 281*, 163–168.

Slomka, J. (2003). Withholding nutrition at the end of life: Clinical and ethical issues. *Cleveland Clinic Journal of Medicine, 70*, 548–552.

Snyder, L., Leffler, C., & the Ethics and Human Rights Committee, American College of Physicians. (2005). Ethics manual. *Annals of Internal Medicine, 142*, 560–582.

Solomon, M. Z., O'Donnell, L., Jennings, B., Guilfoy, V., Wolf, S. M., Nolan, K., et al. (1993). Decisions near the end of life: Professional views on sustaining treatments. *American Journal of Public Health, 83*, 14–23.

Sullivan, R. J. (1993). Accepting death without artificial nutrition or hydration. *Journal of General Medicine, 8*, 220–224.

Tulsky, J. A., Fischer, G. S., Rose, M. R., & Arnold, R. M. (1998). Opening the black box: How do physicians communicate about advance directives? *Annals of Internal Medicine, 129*, 441–449.

Viola, R. A., Wells, G. A., & Peterson, J. (1997). The effects of fluid status and fluid therapy on the dying: A systematic review. *Journal of Palliative Care, 13*, 41–52.

APPENDIX 1

Centers for Disease Control and Prevention Growth Charts

Birth to 36 months: Boys
Length-for-age and Weight-for-age percentiles

NAME _____

RECORD # _____

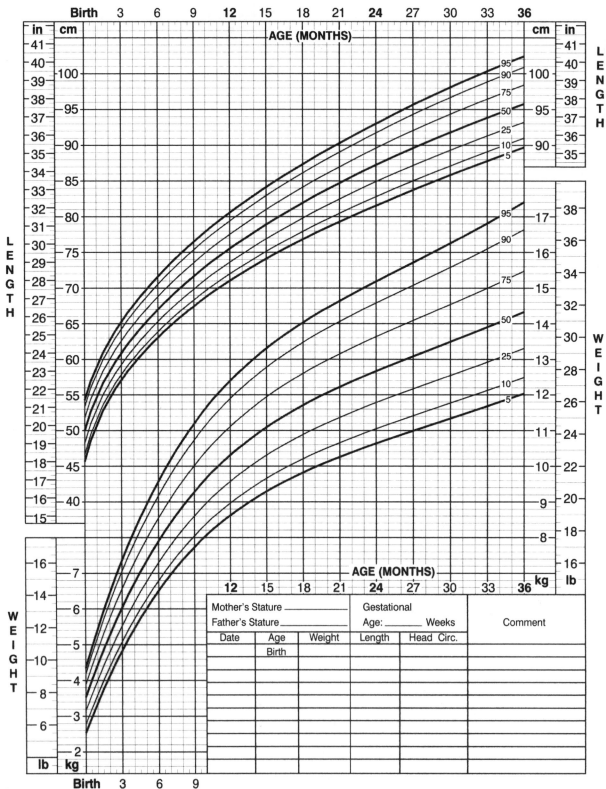

Published May 30, 2000 (modified 4/20/01).
SOURCE: Developed by the National Center for Health Statistics in collaboration with
the National Center for Chronic Disease Prevention and Health Promotion (2000).
http://www.cdc.gov/growthcharts

SAFER · HEALTHIER · PEOPLE™

Birth to 36 months: Girls
Length-for-age and Weight-for-age percentiles

NAME _____

RECORD # _____

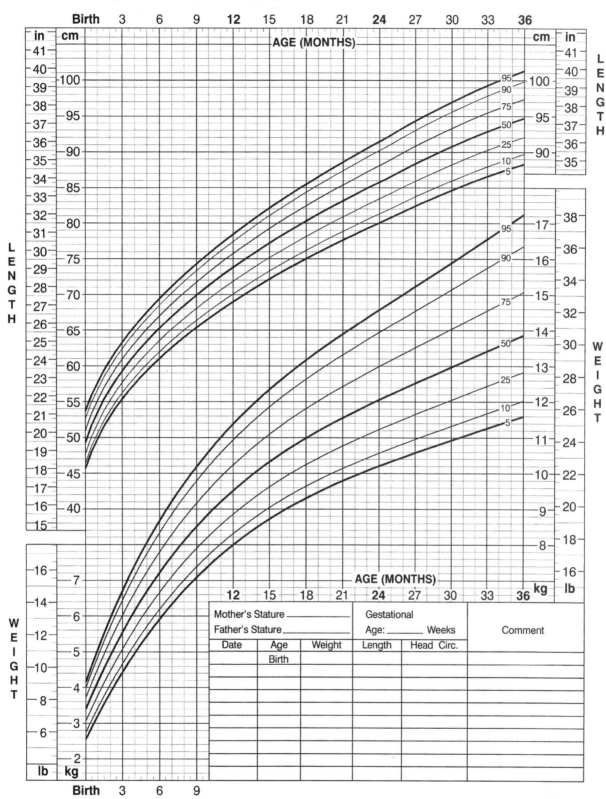

AGE (MONTHS)

Mother's Stature _____
Father's Stature _____

Gestational
Age: _____ Weeks

Comment

Date	Age	Weight	Length	Head Circ.
Birth				

Published May 30, 2000 (modified 4/20/01).
SOURCE: Developed by the National Center for Health Statistics in collaboration with
the National Center for Chronic Disease Prevention and Health Promotion (2000).
http://www.cdc.gov/growthcharts

SAFER · HEALTHIER · PEOPLE™

APPENDIX

2

Dietary Reference Intakes (DRIs)

Dietary Reference Intakes (DRIs): Recommended Intakes for Individuals, Vitamins

Food and Nutrition Board, Institute of Medicine, National Academies

Life Stage Group	Vit A (μg/d)[a]	Vit C (mg/d)	Vit D (μg/d)[b,c]	Vit E (mg/d)[d]	Vit K (μg/d)	Thiamin (mg/d)	Riboflavin (mg/d)	Niacin (mg/d)[e]	Vit B$_6$ (mg/d)	Folate (μg/d)[f]	Vit B$_{12}$ (μg/d)	Pantothenic Acid (mg/d)	Biotin (μg/d)	Choline (mg/d)[g]
Infants														
0–6 mo	400*	40*	5*	4*	2.0*	0.2*	0.3*	2*	0.1*	65*	0.4*	1.7*	5*	125*
7–12 mo	500*	50*	5*	5*	2.5*	0.3*	0.4*	4*	0.3*	80*	0.5*	1.8*	6*	150*
Children														
1–3 y	300	15	5*	6	30*	0.5	0.5	6	0.5	150	0.9	2*	8*	200*
4–8 y	400	25	5*	7	55*	0.6	0.6	8	0.6	200	1.2	3*	12*	250*
Males														
9–13 y	600	45	5*	11	60*	0.9	0.9	12	1.0	300	1.8	4*	20*	375*
14–18 y	900	75	5*	15	75*	1.2	1.3	16	1.3	400	2.4	5*	25*	550*
19–30 y	900	90	5*	15	120*	1.2	1.3	16	1.3	400	2.4	5*	30*	550*
31–50 y	900	90	5*	15	120*	1.2	1.3	16	1.3	400	2.4	5*	30*	550*
51–70 y	900	90	10*	15	120*	1.2	1.3	16	1.7	400	2.4[i]	5*	30*	550*
>70 y	900	90	15*	15	120*	1.2	1.3	16	1.7	400	2.4[i]	5*	30*	550*
Females														
9–13 y	600	45	5*	11	60*	0.9	0.9	12	1.0	300	1.8	4*	20*	375*
14–18 y	700	65	5*	15	75*	1.0	1.0	14	1.2	400[i]	2.4	5*	25*	400*
19–30 y	700	75	5*	15	90*	1.1	1.1	14	1.3	400[i]	2.4	5*	30*	425*
31–50 y	700	75	5*	15	90*	1.1	1.1	14	1.3	400[i]	2.4	5*	30*	425*
51–70 y	700	75	10*	15	90*	1.1	1.1	14	1.5	400	2.4[h]	5*	30*	425*
>70 y	700	75	15*	15	90*	1.1	1.1	14	1.5	400	2.4[h]	5*	30*	425*
Pregnancy														
14–18 y	750	80	5*	15	75*	1.4	1.4	18	1.9	600[i]	2.6	6*	30*	450*
19–30 y	770	85	5*	15	90*	1.4	1.4	18	1.9	600[i]	2.6	6*	30*	450*
31–50 y	770	85	5*	15	90*	1.4	1.4	18	1.9	600[i]	2.6	6*	30*	450*
Lactation														
14–18 y	1,200	115	5*	19	75*	1.4	1.6	17	2.0	500	2.8	7*	35*	550*
19–30 y	1,300	120	5*	19	90*	1.4	1.6	17	2.0	500	2.8	7*	35*	550*
31–50 y	1,300	120	5*	19	90*	1.4	1.6	17	2.0	500	2.8	7*	35*	550*

NOTE: This table (taken from the DRI reports, see www.nap.edu) presents Recommended Dietary Allowances (RDAs) in **bold type** and Adequate Intakes (AIs) in ordinary type followed by an asterisk (*). RDAs and AIs may both be used as goals for individual intake. RDAs are set to meet the needs of almost all (97 to 98 percent) individuals in a group. For healthy breast-fed infants, the AI is the mean intake. The AI for other life stage and gender groups is believed to cover needs of all individuals in the group, but lack of data or uncertainty in the data prevent being able to specify with confidence the percentage of individuals covered by this intake.

[a] As retinol activity equivalents (RAEs). 1 RAE = 1 μg retinol, 12 μg β-carotene, 24 μg α-carotene, or 24 μg β-cryptoxanthin. The RAE for dietary provitamin A carotenoids is twofold greater than retinol equivalents (RE), whereas the RAE for preformed vitamin A is the same as RE.

[b] As cholecalciferol. 1 μg cholecalciferol = 40 IU vitamin D.

[c] In the absence of adequate exposure to sunlight.

[d] As α-tocopherol. α-Tocopherol includes *RRR*-α-tocopherol, the only form of α-tocopherol that occurs naturally in foods, and the 2*R*-stereoisomeric forms of α-tocopherol (*RRR*-, *RSR*-, *RRS*-, and *RSS*-α-tocopherol) that occur in fortified foods and supplements. It does not include the 2*S*-stereoisomeric forms of α-tocopherol (*SRR*-, *SSR*-, *SRS*-, and *SSS*-α-tocopherol), also found in fortified foods and supplements.

[e] As niacin equivalents (NE). 1 mg of niacin = 60 mg of tryptophan; 0–6 months = preformed niacin (not NE).

[f] As dietary folate equivalents (DFE). 1 DFE = 1 µg food folate = 0.6 µg of folic acid from fortified food or as a supplement consumed with food = 0.5 µg of a supplement taken on an empty stomach.

[g] Although AIs have been set for choline, there are few data to assess whether a dietary supply of choline is needed at all stages of the life cycle, and it may be that the choline requirement can be met by endogenous synthesis at some of these stages.

[h] Because 10 to 30 percent of older people may malabsorb food-bound B_{12}, it is advisable for those older than 50 years to meet their RDA mainly by consuming foods fortified with B_{12} or a supplement containing B_{12}.

[i] In view of evidence linking folate intake with neural tube defects in the fetus, it is recommended that all women capable of becoming pregnant consume 400 µg from supplements or fortified foods in addition to intake of food folate from a varied diet.

[j] It is assumed that women will continue consuming 400 µg from supplements or fortified food until their pregnancy is confirmed and they enter prenatal care, which ordinarily occurs after the end of the periconceptional period—the critical time for formation of the neural tube.

Copyright 2004 by the National Academy of Sciences. All rights reserved.

Dietary Reference Intakes (DRIs): Recommended Intakes for Individuals, Elements
Food and Nutrition Board, Institute of Medicine, National Academies

Life Stage Group	Calcium (mg/d)	Chromium (µg/d)	Copper (µg/d)	Fluoride (mg/d)	Iodine (µg/d)	Iron (mg/d)	Magnesium (mg/d)	Manganese (mg/d)	Molybdenum (µg/d)	Phosphorus (mg/d)	Selenium (µg/d)	Zinc (mg/d)	Potassium (g/d)	Sodium (g/d)	Chloride (g/d)
Infants															
0–6 mo	210*	0.2*	200*	0.01*	110*	0.27*	30*	0.003*	2*	100*	15*	2*	0.4*	0.12*	0.18*
7–12 mo	270*	5.5*	220*	0.5*	130*	11	75*	0.6*	3*	275*	20*	3	0.7*	0.37*	0.57*
Children															
1–3 y	500*	11*	340	0.7*	90	7	80	1.2*	17	460	20	3	3.0*	1.0*	1.5*
4–8 y	800*	15*	440	1*	90	10	130	1.5*	22	500	30	5	3.8*	1.2*	1.9*
Males															
9–13 y	1,300*	25*	700	2*	120	8	240	1.9*	34	1,250	40	8	4.5*	1.5*	2.3*
14–18 y	1,300*	35*	890	3*	150	11	410	2.2*	43	1,250	55	11	4.7*	1.5*	2.3*
19–30 y	1,000*	35*	900	4*	150	8	400	2.3*	45	700	55	11	4.7*	1.5*	2.3*
31–50 y	1,000*	35*	900	4*	150	8	420	2.3*	45	700	55	11	4.7*	1.5*	2.3*
51–70 y	1,200*	30*	900	4*	150	8	420	2.3*	45	700	55	11	4.7*	1.3*	2.0*
>70 y	1,200*	30*	900	4*	150	8	420	2.3*	45	700	55	11	4.7*	1.2*	1.8*
Females															
9–13 y	1,300*	21*	700	2*	120	8	240	1.6*	34	1,250	40	8	4.5*	1.5*	2.3*
14–18 y	1,300*	24*	890	3*	150	15	360	1.6*	43	1,250	55	9	4.7*	1.5*	2.3*
19–30 y	1,000*	25*	900	3*	150	18	310	1.8*	45	700	55	8	4.7*	1.5*	2.3*
31–50 y	1,000*	25*	900	3*	150	18	320	1.8*	45	700	55	8	4.7*	1.5*	2.3*
51–70 y	1,200*	20*	900	3*	150	8	320	1.8*	45	700	55	8	4.7*	1.3*	2.0*
>70 y	1,200*	20*	900	3*	150	8	320	1.8*	45	700	55	8	4.7*	1.2*	1.8*
Pregnancy															
14–18 y	1,300*	29*	1,000	3*	220	27	400	2.0*	50	1,250	60	12	4.7*	1.5*	2.3*
19–30 y	1,000*	30*	1,000	3*	220	27	350	2.0*	50	700	60	11	4.7*	1.5*	2.3*
31–50 y	1,000*	30*	1,000	3*	220	27	360	2.0*	50	700	60	11	4.7*	1.5*	2.3*
Lactation															
14–18 y	1,300*	44*	1,300	3*	290	10	360	2.6*	50	1,250	70	13	5.1*	1.5*	2.3*
19–30 y	1,000*	45*	1,300	3*	290	9	310	2.6*	50	700	70	12	5.1*	1.5*	2.3*
31–50 y	1,000*	45*	1,300	3*	290	9	320	2.6*	50	700	70	12	5.1*	1.5*	2.3*

NOTE: This table presents Recommended Dietary Allowances (RDAs) in **bold type** and Adequate Intakes (AIs) in ordinary type followed by an asterisk (*). RDAs and AIs may both be used as goals for individual intake. RDAs are set to meet the needs of almost all (97 to 98 percent) individuals in a group. For healthy breast-fed infants, the AI is the mean intake. The AI for other life stage and gender groups is believed to cover needs of all individuals in the group, but lack of data or uncertainty in the data prevent being able to specify with confidence the percentage of individuals covered by this intake.

Sources: *Dietary Reference Intakes for Calcium, Phosphorous, Magnesium, Vitamin D, and Fluoride* (1997); *Dietary Reference Intakes for Thiamin, Riboflavin, Niacin, Vitamin B₆, Folate, Vitamin B₁₂, Pantothenic Acid, Biotin, and Choline* (1998); *Dietary Reference Intakes for Vitamin C, Vitamin E, Selenium, and Carotenoids* (2000); *Dietary Reference Intakes for Vitamin A, Vitamin K, Arsenic, Boron, Chromium, Copper, Iodine, Iron, Manganese, Molybdenum, Nickel, Silicon, Vanadium, and Zinc* (2001); and *Dietary Reference Intakes for Water, Potassium, Sodium, Chloride, and Sulfate* (2004). These reports may be accessed via http://www.nap.edu. Copyright 2004 by the National Academy of Sciences. All rights reserved.

Dietary Reference Intakes (DRIs): Tolerable Upper Intake Levels (UL[a]), Vitamins

Food and Nutrition Board, Institute of Medicine, National Academies

Life Stage Group	Vitamin A (µg/d)[b]	Vitamin C (mg/d)	Vitamin D (µg/d)	Vitamin E (mg/d)[c,d]	Vitamin K	Thiamin	Riboflavin	Niacin (mg/d)[d]	Vitamin B$_6$ (mg/d)	Folate (µg/d)[d]	Vitamin B$_{12}$	Pantothenic Acid	Biotin	Choline (g/d)	Carotenoids[e]
Infants															
0-6 mo	600	ND[f]	25	ND	ND	ND	ND	ND	ND	ND	ND	ND	ND	ND	ND
7-12 mo	600	ND	25	ND	ND	ND	ND	ND	ND	ND	ND	ND	ND	ND	ND
Children															
1-3 y	600	400	50	200	ND	ND	ND	10	30	300	ND	ND	ND	1.0	ND
4-8 y	900	650	50	300	ND	ND	ND	15	40	400	ND	ND	ND	1.0	ND
Males, Females															
9-13 y	1,700	1,200	50	600	ND	ND	ND	20	60	600	ND	ND	ND	2.0	ND
14-18 y	2,800	1,800	50	800	ND	ND	ND	30	80	800	ND	ND	ND	3.0	ND
19-70 y	3,000	2,000	50	1,000	ND	ND	ND	35	100	1,000	ND	ND	ND	3.5	ND
>70 y	3,000	2,000	50	1,000	ND	ND	ND	35	100	1,000	ND	ND	ND	3.5	ND
Pregnancy															
14-18 y	2,800	1,800	50	800	ND	ND	ND	30	80	800	ND	ND	ND	3.0	ND
19-50 y	3,000	2,000	50	1,000	ND	ND	ND	35	100	1,000	ND	ND	ND	3.5	ND
Lactation															
14-18 y	2,800	1,800	50	800	ND	ND	ND	30	80	800	ND	ND	ND	3.0	ND
19-50 y	3,000	2,000	50	1,000	ND	ND	ND	35	100	1,000	ND	ND	ND	3.5	ND

[a]UL = The maximum level of daily nutrient intake that is likely to pose no risk of adverse effects. Unless otherwise specified, the UL represents total intake from food, water, and supplements. Due to lack of suitable data, ULs could not be established for vitamin K, thiamin, riboflavin, vitamin B12, pantothenic acid, biotin, carotenoids. In the absence of ULs, extra caution may be warranted in consuming levels above recommended intakes.

[b]As preformed vitamin A only.

[c]As α-tocopherol; applies to any form of supplemental α-tocopherol.

[d]The ULs for vitamin E, niacin, and folate apply to synthetic forms obtained from supplements, fortified foods, or a combination of the two.

[e]β-Carotene supplements are advised only to serve as a provitamin A source for individuals at risk of vitamin A deficiency.

[f]ND = Not determinable due to lack of data of adverse effects in this age group and concern with regard to lack of ability to handle excess amounts. Source of intake should be from food only to prevent high levels of intake.

Sources: *Dietary Reference Intakes for Calcium, Phosphorous, Magnesium, Vitamin D, and Fluoride* (1997); *Dietary Reference Intakes for Thiamin, Riboflavin, Niacin, Vitamin B$_6$, Folate, Vitamin B$_{12}$, Pantothenic Acid, Biotin, and Choline* (1998); *Dietary Reference Intakes for Vitamin C, Vitamin E, Selenium, and Carotenoids* (2000); *and Dietary Reference Intakes for Vitamin A, Vitamin K, Arsenic, Boron, Chromium, Copper, Iodine, Iron, Manganese, Molybdenum, Nickel, Silicon, Vanadium, and Zinc* (2001). These reports may be accessed via http://www.nap.edu.

Dietary Reference Intakes (DRIs): Tolerable Upper Intake Levels (UL^a), Elements

Food and Nutrition Board, Institute of Medicine, National Academies

Life Stage Group	Arsenic^b	Boron (mg/d)	Calcium (g/d)	Chromium	Copper (μg/d)	Fluoride (mg/d)	Iodine (μg/d)	Iron (mg/d)	Magnesium (mg/d)^c	Manganese (mg/d)	Molybdenum (μg/d)	Nickel (mg/d)	Phosphorus (g/d)	Potassium	Selenium (μg/d)	Silicon^d	Sulfate	Vanadium (mg/d)^e	Zinc (mg/d)	Sodium (g/d)	Chloride (g/d)
Infants																					
0–6 mo	ND^f	ND	ND	ND	ND	0.7	ND	40	ND	ND	ND	ND	ND	ND	45	ND	ND	ND	4	ND	ND
7–12 mo	ND	ND	ND	ND	ND	0.9	ND	40	ND	ND	ND	ND	ND	ND	60	ND	ND	ND	5	ND	ND
Children																					
1–3 y	ND	3	2.5	ND	1,000	1.3	200	40	65	2	300	0.2	3	ND	90	ND	ND	ND	7	1.5	2.3
4–8 y	ND	6	2.5	ND	3,000	2.2	300	40	110	3	600	0.3	3	ND	150	ND	ND	ND	12	1.9	2.9
Males,																					
Females																					
9–13 y	ND	11	2.5	ND	5,000	10	600	40	350	6	1,100	0.6	4	ND	280	ND	ND	ND	23	2.2	3.4
14–18 y	ND	17	2.5	ND	8,000	10	900	45	350	9	1,700	1.0	4	ND	400	ND	ND	ND	34	2.3	3.6
19–70 y	ND	20	2.5	ND	10,000	10	1,100	45	350	11	2,000	1.0	4	ND	400	ND	ND	1.8	40	2.3	3.6
>70 y	ND	20	2.5	ND	10,000	10	1,100	45	350	11	2,000	1.0	3	ND	400	ND	ND	1.8	40	2.3	3.6
Pregnancy																					
14–18 y	ND	17	2.5	ND	8,000	10	900	45	350	9	1,700	1.0	3.5	ND	400	ND	ND	ND	34	2.3	3.6
19–50 y	ND	20	2.5	ND	10,000	10	1,100	45	350	11	2,000	1.0	3.5	ND	400	ND	ND	ND	40	2.3	3.6
Lactation																					
14–18 y	ND	17	2.5	ND	8,000	10	900	45	350	9	1,700	1.0	4	ND	400	ND	ND	ND	34	2.3	3.6
19–50 y	ND	20	2.5	ND	10,000	10	1,100	45	350	11	2,000	1.0	4	ND	400	ND	ND	ND	40	2.3	3.6

^{a}UL = The maximum level of daily nutrient intake that is likely to pose no risk of adverse effects. Unless otherwise specified, the UL represents total intake from food, water, and supplements. Due to lack of suitable data, ULs could not be established for arsenic, chromium, silicon, potassium, and sulfate. In the absence of ULs, extra caution may be warranted in consuming levels above recommended intakes.

^{b}Although the UL was not determined for arsenic, there is no justification for adding arsenic to food or supplements.

^{c}The ULs for magnesium represent intake from a pharmacological agent only and do not include intake from food and water.

^{d}Although silicon has not been shown to cause adverse effects in humans, there is no justification for adding silicon to supplements.

^{e}Although vanadium in food has not been shown to cause adverse effects in humans, there is no justification for adding vanadium to food and vanadium supplements should be used with caution. The UL is based on adverse effects in laboratory animals and this data could be used to set a UL for adults but not children and adolescents.

^{f}ND = Not determinable due to lack of data of adverse effects in this age group and concern with regard to lack of ability to handle excess amounts. Source of intake should be from food only to prevent high levels of intake.

Sources: *Dietary Reference Intakes for Calcium, Phosphorous, Magnesium, Vitamin D, and Fluoride* (1997); *Dietary Reference Intakes for Thiamin, Riboflavin, Niacin, Vitamin B$_6$, Folate, Vitamin B$_{12}$, Pantothenic Acid, Biotin, and Choline* (1998); *Dietary Reference Intakes for Vitamin C, Vitamin E, Selenium, and Carotenoids* (2000); *Dietary Reference Intakes for Vitamin A, Vitamin K, Arsenic, Boron, Chromium, Copper, Iodine, Iron, Manganese, Molybdenum, Nickel, Silicon, Vanadium, and Zinc* (2001); and *Dietary Reference Intakes for Water, Potassium, Sodium, Chloride, and Sulfate* (2004). These reports may be accessed via http://www.nap.edu.

Dietary Reference Intakes (DRIs): Estimated Energy Requirements (EER) for Men and Women 30 Years of Age[a]

Food and Nutrition Board, Institute of Medicine, National Academies

Height (m [in])	Weight for BMI[c] of 18.5 kg/m2 (kg [lb])	Weight for BMI of 24.99 kg/m2 (kg [lb])	PAL[b]	EER, Men[d] (kcal/day) BMI of 18.5 kg/m2	EER, Men[d] (kcal/day) BMI of 24.99 kg/m2	EER, Women[d] (kcal/day) BMI of 18.5 kg/m2	EER, Women[d] (kcal/day) BMI of 24.99 kg/m2
1.50 (59)	41.6 (92)	56.2 (124)	Sedentary	1,848	2,080	1,625	1,762
			Low active	2,009	2,267	1,803	1,956
			Active	2,215	2,506	2,025	2,198
			Very active	2,554	2,898	2,291	2,489
1.65 (65)	50.4 (111)	68.0 (150)	Sedentary	2,068	2,349	1,816	1,982
			Low active	2,254	2,566	2,016	2,202
			Active	2,490	2,842	2,267	2,477
			Very active	2,880	3,296	2,567	2,807
1.80 (71)	59.9 (132)	81.0 (178)	Sedentary	2,301	2,635	2,015	2,211
			Low active	2,513	2,884	2,239	2,459
			Active	2,782	3,200	2,519	2,769
			Very active	3,225	3,720	2,855	3,141

[a]For each year below 30, add 7 kcal/day for women and 10 kcal /day for men. For each year above 30, subtract 7 kcal/day for women and 10 kcal/day for men.

[b]PAL = physical activity level.

[c]BMI = body mass index.

[d]Derived from the following regression equations based on doubly labeled water data:

Adult man: $EER = 662 - 9.53 \times age (y) + PA \times (15.91 \times wt [kg] + 539.6 \times ht [m])$

Adult woman: $EER = 354 - 6.91 \times age (y) + PA \times (9.36 \times wt [kg] + 726 \times ht [m])$

Where PA refers to coefficient for PAL

PAL = total energy expenditure ÷ basal energy expenditure PA = 1.0 if PAL ≥ 1.0 < 1.4 (sedentary) PA = 1.12 if PAL ≥ 1.4 < 1.6 (low active) PA = 1.27 if PAL ≥ 1.6 < 1.9 (active) PA = 1.45 if PAL ≥ 1.9 < 2.5 (very active)

Dietary Reference Intakes (DRIs): Acceptable Macronutrient Distribution Ranges
Food and Nutrition Board, Institute of Medicine, National Academies

Range (percent of energy)

Macronutrient	Children, 1–3 y	Children, 4–18 y	Adults
Fat	30–40	25–35	20–35
n-6 polyunsaturated fatty acids[a] (linoleic acid)	5–10	5–10	5–10
n-3 polyunsaturated fatty acids[a] (α-linolenic acid)	0.6–1.2	0.6–1.2	0.6–1.2
Carbohydrate	45–65	45–65	45–65
Protein	5–20	10–30	10–35

[a]Approximately 10% of the total can come from longer-chain n-3 or n-6 fatty acids.

Source: *Dietary Reference Intakes for Energy, Carbohydrate, Fiber, Fat, Fatty Acids, Cholesterol, Protein, and Amino Acids* (2002).

Dietary Reference Intakes (DRIs): Recommended Intakes for Individuals, Macronutrients
Food and Nutrition Board, Institute of Medicine, National Academies

Life Stage Group	Total Water[a] (L/d)	Carbohydrate (g/d)	Total Fiber (g/d)	Fat (g/d)	Linoleic Acid (g/d)	α-Linolenic Acid (g/d)	Protein[b] (g/d)
Infants							
0–6 mo	0.7*	60*	ND	31*	4.4*	0.5*	9.1*
7–12 mo	0.8*	95*	ND	30*	4.6*	0.5*	11.0[c]
Children							
1–3 y	1.3*	130	19*	ND	7*	0.7*	13
4–8 y	1.7*	130	25*	ND	10*	0.9*	19
Males							
9–13 y	2.4*	130	31*	ND	12*	1.2*	34
14–18 y	3.3*	130	38*	ND	16*	1.6*	52
19–30 y	3.7*	130	38*	ND	17*	1.6*	56
31–50 y	3.7*	130	38*	ND	17*	1.6*	56
51–70 y	3.7*	130	30*	ND	14*	1.6*	56
>70 y	3.7*	130	30*	ND	14*	1.6*	56
Females							
9–13 y	2.1*	130	26*	ND	10*	1.0*	34
14–18 y	2.3*	130	26*	ND	11*	1.1*	46
19–30 y	2.7*	130	25*	ND	12*	1.1*	46
31–50 y	2.7*	130	25*	ND	12*	1.1*	46
51–70 y	2.7*	130	21*	ND	11*	1.1*	46
>70 y	2.7*	130	21*	ND	11*	1.1*	46
Pregnancy							
14–18 y	3.0*	175	28*	ND	13*	1.4*	71
19–30 y	3.0*	175	28*	ND	13*	1.4*	71
31–50 y	3.0*	175	28*	ND	13*	1.4*	71
Lactation							
14–18 y	3.8*	210	29*	ND	13*	1.3*	71
19–30 y	3.8*	210	29*	ND	13*	1.3*	71
31–50 y	3.8*	210	29*	ND	13*	1.3*	71

NOTE: This table presents Recommended Dietary Allowances (RDAs) in **bold** type and Adequate Intakes (AIs) in ordinary type followed by an asterisk (*). RDAs and AIs may both be used as goals for individual intake. RDAs are set to meet the needs of almost all (97 to 98 percent) individuals in a group. For healthy infants fed human milk, the AI is the mean intake. The AI for other life stage and gender groups is believed to cover the needs of all individuals in the group, but lack of data or uncertainty in the data prevent being able to specify with confidence the percentage of individuals covered by this intake.

[a]*Total* water includes all water contained in food, beverages, and drinking water.
[b]Based on 0.8 g/kg body weight for the reference body weight.
[c]Change from 0.8 g/kg body weight/d in prepublication copy due to calculation error.

Dietary Reference Intakes (DRIs): Additional Macronutrient Recommendations

Food and Nutrition Board, Institute of Medicine, National Academies

Macronutrient	Recommendation
Dietary cholesterol	As low as possible while consuming a nutritionally adequate diet
Trans fatty acids	As low as possible while consuming a nutritionally adequate diet
Saturated fatty acids	As low as possible while consuming a nutritionally adequate diet
Added sugars	Limit to no more than 25% of total energy

Source: *Dietary Reference Intakes for Energy, Carbohydrate, Fiber, Fat, Fatty Acids, Cholesterol, Protein, and Amino Acids* (2002).

Dietary Reference Intakes (DRIs): Estimated Average Requirements for Groups
Food and Nutrition Board, Institute of Medicine, National Academies

Life Stage Group	CHO (g/d)	Protein (g/d)[a]	Vit A (µg/d)[b]	Vit C (mg/d)	Vit E (mg/d)[c]	Thiamin (mg/d)	Riboflavin (mg/d)	Niacin (mg/d)[d]	Vit B6 (mg/d)	Folate (µg/d)[b]	Vit B12 (µg/d)	Copper (µg/d)	Iodine (µg/d)	Iron (mg/d)	Magnesium (mg/d)	Molybdenum (µg/d)	Phosphorus (mg/d)	Selenium (µg/d)	Zinc (mg/d)
Infants																			
7–12 mo		9*												6.9					2.5
Children																			
1–3 y	100	11	210	13	5	0.4	0.4	5	0.4	120	0.7	260	65	3.0	65	13	380	17	2.5
4–8 y	100	15	275	22	6	0.5	0.5	6	0.5	160	1.0	340	65	4.1	110	17	405	23	4.0
Males																			
9–13 y	100	27	445	39	9	0.7	0.8	9	0.8	250	1.5	540	73	5.9	200	26	1,055	35	7.0
14–18 y	100	44	630	63	12	1.0	1.1	12	1.1	330	2.0	685	95	7.7	340	33	1,055	45	8.5
19–30 y	100	46	625	75	12	1.0	1.1	12	1.1	320	2.0	700	95	6	330	34	580	45	9.4
31–50 y	100	46	625	75	12	1.0	1.1	12	1.1	320	2.0	700	95	6	350	34	580	45	9.4
51–70 y	100	46	625	75	12	1.0	1.1	12	1.4	320	2.0	700	95	6	350	34	580	45	9.4
.70 y	100	46	625	75	12	1.0	1.1	12	1.4	320	2.0	700	95	6	350	34	580	45	9.4
Females																			
9–13 y	100	28	420	39	9	0.7	0.8	9	0.8	250	1.5	540	73	5.7	200	26	1,055	35	7.0
14–18 y	100	38	485	56	12	0.9	0.9	11	1.0	330	2.0	685	95	7.9	300	33	1,055	45	7.3
19–30 y	100	38	500	60	12	0.9	0.9	11	1.1	320	2.0	700	95	8.1	255	34	580	45	6.8
31–50 y	100	38	500	60	12	0.9	0.9	11	1.1	320	2.0	700	95	8.1	265	34	580	45	6.8
51–70 y	100	38	500	60	12	0.9	0.9	11	1.3	320	2.0	700	95	5	265	34	580	45	6.8
.70 y	100	38	500	60	12	0.9	0.9	11	1.3	320	2.0	700	95	5	265	34	580	45	6.8
Pregnancy																			
14–18 y	135	50	530	66	12	1.2	1.2	14	1.6	520	2.2	785	160	23	335	40	1,055	49	10.5
19–30 y	135	50	550	70	12	1.2	1.2	14	1.6	520	2.2	800	160	22	290	40	580	49	9.5
31–50 y	135	50	550	70	12	1.2	1.2	14	1.6	520	2.2	800	160	22	300	40	580	49	9.5
Lactation																			
14–18 y	160	60	885	96	16	1.2	1.3	13	1.7	450	2.4	985	209	7	300	35	1,055	59	10.9
19–30 y	160	60	900	100	16	1.2	1.3	13	1.7	450	2.4	1,000	209	6.5	255	36	580	59	10.4
31–50 y	160	60	900	100	16	1.2	1.3	13	1.7	450	2.4	1,000	209	6.5	265	36	580	59	10.4

NOTE: This table presents Estimated Average Requirements (EARs), which serve two purposes: for assessing adequacy of population intakes, and as the basis for calculating Recommended Dietary Allowances (RDAs) for individuals for those nutrients. EARs have not been established for vitamin D, vitamin K, pantothenic acid, biotin, choline, calcium, chromium, fluoride, manganese, or other nutrients not yet evaluated via the DRI process.

[a] For individual at reference weight (Table 1-1). *indicates change from prepublication copy due to calculation error.

[b] As retinol activity equivalents (RAEs). 1 RAE = 1 µg retinol, 12 µg β-carotene, 24 µg α-carotene, or 24 µg β-cryptoxanthin. The RAE for dietary provitamin A carotenoids is twofold greater than retinol equivalents (RE), whereas the RAE for preformed vitamin A is the same as RE.

[c] As α-tocopherol. α-Tocopherol includes RRR-α-tocopherol, the only form of α-tocopherol that occurs naturally in foods, and the 2R-stereoisomeric forms of α-tocopherol (RRR-, RSR-, RRS-, and RSS-α-tocopherol) that occur in fortified foods and supplements. It does not include the 2S-stereoisomeric forms of α-tocopherol (SRR-, SSR-, SRS-, and SSS-α-tocopherol), also found in fortified foods and supplements.

[d] As niacin equivalents (NE). 1 mg of niacin = 60 mg of tryptophan.

[e] As dietary folate equivalents (DFE). 1 DFE = 1µg food folate = 0.6 µg of folic acid from fortified food or as a supplement consumed with food = 0.5 µg of a supplement taken on an empty stomach.

Sources: *Dietary Reference Intakes for Calcium, Phosphorous, Magnesium, Vitamin D, and Fluoride* (1997); *Dietary Reference Intakes for Thiamin, Riboflavin, Niacin, Vitamin B₆, Folate, Vitamin B₁₂, Pantothenic Acid, Biotin, and Choline* (1998); *Dietary Reference Intakes for Vitamin C, Vitamin E, Selenium, and Carotenoids* (2000); *Dietary Reference Intakes for Vitamin A, Vitamin K, Arsenic, Boron, Chromium, Copper, Iodine, Iron, Manganese, Molybdenum, Nickel, Silicon, Vanadium, and Zinc* (2001), and *Dietary Reference Intakes for Energy, Carbohydrate, Fiber, Fat, Fatty Acids, Cholesterol, Protein, and Amino Acids* (2002). These reports may be accessed via www.nap.edu.

APPENDIX

3

Body Mass Index for Adults

	Normal						Overweight					Obese										Extreme Obesity															
BMI	19	20	21	22	23	24	25	26	27	28	29	30	31	32	33	34	35	36	37	38	39	40	41	42	43	44	45	46	47	48	49	50	51	52	53	54
Height (inches)															Body Weight (pounds)																					
58	91	96	100	105	110	115	119	124	129	134	138	143	148	153	158	162	167	172	177	181	186	191	196	201	205	210	215	220	224	229	234	239	244	248	253	258
59	94	99	104	109	114	119	124	128	133	138	143	148	153	158	163	168	173	178	183	188	193	198	203	208	212	217	222	227	232	237	242	247	252	257	262	267
60	97	102	107	112	118	123	128	133	138	143	148	153	158	163	168	174	179	184	189	194	199	204	209	215	220	225	230	235	240	245	250	255	261	266	271	276
61	100	106	111	116	122	127	132	137	143	148	153	158	164	169	174	180	185	190	195	201	206	211	217	222	227	232	238	243	248	254	259	264	269	275	280	285
62	104	109	115	120	126	131	136	142	147	153	158	164	169	175	180	186	191	196	202	207	213	218	224	229	235	240	246	251	256	262	267	273	278	284	289	295
63	107	113	118	124	130	135	141	146	152	158	163	169	175	180	186	191	197	203	208	214	220	225	231	237	242	248	254	259	265	270	278	282	287	293	299	304
64	110	116	122	128	134	140	145	151	157	163	169	174	180	186	192	197	204	209	215	221	227	232	238	244	250	256	262	267	273	279	285	291	296	302	308	314
65	114	120	126	132	138	144	150	156	162	168	174	180	186	192	198	204	210	216	222	228	234	240	246	252	258	264	270	276	282	288	294	300	306	312	318	324
66	118	124	130	136	142	148	155	161	167	173	179	186	192	198	204	210	216	223	229	235	241	247	253	260	266	272	278	284	291	297	303	309	315	322	328	334
67	121	127	134	140	146	153	159	166	172	178	185	191	198	204	211	217	223	230	236	242	249	255	261	268	274	280	287	293	299	306	312	319	325	331	338	344
68	125	131	138	144	151	158	164	171	177	184	190	197	203	210	216	223	230	236	243	249	256	262	269	276	282	289	295	302	308	315	322	328	335	341	348	354
69	128	135	142	149	155	162	169	176	182	189	196	203	209	216	223	230	236	243	250	257	263	270	277	284	291	297	304	311	318	324	331	338	345	351	358	365
70	132	139	146	153	160	167	174	181	188	195	202	209	216	222	229	236	243	250	257	264	271	278	285	292	299	306	313	320	327	334	341	348	355	362	369	376
71	136	143	150	157	165	172	179	186	193	200	208	215	222	229	236	243	250	257	265	272	279	286	293	301	308	315	322	329	338	343	351	358	365	372	379	386
72	140	147	154	162	169	177	184	191	199	206	213	221	228	235	242	250	258	265	272	279	287	294	302	309	316	324	331	338	346	353	361	368	375	383	390	397
73	144	151	159	166	174	182	189	197	204	212	219	227	235	242	250	257	265	272	280	288	295	302	310	318	325	333	340	348	355	363	371	378	386	393	401	408
74	148	155	163	171	179	186	194	202	210	218	225	233	241	249	256	264	272	280	287	295	303	311	319	326	334	342	350	358	365	373	381	389	396	404	412	420
75	152	160	168	176	184	192	200	208	216	224	232	240	248	256	264	272	279	287	295	303	311	319	327	335	343	351	359	367	375	383	391	399	407	415	423	431
76	156	164	172	180	189	197	205	213	221	230	238	246	254	263	271	279	287	295	304	312	320	328	336	344	353	361	369	377	385	394	402	410	418	426	435	443

Source: http://www.nhlbi.nih.gov/guidelines/obesity/bmi_tbl.htm

APPENDIX 4

Review for the Registered Dietitian Examination: Medical Nutrition Therapy for Various Chronic Diseases and Conditions in the Life Cycle

Karlyn Grimes, MS, MPH, RD

The following list of common chronic diseases and medical conditions are well known to the world of medical nutrition therapy. You may encounter a number of these conditions throughout your career in the field of dietetics. Hence, it is recommended that you become familiar with the basic nutritional recommendations for these conditions.

Concepts to Consider When Applying Medical Nutrition Therapy to Chronic Disease

- Knowledge of the etiology and physiology of the disease or condition
- Side effects or complications that can influence the nutritional status of individuals possessing a particular condition
- Potential side effects from drugs commonly used for a particular disease or condition
- Medical nutrition therapy recommendations for the disease (i.e., adjustments in calorie, carbohydrate, protein, fat, and vitamin and mineral recommendations)

Common Chronic Diseases and Conditions

- AIDS/HIV infection
- Food allergies
- Burns
- Cancer (all types)
- Cerebrovascular accident (stroke)
- Celiac disease
- Chronic obstructive pulmonary disease

- Congestive heart failure
- Coronary artery disease, arteriosclerosis, atherosclerosis
- Crohn's disease
- Cystic fibrosis
- Diabetes
- Diverticular disease
- Disordered eating, such as anorexia and bulimia nervosa
- Gastrectomy
- Gastroesophageal reflux disease
- Hepatic cirrhosis hepatitis
- Hypercholesterolemia/hyperlipidemia
- Hypertension
- Hyperthyroidism/hypothyroidism
- Lactose intolerance
- Myocardial infarction
- Osteoporosis
- Pancreatitis
- Peripheral vascular disease
- Renal disease, acute, chronic, end stage
- Short bowel syndrome
- Trauma
- Ulcerative colitis

Medical Terminology Worksheet

Abbreviation	Meaning	Abbreviation	Meaning
a	Before	ESRD	End-stage renal disease
a.c.	Before meals	FBS	Fasting blood sugar
ad lib	As desired	FTT	Failure to thrive
ADL	Activities of daily living	F/U	Follow-up
AF	Osmotic fluid, acid fat	FUO	Fever of undetermined origin
AKA	Above knee amputation	Fx	Fracture
Alb	Albumin	GI	Gastrointestinal
Amb	Ambulate, ambulatory	H/H	Hematocrit/hemoglobin
AODM	Adult onset diabetes mellitus	Hct	Hematocrit
AP	Anteroposterior	Hb	Hemoglobin
ARF	Acute renal failure	HBP	High blood pressure
ASCVD	Arteriosclerotic cardiovascular disease	HEENT	Head, ears, eyes, nose, throat
ASHD	Arteriosclerotic heart disease	HOB	Head of bed
BEE	Basal energy expenditure	H&P	History & physical examination
b.i.d.	Twice a day	HR	Heart rate
BKA	Below knee amputation	HS	Hour of sleep (bedtime)
BMR	Basal metabolic rate	HTN	Hypertension
BP	Blood pressure	IBW	Ideal body weight
Bx	Biopsy	ICU	Intensive care unit
CAD	Coronary artery disease	IDDM	Insulin-dependent diabetes mellitus
CAT, CT	Computed tomography	i.e.	That is
CBC	Complete blood count	I&O	Intake & output
CCU	Coronary care unit	IVF	Intravenous fluid
CF	Cystic fibrosis	kg	Kilogram
CHD	Coronary heart disease	KUB	Kidney, ureter, bladder
CHF	Congestive heart failure	LBW	Low body weight
COPD	Chronic obstructive pulmonary disease	LLE	Left lower extremity
CRF	Chronic renal failure	LLL	Left lower lobe
CVA	Cerebrovascular accident	LLQ	Left lower quadrant
CXR	Chest x-ray	LML	Left mid lobe
DAT	Diet as tolerated	LMP	Last menstrual period
DKA	Diabetic ketoacidosis	LUE	Left upper extremity
DM	Diabetes mellitus	MAC	Mid arm circumference
DOB	Date of birth	MCH	Mean corpuscular volume
DOE	Dyspnea on exertion	MI	Myocardial infarction
Dx	Diagnosis	MCH	Mean corpuscular hemoglobin
ECG, EKG	Electrocardiogram	MCHC	Mean corpuscular hemoglobin concentration
EEG	Electroencephalogram	NAD	No active disease
e.g.	For example	NIDDM	Non–insulin-dependent diabetes mellitus
ETOH	Ethanol	NKA	No known allergies

Medical Terminology Worksheet (continued)

Abbreviation	Meaning	Abbreviation	Meaning
NKDA	No known drug allergies	RUL	Right lower lobe
NPO	Nothing by mouth	RUQ	Right upper quadrant
N&V	Nausea and vomiting	Rx	Prescription
OB	Obstetrics	s	Without
OOB	Out of bed	SBS	Short bowel syndrome
OR	Operating room	SGA	Small for gestational age
OS	Left eye	SOAP	Subjective, objective, assessment, plan
OU	Both eyes, each eye		
p.c.	After meals	SOB	Shortness of breath
PCM	Protein calorie malnutrition	S/P	Status post
PID	Pelvic inflammatory disease	S&S	Signs & symptoms
PKU	Phenylketonuria	Sx	Symptoms
PMH	Past medical history	TB	Tuberculosis
p.o.	By mouth, orally, post operative, phone order	TF	Tube feeding
PPN	Peripheral parenteral nutrition	TG, trig.	Triglycerides
p.r.n.	As needed, whenever necessary	TIA	Transient ischemic attack
PTA	Prior to admission	TIBC	Total iron binding capacity
PUD	Peptic ulcer disease	t.i.d.	Three times a day
PVD	Peripheral vascular disease	TPN	Total parenteral nutrition
q	Every	TPR	Temperature, pulse, respiration
q.d.	Every day	TSH	Thyroid-stimulating hormone
q.h.	Every hour	Tx	Treatment
q.i.d.	Four times a day	UBW	Usual body weight
q.o.d.	Every other day	URI	Upper respiratory infection
RDA	Recommended dietary allowance	US	Ultrasound
RLE	Right lower extremity	UTI	Urinary tract infection
RLL	Right lower lobe	VS	Vital signs
RLQ	Right lower quadrant	WDWN	Well developed well nourished
RO, R/O	Rule out	WNL	Within normal limits
ROM	Range of motion	w/o	Without
RUE	Right upper extremity	#	Number or pounds

Note: Abbreviations vary in different institutions.

Summary of Common Modified and Mechanically Altered Diets

Diet	Description	Indications	Diet Principles/Comments
		Modified Diets	
Regular/house	Provides a well-balanced diet without restrictions or texture modifications. This diet can be adjusted to provide small or large portions.	Postoperative progression diet from a full liquid diet or for otherwise healthy persons with no health or medical contraindications.	Nutritionally adequate diet providing the amounts of energy, protein, vitamins, minerals, and other nutrients sufficient to meet the needs of the average healthy adult.
No added salt (NAS)	Based on the house diet with moderate restrictions in the sodium content of the meals. The diet eliminates or limits foods high in sodium, including processed foods. Generally, this diet provides a maximum of 4 grams of sodium per day.	This diet is recommended for residents with essential hypertension, fluid retention, impaired liver or kidney function, and cardiovascular disease. The appropriate degree of sodium restriction depends on disease severity, presence and amount of edema, and drug therapy.	The primary purpose of a sodium-restricted diet is to restore normal sodium balance to the body by effecting loss of excess sodium and water from extracellular compartments.

continues

Diet	Description	Indications	Diet Principles/Comments
		Modified Diets	
Two-gram sodium	Based on the NAS diet with greater restrictions on the sodium content of the diet. The diet generally eliminates or limits foods high in sodium, including processed foods, fast foods, convenience foods, canned foods, and sodium-containing compounds used in food manufacturing, such as monosodium glutamate (MSG), baking powder, sodium chloride, baking soda, disodium phosphate, sodium propionate, and sodium benzoate, and salt packets are usually eliminated from all trays.	This diet is recommended for individuals with the conditions above that have advanced to a more severe state and is also beneficial to individuals with ascites associated with liver disease, receiving adrenocortical therapy, and with congestive heart failure. The appropriate degree of sodium restriction depends on disease severity, presence and amount of edema, and drug therapy.	The primary purpose of a sodium-restricted diet is to restore normal sodium balance to the body by effecting loss of excess sodium and water from extracellular compartments.
Calorie-controlled diets (1,200-, 1,500-, or 1,800-calorie diets)	A calorie-restricted version of the house diet providing ~50–55% of total calories from carbohydrates, 15–25% of total calories from protein, and 30% of total calories from fat. These diets generally provide limitations in the fat and sugar content of the meals to help with calorie control. These diet plans follow dietary guidelines developed by the American Diabetes Association.	Overweight, obesity, cardiovascular disease, and prediabetes or type 2 diabetes.	Nutritionally adequate except for energy, which is decreased so that the body will utilize fat stores to meet daily energy needs. Generally, vitamin and mineral supplements are recommended for the diets with less than 1,500 calories.
No concentrated sweets (NCS)	Includes most foods allowed on the house diet except diet items are provided whenever possible, including desserts, sugar substitute, diet syrup, and diet jelly. In most cases this diet also provides skim milk instead of whole milk.	Diabetes mellitus, types 1 and 2; gestational diabetes; impaired glucose tolerance or impaired fasting glucose.	For individuals with a stable diabetic condition or with a need for a mild calorie restriction. The goal of the diet is to achieve and maintain optimal blood glucose levels through appropriate food choices.
Renal diet: predialysis	A renal diet is geared to reduce the workload of diseased kidneys, replace substances lost during dialysis, prevent acceleration of nephron damage produced by excessive protein intake, prevent renal osteodystrophy, control dietary phosphorus intake and maintain a normal serum calcium–phosphorous product, maintain lean body mass and optimal nutritional status, maintain normal extracellular fluid volume, pH, and osmolality, postpone initial dialysis, control blood pressure, and manage glucose intolerance.	Chronic renal insufficiency: predialysis	The goals of this diet are to meet nutritional requirements and prevent malnutrition in patients with impaired renal function, to maintain acceptable blood chemistries, blood pressure, and fluid status, and to control edema and electrolyte balance. Basic dietary guidelines: *Energy,* 30–40 kcal/kg; *Protein,* 0.6–0.8 g/kg; *Fluid,* 500 mL + previous days urinary and other losses; *Sodium,* 1–3 g/ day; *Potassium,* unrestricted unless serum K > 5.5 mEq/L; *Phosphorus,* 600–800 mg/day (Ca/K product no higher than 70); *Calcium,* 1,200–1,600 mg/day.

continues

Diet	Description	Indications	Diet Principles/Comments

Modified Diets

Diet	Description	Indications	Diet Principles/Comments
Renal diet: hemodialysis	A renal diet is geared to reduce the workload of diseased kidneys, replace substances lost during dialysis, prevent acceleration of nephron damage produced by excessive protein intake, prevent renal osteodystrophy, control dietary phosphorus intake and maintain a normal serum calcium–phosphorous product, maintain lean body mass and optimal nutritional status, maintain normal extracellular fluid volume, pH, and osmolality, postpone initial dialysis, control blood pressure, and manage glucose intolerance.	End-stage renal disease requiring hemodialysis.	The goals of this diet are to meet nutritional requirements and prevent malnutrition in patients with impaired renal function, to maintain acceptable blood chemistries, blood pressure, and fluid status, and to control edema and electrolyte balance. Nutrients of top nutritional concern include protein (higher intakes are recommended once hemodialysis is initiated), phosphorus, potassium, sodium, and fluids. Basic dietary guidelines: *Energy,* 30–35 kcal/kg if 60+ years and 35 kcal/kg if less than 60 years; *Protein,* 1.0–1.2 g/kg at least 50% biological value; *Fluid,* 750–1,500 mL/day or 500 mL and urinary losses; *Sodium,* 1–3 g/day; *Potassium,* 1,500–3,000 mg/day; *Phosphorus,* 600–1,200 mg/day (Ca/P product no higher than 70); *Calcium,* 1–2 g/day.
High fiber	A general diet with emphasis on fiber-rich foods, which include fruits, vegetables, legumes, and whole grain rice, breads, and cereals. Intake of 20–35 g of fiber is recommended each day. When increasing fiber intake it is recommended that it is done gradually and plenty of fluids are emphasized.	Prevention or treatment of various gastrointestinal, cardiovascular, and metabolic conditions, including diverticular disease, colon cancer, diabetes, constipation, irritable bowel syndrome, Crohn's disease, hypercholesterolemia, and obesity.	To increase fecal bulk, promote regularity, normalize serum lipid level, and blunt the postprandial blood glucose response.
Low fiber/low residue	To prevent the formation of an obstructing bolus of high-fiber foods in patients with narrowed intestinal or esophageal lumens or to reduce the frequency of painful stools in acute phases of diverticulitis or inflammatory bowel disease. Also, used as a postoperative diet as a step toward a general diet.	Low-fiber diets are indicated during acute phases of diverticulosis, infectious enterocolitis, ulcerative colitis, or Crohn's disease when the bowel is markedly inflamed, fixed radiologic strictures are present, or the intestinal lumen is narrowed. The diet may also be useful for a short period in the transition between a completely liquid diet with patients convalescing from surgery, trauma, or other illnesses.	Fiber-rich foods are avoided in this diet, including fruits, vegetables, legumes, and whole-grain rice, breads, and cereals. If a low residue diet is indicated, all fruits and vegetables, including prune juice, should be eliminated except white potatoes without skin and strained fruit and vegetable juices. Because milk may contribute to fecal residue, certain patients may benefit from restricting their milk intake to 2 cups per day.
Fat and cholesterol controlled (step 1 and step 2 diets)	A diet that limits total fat intake to less than 30% of total calories and that limits saturated fat and cholesterol in two phases, known as step 1 and step 2 diets.	For individuals with coronary heart disease, hypercholesterolemia, hyperlipidemia, dyslipidemia, dysbetalipoproteinemia, gallbladder disease, abnormalities in fat digestion and absorption, and/or obesity in an attempt to normalize blood lipid levels, reduce gallbladder exacerbations, and manage excess body weight.	*Step 1:* less than 30% of kcal from fat, 8–10% from saturated fatty acids (SFA), and 300 mg/day from cholesterol. *Step 2:* same as step 1, but 7% from SFA and 200 mg/day from cholesterol. Emphasis on grains, cereals, legumes, vegetables, fruits, lean meats, poultry, fish, and nonfat dairy products. Restriction of animal fats recommended, meat is limited to 5–6 oz/day and eggs 4x/wk. Sodium restricted to 2,400 mg/day.

continues

Diet	Description	Indications	Diet Principles/Comments
		Modified Diets	
Lactose restricted/ lactose free	A diet limited in its content of the disaccharide lactose. It provides an amount of lactose small enough to avoid recurrence of symptoms in mild forms of lactose intolerance, usually less than 8 to 12 g lactose daily.	Intended for lactose-deficient individuals to prevent excess gas, bloating, cramping, and diarrhea caused by foods containing the simple sugar lactose. A patient with proven lactose intolerance who does not experience relief of abdominal pain and diarrhea may have lactose intolerance secondary to another disorder that requires treatment, such as celiac disease, regional enteritis, or postgastrectomy dumping syndrome.	Small amounts of dairy foods in divided doses are recommended because individuals vary in their tolerance of lactose-containing foods. Tolerance for lactose may decrease with age and degree of gastrointestinal disease. Nutritionally adequate as long as dairy foods are not avoided or lactose-free or lactase-containing products are used.
High calorie, high protein	To provide energy and nutrients in excess of usual requirements to improve overall nutritional status, prevent malnutrition, promote weight gain, meet need for increased nutrients, and optimize the ability to respond to medical treatment.	Persons with wasting acute or chronic conditions such as cancer, HIV infection/AIDS, chronic gastrointestinal problems, burns, wounds, trauma, renal disease (dialysis), protein–calorie malnutrition, cystic fibrosis, failure to thrive, and in preparation for and recovery from surgery.	Focuses on calorie-dense and protein-dense foods. The diet often exceeds 30% of total calories from fat to increase calorie density of the total diet. Generally, the diet should provide at least 120–150% of Recommended Daily Allowance for energy and protein. Small frequent feedings of calorie- and nutrient-dense foods are recommended.

Diet	Description	Indications	Diet Principles/ Nutritional Adequacy
		Modified Diets	
Phenylalanine restricted	A diet in which the intake of phenylalanine is limited to a prescribed level governed by individual tolerance. Blood levels of phenylalanine rise because of a defect in or absence of the enzyme phenylalanine hydroxylase.	For individuals with phenylketonuria (PKU) in an attempt to control blood phenylalanine levels to allow the greatest development of intellectual potential.	The goal of this diet is to provide enough protein, tyrosine, and energy for the promotion of growth and development and to meet vitamin, mineral, and fluid needs of the individual.
Gluten free	The diet is intended to eliminate toxic glutens or, more specifically, the toxic fraction, gliadin. Its aim is to ameliorate the symptoms of diarrhea, abdominal distention, flatulence, steatorrhea, failure to thrive, chronic pain, and anemia associated with gluten/gliadin intolerance.	For individuals with celiac disease, nontropical sprue, or gluten-sensitive enteropathy.	A diet free of gliadin or glutens, such as those in wheat, rye, oat, and barley protein, and malt. Gliadin and glutens are toxic to individuals with gluten-sensitive enteropathy. Constipation may be encountered on this diet because wheat fiber is excluded from the diet. Alternative sources of insoluble fiber and roughage are needed to prevent the problem.

Diet	Description	Indications	Diet Principles/ Nutritional Adequacy
		Transitional Diets	
Clear liquid	A diet that includes only foods that are clear and liquid at body temperature, such as fat-free broth,	The diet is intended to provide an oral source of fluids and a small amount of energy and electrolytes.	This diet should not be used for more than 24 hours, because it is inadequate in calories and most

continues

Diet	Description	Indications	Diet Principles/ Nutritional Adequacy

Transitional Diets

Diet	Description	Indications	Diet Principles/ Nutritional Adequacy
	bouillon, coffee, tea, decaffeinated coffee, strained fruit juices, flavored gelatin, carbonated beverages, Popsicles, fruit ices, and hard candies.	It is used to prevent dehydration and to reduce colonic residue to a minimum and in preparation for bowel surgery or before colonoscopic examination, or a transitional diet from intravenous feeding or acute gastrointestinal disturbances.	nutrients even when supplemented with low-residue, liquid-protein products.
Full liquid	A diet consisting of foods that are liquid at body temperature, supplemented with commercial liquid supplements.	A full liquid diet is indicated after oral or plastic surgery of the face and neck or in other postoperative states such as in esophageal surgery. It may also be used as a transition between a clear liquid diet and a fiber-restricted or regular diet. It is used in conjunction with dilatation procedures in the management of esophageal stricture, after mandibular fractures, or with any patient who cannot chew properly or who has an esophageal or pharyngeal disorder that interferes with the normal handling of solid foods.	If planned properly, the diet can be nutritionally adequate. A variety of foods may be included, such as fruit and vegetable juices, strained hot cereals, broths, milk, eggs, egg substitutes, commercial liquid formulas, high-protein broths, high-protein cereals, puddings, and gelatins.

Diet	Description/ Nutritional Adequacy	Indications	Diet Principles

Texture-Modified Diets

Diet	Description/ Nutritional Adequacy	Indications	Diet Principles
Mechanical soft/ground	To provide texture-modified food that requires minimal chewing.	This texture-modified diet is indicated for individuals with compromised chewing and/or swallowing ability, dental problems, and/or an edentulous status. This diet is often well tolerated by individuals after head and neck surgery as they transition back to a regular diet.	This diet includes foods modified in texture, such as chopped, ground, mashed, and pureed foods, that allow for ease of mastication. Certain raw and hard foods are eliminated from this diet. Gravies and sauces are recommended to moisten the foods.
Dysphagia (dysphagia regular, dysphagia ground, dysphagia puree)	A diet intended to provide nutrition in a form that fits the specific anatomic and functional needs of the patient, to maintain or improve nutritional status, to avoid or limit possible adverse reactions such as aspiration that result from attempts to feed the dysphagic patient, to provide adequate hydration in the patient who cannot handle thin liquids, and to help the patient achieve the highest level of consistency tolerance possible.	For individuals with dysphagia, swallowing impairment, neurologic illness, and receiving surgical procedures and anticancer therapy that may cause dysphagia.	Semisolid foods that form a cohesive bolus, spoon-thick liquids, and medium-thick liquids are most likely to be tolerated. The best consistency depends on the individual patient. Thin liquids, foods that fall apart, and sticky or bulky foods are poorly tolerated. Generally, a speech language pathologist performs a speech evaluation and uses a test tray containing foods of varying consistency to determine which foods and textures are best tolerated by the individual.
Pureed	Same as above. Thick, smooth, homogenous, semi-liquid textures.	Same as above. Severely reduced oral preparatory stage abilities, impaired lip and tongue control, delayed swallowing reflex triggering, oral hypersensitivity, reduced pharyngeal peristalsis, and/or cricopharyngeal dysfunction.	Same as above. Spoon-like or pudding-like consistency. No coarse textures, nuts, or raw fruits and vegetables.

Analysis of Protein and/or Calorie Supplements

Product*	Indications for Use	Caloric Density (kcal/cc)†	Carbohydrate (g/1,000 cc)	Protein (g/1,000 cc)	Fat (g/1,000 cc)
Ensure™	Complete balanced nutrition	1.06 kcal/mL	169 g/L	37.2 g/L	25.9 g/L
Ensure Plus™	High-calorie liquid nutrition	1.5 kcal/mL	200 g/L	54.9 g/L	53.3 g/L
Carnation Instant Breakfast™	Supplement	0.93 kcal/mL	167 g/L	51 g/L	21 g/L
Diet Carnation Instant Breakfast™	General nutrition	0.7 kcal/mL	136 g/L	68 g/L	28 g/L
Glucerna™	Glucose intolerance	1.0 kcal/mL	100 g/L	45 g/L	47.5 g/L
Healthshakes™	Supplement	280 (6 oz)		9 (6 oz)	
Jevity™	Isotonic with fiber	1.06 kcal/mL	154.4 g/L	44.3 g/L	34.7 g/L
Nepro™	Dialysis patient, chronic/acute renal failure	2 kcal/mL	215.2 g/L	69.9 g/L	95.6 g/L
Osmolite™	Isotonic	1.06 kcal/mL	151 g/L	37.1 g/L	34.7 g/L
Osmolite HN™	High nitrogen, isotonic	1.06 kcal/mL	143.9 g/L	44.3 g/L	34.7 g/L
PediaSure™	Children	1.0 kcal/mL	109 g/L	30 g/L	49.7 g/L
Promote™	High protein	1.0 kcal/mL	130 g/L	62.5g/L	26 g/L
Pulmocare™	Cardiac patient	1.5 kcal/mL	105 g/L	62.6 g/L	93.3 g/L
2 Cal HN™	High kcal, high protein	2.0 kcal/mL	217.3 g/L	83.7 g/L	90.9 g/L
Suplena™	Low protein, complete, for dialyzed patient with renal failure	2.0 kcal/mL	256 g/L	30 g/L	96 g/L

*Most of these products are manufactured by Mead Johnson or Novartis. Information about these products can be obtained by visiting the manufacturers' Websites.

†Remember when calculating grams per cc that 1,000 cc = 1,000 mL = 1 liter; 1 oz = 30 cc or 30 mL; 120 cc = 4 oz; 240 cc = 8 oz.

Review of Common Laboratory Values

The following chart presents common laboratory values that you will encounter during your internship experience. Please record the significance of the particular laboratory measurement, the normal laboratory value range, and what may be the problem when these laboratory values are above or below the norm.

Laboratory Measurement	Significance of the Measurement	Normal Laboratory Value Range	Conditions Related to Elevated Readings	Conditions Related to Low Readings
Albumin, serum	Chief blood protein used to assess protein and nutritional status. Also used as a measure of hepatic function.	Adult: 3.5–5 g/dL *Or* 35–50 g/L	Dehydration; albumin in urine signals kidney disease.	Malnutrition, pregnancy, liver disease, protein-losing enteropathy, protein-losing nephropathy, overhydration, increased capillary permeability, inflammatory disease, B_{12} and familial idiopathic dysproteinemia.

continues

Laboratory Measurement	Significance of the Measurement	Normal Laboratory Value Range	Conditions Related to Elevated Readings	Conditions Related to Low Readings
Vitamin B_{12}, serum	To assess vitamin B_{12} status.	100–700 pg/mL Or 74–517 pmol/L	Leukemia, polycythemia vera, severe liver dysfunction, myeloproliferative disease.	Pernicious anemia, malabsorption syndrome, inflammatory bowel disease, intestinal worm infestation, atopic gastritis, Zollinger-Ellison syndrome, large proximal gastrectomy, resection of terminal ileus, achlorhydria, pregnancy, folic acid deficiency, and vitamin C deficiency.
Blood urea nitrogen (BUN)	Measures the amount of urea nitrogen. Directly related to the metabolic function of the liver and the excretory function of the kidney.	Adult: 10–20 mg/dL Or 3.6–7.1 mmol/L Child: 5–18 mg/dL Elderly: may be slightly higher than adult.	Possible renal failure/disease, gastrointestinal bleeding, congestive heart failure, increased protein intake, sepsis, insufficient renal blood supply, blocked urinary tract, or dehydration.	Possible liver disease, malnutrition, anabolic steroids, overhydration, negative N balance, pregnancy, or nephrotic syndrome.
Chloride, serum	Performed as part of multiphasic testing of electrolyte status. Provides feedback on acid-base balance and hydration status.	Adult/elderly: 90–110 mEq/L Or 98–106 mmol/L Children: 90–110 mEq/L	Dehydration, renal tubular acidosis, Cushing syndrome, eclampsia, multiple myeloma, kidney dysfunction, metabolic acidosis, anemia, hyperventilation, or hyperparathyroidism.	Overhydration, congestive heart failure, vomiting, chronic respiratory acidosis, Addison disease, burns, metabolic alkalosis, diuretic therapy, hypokalemia, aldosteronism, respiratory acidosis, or salt-losing nephritis.
Cholesterol, serum	To help assess the risk of arteriosclerotic heart disease. Done as part of lipid profile testing.	< 200 mg/dL Or < 5.2 mmol/L Less than age 20 years: < 180 mg/dL	Hypercholesterolemia, hyperlipidemia, hypothyroidism, uncontrolled diabetes, pregnancy, nephrotic syndrome, high-cholesterol diet, stress, hypertension, or myocardial infarction.	Heredity, malnutrition.
Creatinine, serum	Allows for assessment of the amount of lean body mass (fat-free mass) and can identify impaired renal function.	Female: 0.5–1.1 mg/dL Or 44–97 mmol/L Male: 0.6–1.2 mg/dL	Glomerulonephritis, acute tubular necrosis, urinary tract obstruction, reduced renal blood flow, shock, dehydration, atherosclerotic, diabetic nephropathy, nephritis, or acromegaly.	Debilitation, decreased muscle mass, muscular dystrophy, or myasthenia gravis.
Ferritin, serum	A test for iron status, considered the best test for detecting the early stages of anemia because it is an indicator of an individual's iron stores.	Male: 12–300 µg/mL Female: 10–150 µg/mL	Hemochromatosis, hemosiderosis, megaloblastic anemia, hemolytic anemia, alcoholic/inflammatory hepatocellular disease, or advanced cancer.	Severe protein deficiency, iron deficiency anemia, or hemodialysis.

continues

Laboratory Measurement	Significance of the Measurement	Normal Laboratory Value Range	Conditions Related to Elevated Readings	Conditions Related to Low Readings
Folic acid, serum	To identify hemolytic disorders and detect anemia caused by folic acid deficiency.	5–20 µg/mL	Pernicious anemia, vegetarianism, or recent massive blood transfusion.	Folic acid deficiency anemia, hemolytic anemia, malnutrition, malabsorption syndrome, malignancy, pregnancy, alcoholism, liver disease, anorexia, or chronic renal disease.
Glucose, serum	Measurement of the amount of glucose in the blood. A true elevation indicates diabetes.	2 yr to adult: 70–105 mg/dL *Or* 3.9–5.8 mmol/L	Diabetes mellitus, acute stress response, Cushing syndrome, chronic renal failure, glucagonoma, acute pancreatitis, diuretic therapy, or corticosteroid therapy.	Insulinoma, hypothyroidism, hypopituitarism, Addison disease, extensive liver disease, insulin overdose, or starvation.
Glycosylated hemoglobin (HbAIc)	Test used to monitor diabetes treatment and dietary compliance over the previous 3 months. Provides an accurate long-term index of the patient's average blood glucose levels.	Good: 7% Fair: 10% Poor: 13–20%	Newly diagnosed diabetes patient, poorly controlled diabetes, acute stress response, Cushing syndrome, pregnancy, glucagonoma, corticosteroid therapy, or splenectomized patient.	Hemolytic anemia, chronic blood loss, or chronic renal failure.
Hematocrit (Hct)	Measure of the percentage of the total blood volume that is made by the red blood cell.	Men: 42–52% Women: 37–47% Pregnant women: > 33%	Congential heart disease, polycythemia vera, severe dehydration, erythrocytosis, severe diarrhea, eclampsia, burns, dehydration, or chronic obstructive pulmonary disease.	Anemia, hyperthyroidism, cirrhosis, hemolytic reaction, hemorrhage, dietary deficiency, bone marrow failure, normal pregnancy, rheumatoid arthritis, multiple myeloma, malnutrition, leukemia, or hemoglobinopathy.
Hemoglobin (Hb)	Measure of total amount of hemoglobin in the peripheral blood, which reflects the number of red blood cells.	Men: 14–18 g/dL Women: 12–16 g/dL	Congenital heart disease, polycythemia vera, hemoconcentration of the blood, chronic obstructive pulmonary disease, congestive heart failure, high altitudes, severe burns, or dehydration.	Anemia, severe hemorrhage, hemolysis, cancer, nutritional deficiencies, lymphomas, systemic lupus erythematosus, sarcoidosis, kidney disease, sickle cell anemia, or neoplasia.
High-density lipoprotein (HDL) ("healthy") cholesterol	Measurement identifying persons at risk for developing heart disease and to monitor therapy effectiveness if abnormalities are found.	Male: > 45 mg/dL Female: > 55 mg/dL	Familial HDL, lipoproteinemia, or excessive exercise.	Familial low HDL, hepatocellular disease, hepatitis, cirrhosis, hypoproteinemia, nephrotic syndrome, or malnutrition.
Low-density lipoprotein (LDL) ("lethal") cholesterol	Same as above.	60–80 mg/dL	Familial LDL, lipoproteinemia, nephrotic syndrome, glycogen storage disease, hypothyroidism, alcohol consumption, or chronic liver disease.	Familial hypolipoproteinemia, hypoproteinemia, malabsorption, severe burns, malnutrition, or hyperthyroidism.

continues

Laboratory Measurement	Significance of the Measurement	Normal Laboratory Value Range	Conditions Related to Elevated Readings	Conditions Related to Low Readings
Mean corpuscular volume (MCV)	A test routinely performed as part of complete blood cell count (CBC). Detects anemia and provides information about red blood cell size.	Adult/elderly/child: 80–90 μm^3	Liver disease, antimetabolic therapy, alcoholism, pernicious anemia, or folic acid deficiency.	Iron deficiency anemia or thalassemia.
Mean corpuscular hemoglobin (MCH)	Routinely performed as part of complete blood count. Provides information about the weight of the red blood cell.	Adult/elderly/child: 27–31 pg	Macrocytic anemia.	Microcytic anemia or hypochromic anemia.
Mean corpuscular hemoglobin concentration (MCHC)	Routinely performed as part of complete blood cell count. Provides information on the hemoglobin concentration of red blood cells.	Adult/elderly/child: 32–36 g/dL *Or* 32–36%	Spherocytosis, intravascular hemolysis, or cold agglutinins.	Iron deficiency anemia or thalassemia.
Potassium, serum	Indicator of hyperkalemia and hypokalemia.	Adults/elderly: 3.5–5 mEq/L Child: 3.4–7 mEq/L	Excessive dietary intake or intravenous intake, acute or chronic renal failure, hypoaldosteronism, aldosterone-inhibiting diuretics, crush injuries, hemolysis, transfusion of hemolyzed blood, infection, acidosis, or dehydration.	Inadequate dietary intake, suboptimal intravenous intake, burns, diuretics, gastrointestinal disorders, diarrhea, vomiting, hyperaldosteronism, Cushing syndrome, renal tubular acidosis, licorice ingestion, insulin administration, glucose administration, ascites, renal artery stenosis, or cystic fibrosis.
Sodium, serum	A measurement used to determine extracellular osmolality.	Adults/elderly: 136–145 mEq/L Child: 136–145 mEq/L	Excessive dietary intake, excessive sodium in intravenous fluids, Cushing syndrome, hyperaldosteronism, excessive sweating, extensive thermal burns, diabetes insipidus, or osmotic diuresis.	Inadequate dietary intake, suboptimal intravenous intake, Addison disease, diarrhea, vomiting, diuretic administration, chronic renal insufficiency, excessive oral water intake, or congestive heart failure.
Thyroid-stimulating hormone (TSH)	A measurement used to differentiate primary hypothyroidism from secondary hypothyroidism.	Increased thyroid function with administration of exogenous TSH. Adult: 0.4–5 mIU/L	Abnormal findings are primary (thyroidal) hypothyroidism and secondary (hypothalamic-pituitary) hypothyroidism.	Hyperthyroidism caused by Graves disease, a type of goiter, or a noncancerous tumor or by damage to the pituitary gland, and in individuals with an underactive thyroid gland but receiving too much thyroid hormone medication.

continues

Laboratory Measurement	Significance of the Measurement	Normal Laboratory Value Range	Conditions Related to Elevated Readings	Conditions Related to Low Readings
Thyroxine (T_4)	A direct measurement of the total amount of T_4 present in an individuals' blood. T4 makes up nearly all of what we call thyroid, the hormone.	Adult male: 4–12 µg/dL Adult female: 5–12 µg/dL Adult > age 60: 5–11 µg/dL	Graves disease, Plummer disease, acute thyroiditis, pregnancy, hepatitis, congenital hyperproteinemia, familial dysalbuminemia, or hyperthyroxinemia.	Cretinism, surgical ablation, myxedema, pituitary insufficiency, hypothalamic failure, protein malnutrition, iodine insufficiency, renal failure, Cushing syndrome, or cirrhosis.
Total iron, serum	Measurement of the quantity of iron bound to transferring in the blood.	Males: 65–175 µg/dL Females: 50–170 µg/dL	Hemosiderosis, hemochromatosis, hemolytic anemia, hepatitis, hepatic necrosis, lead toxicity, iron poisoning, or massive transfusion.	Insufficient dietary iron, chronic blood loss, inadequate iron absorption, pregnancy (late), iron deficiency anemia, neoplasia, chronic gastrointestinal blood loss, chronic hematuria, or chronic heavy physiologic or pathologic menstruation.
Total iron binding capacity (TIBC)	A measurement of all proteins available for binding mobile iron.	250–420 µg/dL	Oral contraceptives, late pregnancy, polycythemia vera, or iron deficiency anemia.	Hypoproteinemia, inflammatory diseases, cirrhosis, hemolytic anemia, pernicious anemia, or sickle cell anemia.
Total protein, serum	Measurement to help determine osmotic pressure within the vascular space. A measure of nutritional status.	Adult/elderly: 6.4–8.3 g/dL	Dehydration, possibly leukemia, an autoimmune disease, cirrhosis, kidney disease, chronic infection, hemolytic anemia, or Hodgkin's disease.	Malnutrition, pregnancy, liver disease, protein-losing enteropathies, protein-losing nephropathies, overhydration, or inflammatory disease.
Transferrin, serum	Transferrin is a globulin protein bound to iron. Determines the amount of iron-binding proteins.	Adult male: 215–365 mg/dL Adult female: 250–380 mg/dL	Pregnancy, estrogen therapy, inadequate iron stores, iron deficiency anemia, acute hepatitis, polycythemia, or oral contraceptive use.	Malignancy, collagen vascular disease, liver disease, infection, malnutrition, iron deficiency sickle cell anemia, pernicious anemia, or hypoproteinemia.
Triglycerides, serum	Part of a lipid profile to assess risk of coronary and vascular disease.	Male: 40–160 mg/dL Female: 35–135 mg/dL	Glycogen storage disease, hyperlipidemias, hypothyroidism, diet high in carbohydrates, poorly controlled diabetes, nephrotic syndrome, alcoholic cirrhosis, pregnancy, or cirrhosis.	Malabsorption syndrome, malnutrition, or hyperthyroidism.
Triiodothyronine (T_3)	Accurate measure of thyroid function.	Aged 20–50 years: 70–205 ng/dL Over age 50: 40–180 ng/dL	Graves' disease, Plummer disease, toxic thyroid adenoma, pregnancy, hepatitis, acute thyroiditis, or congenital hyperproteinemia.	Hypothyroidism, cretinism, myxedema, pituitary insufficiency, hypothalamic failure, protein malnutrition, iodine deficiency, or renal failure.

Review of Common Medications

Medication	Intended Use	Common Side Effects	Drug–Nutrient Interactions or Dietary Considerations
Aldactone™ (spironolactone)	Diuretic, antihypertensive	Anorexia, thirst, dry mouth, nausea, vomiting, cramps, diarrhea.	Take with food, avoid excessive potassium intake, avoid natural licorice.
Aricept™	Anti-Alzheimer's, cholinesterase inhibitor	Anorexia, decreased weight, nausea and vomiting, bloating, diarrhea, gastrointestinal bleeding.	N/A
Atenolol™	Antihypertensive, antiangina	Nausea, diarrhea.	Avoid natural licorice, take with food.
AZT™ Retrovir™ (zidovudine)	Anti-HIV medications that stop HIV from infecting uninfected cells but do not help infected cells	Long-term use associated with muscle loss. Other side effects include anemia, white blood cell depression, lip, mouth and tongue sores, bone marrow damage, headaches, skin rash, itching, weakness, nervousness, dizziness, nausea, stomach pain, confusion, loss of speech or appetite, muscle aches, fever or sweating, sore throat, or abnormal bruising or bleeding.	Best taken on an empty stomach, but may be taken with food. Recommended that users take manganese, B vitamins, and vitamin E with Retrovir.
BuSpar™	Antianxiety	Nausea, diarrhea.	Caution with grapefruit juice. Avoid alcohol.
Calcijex™/ Calcitriol™	Calcium regulator	Increases calcium absorption, anorexia, decreased weight, increased thirst, dry mouth, metallic taste, nausea and vomiting, constipation, diarrhea.	Dialysis, low phosphorus diet.
Cholestyramine™	Antihyperlipidemic, antidiarrheal	May decrease absorption of fat, Ca, Fe, Zn, Mg, vitamins A, D, E, and K, medium-chain triglycerides, and folate. Anorexia, increased or decreased weight, belching, nausea and vomiting, dyspepsia, constipation, diarrhea.	Decrease dietary fat and cholesterol intake, increase fluids, increase fiber, decrease calcium, if needed. Take before meals. Never take powder dry.
Cimetidine™	Antisecretory, antiulcer, anti-GERD	Decreased Fe and B_{12} absorption. Decreased gastric acid secretions, increased gastric pH, nausea and vomiting, diarrhea.	May need bland diet, limit caffeine, caution with alcohol.
Cipro™	Antibiotic	Nausea and vomiting, abdominal pain, diarrhea.	Milk or yogurt decreases absorption and availability. Take with meals. Avoid milk, yogurt, and caffeine.
Colchicine™	Used to prevent or treat attacks of gout (also called gouty arthritis).	*Common:* diarrhea, nausea, vomiting, stomach pain. *Rare:* black tarry stools, blood in urine or stools, difficulty in breathing when exercising, fever with or without chills,	Limit alcohol intake. Monitor appetite.

continues

Medication	Intended Use	Common Side Effects	Drug–Nutrient Interactions or Dietary Considerations
		headache, large hive-like swellings on the face, eyelids, mouth, lips, and/or tongue, pinpoint red spots on skin, sores, ulcers, or white spots on lips or in mouth, sore throat, unusual bleeding or bruising, unusual tiredness or weakness.	
Cozaar™	Antihypertensive	N/A	Decrease sodium intake, decreased calcium intake may be recommended. Avoid natural licorice.
Corticosteroids (Prednisone™)	Antiinflammatory, immunosuppressant	Increased appetite, increased weight, anorexia, calcium wasting-osteoporosis/necrosis, edema, increased blood pressure.	Take with food, decrease sodium intake and increase protein intake, avoid alcohol.
Coumadin™ (Warfarin™)	Anticoagulant	Nausea and vomiting, cramps, diarrhea.	Consistent intake of potassium essential. Caution with vitamin C, caution with > 60 g raw or boiled onions. Avoid/limit garlic, ginger, Ginkgo, and avocado.
Digoxin™	Cardiotonic, antiarrhythmic, anti–congestive heart failure	Anorexia, decreased weight, nausea and vomiting, diarrhea.	Increase potassium intake, decrease sodium intake, and ensure adequate magnesium and calcium intake. Take separately from high-fiber foods or foods high in pectin.
DiaBeta™	Oral hypoglycemic	Increased or decreased appetite, increased weight, dyspepsia, nausea, diarrhea, constipation.	Avoid alcohol.
Elavil™	Antidepressant	Dry mouth, nausea, vomiting, anorexia, taste changes, epigastric distress, diarrhea, constipation, paralytic ileus.	Take with food, high-fiber intake may decrease the drug's effectiveness. Limit caffeine, avoid alcohol, St. John's wort, SAM-e, and yohimbe.
Eldepryl™	Anti-Parkinson, MAO inhibitor	Dry mouth, dysphagia, nausea, abdominal pain.	Take with breakfast and lunch, avoid foods high in tyramine.
Erythromycin™	Antibiotic	Anorexia, epigastric distress, nausea and vomiting, abdominal cramps, diarrhea.	Avoid concurrent alcohol use.
Ferrous sulfate, Fumerin™ and Gluconate™	Hematinic, antianemic	Anorexia, nausea and vomiting, dyspepsia, bloating, constipation, diarrhea, dark stools.	Take with 8 oz water or juice on an empty stomach. Limit alcohol.
Flagyl™	Antibiotic, amebicide, antitrichomonal	Anorexia, dry mouth, stomatitis, metallic taste, nausea and vomiting, epigastric distress, diarrhea, constipation.	Take with food. Avoid alcohol.

continues

Medication	Intended Use	Common Side Effects	Drug–Nutrient Interactions or Dietary Considerations
Glipizide™	Oral hypoglycemic	Increased or decreased appetite, increased weight, dyspepsia, nausea, diarrhea, constipation.	Take 30 min before first meal of the day. Limit alcohol.
Glucophage™	Oral hypoglycemic	Anorexia.	Take with food. Avoid alcohol.
Glyburide™	Oral hypoglycemic	Increased or decreased appetite, increased weight, dyspepsia, nausea, diarrhea, constipation.	If once a day, take with first meal of the day. Avoid alcohol.
Haldol™	Antipsychotic	Increased appetite, weight gain, anorexia, dry mouth, increased salivation, dyspepsia, nausea, vomiting, constipation, diarrhea.	Take with food. Avoid alcohol.
Hydrochlorothiazide (HCTZ)	Antihypertensive, diuretic	Anorexia, increased thirst, dry mouth, nausea and vomiting, gastrointestinal irritation, diarrhea, constipation.	Take in the morning with food or milk. Limit alcohol.
Insulin (Novolin™, Humulin™)	Antidiabetic, hypoglycemic	Increased weight.	Limit alcohol. Follow a diabetic meal plan to balance food with insulin.
Isoniazid™	Antituberculosis	Dry mouth, nausea and vomiting, epigastric distress, constipation, diarrhea.	Take 1 hr before or 2 hr after meals. Pyr supplement. Avoid foods high in tyramine or histamine.
Klonopin™	Anticonvulsant	Dry/sore mouth, constipation, abdominal cramps, gastritis, changes in appetite, nausea, anorexia, diarrhea, increased salivation.	Take with food, limit caffeine, avoid alcohol, caution with some herbal products.
Lasix™ (furosemide)	Diuretic, antihypertensive	Anorexia, increased thirst, oral irritation, stomach cramps, nausea and vomiting, diarrhea, constipation.	Take with food. Increase potassium and magnesium. Decrease caloric and sodium intake. Avoid natural licorice.
Levodopa™	Anti-Parkinson	Dry mouth, bitter taste, nausea, vomiting, anorexia, constipation, diarrhea, abdominal pain, excessive salivation, increased or decreased weight, epigastric distress.	May take with low-protein foods or juices but not with high-protein foods.
Lipitor™	Antihyperlipidemia	Nausea, dyspepsia, abdominal pain, constipation.	Avoid grapefruit juice and alcohol. Decrease fat and cholesterol intake.
Methotrexate™	Antineoplastic, antipsoriatic, antiarthritic	Stomatitis, altered taste, nausea and vomiting, diarrhea, anorexia, decreased weight, dehydration.	Encourage fluid intake. Avoid alcohol.
Micronase™	Oral hypoglycemic	Increased or decreased appetite, increased weight, dyspepsia, nausea, diarrhea, constipation.	If once a day, take with first meal of the day. Avoid alcohol.

continues

Medication	Intended Use	Common Side Effects	Drug–Nutrient Interactions or Dietary Considerations
Monoamine oxidase (MAO) inhibitors (isocarboxazid)	Antidepressant, MAO inhibitor	Possible B_6 deficiency, increased appetite, increased weight.	Avoid foods high in tyramine and tryptophan such as cheese, yogurt, and pickled, fermented, and smoked foods. Limit caffeine, avoid tryptophan supplements, may need B_6 supplement, avoid St. John's wort and alcohol. Caution with diabetes—may decrease serum glucose.
Monopril™	Antihypertensive, angiotensin-converting enzyme inhibitor	N/A	Decreased calcium and sodium intake may be recommended. Avoid salt substitutes. Caution with potassium supplements, Ensure adequate fluid intake. Avoid natural licorice and alcohol.
Oral contraceptives	Used to prevent pregnancy and regulate the menstrual cycle	Increased or decreased appetite, decrease in loss of calcium from the bones, increased absorption of calcium into the bones, nausea and vomiting, bloating, cramps, diarrhea, edema, increased blood pressure.	Take with food the same time each day. Limit alcohol. Increase foods high in Mg, folate, Pyr, and vitamin B_{12}.
Ofloxacin™	Antibiotic	Dry mouth, taste loss, nausea and vomiting, abdominal pain, diarrhea, decreased appetite, constipation, headache, insomnia, dizziness, vaginitis.	Take with 8 oz water. Ensure adequate fluid intake.
Paxil™	Antidepressant, anti–obsessive-compulsive disorder, anti-panic disorder	Decreased appetite, increased or decreased weight, dry mouth, taste changes, nausea, dyspepsia, constipation, diarrhea.	Avoid St. John's wort, SAM-e, and yohimbe.
Phenobarbital™	Sedative, hypnotic, anticonvulsant	Nausea and vomiting, constipation, increased rate of metabolism of vitamins D and K.	Avoid alcohol and caffeine. Increase consumption of vitamin C and calcium.
Phenytoin (Dilantin™)	Anticonvulsant	Taste changes, dysphagia, nausea, vomiting, constipation.	Take with food or milk, avoid alcohol, caution with diabetes—may increase serum glucose. Folate supplement needed. May need vitamin D supplement.
Phos-Lo™	Phosphate binder	Decrease iron absorption, anorexia, nausea and vomiting, constipation.	Take with meals. Avoid calcium supplements.
Prilosec	Antiulcer, antisecretory, anti-GERD	May decrease iron and B_{12} absorption, decreased gastric acid secretion, increase gastric pH, abdominal pain, constipation, diarrhea.	Take just before a meal, preferably in the morning. Swallow whole, do not crush.
Probenecid™	Used in the treatment of chronic gout or gouty arthritis	Fast or irregular breathing; puffiness or swellings of the eyelids or around the eyes; shortness of breath,	Do not take aspirin or other salicylates or drink alcoholic beverages while taking this medicine, unless

continues

Medication	Intended Use	Common Side Effects	Drug–Nutrient Interactions or Dietary Considerations
		troubled breathing, tightness in chest, or wheezing; changes in the skin color of the face occurring together with any of the other side effects listed here; or skin rash, hives, or itching occurring together with any of the other side effects listed here.	you have first checked with your doctor.
Prozac™	Antidepressant, selective serotonin reuptake inhibitor	Anorexia, decreased weight, dry mouth, taste changes, dyspepsia, nausea, vomiting, diarrhea, constipation.	Take in morning with meals. No tryptophan supplements. Avoid alcohol and St. John's wort. Caution with diabetes—may cause hypoglycemia.
Remeron™	Antidepressant	Increased appetite, increased weight, increased thirst, dry mouth, nausea and vomiting, abdominal pain, constipation.	Avoid St. John's wort and alcohol.
Synthroid™	Thyroid preparation	Appetite changes, weight loss.	Take on an empty stomach before breakfast to increase absorption.
Tegretol™	Anticonvulsant	Anorexia, dry mouth, decreased appetite, stomatitis, glossitis, nausea, vomiting, abdominal pain, constipation, diarrhea.	Take with food, avoid alcohol and psyllium seed. Caution with grapefruit juice.
Tetracycline™ (doxycycline minocycline)	Antibiotic	Anorexia, stomatitis, nausea and vomiting, cramps, diarrhea.	Take with 8 oz water 1 hr before or 2 hr after food or milk.
Thiazide diuretics	Diuretic used to treat high blood pressure and to decrease the amount of water held within the body	*Rare:* black tarry stools, blood in urine or stools, cough or hoarseness, fever or chills, joint pain, lower back or side pain, painful or difficult urination, pinpoint red spots on skin, skin rash or hives, stomach pain (severe) with nausea and vomiting, unusual bleeding or bruising, yellow eyes or skin.	Weight control and a low sodium diet are recommended. Consume foods high in potassium. *Signs and symptoms of too much potassium loss:* dry mouth, increased thirst, irregular heartbeat, mood or mental changes, muscle cramps or pain, nausea or vomiting, unusual tiredness or weakness, weak pulse. *Signs and symptoms of too much sodium loss:* confusion, convulsions, decreased mental activity, irritability, muscle cramps, unusual tiredness or weakness.
Vasotec™	Antihypertensive, angiotensin-converting enzyme inhibitor, anti–congestive heart failure	Stomatitis, nausea and vomiting, abdominal pain, diarrhea.	Decreased sodium and calorie intake may be recommended. Avoid salt substitutes, natural licorice, and alcohol. Caution with potassium supplements.
Wellbutrin™	Antidepressant	Anorexia, increased or decreased weight, increased appetite, dry mouth, stomatitis, dyspepsia, nausea, diarrhea, vomiting, constipation.	Take with food; avoid alcohol and St. John's wort. May lead to anemia.
Zoloft™	Antidepressant, selective serotonin reuptake inhibitor	Increased or decreased appetite, dry mouth, nausea, vomiting, diarrhea, constipation, dyspepsia.	Take consistently with or without food, avoid alcohol, anemia.

Individual and Group Assessment, Education, and Counseling Worksheets

Pregnancy and Lactation Worksheets

1. *Provide user-friendly dietary recommendations for ways to increase dietary calcium, iron, and folic acid intake. Why do pregnant women require extra quantities of these three nutrients?*

Calcium: During pregnancy the rate of bone turnover increases. Adequate calcium and vitamin D is required to minimize osteoporosis in the later life. Calcium is also essential for fetal development of bones and teeth.

Iron: Extra iron is required during pregnancy to support the formation of the placenta and the formation of the hemoglobin required by the expansion of the blood volume and to compensate for the loss of the blood during delivery. Adequate iron intake is also essential for preventing the depletion of the maternal stores and the development of iron deficiency anemia. Iron deficiency in the mother does not lead to a deficiency in the infant but may increase the risk of a low birth weight infant, premature delivery, or prenatal mortality.

Folic acid: The presence of a folic acid deficiency can lead to a reduced rate of DNA synthesis and mitotic activity in the individual cells. This can lead to congenital malformations and neural tube defects such as spina bifida, anencephaly, premature detachment of the placenta, hemorrhage, and low birth weight.

2. *Briefly describe what nutritional recommendations you would provide for a newly pregnant women whose prepregnancy weight is within normal limits. Include calorie recommendations, specific nutrients this individual should emphasize in her diet, foods to avoid during pregnancy, and so on.*

> Adequate energy intake is necessary to satisfy the pregnant mother's nutritional needs and to allow for about a 0.4-kg weight gain per week during the final 30 weeks of pregnancy. To meet nutritional needs, an additional 10 to 16 g/day of protein intake is needed. Sodium intake should not be excessive but should be no less than 2 g/day. Vitamin and mineral intake should meet the Recommended Daily Allowance for pregnant women. Adequate folic acid intake requires supplementation. Calcium needs are 1,000 mg/day. Caffeine intake should be limited to less than 200 mg/day (about two cups of coffee). Heartburn is common during pregnancy and can be alleviated by limiting the amount of food consumed at one time, consuming fluids between meals, wearing loose clothing, and sitting upright after meals for 3 hours before lying down. If constipation exists, a pregnant woman should consume fiber-rich foods and increase fluid intake.

3. *How do nutritional needs differ during pregnancy versus lactation? Why are each of the following substances not recommended during pregnancy and lactation: alcohol, tobacco, artificial sweeteners, and caffeine?*

Alcohol: Alcohol exposure to the developing fetus can trigger fetal alcohol syndrome, causing malformations such as facial malformations, low weight and height, smaller than normal head circumference, and mental and physical retardation. Excessive alcohol intake during pregnancy may also lead to a stillbirth.

Tobacco: Exposure to tobacco in utero has been shown to decrease infant birth weight and increase the risk of perinatal morbidity and mortality. Tobacco can cause a reduced blood flow to the uterus and often blunts appetite, potentially leading to a reduced food intake by the mother.

Artificial sweeteners: The use of saccharin is not recommended during pregnancy. Use of aspartame should also be restricted to less than 50 mg/kg body weight. Aspartame can lead to an increase in blood phenylalanine in women with phenylketonuria, which can lead to fetal brain damage.

Caffeine: Excessive caffeine consumption in pregnancy may produce problems with bone formation, causing deformed fingers, toes, and cleft palate. Also, excessive caffeine intake can lead to overstimulation of the mother and fetus.

4. *The following table shows recommended weight gain:*

Prepregnancy Weight	Recommended Weight Gain (lb)
Underweight (< = 85% ideal body weight)	28–40
Normal body weight	25–35
Overweight (> =120% ideal body weight)	15–25
Twin pregnancy	40–45

5. *The following table shows nutritional remedies for conditions common to pregnancy:*

Symptom/Condition	Description/Cause	Nutritional Intervention
Constipation	Usually occurs during the latter part of pregnancy due to reduced gut motility, physical inactivity, and pressure exerted on the bowel by the enlarged uterus.	Increase fluids and fiber. If necessary, add stool softeners.
Fluid retention/edema	Usually present in the third trimester. May be caused by the pressure of the enlarging uterus on the veins returning fluid from the legs.	Normal edema does not require sodium restriction or dietary change.
Gestational diabetes	Glucose intolerance, the onset or first recognition of which occurs during pregnancy. Diagnosis is made during the second or third trimester.	Limit intake of high-carbohydrate foods. Eat small, frequent meals. Perform self-monitoring of blood glucose levels, ketones, appetite, and weight gain. Ensure adequate calories and nutrition.
Heartburn	Usually occurs during latter part of pregnancy due to pressure of the enlarged uterus on the stomach in combination with the relaxation of the esophageal sphincter.	Limit the amount of food consumed at one time. Drink fluids between meals. Wear loose clothing around waist, eat slowly, and remain upright for at least 3 hr after meals.
Hyperemesis	Severe and continued nausea and vomiting	Hospitalization to control dehydration, correct electrolyte imbalances, or excessive weight loss. Encourage small, frequent meals and lots of fluids. Eat foods, as tolerated.
Leg cramps	Usually occurs at night. Sudden contractions of the gastrocnemius muscles.	Increase calcium intake.
Nausea/morning sickness	Common during the early months. May cause acute protein/energy deficit and aberrations in some vitamins, minerals, and electrolytes.	Encourage small, frequent, dry meals of easily digested carbohydrate-containing foods. Liquids are best tolerated between meals. Avoid foods/odors that trigger nausea.
Pica	Cravings for persistent ingestion of nonfood items that have little nutritional value. Poorly understood. Certain foods may relieve nausea and vomiting or compensate for a nutritional deficiency.	Ensure adequate calories and optimal nutrition.
Pregnancy induced hypertension	Characterized by hypertension, proteinuria, and edema. Hypoalbuminemia, hypovolemia, and subsequent hemoconcentration are also present. Generally occurs in the third trimester. Associated with poverty, lack of prenatal care, and poor nutritional status (i.e., protein and calcium deficiency).	Calcium and magnesium supplementation may help. Restriction of sodium consumption is recommended.

continues

6. *The following table shows common tests performed during pregnancy:*

Test	Description
Alpha-fetoprotein screening	Alpha-fetal protein normally produced by the fetal liver and yolk sac. Helpful in the diagnosis of fetal body wall defects. The most notable of these are neural tube defects.
Amniocentesis	To determine fetal maturity status, sex of fetus, genetic and chromosomal aberrations, fetal status affected by Rh isoimmunization, hereditary metabolic disorders, anatomic abnormalities, and fetal distress.
Chorionic villi sampling	Performed on women whose unborn child may be at risk for life-threatening or significant genetic defects (i.e., older age at time of pregnancy, frequent spontaneous abortions, pregnancies with fetuses with genetic defects, and women identified as having a genetic defect themselves).
Fetal heart rate monitoring	Part of the fetal biophysical profile. Ultrasound, fetal activity study, nonstress test (noninvasive) that monitors acceleration of the fetal heart rate.
Glucose tolerance test	For women who have a history of delivering large infants, stillbirths, or neonatal births. Also for women who have transient glycosuria or hyperglycemia during pregnancy.
Hemoglobin (Hb)	Refer to preceding Review of Common Laboratory Values.
Hematocrit (Hct)	Refer to preceding Review of Common Laboratory Values.
Oral glucose test	A test in which a pregnant women consumes a predetermined amount of a sugary drink and then has their blood sugar levels measured 1 hr after they finish consuming the liquid to determine whether they have elevated blood sugar levels that need to be monitored in case gestational diabetes develops.
Ultrasound	Provides accurate visualization of the fetus' abdominal aorta, liver, gallbladder, pancreas, bile ducts, kidneys, ureters, bladder, spine, and other important organs to ensure that development of the fetus and its systems are normal. Also used to determine the age of the fetus.

7. *Describe the advantages of breast-feeding versus bottle-feeding, especially during an infant's first 4 to 6 months. What are common barriers to initiation and continuation of breast-feeding? What are solutions to these barriers?*

Breast-feeding has many advantages. First, it provides the newborn with important immunologic factors, with the highest concentrations occurring in the colostrum provided during the first few days after birth before the mother's milk comes in. These immunologic factors can protect infants against life-threatening diseases, result in fewer respiratory and intestinal infections, and may protect against illness later in life (diabetes, lymphoma, celiac disease, and Crohn's disease). Second, the child and mother benefit psychologically and emotionally from the breast-feeding experience. The infant derives a sense of security and belonging from the warmth of the mother's body and being held. Breast-feeding increases the mother's feelings of competence in dealing with her child. Third, breast-feeding protects against the development of obesity in the child and, to a lesser degree, in the mother, reduces the risk of breast cancer in the mother, and promotes the contraction of the uterus after childbirth so it can return it to its normal size.

Breast milk is nutritionally superior to any alternative, is bacteriologically safe, always fresh, contains a variety of antiinfectious factors and immune cells, is least allergenic of any infant food, promotes good jaw and tooth development in the newborn, costs less than commercial formulas, automatically promotes close mother–child contact, and is more convenient once the process is established.

Common barriers to breast-feeding are constant fatigue, lack of freedom to return to work and social life, possibility of breast infection, mother's desire to quickly restore her figure to normal, concerns about being unable to secrete sufficient milk, concerns about environmental contaminants being passed to infant, and economic factors (the need to work for income).

Solutions to the common barriers to long-term breast-feeding are as follows: have written breast-feeding policy at health centers, train health care workers in breast-feeding, inform all pregnant women about the benefits of breast-feeding, have mother initiate breast-feeding during the first half hour of birth, have nurses or lactation consultants show mothers how to breast-feed properly, provide newborns no food or drink other than breast milk unless medically indicated, practice rooming-in, allow mothers and infants to remain together for at least 24 hours after birth, discourage use of artificial pacifiers/teats, and establish breast-feeding support groups and refer mothers upon discharge.

8. *The following table compares the various infant formulas:*

Formula	Indications
Alimentum™	For food allergies and colic (due to protein sensitivity): • Hypoallergenic • Nutritionally complete formula for infants and children with severe food allergies and colic due to protein sensitivity • Provides an easily digested and absorbed fat blend • Provides predigested protein to avoid symptoms of milk allergy in most infants and children
Enfamil with iron™	Enfamil with iron is designed to provide complete nutrition to the infant. Enfamil with iron has a protein blend that is easy to digest, has a 60:40 whey-to-casein protein ratio, is similar to breast milk, has calcium to help build strong bones as happens with breast-fed infants, and about 50% of the calories in both breast milk and Enfamil with iron come from fat.
Enfamil Premature™	Enfamil Premature LIPIL is designed for use in the hospital as a sole source of nutrition for premature infants who are not breast-fed. It is enriched to provide added nutrition that premature infants need. Enfamil Premature LIPIL also has a unique blend of DHA and ARA, ingredients that are important building blocks for an infant's brain and eyes.
Isomil Advance™	This formula is used when DHA and ARA are recommended. It is milk-free and lactose-free. DHA and ARA are special nutrients found in breast milk that are important for mental and visual development.
Isomil 2™	For infants 6–18 mo, eating cereal and baby foods. Milk-free and lactose-free. As infants grow their nutritional needs change. For example, the amount of calcium infants need doubles by the time they reach age 1. Cereals and other foods alone may not provide all the calcium an infant needs during this time of rapid growth. Isomil 2 has been specially designed to help meet the nutritional requirements of older infants and toddlers. Isomil 2 provides calcium to help support developing bones and is fortified with iron, which is important for brain development.
Nutramigen™	This formula is used for those infants with colic, often indicated by an infant who screams and cries. Even the most experienced parents do not always know what to do. Calling the infant's doctor is always the best place to start to determine whether medical attention is required. When colic is the reason for the infant's distress, his or her doctor may suspect protein allergy, a reaction that can occur to the protein in either milk-based or soy-based formulas. Protein allergy is serious business. In infants it can cause a variety of problems, such as diarrhea, difficulty breathing, hives, a kind of rash known as atopic eczema, and the uncontrollable screaming and crying that is often termed "colic." If a protein-related problem is suspected, a special formula, such as Nutramigen, is prescribed. This member of the Enfamil Family of Formulas™ is the only infant formula that clinical studies have proven to be effective for managing colic due to cow's milk protein allergy. In fact, Nutramigen has been trusted for more than 50 years to help manage infants with protein allergy.

continues

Formula	Indications
PediaSure™	• Milk-based complete balanced nutrition: 1.0 Cal per mL, 237 Cal per 8 fl oz, from a balanced distribution of protein, fat, and carbohydrate (caloric distribution: protein, 12%; fat, 44%; carbohydrate, 44%). • Comes in four "kid-approved" flavors: chocolate, strawberry, vanilla, and banana cream. • Potential renal solute load: close to that of infant formulas. • High-quality protein: 82% casein, 18% whey. Amino acid profile meets NAS-NRC standards for high-quality proteins. • Gluten-free and lactose-free. • Fat content, 50 g/L: 50% high oleic safflower oil, 30% soy oil, and 20% medium chain triglycerides. • Contains selenium, chromium, molybdenum, inositol, taurine, and carnitine. • Calcium-to-phosphorus ratio of 1.2:1. Conforms to AAPCON recommendations for growing children. • Iron concentration of 1.4 mg/100 Cal. Meets NAS-NRC recommendations for children 1–10 years old in 1,000 Cal. • Appropriate vitamin D content: 51 IU/100 Cal meets children's needs better than most adult enteral products.
PediaSure With Fiber™	PediaSure With Fiber enteral formula is designed to provide a source of complete balanced nutrition for children aged 1–10 years who may benefit from fiber. It is a lower osmolality formula than PediaSure. PediaSure With Fiber enteral formula is designed for children who are fed by tube and contains soy fiber at a level shown to be well tolerated by children. It also is appropriate for oral feeding. Not approved for children with galactosemia.
Peptamen™	Peptamen® Complete Isotonic Liquid Elemental Diet is formulated to provide complete or supplemental nutritional support in an easily absorbed form for patients with impaired gastrointestinal function. Patients benefiting from Peptamen Diet may include those with short bowel syndrome, inflammatory bowel disease, malabsorption syndromes, pancreatic insufficiency, chronic diarrhea, radiation enteritis, and delayed gastric emptying. Peptamen Diet may also be useful as a dual feeding with total parenteral nutrition or as a transition diet from total parenteral nutrition. *Note:* Peptamen Diet contains ingredients (i.e., partially hydrolyzed whey protein, from cow's milk protein) that may not be appropriate for individuals with food allergies.
Portagen™	Portagen provides complete nutrition for infants and toddlers under 2 years of age who do not efficiently digest or absorb conventional fat. Portagen contains appropriate levels of readily digestible protein, fat, and carbohydrate for infants and toddlers less than 2 years of age and is iron-fortified, lactose-free, and gluten-free. Available as an unflavored powder that may be flavored or sweetened to taste, Portagen provides 86% of its fat as medium chain triglycerides (MCT oil), a type of fat that is easily digested and absorbed. Linoleic acid is provided through corn oil. Portagen should be used only under a physician's supervision.
Pregestimil™	Pregestimil infant formula is rarely used without a doctor's recommendation. It provides the same extensively predigested protein as Nutramigen, but it differs from Nutramigen in its source of fat. The fat blend in Pregestimil consists mostly of a special type of fat, MCT oil, that is more easily digested and absorbed than the close-to-breast-milk fat blend in Enfamil, LactoFree, Nutramigen, and ProSobee. The unique formulation of Pregestimil is designed for feeding infants with diseases or disorders that make it difficult for them to absorb the fat blend in most other formulas. These conditions include short bowel syndrome, steatorrhea (fat in the stool), cystic fibrosis, or persistent diarrhea that does not respond to treatment.
ProSobee™ (Enfamil™)	Iron-fortified powder specially designed for infants in the first 12 months needing a soy formula. It is milk-free and lactose-free and easy to digest.

continues

Formula	Indications
Similac with Iron™	Excellent nutrition for infants aged 0–12 mo: • When DHA and ARA, special nutrients found in breast milk, are recommended. • DHA and ARA are special nutrients found in breast milk that are important for mental and visual development. Similac Advance is an excellent choice when DHA and ARA are recommended. • Ideal for supplementation. • Provides calcium for growing bones. • Designed to be gentle on the infant's developing digestive system.
Similac NeoSure™	NeoSure Advance contains DHA and ARA, special nutrients found in breast milk that are important for brain and eye development. DHA and ARA have been clinically shown to improve visual development in preterm infants.

ARA, arachidonic acid; DHA, docosahexaenoic acid.

9. *The following table provides pregnancy and lactation medical terminology:*

Abbreviation or Term	Meaning
AFP	Alpha-fetoprotein screening
BF	Breast-feed
Colostrum	A milk-like secretion from the breast, present during the first day or so after delivery before milk appears; rich in protective factors
DOB	Date of birth
Eclampsia	A severe stage of preeclampsia characterized by convulsions
EDC	Estimated date of confinement
FTT	Failure to thrive
G	Gravida
Gest	Gestation
GYN	Gynecology
Hyperemesis	Severe and continued nausea and vomiting
LBW	Low birth weight < 5.5 lb
LMP	Last menstrual period
Mature milk	Milk that comes in after the colostrum
NICU	Neonatal intensive care unit
OB	Obstetrics
Parity	The number of children borne by one woman
PIH	Pregnancy induced hypertension
Postpartum	After birth
Preeclampsia	A condition characterized by hypertension, fluid retention, and protein in the urine; formerly known as pregnancy induced hypertension
SGA	Small for gestational weight
SRM	Spontaneous rupture of membranes
Toxemia	Hypertensive disease of pregnancy
VLBW	Very low birth weight

Diabetes Worksheets

1. *Define diabetes mellitus. What is the incidence of all types of diabetes in the United States? Are diabetes or the complications from this disease one of the leading causes of death in the United States?*

Definition

Diabetes mellitus is a group of genetically and clinically related disorders characterized by blood glucose levels above defined limits. Diverse etiologic and pathologic mechanisms contribute to a relative or absolute deficiency in insulin, a hormone secreted by pancreatic beta cells. Significant clinical complications are associated with the hyperglycemia of diabetes:

- Macrovascular disease (two to six times greater risk than in the general population)
- Heart disease
- Stroke
- Peripheral vascular disease
- Microvascular disease
- Nephropathy
- Retinopathy
- Neuropathy
- Peripheral
- Autonomic

Overall, the risk for death among people with diabetes is about two times that of people without diabetes. However, the increased risk associated with diabetes is greater for younger people (i.e., 3.6 times for people aged 25 to 44 years versus 1.5 for those aged 65 to 74 years) and women (i.e., 2.7 times for women aged 45 to 64 years versus 2.0 for men in the same age group). Heart disease is the leading cause of diabetes-related deaths. Adults with diabetes have heart disease death rates about two to four times higher than adults without diabetes (American Diabetes Association, 2002).

The development of these complications is believed to be correlated to the level of blood glucose control maintained throughout the diabetic individual's life span. This assumption continues to be investigated. However, even individuals with impaired glucose tolerance are subject to increased incidence of macrovascular complications. Generally, complications do not appear until diabetes has been present for more than 15 to 20 years. Genetic and environmental factors play a role in the development of the complications associated with disease.

Individuals with diabetes are classified into two primary categories according to their etiology and subsequent treatment needs. Nearly 90% of individuals with diabetes have non–insulin-dependent diabetes mellitus (NIDDM); 5% to 10% have insulin-dependent diabetes mellitus (IDDM). Other classifications of glucose intolerance include gestational diabetes and impaired glucose tolerance.

Prevalence of Diabetes

Total: 17 million people, 6.2% of the population have diabetes
Diagnosed: 11.1 million people
Undiagnosed: 5.9 million people
New cases diagnosed per year: 1 million people aged 20 years or older

Diabetes was the sixth leading cause of death listed on U.S. death certificates in 1999 (American Diabetes Association, 2002).

2. *Common characteristics of Types 1 and 2 diabetes: complete the following chart describing the differences between Type 1 and Type 2.*

Characteristics	Type 1 Diabetes (IDDM)	Type 2 Diabetes (NIDDM)
Percentage of diabetics	May account for 5–10% of all diagnosed cases of diabetes.	May account for about 90–95% of all diagnosed cases of diabetes.
Insulin production	Body's immune system destroys pancreatic beta cells, the only cells in the body that make the hormone insulin that regulates blood glucose.	Begins as insulin resistance. As the need for insulin rises, the pancreas gradually loses its ability to produce insulin.
Status of insulin receptors	Nonfunctional.	May be nonfunctional.
Age at onset	Childhood to young adult.	Childhood to older adulthood.
Etiology/metabolic abnormalities	Cell-mediated autoimmune destruction of the beta cells of the pancreas; idiopathic.	Abnormal pattern of insulin secretion and action; decreased cellular uptake of glucose and increased postprandial glucose, increased release of glucose by liver. Etiology mostly unknown.
Genetic influences on disease development	Genetic predisposition.	Genetic and environmental factors.
Common disease-related symptoms	Skin conditions, gum disease, retinopathy, kidney disease, transplantation, neuropathy, cardiovascular disease, feet complications.	
Rate at which symptoms appear	Variable: some rapidly, some slowly.	Gradual.
Associated conditions	Skin conditions, gum disease, retinopathy, kidney disease, transplantation, neuropathy, cardiovascular disease, feet complications.	
Risk of metabolic ketoacidosis	High.	Nonketotic.
Possibility of elimination of the disease from one's life	None.	Poor to good.
Medications	Insulin therapy, oral hypoglycemic agents.	
Primary dietary objectives	Maintain optimal blood glucose levels.	

3. *Laboratory tests important to the diagnosis and management of diabetes mellitus: describe the following laboratory tests, including acceptable ranges for the laboratory measurement.*

Laboratory Measurement	Description and Significance	Accepted Laboratory Value Range
Blood urea nitrogen (BUN)	Measures the amount of urea nitrogen in the blood which is formed in the liver as the end product of protein metabolism. Measurements of BUN and creatinine are the two most commonly ordered tests of the kidney's ability to excrete metabolic waste. Individuals with diabetes are at a greater risk of possessing compromised renal function.	10–12 mg/dL (adult)

continues

Laboratory Measurement	Description and Significance	Accepted Laboratory Value Range
Creatinine	Creatinine is correlated with changes in the serum urea nitrogen (BUN) for diagnostic purposes but is more accurate as an index of the glomerular filtration rate. It is therefore used to test the kidney's ability to excrete metabolic wastes or in those instances where the cause of an elevated BUN value is uncertain.	0.5–1.1 mg/dL (female) 0.6–1.2 mg/dL (male)
Fasting blood glucose	Measurement of blood glucose levels after fasting for ~8 hr. In the fasting state, glucose levels, tend to be at their lowest.	70–105 mg/dL Critical values: < 50 and > 400 mg/dL (male) < 40 and > 400 mg/dL (female)
Fingerstick blood sugar evaluations	Random measurements of blood glucose levels obtained by pricking one's finger.	70–105 mg/dL Critical values: < 50 and > 400 mg/dL (male) < 40 and > 400 mg/dL (female)
Glucose tolerance test (GTT)	GTTs are provocative, or stimulating, tests in which large doses of glucose are given, orally or by intravenous injection, and the rise and fall of the blood glucose level, and in many cases urine glucose, are checked at timed intervals.	Fasting: 70–115 mg/dL 30 min: < 200 1hr: < 200 2 hr: < 140 3 hr: 70–115 4 hr: 70–115
Glycosylated hemoglobin (HbAlc)	Measurement of HbAlc provides a picture of the state of hyperglycemia over time in an individual (the 120-day life span of the red blood cell), and elevated levels correlate with glucose intolerance in diabetics.	Good diabetic control: 6.0–8.0% Poor diabetic control: 10%+
Total cholesterol, including HDL and LDL components	Individuals with diabetes are at a greater risk for cardiovascular complications, including elevated blood lipid levels. These measurements are performed regularly to minimize diabetes-related cardiovascular complications.	HDL: Male: >45 mg/dL Female: >55 mg/dL LDL: 60–80 mg/dL Cholesterol: < 200 mg/dL Or < 5.2 mmol/L Under age 20 years: < 180 mg/dL
Triglycerides	Generally included as part of a lipid profile along with HDL and LDL cholesterol but has little predictive value by itself and increases after fat consumption.	Male: 40–160mg/dL Female: 35–135 mg/dL
Urine glucose tests	A measure of the amount of glucose in the urine. Urinary threshold maximums vary among individuals, and glucosuria is not a true indicator of serum glucose levels.	Urinary threshold levels vary among individuals. Changes in normal urine glucose levels are sometimes monitored in diabetics. Random: Negative 24 hr: < equal sign0.5 g/day
Urine ketone tests	Ketonuria of sufficient concentration to produce a positive response in testing reflects an alteration in carbohydrate metabolism with secondary disturbance in lipid metabolism. Diabetes is the only disease in which ketonuria has a true diagnostic importance. The presence of ketonuria in diabetes is a major indicator of impending or established ketoacidosis.	Normal: Negative for all age groups

4. *Diabetes-related complications and symptoms: describe the following potential complications related to diabetes mellitus and provide solutions for each dilemma.*

Diabetes-Related Symptoms	Symptoms and Causes	Dietary and Medical Solutions
Diabetic coma	A coma in a diabetic due to the buildup of ketones in the bloodstream. Ketones are a product of metabolizing (using) fats rather than the sugar glucose for energy.	The best approach to diabetic coma is prevention. Careful diet, medication, and insulin dosing as needed should prevent ketone buildup. Patients with diabetes and their family members should be aware of the early signs of ketone buildup. These include weight loss, nausea, confusion, gasping for breath, and a characteristically sweet chemical odor similar to that of acetone or alcohol ("acetone breath") to the patient's breath and sometimes sweat. Diabetic coma may be presaged (heralded) by confusion and convulsions.
Glycosuria	Elevated blood glucose leads to spillage of glucose into the urine (glucosuria) so that the urine is sugary. (The term *diabetes mellitus* means "sweet urine.") Aside from diabetes, the many other causes of high blood sugar include just eating more sugar (or food) than usual, the presence of an infection or another illness, an injury, and the stress of surgery.	High blood sugar may produce few or no symptoms. When there are symptoms, they may be dry mouth, thirst, frequent urination, urination during the night, blurry vision, fatigue or drowsiness, weight loss, or increased appetite. An individual with any of these symptoms needs to see their health care provider for a thorough medical assessment.
Hyperglycemia	Hyperglycemia is often found in diabetes mellitus. It occurs when the body does not have enough insulin or cannot use the insulin it has to turn glucose into energy. Hyperglycemia may also occur in Cushing syndrome and other conditions. The signs of hyperglycemia are polydipsia (a great thirst), polyuria (a need to urinate often), and a dry mouth.	Individual meal management and possible drug therapy. See the following sections.
Hypoglycemia	Low blood sugar (glucose). When symptoms of hypoglycemia occur together with a documented blood glucose under 45 mg/dL, and the symptoms promptly resolve with the administration of glucose, the diagnosis of hypoglycemia can be made with some certainty. The causes of hypoglycemia include drugs (such as insulin), liver disease, surgical absence of the stomach, tumors that release excess amounts of insulin, and prediabetes. In some patients, symptoms of hypoglycemia occur during fasting (fasting hypoglycemia). In others, symptoms of hypoglycemia occur after meals (reactive hypoglycemia).	Hypoglycemia is only significant when it is associated with symptoms. The symptoms may include anxiety, sweating, tremor, palpitations, nausea, pallor, headache, mild confusion, abnormal behavior, loss of consciousness, seizure, and coma. Immediate treatment of severe hypoglycemia consists of administering large amounts of glucose, and repeating this treatment at intervals if the symptoms persist. Treatment must also be directed at the underlying cause. Patients with diabetes mellitus who develop low blood glucose from their medicines require medication adjustments. Treatment of reactive hypoglycemia consists of dietary measures, including fewer concentrated sweets and the ingestion of multiple small meals throughout the day.

continues

Diabetes-Related Symptoms	Symptoms and Causes	Dietary and Medical Solutions
Ketoacidosis	A feature of uncontrolled diabetes mellitus characterized by a combination of ketosis and acidosis. Ketosis is the accumulation of substances called ketone bodies in the blood. Acidosis is increased acidity of the blood. Symptoms of ketoacidosis include slow deep breathing with a fruity odor to the breath, confusion, frequent urination (polyuria), poor appetite, and eventually loss of consciousness.	The treatment of ketoacidosis is a matter of urgency and is usually done in a hospital. It may require the administration of intravenous fluids, insulin, and glucose and the institution of changes in the person's diet.
Nephropathy	Kidney disease associated with long-standing diabetes. It affects the network of tiny blood vessels (the microvasculature) in the glomerulus, a key structure in the kidney that is composed of capillary blood vessels and that is critically necessary for the filtration of the blood. Features of diabetic nephropathy include the nephrotic syndrome with excessive filtration of protein into the urine (proteinuria), high blood pressure (hypertension), and progressively impaired kidney function. When severe, diabetic nephropathy leads to kidney failure, end-stage renal disease, and the need for chronic kidney dialysis or a kidney transplant.	0.8 g/kg of protein, if glomerular filtration rate normal. 0.6 g/kg if glomerular filtration rate declines.
Polydipsia	Excessive thirst all the time. Polydipsia occurs, for example, in untreated or poorly controlled diabetes mellitus.	Can be alleviated by treating elevated blood sugar levels.
Polyphagia	Frequent hunger and eating.	Management of blood sugar levels can help manage appetite. When insulin is not functioning well or is not produced in the body at all, the glucose in the blood cannot get into the body cells to feed them. As a result, the cells are starving and send a message to the brain to increase appetite.
Polyuria	The passage of an abnormally large amount of urine. Someone with polyuria passes too much urine and so may have frequency, the need to urinate frequently. Polyuria is a "classic textbook" sign of diabetes mellitus that is under poor control or not yet under treatment.	Treatment of hyperglycemia will alleviate polyuria.
Retinopathy	A common complication of diabetes affecting the blood vessels in the retina (the thin light-sensitive membrane that covers the back of the eye). If untreated, it may lead to blindness. If diagnosed and treated promptly, blindness is usually preventable. Diabetic retinopathy begins without any noticeable change in vision. But even then there often are extensive changes in the retina visible to an ophthalmologist (eye doctor). It is therefore important for a diabetic to have an eye examination at least once (ideally twice) a year.	Treatment is by laser surgery, usually on an outpatient basis. The nature of the laser treatment depends on the stage of the retinopathy. Laser therapy can only stop the progression of diabetic retinopathy. It cannot reverse the damage already done. The progression of the retinopathy can be slowed down by careful control of the diabetes, effective reduction of high blood pressure together with regular eye exams, and, if needed, prompt laser therapy.

5. *Define and describe the role of insulin and oral hypoglycemic medications in the treatment of Type 1 and Type 2 diabetes.*

The major goal in treating diabetes mellitus is controlling elevated blood sugars (glucose) without causing abnormally low levels of blood sugar. Type 1 diabetes mellitus is treated with insulin, exercise, and a diabetic diet. Insulin is the mainstay of treatment for patients with type 1 diabetes mellitus. Insulin is also important in Type 2 diabetes when blood glucose levels cannot be controlled by diet, weight loss, exercise, and oral medications.

Ideally, insulin medication should be administered in a manner that mimics the natural pattern of insulin secretion by a healthy pancreas. The complex pattern of insulin secretion by the pancreas is difficult to duplicate. Still, adequate blood glucose control can be achieved with careful attention to diet, regular exercise, home blood glucose monitoring, and multiple insulin injections throughout the day.

Type 2 diabetes mellitus is first treated with weight reduction, a diabetic diet, and exercise. When these measures fail to control the elevated blood sugars, oral medications are used. If oral medications are still insufficient, insulin medications are considered. Based on what is known, medications for Type 2 diabetes are designed to

- Increase the insulin output by the pancreas
- Decrease the amount of glucose released from the liver
- Increase the sensitivity (response) of cells to insulin
- Decrease the absorption of carbohydrates from the intestine

Adherence to a diabetic diet is an important aspect of controlling elevated blood sugar in patients with diabetes mellitus. The American Diabetes Association has provided guidelines for a diabetic diet that is a balanced, nutritious diet low in fat, cholesterol, and simple sugars. The total daily calories are evenly divided into three meals. In the past 2 years, the American Diabetes Association has lifted the absolute ban on simple sugars. Small amounts of simple sugars are allowed when consumed with a complex meal.

Weight reduction and exercise are important treatments of diabetes. Weight reduction and exercise increase the body's sensitivity to insulin, thus helping to control blood sugar elevations.

6. *Diabetes specific medications: fill in the following chart to outline some of the characteristics of insulin and some common oral hypoglycemic agents. This information should be considered when planning meal and medication times.*

Characteristics of Insulin

Generic Name (Brand)	Onset	Peak	Duration
Rapid acting (Lispro™)	5–15 min	30–60 min	2–4 hr
Short acting (regular)	30 min	2–5 hr	6–8 hr
Intermediate acting (NPH™, Lente™)	1–2½ hr	8–14 hr	22 hr
Long acting (Ultralente™)	4–6 hr	10–18 hr	24–36 hr

Common Oral Hypoglycemic Agents

Agent	Information
Precose™	The name of the alpha-glucosidase inhibitor available in the United States is Precose. Because Precose works on the intestine, its effects are additive to diabetic medications that work at other sites, such as sulfonylureas. Clinical studies have shown statistically better blood glucose control in patients treated with Precose and a sulfonylurea versus the sulfonylurea alone. Precose is currently used alone or in combination with a sulfonylurea. Precose is taken three times a day at the beginning of meals. The dosage varies from 25 to 100 mg with each meal. The maximum recommended dose is 100 mg three times a day. At doses greater than this, reversible liver abnormalities may be seen. Because of its mechanism of action, Precose has significant gastrointestinal side effects. Abdominal pain, diarrhea, and gas are common and are seen in up to 75% of patients taking Precose. For this reason, Precose is administered using a low initial dose that is increased over weeks depending on the patient's tolerance.
Sulfonylureas	Historically, increasing the insulin output by the pancreas has been the major area targeted by medications used to treat Type 2 diabetes. These medications belong to a class of drugs called sulfonylureas. Sulfonylureas primarily lower blood glucose levels by increasing the release of insulin from the pancreas. Older generations of these drugs include chlorpropamide and tolbutamide, whereas newer drugs include glyburide (DiaBeta™), glipizide (Glucotrol™), and glimepiride (Amaryl™). These drugs are effective in rapidly lowering blood sugars but run the risk of causing hypoglycemia. In addition, they are sulfa compounds and should be avoided in patients with sulfa allergies.
Meglitinides	Recently, a new class of drugs that affect insulin release has been approved by the U.S. Food and Drug Administration (FDA) for use in Type 2 diabetes. Known as meglitinides, these drugs also work on the pancreas to promote insulin secretion. Unlike sulfonylureas that bind to receptors on the insulin producing cells, meglitinides work through a separate potassium based channel on the cell surface. Repaglinide (Prandin™) and nateglinide (Starlix™) are short-acting agents that are taken 30 min before meals. Unlike the sulfonylureas, which last longer in the body, Prandin and Starlix are very short acting, with peak effects within 1 hr. For this reason they are given up to three times a day just before meals. Because these drugs also increase circulating insulin levels, they may also cause hypoglycemia, but the literature suggests this is less frequent than the hypoglycemia seen with sulfonylurea agents.
Biguanides	A class of drugs called biguanides has been used for many years in Europe and Canada. In 1994 the FDA approved the use of metformin (Glucophage™) for the treatment of Type 2 diabetes in the United States. Glucophage™ is unique in its ability to decrease glucose production from the liver. Briefly, because metformin does not increase insulin levels, when used alone it does not usually cause hypoglycemia. In addition, metformin has an effect whereby it tends to suppress appetite, which may be beneficial in this population. Metformin may be used by itself or in conjunction with other oral agents or insulin. It should not be used in patients with kidney impairment and should be used with caution in those with liver impairment. The older parent compounds of metformin were associated with a serious condition called lactic acidosis with a dangerous acid buildup in the blood resulting from accumulation of the drug and its breakdown products. Although metformin is safer in this regard, it is recommended that the drug be discontinued for 24 hr before any dye-related procedure (such as intravenous pyelogram kidney study) or surgery is performed. The dyes may impair kidney function and cause a buildup of the drug in the blood. Metformin can be restarted after these procedures once the patient has urinated normally.
Thiazolidinediones	At present in the United States, the class of drugs known as thiazolidinediones lowers blood glucose by improving target cell response to insulin (increasing the sensitivity of the cells to insulin). Troglitazone (Rezulin™) was the first of this type of compound introduced in the United States. Sister compounds are now available with a better safety profile. These drugs include pioglitazone (Actos™) and rosiglitazone (Avandia™).

Pioglitazone (Actos™) and rosiglitazone (Avandia™) are new thiazolidinediones that have been approved for use in the United States. Although they are sister compounds to Rezulin, extensive studies failed to show any liver problems associated with these particular drugs. Both Avandia and Actos act by increasing the sensitivity (responsiveness) of cells to insulin. They improve sensitivity to insulin in muscle and fat tissue. These drugs have been effective in lowering blood sugars in patients with Type 2 diabetes; Actos and Avandia act within 1 hr of administration and are dosed daily. It is important to note that it takes up |

continues

to 6 weeks to see a drop in blood glucose levels on these agents and up to 12 weeks to see a maximum benefit. Actos™ and Avandi™ have been approved as first-line therapy in diabetes and for use in combination. Both medications may be used in patients taking other oral agents as well as those using insulin.

As an aside, Actos and Avandia have an added benefit of changing cholesterol patterns in diabetes. HDL, or good, cholesterol increases on these medications and triglycerides often decrease, but there is some controversy regarding what happens to LDL, or bad, cholesterol.

7. Briefly describe the rationale for use of insulin pumps, intensive insulin therapy, and multiple daily insulin injections.

Prefilled insulin pens: In the past, insulin was available only in an injectable form. This involved carrying syringes (which a few decades ago were made of glass and required sterilization), needles, vials of insulin, and alcohol swabs. Needless to say, patients often found it difficult to take multiple shots a day, and as a result good blood sugar control was often compromised. Many pharmaceutical companies are now offering discreet and convenient methods of insulin delivery. Both Novo Nordisk and Lily have an insulin pen delivery system. This system is similar to an ink cartridge in a fountain pen. A small pen-sized device holds an insulin cartridge (usually containing 300 units). Cartridges are available in the most widely used insulin formulations, such as those listed in the preceding table. The amount of insulin to be injected is dialed in by turning the bottom of the pen until the required number of units is seen in the dose-viewing window. The tip of the pen consists of a needle that is replaced with each injection. A release mechanism allows the needle to penetrate just under the skin and deliver the required amount of insulin. The cartridges and needles are disposed of when finished and new ones are simply inserted. These insulin-delivery devices are discreet and less cumbersome than traditional methods.

Insulin pump: The most recently available advance in insulin delivery is the insulin pump. In the United States, MiniMed™, Deltec™, and Disetronic™ market the insulin pump. An insulin pump is composed of a pump reservoir similar to that of an insulin cartridge, a battery-operated pump, and a computer chip that allows the user to control the exact amount of insulin delivered. Currently, pumps on the market are about the size of a beeper. The pump is attached to a thin plastic tube (an infusion set) that has a soft cannula (or needle) at the end through which insulin passes. This cannula is inserted under the skin, usually on the abdomen. The cannula is changed every 2 days. The tubing can be disconnected from the pump while showering or swimming. The pump is used for continuous insulin delivery, 24 hours a day. The amount of insulin is programmed and is administered at a constant rate (basal rate). Often, the amount of insulin needed over the course of 24 hours varies, depending on factors like exercise, activity level, and sleep. The insulin pump allows for the user to program many different basal rates to allow for this variation in life-style. In addition, the user can program the pump to deliver a "bolus" during meals to cover the excess demands of carbohydrate ingestion. Over 50,000 people worldwide are using an insulin pump. This number is growing dramatically as these devices become smaller and more user-friendly. Insulin pumps allow for tight blood sugar control and life-style flexibility while minimizing the effects of low blood sugar (hypoglycemia). At present, the pump is the closest device on the market to an artificial pancreas. Naturally, the next step would be a pump that can also sense blood sugar levels and adjust the insulin delivery accordingly. Much effort is being concentrated on this area of research, and possibly, even within the next year, a prototype device may be available for trial.

Inhalation: Another promising route of insulin administration is through inhalation. Inhaled insulin is currently being tested but has not been approved by the U.S. Food and Drug Administration. Many devices are available that allow for other medications to be used in this manner, the best example of which is asthma therapy. Insulin is not absorbed through the bronchial tubes (airways) and must reach the air sacks at the end of the bronchial tubes (alveoli) to be absorbed. Once at the alveoli, insulin can be absorbed and enter the bloodstream. Currently, powdered inhalers and nebulizers are being studied to determine which delivery system is the most reliable. The safety of inhaled insulin still needs to be established before a product for consumer use can be made available. Trials are currently underway to establish the safety of inhaled insulin.

8. *Explain the importance and/or provide solutions for the following issues commonly addressed as part of the dietary management of Type 1 and Type 2 diabetes.*

Timing and frequency of meals and snacks: This prevents spikes in blood glucose levels and maintains normal blood glucose levels. Eating meals at about the same time every day helps keep blood sugar levels in the target range. Eating snacks during the day and before, during, or after exercise is necessary as well. This prevents or delays the start of diabetes complications such as nerve, eye, kidney, and blood vessel damage.

Managing sick days: When sick, stress levels are increased. To deal with this stress, the body releases hormones that help it fight disease. These hormones have side effects. Blood sugar levels increase and interfere with the blood sugar–lowering effects of insulin. Usual doses of insulin should be taken when sick. Monitoring of blood glucose levels and urine testing for ketones should be done four times daily. If regular foods are not tolerated, liquid or soft cholesterol-containing foods should be eaten. At least 50 g of cholesterol should be consumed every 3 to 4 hours in small frequent feedings. Ample amounts of liquid should be consumed every hour. The health care team should be called if illness continues for more than 1 day.

Necessary changes to medication administration and food choices when physical activity is added to the equation: Blood glucose should be checked twice before exercise. If insulin or diabetes pills are taken, blood glucose monitoring is important to avoid low blood glucose levels. Blood glucose should be monitored 30 minutes before and again just before exercise. Check during and after exercise also. Plan exercise and diabetes care to avoid levels that are too low or too high. It is best to exercise 1 to 3 hours after a meal. Avoid exercising when insulin is at peak. Check for ketones whenever blood glucose levels are too high.

Alcohol consumption and its influence on the diabetic condition: The risk of low blood sugars is greater when alcohol is consumed. Alcohol should not be consumed on an empty stomach but with a meal or after eating a snack. Drinking as little as 2 ounces of alcohol on an empty stomach can lead to very low blood glucose. It is important to check blood glucose before sleep. A snack should be eaten to avoid hypoglycemia while sleeping.

The use of artificial sweeteners in the dietary treatment of diabetes: This can be part of a healthful eating plan, but it must be included as part of the daily carbohydrate allowance. Sucrose and sucrose-containing foods may be used in moderation as part of a balanced meal plan. Fructose appears to produce a lower glycemic response than the same amounts of sucrose or other cholesterol but should be consumed in moderation. The common sugar alcohols (polyols), sorbitol, mannitol, and xylitol produce a lower glycemic response than sucrose and other carbohydrates.

9. *Diet planning with the exchange system:* Use the "Exchange Lists for Meal Planning" found on http://www.diabetes.org/nutrition-and-recipes/nutrition/exchangelist.jsp. Fill in the number of servings you would recommend from each food group for each calorie level. Use the following guidelines to calculate the following meal patterns:

1. Determine caloric needs based on usual eating habits, medications, medical condition(s), and activity level.
2. Distribute calories as follows: carbohydrate (g) = 55% to 60% total calories, 4 kcal/g; protein (g) = 10% to 20% total calories, 4 kcal/g; fat (g) = 25% to 30% total calories, 9 kcal/g.
3. Convert carbohydrate, protein, and fat into exchanges according to individual preferences.
4. Distribute exchanges into meals and snacks according to medication and life-style.

Food Group	1,200 Calories	1,500 Calories	1,800 Calories	2,000 Calories	2,200 Calories
Starch/bread					
Vegetable					
Fruit					
Meat					
Milk					
Fat					

10. *Describe the concept of carbohydrate counting used in diabetes management. What is the rationale for this method? What are the advantages and disadvantages of this method versus the exchange system?*

Carbohydrate counting, or carb counting, is a meal planning system in which you eat a specific number of carbohydrate grams at each meal or snack. Although it is an effective plan for anyone with an eye on their diet, it is especially helpful for people with diabetes.

Carb counting is easy to learn. Most people believe it gives them flexibility in food choices, making social situations and eating out easier. The most compelling reason to use carb counting is simply because it can improve blood glucose control. Before you start consult your dietitian or health care provider. There is no meal planning approach that is right for everyone—each person needs an individualized plan.

Carbohydrates are the basis of all the food groups, so you'll find them in nearly every food. With carb counting, the source of the carbohydrate is not as important as how much of it you eat. That is good news for people with diabetes because carbohydrates are in starches, fruits, dairy products, vegetables, and, dare we say it, sugary sweets. This plan lets you eat a wide variety of foods, as long as you stay within your per-meal allowances of carbohydrates.

How Carb Counting Works

Make a plan: Determine the number of carbohydrate grams you should have at each meal or snack and whether to count "grams" or "choices." Grams are counted simply by adding the total carbohydrate content in each food serving. Choices, like the familiar exchanges, are selections from food groups. One choice equals 15 grams of carbohydrates. Choices are less precise than grams but easier to use and accurate enough for people who do not take insulin.

Each person's plan differs, and the following chart shows just one example:

	Choices	Grams
Breakfast	3–4	45–60
Lunch	4–5	60–75
Dinner	5–6	75–90
Snacks	0–1	0–15

Learn the carbohydrate counts of foods: You will need your blood glucose meter, a food scale, measuring cups and spoons, carbohydrate content guidebooks, and the Nutrition Facts on food labels. You will use these essential tools at every meal while learning the system and then only at a few meals each week once you become comfortable with measuring.

If you are counting choices and are familiar with the exchange system, you can easily memorize these converted measurements:

> 1 starch exchange = 15 grams = 1 choice
> 1 fruit exchange = 15 grams = 1 choice
> 1 milk exchange = 12 grams = 1 choice
> 3 vegetable exchanges = 15 grams = 1 choice
> 1 meat exchange = 0 grams = 0 choice
> 1 fat exchange = 0 grams = 0 choice

In a typically healthy diet 50% to 60% of your day's total calories come from carbohydrates. The rest come from protein and fat, which do not contain any carbohydrates and therefore are not added to the total carbohydrate gram count.

Anemia Worksheets

1. *What nutrients are required for red blood cell formation and maturation, other than protein?*
   Folic acid (folate), with vitamin B_{12}, is necessary for the formation of normal red blood cells and the synthesis of DNA, the genetic material of cells. Iron is also essential for allowing red blood cells to carry oxygen properly.
2. *How does a deficiency of folic acid lead to anemia?*
   Folic acid deficiency causes macrocytic anemia in which the red blood cells are fewer in number, larger in size, and contain less oxygen-carrying hemoglobin than normal. The symptoms of anemia are lethargy, apathy, breathlessness, poor body temperature regulation, pallor, forgetfulness, irritability, and stomach disorders.
3. *What is the name for folic acid deficiency anemia?*
   Megaloblastic anemia.
4. *What other nutrient deficiency can cause this type of anemia?*
   Vitamin B_{12}.
5. *What are the best sources of folic acid?*
   Most of the folic acid in foods (with the exception of the folic acid added to enriched flour and breakfast cereals) occurs as folate. Folate is only about half as available for the body to use as is the folic acid

in pills and supplements. Folate also is easily destroyed by sunlight, overcooking, or the storing of foods at room temperature for an extended period of time.

Good dietary sources of folate include

Leafy green vegetables
Liver
Mushrooms
Oatmeal
Peanut butter
Red beans
Soy
Wheat germ
Enriched grain products
Citrus fruits (orange juice, grapefruit, etc.)

6. *Why is there an expanded need for folate during pregnancy?*
Folic acid deficiency has been implicated as a cause of neural tube defects in the developing fetus. Recent research has shown that adequate amounts of folic acid can prevent up to half of these birth defects if women start taking folic acid supplements shortly before conception. It is important for all women attempting to become pregnant to take folic acid supplementation. It is best to begin taking supplements 3 months before attempting pregnancy; if already pregnant, begin immediately. Folic acid is contained in almost all prenatal vitamins.

Besides helping to prevent certain birth defects, folic acid plays other important roles during pregnancy. A pregnant woman needs extra folic acid to help her to produce the additional blood cells she needs. Folic acid also is crucial to support the rapid growth of the placenta and fetus. This vitamin is needed to produce new DNA (genetic material) as cells multiply. Without adequate amounts of folic acid, cell division could be impaired, possibly leading to poor growth in the fetus or placenta.

7. *What is the Recommended Daily Allowance for folic acid in pregnancy?*
The March of Dimes recommends that all women who can become pregnant take a multivitamin that contains 400 μg of folic acid every day and eat a healthy diet. This is the only sure way a woman can get all the folic acid and other vitamins she needs. Most women get less than half of the recommended amount of folic acid daily. The Institute of Medicine recommends that women increase their intake of synthetic folic acid to 600 μg/day once their pregnancy is confirmed. Most doctors recommend a prenatal vitamin that contains at least this amount of folic acid. However, women should not take more than 1,000 μg (or 1 mg) without their doctor's advice.

The Institute of Medicine also recommends that women eat a diet rich in foods that contain folate or folic acid. Folate is the natural form of folic acid that is found in foods. Orange juice, other citrus fruits and juices, leafy green vegetables, beans, peanuts, broccoli, asparagus, peas, lentils, and whole-grain products all contain folate. Synthetic (manufactured) folic acid is added to certain grain products, including flour, rice, pasta, cornmeal, bread, and cereals. These foods are considered to be "fortified" with folic acid.

8. *Women who have prolonged use of oral contraceptives before pregnancy may have low serums levels of folate. Why?*
In several cases women taking oral contraceptives developed folic acid deficiency. However, it appears that many of these women had low intake of folic acid or problems with intestinal absorption before taking birth control pills. Again, women on birth control pills should regularly eat good sources of folic acid. Good folate nutrition is especially important for women who become pregnant shortly after they stop taking oral contraceptives.

9. *Vitamin B$_{12}$ deficiency is rare. Why?*
Unlike other water-soluble nutrients, vitamin B$_{12}$ is stored in the liver, kidneys, and other body tissues. It can take several years before signs of the deficiency appear, all because of poor dietary intake, so nutritional deficiency of this vitamin is extremely rare.

10. *When is a deficiency of vitamin B$_{12}$ likely to occur?*
Diets of most adult Americans provide recommended intakes of vitamin B$_{12}$, but deficiency may still occur as a result of an inability to absorb B$_{12}$ from food. It can also occur in individuals with dietary patterns that exclude animal or fortified foods. As a general rule, most individuals who develop a vitamin B$_{12}$ deficiency have an underlying stomach or intestinal disorder that limits the absorption of vitamin B$_{12}$. Sometimes the only symptom of these intestinal disorders is anemia resulting from B$_{12}$ deficiency.

Characteristic signs of B$_{12}$ deficiency include fatigue, weakness, nausea, constipation, flatulence, loss of appetite, and weight loss. Deficiency also can lead to neurologic changes such as numbness and tingling in the hands and feet. Additional symptoms of B$_{12}$ deficiency are difficulty in maintaining balance, depression, confusion, poor memory, and soreness of the mouth or tongue. Some of these symptoms can also result from a variety of medical conditions other than vitamin B$_{12}$ deficiency. It is important to have a physician evaluate these symptoms so that appropriate medical care can be given.

11. *Maternal iron deficiency does not usually result in an infant who is anemic at birth. Why?*
An infant gets all the iron he or she needs from the mother's iron stores. The only way an infant may be anemic at birth is if the mother is severely anemic and has minimal iron to offer the fetus. Iron deficiency anemia is a risk for the mother during pregnancy because the infant draws on the mother's iron stores and also the mother requires more iron to support her expended blood volume. It is important to note that iron deficiency during pregnancy is associated with an increased risk of preterm delivery and low birth weight infants.

12. *What role does hemoglobin play in the body?*
Hemoglobin is the protein molecule in red blood cells that carries oxygen from the lungs to the body's tissues and returns carbon dioxide from the tissues to the lungs. The iron contained in hemoglobin is responsible for the red color of blood.

13. *What is hematocrit?*
The hematocrit is the percent of whole blood that is composed of red blood cells. The hematocrit is a measure of both the number of red blood cells and the size of red blood cells.

The hematocrit is almost always ordered as part of a complete blood count, which measures the number of red blood cells, the number of white blood cells, the total amount of hemoglobin in the blood, and the fraction of the blood composed of red blood cells (hematocrit).

14. *Around 3 to 5 months, lower levels of hemoglobin are normal in the pregnant women. Why?*
Anemia in pregnancy is very common and is present in almost 80% of pregnant women. Because the volume of blood increases during pregnancy (hemodilution), a moderate decrease in the concentration of red blood cells and hemoglobin is normal. The hematocrit value (the percentage of red blood cells relative to plasma volume) in nonpregnant women ranges from 38% to 45%. However, in pregnant women, because of hemodilution normal values can be much lower, for example, 34% in single and 30% in twin or multiple pregnancy even with normal stores of iron, folic acid, and vitamin B$_{12}$. This lower range simply reflects "the physiologic hemodilution of pregnancy" and does not indicate a decrease in oxygen-carrying capacity or true anemia.

15. *What are acceptable levels of hematocrit and hemoglobin in pregnancy? In nonpregnant women?*
Nonpregnant: Hb 12.0, Hct 36

Pregnant first trimester: Hb 11.0, Hct 33
Pregnant second trimester: Hb 10.5, Hct 32
Pregnant third trimester: Hb 11.0, Hct 33

During the third trimester it is almost impossible to get enough iron from the diet, which means that the mother's iron stores will be drawn on to meet the demand.

16. *What is the recommended level of iron supplementation in pregnancy?*
    30 mg/day

17. *How much iron is typically found in breast milk?*
    Breast milk is a complex composition of important proteins, fatty acids, sugars, amino acids, iron, and many other nutrients that are tailored to meet an infant's specific and changing needs. By 6 months of age, though breast milk is still an excellent source of nutrition for the infant, it no longer provides the entire range of nutrients needed for continued growth. Between the fourth and the sixth month an infant's diet should begin to include solid foods that provide the extra calories and nutrients (especially iron) that breast milk alone cannot. When taken in combination with solid foods, breast milk remains an excellent source of nutrition for infants for as long as breast-feeding continues.

18. *To diagnose iron deficiency anemia, what signs and symptoms would you look for both physically and from a laboratory standpoint?*
    With iron deficiency anemia there is a history of weakness, fatigue, tachycardia, dyspnea, and pallor from anemia and tissue iron depletion. Physical findings include pallor, tachycardia, glossitis, koilonychia (spoon nails), and angular stomatitis. Signs and symptoms of an underlying disease may be present. Laboratory studies reveal (1) decreased reticulocyte count and mean corpuscular volume, (2) hypochromic microcytic cells on blood smears, (3) low serum ferritin, and (4) hypercellular marrow with absent sideroblasts and storage iron.

19. *How long does it take for a woman to replace iron stores after pregnancy?*
    Birth is associated with blood loss. If a woman is anemic during pregnancy, she should take iron for several months after delivery to help the body replace the lost blood cells and iron stores. Breast-feeding women may also need to take iron because iron is lost in breast milk. How long it takes a woman to replace her iron stores depends on how deficient she became during pregnancy, but generally between 3 and 6 months postpregnancy a woman's iron stores should be back to normal.

20. *List the three most common causes of anemia.*
    There are a number of different causes and types of anemia. Some of the more common causes of anemia include the following:

    - Increased loss of red blood cells
      - Increased blood loss from specific diseases (ulcers, cancers, certain types of infection)
      - Menstruation, trauma, or hemorrhoids
      - Certain medications that increase or cause bleeding, such as aspirin or nonsteroidal antiinflammatory drugs (e.g., ibuprofen, naproxen, and others)
    - Increased need for hemoglobin or red blood cells
      - Chronic diseases, such as arthritis, kidney failure, inflammatory bowel disease, and liver disease
      - Specific vitamin/mineral deficiencies, such as iron, vitamin B_{12}, and folic acid
      - Conditions where nutrient absorption is a problem, such as with celiac disease
      - Excessive alcohol ingestion
      - Decreased activity of the bone marrow
      - Kidney disease or kidney failure
      - Chemotherapy medications

- Increased destruction of the red blood cells in the body (hemolysis)
  - Inherited (genetic) conditions, such as sickle cell disease
  - Conditions where the body's defense (immune system) causes destruction of the red blood cells

Nutrition Research and Programs Worksheets

1. *Describe the difference between a nutritional survey and nutritional surveillance.*

   A *surveillance* is an approach to collecting data on a population's health and nutritional status in which data collection occurs regularly and repeatedly.

   A *survey* is a systematic study of a cross-section of individuals who represent the target population.

2. *Describe the following nutritional surveys (i.e., goals for data collection, past survey results, significance of the results to the field of dietetics).*

- *Ten State Survey (1970):* In the late 1960s concerns about the nutritional status of Mississippi school-children and widespread hunger and malnutrition led to the nation's first comprehensive nutrition survey. This survey was conducted between 1968 and 1970 in 10 states.
- *National Health and Nutrition Examination Survey (NHANES):* This survey is ongoing. The NHANES target population is the civilian, noninstitutionalized, U.S. population. NHANES 1999–2000 includes over-sampling of low-income persons, adolescents aged 12 to 19 years, persons 60+ years of age, African-Americans, and Mexican-Americans. The major objectives of the NHANES are (1) to estimate the number and percent of persons in the U.S. population and designated subgroups with selected disease and risk factors; (2) to monitor trends in the prevalence, awareness, treatment, and control of selected diseases; (3) to monitor the trends in risk behaviors and environmental exposures; (4) to analyze risk factors for selected diseases; (5) to study the relationship between diet, nutrition, and health; and (6) to explore emerging public health issues and new technologies.
- *USDA Household Food Consumption Surveys:* These ongoing surveys collect data that are used to describe food consumption behavior and to evaluate the nutritional content of diets for their implications for food policies, marketing, food safety, food assistance, and nutrition education. Target population consists of private households of all income levels.

3. *Describe the following federal programs. Consider the following questions as you describe each program.*

- What federal organization supports the program?
- What is the programs' target population?
- What are the programs' eligibility guidelines?
- What nutritional services does the program provide?
- If supplemental foods are distributed, where are they obtained and what types of foods are generally provided?

   A. School Breakfast and Lunch Programs (Child Nutrition Act)

   Breakfast: Permanently authorized by the Child Nutrition Act of 1966. Federal funding is provided in the form of cash reimbursements for each breakfast served, varied in amount by the family income of the participating child. All children in participating schools and residential institutions are eligible for a federally subsidized meal, regardless of family income. However, free meals must be offered to children from families with incomes below 130% of the federal poverty income level and reduced price meals to those with family incomes between 130% and 185% of the poverty level. The program is administered by the Food and Nutrition Service and funded by annual agricultural appropriations.

   Some 6.9 million children in more than 68,000 schools participated in the School Breakfast Program every day in fiscal year 1997. As in the school lunch program, low-income children may qualify to receive school breakfast free or at a reduced price, and states are reimbursed according to the number of meals served in each category. Meals must meet nutritional standards similar to those in the National School Lunch Program. Congress appropriated $1.3 billion for the School Breakfast Program for fiscal year 1998.

Lunch: The National School Lunch Program is a federally assisted meal program operating in more than 99,800 public and nonprofit private schools and residential child care institutions. It provides nutritionally balanced, low-cost, or free lunches to more than 26 million children each school day. In 1998 Congress expanded the National School Lunch Program to include reimbursement for snacks served to children in after-school educational and enrichment programs to include children through 18 years of age.

The Food and Nutrition Service administers the program at the federal level. At the state level, the National School Lunch Program is usually administered by state education agencies, which operate the program through agreements with school food authorities.

Generally, public or nonprofit private schools of high school grade or under and public or nonprofit private residential child care institutions may participate in the school lunch program. School districts and independent schools that choose to take part in the lunch program get cash subsidies and donated commodities from the U.S. Department of Agriculture (USDA) for each meal they serve. In return they must serve lunches that meet federal requirements, and they must offer free or reduced-price lunches to eligible children. School food authorities can also be reimbursed for snacks served to children through age 18 in after school educational or enrichment programs.

Any child at a participating school may purchase a meal through the National School Lunch Program. Children from families with incomes at or below 130% of the poverty level are eligible for free meals. Those with incomes between 130% and 185% of the poverty level are eligible for reduced price meals, for which students can be charged no more than 40 cents. (For the period July 1, 2003 through June 30, 2004, 130% of the poverty level is $23,920 for a family of four; 185% is $34,040.)

Children from families with incomes over 185% of poverty pay full price, though their meals are still subsidized to some extent. Local school food authorities set their own prices for full-price (paid) meals but must operate their meal services as nonprofit programs.

After-school snacks are provided to children on the same income eligibility basis as school meals. However, programs that operate in areas where at least 50% of students are eligible for free or reduced price meals serve all snacks free.

B. Special Milk Program

Offers federal reimbursements for each half pint of milk served to a child in a participating outlet, which generally is any school or facility caring for children that does not participate in other federally subsidized meal programs. There is an exception from this limitation for kindergarten children in split session programs. The program is permanently authorized under the Child Nutrition Act of 1966. Schools may offer free milk to children meeting free lunch income requirements, if they choose, and this milk is reimbursed at full cost. Otherwise, children buy so-called paid milk, which is subsidized at a legislatively set rate for each half pint served. This program is administered by the Food and Nutrition Service and funded by annual agricultural appropriations.

C. Child and Adult Care Food Program

USDA's Child and Adult Care Food Program (CACFP) plays a vital role in improving the quality of day care and making it more affordable for many low-income families. Each day, 2.6 million children receive nutritious meals and snacks through CACFP. The program also provides meals and snacks to 74,000 adults who receive care in nonresidential adult day care centers. CACFP reaches even further to provide meals to children residing in homeless shelters and snacks and suppers to youths participating in eligible after-school-care programs.

Section 226.2 of the regulations describes who may receive CACFP meal benefits. *Children* means "(a) persons 12 years of age and under, (b) children of migrant workers 15 years of age and under, and (c) persons with mental or physical handicaps, as defined by the State, enrolled in an institution or a child care facility serving a majority of persons 18 years of age and under." Provider's own children are eligible only in tier I day care homes, when other nonresidential children are enrolled in the day care home and are participating in the meal service. *Adult participant* means "a person enrolled in an adult day care center who is functionally impaired . . . or 60 years of age or older." The adult component of CACFP is targeted to individuals who remain in the community and reside with family members. Individuals who reside in institutions are not eligible for CACFP benefits.

In addition, Public Law 105-336 makes CACFP snacks available to children and youths through age 18 in eligible after-school-care programs.

D. Head Start

Head Start and Early Head Start are comprehensive child development programs that serve children from birth to age 5, pregnant women, and their families. They are child-focused programs and have the overall goal of increasing the school readiness of young children in low-income families.

The Head Start program is administered by the Head Start Bureau, the Administration on Children, Youth and Families, Administration for Children and Families, Department of Health and Human Services. Grants are awarded by the Administration on Children, Youth and Families Regional Offices and the Head Start Bureau's American Indian–Alaska Native and Migrant and Seasonal Program branches directly to local public agencies, private organizations, Native American tribes, and school systems for the purpose of operating Head Start programs at the community level.

The Head Start program has a long tradition of delivering comprehensive and high-quality services designed to foster healthy development in low-income children. Head Start grantee and delegate agencies provide a range of individualized services in the areas of education and early childhood development; medical, dental, and mental health; nutrition; and parent involvement. In addition, the entire range of Head Start services is responsive and appropriate to each child's and family's developmental, ethnic, cultural, and linguistic heritage and experience.

All Head Start programs must adhere to Program Performance Standards. The Head Start Program Performance Standards define the services that Head Start programs are to provide to the children and families they serve. They constitute the expectations and requirements that Head Start grantees must meet. They are designed to ensure that the Head Start goals and objectives are implemented successfully, that the Head Start philosophy continues to thrive, and that all grantee and delegate agencies maintain the highest possible quality in the provision of Head Start services.

E. Women, Infants, and Children Program (WIC)

Population served: The WIC target population are low-income, nutritionally at risk:
- Pregnant women (through pregnancy and up to 6 weeks after birth or after pregnancy ends)
- Breast-feeding women (up to infant's first birthday)
- Non–breast-feeding postpartum women (up to 6 months after the birth of an infant or after pregnancy ends)
- Infants (up to first birthday): WIC serves 45% of all infants born in the United States.
- Children up to their fifth birthday

Benefits: The following benefits are provided to WIC participants:
- Supplemental nutritious foods
- Nutrition education and counseling at WIC clinics
- Screening and referrals to other health, welfare, and social services

Program delivery: WIC is not an entitlement program because Congress does not set aside funds to allow every eligible individual to participate in the program. WIC is a federal grant program for which Congress authorizes a specific amount of funds each year for the program. WIC is administered at the federal level by Food and Nutrition Service by 87 WIC state agencies, through approximately 46,000 authorized retailers. WIC operates through 2,000 local agencies in 10,000 clinic sites, in 50 state health departments, 32 Indian tribal organizations, American Samoa, District of Columbia, Guam, Puerto Rico, and the Virgin Islands.

Nutritional resources provided: In most WIC state agencies, WIC participants receive checks or food instruments to purchase specific foods each month that are designed to supplement their diets. WIC food is high in one or more of the following nutrients: protein, calcium, iron, and vitamins A and C. These are the nutrients frequently lacking in the diets of the program's low-income target population. Different food packages are provided for different categories of participants. A few WIC state agencies distribute WIC foods through warehouses or deliver WIC foods to participants.

WIC foods include iron-fortified infant formula and infant cereal, iron-fortified adult cereal, vitamin C-rich fruit and/or vegetable juice, eggs, milk, cheese, peanut butter, dried beans or peas, tuna, and carrots. Special infant formulas and certain medical foods may be provided when prescribed by a physician or health professional for a specified medical condition.

F. Expanded Food and Nutrition Education Program (EFNEP)

The Cooperative State Research, Education, and Extension Service's Expanded Food and Nutrition Education Program (EFNEP) is a unique program that currently operates in all 50 states and in American Samoa, Guam, Micronesia, Northern Marianas, Puerto Rico, and the Virgin Islands. It is designed to assist limited resource audiences in acquiring the knowledge, skills, attitudes, and changed behavior necessary for nutritionally sound diets and to contribute to their personal development and the improvement of the total family diet and nutritional well-being.

Adult EFNEP: Through an experiential learning process, adult program participants learn how to make food choices to improve the nutritional quality of the meals they serve their families. They increase their ability to select and buy food that meets the nutritional needs of their family. They gain new skills in food production, preparation, storage, safety, and sanitation, and they learn to better manage their food budgets and related resources such as Food Stamps. EFNEP is delivered as a series of 10 to 12 or more lessons, often over several months, by paraprofessionals and volunteers, many of whom are indigenous to the target population. The hands-on, learn-by-doing approach allows the participants to gain the practical skills necessary to make positive behavior changes. Through EFNEP, participants learn self-worth, that they have something to offer their families and society.

Youth EFNEP: The delivery of EFNEP youth programs takes on various forms. EFNEP provides nutrition education at schools as an enrichment of the curriculum, in after-school-care programs, through 4-H EFNEP clubs, day camps, residential camps, community centers, neighborhood groups, and home gardening workshops. In addition to lessons on nutrition, food preparation, and food safety, youth topics may also include fitness, avoidance of substance abuse, and other health-related topics.

Program delivery: County Extension home economists provide on-the-job training and supervise paraprofessionals and volunteers, who teach EFNEP. Paraprofessionals usually live in the communities where they work. They recruit families and receive referrals from neighborhood contacts and community agencies (i.e., Food Stamps, WIC, etc.). Methods for program delivery may include direct teaching in group or one-to-one situations; mailings and telephone teaching to complement other teaching methods; mass media efforts to develop understanding, awareness, and involvement in the educational program; and development and training of volunteers to assist with direct teaching of adults and youth.

G. Maternal and Child Health Bureau

Goal: To improve the health of all mothers and children consistent with the applicable health status goals and national health objectives established by the Secretary of the U.S. Department of Health and Human Services.

History: Has operated as a federal–state partnership for more than 65 years. When the Social Security Act was passed in 1935, the federal government, through Title V, pledged its support of state efforts to extend and improve health and welfare services for mothers and children. Title V has been amended many times over the years to reflect the expansion of the national interest in maternal and child health. It was converted to a block grant program as part of the Omnibus Budget Reconciliation Act of 1981. Congress later sought to balance the flexibility of the block grant with greater accountability by the states. Through the 1989 Omnibus Budget Reconciliation Act states were required to report on progress made toward key maternal and child health indicators and to provide other program information.

States and jurisdictions: States and jurisdictions use Title V funds to design and implement a wide range of maternal and child health programs that meet national and state needs. Although specific initiatives may vary among the 59 states and jurisdictions utilizing Title V funds, all programs work to do the following:
- Reduce infant mortality and incidence of handicapping conditions among children
- Increase the number of children appropriately immunized against disease
- Increase the number of children in low-income households who receive assessments and follow-up diagnostic and treatment services
- Provide and ensure access to comprehensive perinatal care for women; preventative and child care services; comprehensive care, including long-term care services, for children with special health care needs; and rehabilitation services for blind and disabled children under 16 years of age who are eligible for Supplemental Security income
- Facilitate the development of comprehensive, family-centered, community-based, culturally competent, coordinated systems of care for children with special health care needs

H. Older Americans Act, Title IIIC

This Act is intended to improve older people's nutrition status and enable them to avoid medical problems, continue living in communities of their own choice, and stay out of institutions. It provides low-cost nutritious meals, opportunities for social interaction, nutrition education, and shopping assistance, counseling and referral to other social and rehabilitation services, and transportation services. Other programs are the Congregate Meals Program and Home-Delivered Meals Program.

I. Medicare

Assists people 65 years of age or older, people of any age with end-stage renal disease, people on Social Security disability payment programs for more than 2 years, and qualified railroad retirement beneficiaries and merchant seamen. It is administered by the Health Care Financing Administration of the Department of Health and Human Services and consists of two separate parts: hospital insurance (Part A) and medical insurance (Part B)

J. Medicaid

Provides assistance for eligible low-income persons, the aged, blind, people with disabilities, and members of families with dependent children in which one parent is absent, incapacitated, or unemployed. Individual states define eligibility, benefits, and payment schedules.

4. *Describe home-delivered meals. Who is eligible for these meals?*

Home-delivered meals are direct food delivery. Funding source is private. Home meals are delivered to older adults that complement weekday congregate programs. Attention is given to needs of permanently or temporarily home-bound elderly individuals. All persons 60 years and older (and spouses of any age) are eligible to receive meals, regardless of their income level. Priority is given to those who are economically and socially needy.

5. *What are congregate meals? Who is eligible?*

Nutritious meals are served to improve older people's nutrition status and provide social interaction. Congregate meals sites are often community centers, senior citizen centers, religious facilities, schools, extended care facilities, or elderly housing complexes. All persons 60 years and older (and spouses of any age) are eligible to receive meals, regardless of their income level. Priority is given to those who are economically and socially needy.

6. *Describe a food pantry and soup kitchen. How do they fit into the emergency food network? Who is eligible?*

Food pantries, along with food banks, soup kitchens, prepared and perishable food programs, and other emergency food assistance programs, help fill the gaps in the federal programs to provide meals to the hungry. Food pantries are usually attached to existing nonprofit agencies that distribute bags or boxes of groceries to people experiencing food emergencies. Distributed foods are prepared and consumed elsewhere. Pantries often require referrals or proof of need.

Food Stamp Worksheet

1. *After applying for Food Stamps and providing all the required documentation, how long should it take for an eligible applicant to receive the stamps?*

The food stamp office provides an application form on the same day food stamps are requested. They can be asked for in person, over the phone, or by mail. The office will accept the form on the same day it is turned in, even if they cannot interview the applicant on that day. Applicants must fill in their name, address, telephone number, and as much other information as they can on the form and sign it. The form can be hand delivered or sent to the office as soon as possible. (Some states may let applicants fax or e-mail their application form to the office.) A food stamp worker can help applicants fill out the rest of the form during their interview. *All questions must be answered completely and honestly. If applicants fail to do so, they can be removed from the program, fined, put in prison, or all three.*

If applicants qualify for food stamps, they get them no later than 30 days from the date the office received their application. If the household has little or no money and needs help right away, they need to let the food stamp office know and may be able to get food stamps within 7 days.

2. *What are the income requirements for food stamp eligibility? What are the exceptions to this income requirement?*

Households must meet income tests *unless* all members are receiving Title IV (TANF), Social Security income, or in some places general assistance. Most households must meet both the gross and net income tests, but a household with an elderly person or a person who is receiving certain types of disability payments only has to meet the net income test. Gross income means a household's total nonexcluded income before any deductions have been made. Net income means gross income minus allowable deductions.

3. *While receiving food stamps, if you are unemployed or working less than 20 hours a week you must "register" to work. Who are the exceptions to this case?*

With some exceptions, able-bodied adults aged between 16 and 60 must register for work, accept suitable employment, and take part in an employment and training program to which they are referred by the food stamp office. Failure to comply with these requirements can result in disqualification from the program. In addition, able-bodied adults aged between 18 and 50 who do not have any dependent children can get food stamps only for 3 months in a 36-month period if they do not work or participate in a work fare or employment and training program other than job search. This requirement is waived in some locations.

4. *Do you need a permanent address to receive food stamps?*

Yes, so you can be monitored to ensure you are abiding by the rules and regulations established by the Food Stamp Act.

5. *Which members of the family applying for food stamps require Social Security cards? If you do not have proof of citizenship, can you receive food stamps?*

A Social Security number must be provided for every household member, including children. If any household member does not have a Social Security number, he or she must apply for one. If you are otherwise eligible for food stamps, you can get them for a short time while you are waiting for your Social Security number.

U.S. citizens are eligible for the program. Certain noncitizens, such as those admitted for humanitarian reasons and those admitted for permanent residence, are also eligible for the program. Eligible household members can get food stamps even if there are other members of the household that are not eligible.

The 2002 Farm Bill restores food stamp eligibility to most legal immigrants who

- Have lived in the country for 5 years; or
- Are receiving disability-related assistance or benefits, regardless of entry date; or
- Starting 10-1-03, are children regardless of entry date.

6. *Once you become eligible to receive food stamps, how long do you remain certified?*

You are eligible to receive food stamps as long as you meet the eligibility requirements.

7. *List the items you can and cannot purchase with food stamps.*

You can spend food stamps like cash at most stores that sell food. The cashier may ask you to show your food stamp identification. Food stamps can only be used for food and for plants and seeds to grow food for your household to eat. Sales tax cannot be charged on items bought with food stamps.

Food stamps cannot be used to buy any nonfood item, such as pet food; soaps, paper products, and household supplies; grooming items, toothpaste, and cosmetics; alcoholic beverages and tobacco; vitamins and medicines; any food that will be eaten in the store; and hot foods.

Community Case Study

A pregnant Haitian women, age 23, has just arrived in this country with her children, ages 2, 5, and 7. Mrs. Jean-Pierre is staying with her cousin in an uncomfortable living situation. The only provision is shelter because Mrs. Jean-Pierre's cousin can barely feed her family let alone worry about feeding four other mouths.

To which federal programs is Mrs. Jean Pierre eligible? List the potential sources of food and income that Mrs. Jean-Pierre and her children can receive. Plan these foods and resources into a meal plan. Can the food and income resources available to this family ensure proper nutritional status? Will the food or income resources change when the infant is born?

> The federal programs providing eligibility are WIC, Head Start, School Breakfast and Lunch Programs, Medicaid, EFNEP, food pantries, and Food Stamp Program. Meals for school-aged children are provided by School Breakfast and Lunch programs and Head Start. Health care for an entire family is provided by Medicaid. Mother can plan foods around food pantry items and WIC foods and use these foods for snacks for school-aged children to bring to school. EFNEP may help her with ideas on how to effectively budget household resources. She may be eligible for food stamps. However, resources may be inadequate, therefore she may need to work to provide more income. Yes, resources will change but WIC may provide infant formula (if deciding against breast-feeding). Other necessities (diapers, baby clothes, etc.) are needed.

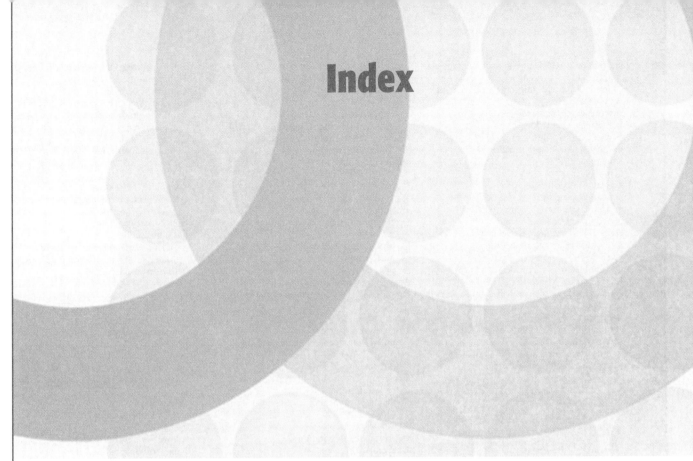

Index

allergies. *See also* food allergies
  allergic disease, explained, 64
  allergic reaction, symptoms of, 247, 248t
  colic, 44
  early diet, effect of, 63–65
alpha-linolenic acid, 233, 235
Alternate Healthy Eating Index, 351
aluminum in parenteral nutrition, 178
amenorrhea, 290
America on the Move, 350
American Cancer Institute, 381
American Cancer Society, 351, 357, 358
American Diabetes Association, 351, 381
American Dietetic Association
  ethical and legal issues in nutrition,
    hydration, and feeding, 446
  website, 329
American Health Care Association, 428
American Heart Association, 351
American Institute of Cancer Research, 351
amino acids
  aromatic, 147–150, 147f
  oxidation of, 186
  vegetarian diets, 231
ammonia accumulation, 152
Amsterdam Growth and Health
  Longitudinal Study, 7t
anaphylaxis, defined, 249
android (apple shape) obesity, 392
anemia
  copper, 176, 201
  explained, 86
  folic acid, 189–190
  hypochromic, 176
  megaloblastic, 188–189
  premature infants, 168, 176
  vitamin B$_6$, 188
anemia, iron deficiency
  infants, 48–49
  older adults, 387
  pediatric public health nutrition services,
    127
anorexia
  appetite assessment, 411
  cancer patients, 333t
anorexia nervosa
  adolescent nutrition, 121
  diagnostic criteria, 299t
  eating disorders, 299, 309
  medical consequences, 302–303, 303t
anthropometrics
  attention deficit hyperactivity disorder,
    218
  autism, 217
  cerebral palsy, 214–215
  malnutrition and nutrient deficits, 417
  Prader-Willi syndrome, 210
  spina bifida, 212–213
antiarrhythmic agents, 399
anticarcinogens, 194
anticholinergic medications, 399
anticipatory guidance, 101–102
anticoagulant agents, 398, 399, 400f
anticonvulsant medications
  nutrients, blood levels of, 205–206
  nutrients, interactions with, 214, 215
antioxidants
  Down syndrome, children with, 208
  older adults, 383, 383f
  vitamin E, 194
anxiety disorders, 300
apoptosis, defined, 381
appetite
  assessment of, 411–412
  conditions affecting, 411t

defined, 411
diet modification, 412–413
impaired, interventions for, 414–417,
  414t, 415t
impairment, age-related, 411–413, 411t
Prader-Willi syndrome, 209, 210, 211
Appetite, Hunger, Sensory Perception
  questionnaire, 412
appetite stimulants
  failure to thrive, 158
  older adults, 414
apple shape (android) obesity, 392
arachidonic acid
  attention deficit hyperactivity disorder,
    219
  phenylketonuria, 149
  postpartum depression, 79, 80
  preterm infant formula, 47–48
Area Agency on Aging, 414
Arnold-Chiari malformation of the brain,
  213
aromatase, 112
aromatic amino acids
  phenylalanine metabolism, 147, 147f
  phenylketonuria, 147–149
  tyrosinemias, 149–150
artificial hydration and nutrition. *See also*
  hydration; tube feeding
  definition, indications, and prevalence, 445
  older adults, 397
ascorbate, oral, 150
ascorbic acid. *See* vitamin C
aspartame, 148
Asperger syndrome, 216
aspiration
  swallowing problems, 416
  tube feeding, 445
assessment methodology for older adults,
  380–381
asthma
  magnesium, 199
  multivitamins, 52
  vitamin C, 190
athletes, dietary guidelines for
  alcohol, caffeine, soda, 287
  body composition, 288
  calcium, 283
  carbohydrates, 279–280
  childhood through adolescence, 290–291
  dietary supplements, 291–293
  eating disorders, 307
  eating disorders and the female athlete
    triad, 289–290
  energy, 279, 279t
  fat, 281
  fluids and electrolytes, 283–285
  iron, 282–283, 282t
  muscle mass, increasing, 288
  nutrition after exercise, 286–287
  nutrition during exercise, 285
  protein, 280–281
  sports beverages, 285–286
  sports during pregnancy, lactation, and
    menopause, 293–294
  vitamins and minerals, 281–283, 282t
  weight cycling, 288–289
atopic dermatitis, 64
attention deficit hyperactivity disorder,
  217–219
authoritarian parenting style, 100
authoritative parenting style, 100
autism
  explained, 216–217
  nutrition assessment, 217
  vitamin B$_6$ therapy, 188

autism spectrum disorders, 216
autoimmunity, 294, 309
autonomy, defined, 450
autosomal recessive genetic inheritance, 143
Avon Longitudinal Study of Parents and
  Children
  described, 12–13
  peanut allergy, 65

B
B vitamins. *See entries at* vitamin B
Babson Benda intrauterine and postnatal
  chart, 165, 166
bacteriostatic, defined, 387
basal metabolic rate
  energy expenditure, total, 369
  older adults, malnutrition in, 418
behaviors, food-related
  early establishment of, 55
  hunger, 89
  Prader-Willi syndrome, 211
Belmont Report, 3, 4
beneficence, defined, 450
beriberi, 186
beta-3 agonists, 401
beta-adrenergic antagonists, 399
beta-carotene, 191, 192. *See also* vitamin A
betaine, 152
beverages. *See also* hydration
  drink, meaning of, 446
  early food trends and preferences, 56
  overweight status in children, 241
binge drinking, defined, 393
binge eating disorder, 300, 301t
binge eating-purging subtype of anorexia
  nervosa, 299, 299t
bioavailability of nutrients, 231
biochemical measures. *See also* laboratory
  tests
  attention deficit hyperactivity disorder, 218
  autism, 217
  cerebral palsy, 215
  children with developmental disabilities,
    205–206
  parenteral nutrition, premature infants,
    177
  Prader-Willi syndrome, 210
  spina bifida, 213
Bland, Anthony, 448
blindness
  vitamin A, 191
  vitamin E, 194
blood cells
  leucopenia, 302
  lymphocytes, 398, 401f
  microcytic, 391f
  normocytic, 391f
  red, 189–190, 390f, 391f
BMI. *See* body mass index (BMI)
body composition
  adolescent physical growth, 109
  athletes, 288
body dissatisfaction, 121–122
body fat. *See* adipose tissue/body fat
body habitus, 389, 392
body mass index (BMI)
  adolescent growth, assessment of, 112
  Ireton-Jones equation, 328
  obesity, 352
  Prader-Willi syndrome, 210
  weight categories, 368–369, 368t
Bogalusa Heart Study, 9, 10, 15–16
bolus feedings
  enteral nutrition, 170
  parenteral nutrition, 175

outcomes management system, 328
outpatient treatment for eating disorders, 304–305
over-the-counter preparations, 398–399, 398f
overfeeding, 56
overweight children
    assessment of, 237–238, 238f
    cultural disparities, 238
    dietary trends affecting, 239–240
    energy balance, 239
    environmental influences, 239–244
    health effects, 237–238
    intervention and prevention, 244–245, 257–258
    physical inactivity, 242–243
    programs and resources for prevention, 245–246
    rates of in the U.S., 237, 238f
    school physical education, 243
    societal factors influencing, 239
    television viewing, 243–244
    websites, 259–260
overweight status
    BMI, 352
    pediatric public health nutrition services, 127
    physical activity and weight management, 368–369, 368t
    prevalence of, 352, 353
    WIC program, 130
oxandrolone, 414
oxidative stress
    alcohol use, 393, 393f
    Down syndrome, children with, 208

P

palatability of food, 436
palmitate, 191
Pancrease MT 4 enzymes, 44
paralysis with spina bifida, 212
parathyroid hormone, 116
parenteral nutrition, premature infants
    biochemical monitoring, 177
    cholestasis, 174–175
    complications, 177–178
    explained, 172
    initiating, 172–176
    nutrition additives, 177
    vitamins and trace elements, 176
parents
    consent for research with children, 4
    eating as learned behavior, 95
    food preferences, development of, 95–102
    influence of parents, 94–95
    neonatal and early infant weight gain, 95
    overweight status in children, 241–242
    parenting styles, 100
    promoting healthy nutrition in early childhood, 94–102
peak bone mass
    adolescent physical growth, 110
    calcium retention, 197
peak height velocity, 109
peanuts
    food allergies, 65
    peanut-free diet, 254t
Pediasure®, 94
Pediatric Nutrition Surveillance System
    infant and child nutrition, 136
    nutrition monitoring, 5, 9
    overweight status, 127
pediatric vegetarianism. See vegetarianism, pediatric

peer groups, 114
pellagra, 187
percutaneous endoscopic gastrostomy (PEG) tubes, 445
percutaneously inserted central catheters (PICC lines), 172–173
periosteal apposition, 109
peripheral parenteral nutrition, 172
peripheral vascular disease, 419
peritoneal dialysis, 337
permanent vegetative state, 447, 448
permissive effect of cellular senescence, 392
permissive parenting style, 100
personality disorders, 300–301
pervasive developmental disorder, 216
pervasive refusal syndrome, 308
pet ownership, 394–395, 394f
phagocytosis, 387
pharmacologic considerations for older adults, 398–400, 398f, 399f, 400f, 401f
phasic biting, 58
phentermine, 400
phenylalanine
    metabolism of, 147, 147f
    phenylketonuria, 147–149
    tyrosinemias, 150
phenylketonuria
    clinical symptoms and diagnosis, 147–148
    explained, 147
    maternal phenylketonuria, 149
    medical nutrition therapy, 148–149
phosphorus
    chronic kidney disease, 338t
    functions, deficiencies, and food sources, 200–201
    supplements, 200–201
    vitamin D, 193
physical activity
    adolescent physical growth, 110
    cancer, 358
    cardiovascular disease, 356
    childhood obesity, prevention of, 245
    Down syndrome, children with, 297
    failure to thrive, assessment of, 157
    guidelines for, 239
    hypertension, 354
    life-style determinants of successful aging, 390–391
    obesity prevention, 370–371, 370–374, 374t
    overweight status in children, 242–243
    Prader-Willi syndrome, 212
    toddlers and school-aged children, normal, 93
    type 2 diabetes, 296
    weight loss interventions, 371–372
    weight loss maintenance, 373–374, 374t
    weight management, 353
physical examination for food allergies, 250
physical fitness, components of, 371
physical growth
    adolescents, 109–110
    zinc, 202
Physicians' Health Studies, 21–22
Physicians' Health Studies II, 26–27
physiologic changes
    adults, 326–327, 327t
    age-related, 413
phytate, 231
PICC lines (percutaneously inserted central catheters), 172–173
"picky eaters", 213
placebo effect of dietary supplements, 292
Pneumocystis carinii pneumonia, 338

polycystic ovary syndrome, 296–297
polypharmacy, 398–399, 398f, 399f
portion sizes. See food portions (serving sizes)
postconceptional age, 166
postdischarge premature infant formulas, 168–169
postmenstrual age, 166
postpartum depression, 79–80
potassium
    chronic kidney disease, 338t
    functions, deficiencies, and food sources, 200
    hypertension, 419
    loss during exercise, 284
    supplements, 200
poverty
    failure to thrive, 156
    older adults, 380
    oral health problems, 415
Prader-Willi syndrome
    appetite and obesity, 209, 210
    described, 209
    genetic basis, 209–210
    glucose tolerance test, 205
    metabolic abnormalities, 210
    nutrition assessment, 210–212
pregnancy
    adolescent nutrition and medical complications, 120–121
    diabetes, 337
    eating disorders, 307
    nutritional requirements during, 41–42
    sports activities, 293
Pregnancy Nutrition Surveillance System, 5, 7–8t, 136
prematurity. *See also* neonatal intensive care nutrition
    defined, 165
    pediatric public health nutrition services, 127
    preterm infants, 200
prenatal and infant nutrition, special topics in. *See also* infants, normal, nutrition for
    failure to thrive, 155–160, 156t, 158t
    genetics and inborn errors of metabolism, 143–155, 144f, 147f, 151f, 153f, 154f
    neonatal intensive care nutrition, 165–179
presbyosmia, 413
preschool, and childhood obesity, 244
prevalence, defined, 323
prevention strategy levels, 348–350
prick-puncture skin tests, 250–251
primary care setting, 372–373
primary prevention strategies, 348–349, 350
private placement long-term care facilities, 427t
pro-oxidant, defined, 387
proactive approach to nutrition care, 430, 433
Produce for Better Health Foundation, 246
progesterone
    eating disorders and female athlete triad, 290
    secondary sex characteristics, 110
prospective cohort studies
    described, 18–19
    explained, 13
    Framingham Heart Study, 19
    Health Professionals Follow-up Study, 21
    Iowa Women's Health Study, 22–23
    Nurses' Health Studies, 19–21
    Physicians' Health Studies, 21–22
protein
    adult nutritional requirements, 325
    athletes, requirements for, 280–281

selenium
  functions, deficiencies, and food sources, 203
  parenteral nutrition, premature infants, 176
self-care by adults, 349
self-harming behaviors, 301
self-regulation of food intake, 98–100
senescence, defined, 379
sensory loss, age-related, 413
serotonin, 385
serotonin reuptake inhibitors
  anorexia nervosa, 306
  obesity, 400–401
sertraline, 400–401
serving sizes. See food portions (serving sizes)
Seventh-Day Adventists, 230
shellfish-free diet, 255t
short bowel syndrome, 174–175
sibutramine, 401
simple carbohydrates, 279–280
Simplified Nutritional Appetite Questionnaire, 412
Sjögren syndrome, 417
skilled nursing facilities
  long-term care facility, type of, 427t
  older adults, 396
skin texture, 191
skinfold thickness measures, 392
small for gestational age
  diabetes in children, 296
  explained, 165
smoking and tobacco
  adolescent nutritional status, 120
  cardiovascular disease, 356–357
  life-style determinants of successful aging, 393
  oral health problems, 415
  psychosocial development during adolescence, 114, 115
snacks for toddlers through school-aged children, 92
social isolation, defined, 411
social programs for prevention of childhood obesity, 244–245
social support
  breast-feeding, 74
  life-style determinants of successful aging, 396
societal influences on overweight children, 239
sociodemographic factors, adolescent dietary intake, 117–118
socioeconomic factors
  life-style determinants of successful aging, 395–396
  protein intake by older adults, 383
soda pop, 285, 287
sodium
  adolescent requirements and consumption, 116
  chronic kidney disease, 338t
  hypertension, 419
  loss during exercise, 284
  postexercise intake, 285
soil, selenium in, 203
solid food, introduction of
  Down syndrome, children with, 208
  premature infants, 171–172
somatic mutation theory of aging, 381
sorbitol intake, 154, 155
soy-free diet, 255t
spastic quadriplegia, 214
Special Milk Program, 133
Special Olympics, 208

Special Supplemental Nutrition Program for Women, Infants, and Children (WIC)
  childhood obesity, prevention of, 244
  Down syndrome, children with, 209
  Farmers' Market Nutrition Program, 129
  federal public health nutrition programs, 129–130
  food packages, 62
  iron deficiency anemia, 48
  postdischarge infant formulas, 169
Special Turku Coronary Risk Factor Intervention Project for Babies, 14
specificity, defined, 387
spina bifida, 212–214
sports beverages, 285–286
staffing requirements for long-term care facilities, 428–429
standardized care, 328
standardized process, 328
staple foods, 435
state survey, 428, 438
statin drugs, 355
stature. See also height
  short, 112–113
  tall, 113
stereotypes, 373
steroid therapy, 191
stress fractures, 290–291
Stress-Free Feeding©, 246
substance misuse and abuse
  bulimia nervosa, 299
  eating disorders, 301
substituted judgment, 447
sucking reflex
  Down syndrome, children with, 208
  feeding skills and neuromuscular development of infants, 58
  Prader-Willi syndrome, 211
sucrose
  carbohydrate requirements for athletes, 279
  fructose intolerance, 154, 155
sugar consumption, adolescent, 117
suicide, 301
sulfur-containing amino acids
  disorders of, 150–152, 151f
  homocystinuria, 150–152
  methionine, homocysteine, and cystathionine, metabolism of, 150, 151f
Summer Food Service for Children, 133, 135
summer food service programs, 245
sun exposure and vitamin D
  adolescents, 116
  infants, 51
  osteoporosis, 361
  toddler and preschooler nutrition, 192–193
  toddlers through school-aged children, 85–86
superoxide dismutase, 194
supplemental nutrients
  normal infant nutrition, 51–52
  toddlers and school-aged children, normal, 94
support groups for celiac disease, 273
surveillance systems for infant, child, and adolescent nutrition, 136
Survey in Europe on Nutrition and the Elderly, a Concerted Action, 412
survey process for long-term care facilities, 437, 438, 438t
swallowing problems, 416–417
"sweaty feet" odor, 146
sympathomimetic effect, 393
syncope, 304

syndromes, defined, 205
synergistic, defined, 393

T
T cells, 52
"tactile defensiveness", 171
Tanner stages of adolescent development, 112
Team Nutrition initiative, 135
teeth. See also oral health
  calcium, 197
  dentition, defined, 413
  dentures, 415
television viewing
  childhood obesity, prevention of, 245–246
  food cravings, influence on, 90–91
  overweight status in children, 243–244
tertiary prevention, defined, 349
testosterone
  age-related risks for malnutrition, 414
  bone, hormonal actions on, 112
  eating disorders and athlete triad, 290
  secondary sex characteristics, 110, 111
tetrabiopterin, 385f
tetrahydrobiopterin, 148
theobromine, 393
theophylline, 393
therapeutic alliance for eating disorders, 305
Therapeutic Lifestyle Changes diet, 330, 331t
thiamin. See vitamin B$_1$
thromboembolism, 151
thyroid
  Down syndrome, 205
  eating disorders and athlete triad, 290
  iodine, 203
  selenium, 203
tobacco. See smoking and tobacco
toddler and preschool nutrition. See disabilities, children with; minerals, for children; vitamins, for children
toddlers through school-aged children, normal nutrition for
  breakfast, 92–93
  children's meals, planning, 88–89
  choking prevention, 91, 91t
  dental health, 92
  eating as learned behavior, 95
  energy and nutrient needs, 83–84, 84t
  failure to thrive, 90
  food preferences, development of, 95–102
  foods at 1 year, 87–88
  grazing, 90
  growth expectations, 83
  high calorie supplements, 94
  hunger and behavior, 89
  Internet resources, 103
  lactose intolerance, 90
  meal participation, 91
  milk, fat content of, 87
  neonatal and early infant weight gain, 95
  new foods, introducing, 88, 89t
  nutrition for, 83–94
  parents' role in healthy nutrition, 94–102
  physical activity, 93
  picky eating, 90
  role models, 92
  school, nutrition at, 93
  snacks, 92
  television and media influence, 90–91
  toddlers, mealtimes with, 88, 88t
  vitamins and minerals, 84–87, 84t, 85t, 86t
  water, 87
  weight gain, excessive, 93–94
total parenteral nutrition, 172
toxicity
  copper, 201

weight loss quality measure, 439
weight management, 352–353
wheat-free diet, 254–255t
WIC. *See* Special Supplemental Nutrition
  Program for Women, Infants, and
  Children (WIC)
Wilson disease, 201
women, older, 420–421
Women's Health Initiative study, 24–26
World Breastfeeding Week, 246
World Health Organization, 43

X
Xenical, 400
xerostomia

cancer patients, 333t
defined, 416

Y
young adult years, 323
Young Finns Study, 12
Youth Risk Behavior Surveillance System
  adolescent nutrition, 136
  alcohol and drug use, 114
  nutrition monitoring, 9, 15
  overweight status in children, 243

Z
z-scores, defined, 155
zinc

copper deficiencies, 201, 202
functions, research, deficiencies, and food
  sources, 202–203
iron intake, excessive, 49
normal infant nutrition, 50
older adults, 387–388, 390f, 391f
parenteral nutrition, premature infants,
  176
vegetarian children, 231–232, 232
Zoloft, 401